NATIONAL ACADEMIES

Sciences
Engineering
Medicine

NATIONAL
ACADEMIES
PRESS
Washington, DC

Sex and Gender Identification and Implications for Disability Evaluation

Hortensia de los Angeles Amaro and
Mary-Beth Malcarney, *Editors*

Committee on Sex and Gender
Identification and Implications for
Disability Evaluation

Board on Health Care Services

Health and Medicine Division

Consensus Study Report

NATIONAL ACADEMIES PRESS 500 Fifth Street, NW Washington, DC 20001

This activity was supported by a contract between the National Academy of Sciences and the Social Security Administration (Contract #: 28321318D00060015; Task Order #28321323FDS030023). Any opinions, findings, conclusions, or recommendations expressed in this publication do not necessarily reflect the views of any organization or agency that provided support for the project.

International Standard Book Number-13: 978-0-309-71931-5
International Standard Book Number-10: 0-309-71931-3
Digital Object Identifier: https://doi.org/10.17226/27775
Library of Congress Control Number: 2024949281

This publication is available from the National Academies Press, 500 Fifth Street, NW, Keck 360, Washington, DC 20001; (800) 624-6242 or (202) 334-3313; http://www.nap.edu.

Suggested citation: National Academies of Sciences, Engineering, and Medicine. 2024. *Sex and gender identification and implications for disability evaluation.* Washington, DC: The National Academies Press. https://doi.org/10.17226/27775.

The **National Academy of Sciences** was established in 1863 by an Act of Congress, signed by President Lincoln, as a private, nongovernmental institution to advise the nation on issues related to science and technology. Members are elected by their peers for outstanding contributions to research. Dr. Marcia McNutt is president.

The **National Academy of Engineering** was established in 1964 under the charter of the National Academy of Sciences to bring the practices of engineering to advising the nation. Members are elected by their peers for extraordinary contributions to engineering. Dr. John L. Anderson is president.

The **National Academy of Medicine** (formerly the Institute of Medicine) was established in 1970 under the charter of the National Academy of Sciences to advise the nation on medical and health issues. Members are elected by their peers for distinguished contributions to medicine and health. Dr. Victor J. Dzau is president.

The three Academies work together as the **National Academies of Sciences, Engineering, and Medicine** to provide independent, objective analysis and advice to the nation and conduct other activities to solve complex problems and inform public policy decisions. The National Academies also encourage education and research, recognize outstanding contributions to knowledge, and increase public understanding in matters of science, engineering, and medicine.

Learn more about the National Academies of Sciences, Engineering, and Medicine at **www.nationalacademies.org**.

COMMITTEE ON SEX AND GENDER IDENTIFICATION AND IMPLICATIONS FOR DISABILITY EVALUATION

KATHRYN WHETTEN, Professor of Public Policy and Global Health,
Director, Center for Health Policy and Inequalities Research,
Codirector, Duke Sexual and Gender Minority Wellness Program;
Research Director, Hart Fellows Program, Duke University
SELMA FELDMAN WITCHEL, Professor Emerita, UPMC Children's
Hospital of Pittsburgh, University of Pittsburgh School of Medicine
NANCY FUGATE WOODS, Professor Emerita, Biobehavioral Nursing
and Health Informatics, University of Washington School of Nursing

Consultants to the Committee

PATRICIA M. OWENS, U.S. Government Accountability Office (*retired*)
DAVID WITTENBURG, Mathematica Policy Research, Inc.

Study Staff

MARY-BETH MALCARNEY, Study Director/Responsible Staff Officer,
Program Officer
KAREN L. HELSING, Senior Program Officer
TAYLOR KING, Associate Program Officer
ADRIENNE FORMENTOS, Associate Program Officer
ADAEZE OKOROAJUZIE, Senior Program Assistant
SHARYL NASS, Senior Director, Board on Health Care Services

Reviewers

This Consensus Study Report was reviewed in draft form by individuals chosen for their diverse perspectives and technical expertise. The purpose of this independent review is to provide candid and critical comments that will assist the National Academies of Sciences, Engineering, and Medicine in making each published report as sound as possible and to ensure that it meets the institutional standards for quality, objectivity, evidence, and responsiveness to the study charge. The review comments and draft manuscript remain confidential to protect the integrity of the deliberative process.

We thank the following individuals for their review of this report:

HENRY AARON, The Brookings Institution
ASH ALPERT, Yale School of Medicine
TANDY AYE, Stanford University School of Medicine
KELLAN E. BAKER, Whitman-Walker Institute
DAVID COLLISTER, University of Alberta, Canada
HOWARD GOLDMAN, University of Maryland School of Medicine
VERONICA GOMEZ-LOBO, Children's National Hospital
KACIE KIDD, West Virginia University School of Medicine
MITCHELL R. LUNN, Stanford University School of Medicine
MARYBETH MUSUMECI, The George Washington University's Milken Institute School of Public Health
G. NIC RIDER, Eli Coleman Institute for Sexual and Gender Health, University of Minnesota Medical School
JAE SEVELIUS, Columbia University
PATRICIA SILVEYRA, Indiana University School of Medicine

Although the reviewers listed above provided many constructive comments and suggestions, they were not asked to endorse the conclusions of this report, nor did they see the final draft before its release. The review of this report was overseen by **ROBERT S. LAWRENCE,** Johns Hopkins Bloomberg School of Public Health, and **WALTER R. FRONTERA,** University of Puerto Rico School of Medicine. They were responsible for making certain that an independent examination of this report was carried out in accordance with the standards of the National Academies and that all review comments were carefully considered. Responsibility for the final content rests entirely with the authoring committee and the National Academies.

Acknowledgments

The committee extends its sincere thanks to the many individuals who shared their time and expertise to support its work and inform its deliberations. This study was sponsored by the Social Security Administration, and we thank Vincent Nibali for his guidance and support of this important project, including verifying relevant technical content pertaining to the disability determination process for accuracy.

The committee benefited greatly from discussions with the individuals who presented at the committee's open sessions: Sofia Ahmed, Ash Alpert, David Collister, Yee Won Chong, Katharine Dalke, Ethan Fechter-Leggett, Louise Fleming, Dinah Foer, Veronica Gomez-Lobo, Rachel Harrington, Noi Liang, Charlie Manzano, Lexi Matza, Alex McConnell, Vincent Nibali, Roman Ruddick, Carl Streed, Jr., Justin Tsang, and Jess Walters. Agendas for the public meetings are provided in Appendix A.

Our appreciation goes to the reviewers for their invaluable feedback on an earlier draft of the report and to the monitor and coordinator who oversaw the report review. The committee acknowledges the many staff within the Health and Medicine Division who provided support in various ways to this project, including Mary-Beth Malcarney (study director), Taylor King (associate program officer), Adrienne Formentos (associate program officer), Adaeze Okoroajuzie (senior program assistant), Karen Helsing (senior program officer), and Julie Wiltshire (senior finance business partner). The committee extends great thanks and appreciation to Sharyl Nass, senior director, Board on Health Care Services, who oversaw the project. The committee also appreciates Christopher Lao-Scott and Rebecca Morgan (senior librarians) for their research assistance and fact checking. The report review, production, and communications staff all provided valuable guidance to ensure the success of the final product. Will Cole, Daniel J. Slack, Jiby Yohannan, Derek Chen, Nithya Krishnamurthy, and Joshua D. Safer drafted papers for the committee, which were valuable contributions to the narrative. Rona Briere and her staff are to be credited for the superb editorial assistance they provided in preparing the final report.

Contents

Boxes, Figures, and Tables

BOXES

FIGURES

TABLES

Acronyms and Abbreviations

AACC	American Association for Clinical Chemistry
AAP	American Academy of Pediatrics
ACA	Affordable Care Act
ACO	accountable care organization
ACOG	American College of Obstetricians and Gynecologists
ACOS	asthma–COPD [chronic obstructive pulmonary disease] overlap syndrome
ACS	American Cancer Society
AHIP	America's Health Insurance Plans
AMA	American Medical Association
AMH	anti-Müllerian hormone
AI/AN	American Indian/Alaska Native
AIS	androgen insensitivity syndrome
ALJ	Administrative Law Judge
AMA	American Medical Association
aOR	adjusted odds ratio
ASD	autism spectrum disorder
BCBSA	Blue Cross Blue Shield Association
BIA	bioelectrical impedance analysis
BMI	body mass index
BRFSS	Behavioral Risk Factor Surveillance System

CAKUT	congenital development anomalies of the kidney and urinary tract
CDC	Centers for Disease Control and Prevention
CDR	continuing disability review
CE	consultative examination
CF	cystic fibrosis
CFF	Cystic Fibrosis Foundation
CHIP	Children's Health Insurance Program
CI	confidence interval
CKD	chronic kidney disease
CKD-EPI	Chronic Kidney Disease Epidemiology Collaboration
CKiD	Chronic Kidney Disease in Children (Study)
CMS	Centers for Medicare & Medicaid Services
COPD	chronic obstructive pulmonary disease
DDS	Disability Determination Services
DE	disability examiner
DLCO	diffusing capacity of the lungs for carbon monoxide
DoD	U.S. Department of Defense
DSD	difference of sex development
eGFR	estimated glomerular filtration rate
EHR	electronic health record
ERS/ATS	European Respiratory Society/American Thoracic Society
ESKD	end-stage kidney disease
FEV_1	forced expiratory volume in the first minute
FFM	Federally Facilitated Marketplace (platform)
FQHC	federally qualified health center
FVC	forced vital capacity
GAHT	gender-affirming hormone therapy
GFR	glomerular filtration rate
GnRH	gonadotropin-releasing hormone
hCG	human chorionic gonadotropin
HHS	U.S. Department of Health and Human Services
HIV	human immunodeficiency virus
HPG	hypothalamic-pituitary-gonadal (axis)
HPS	Household Pulse Survey
HRSA	Health Resources and Services Administration

ICD	International Classification of Diseases and Related Health Problems
IHD	ischemic heart disease
IHS	Indian Health Service
IPF	idiopathic pulmonary fibrosis
IVF	in vitro fertilization
KPMAS	Kaiser Permanente Mid-Atlantic States
LGBTQ+	lesbian, gay, bisexual, transgender, queer, and other sexual orientations and gender identities
MA	Medicare Advantage
MC	medical consultant
MCO	managed care organization
mGFR	measured glomerular filtration rate
MRKH	Mayer-Rokitansky-Küster-Hauser
NAIC	National Association of Insurance Commissioners
NHIS	National Health Interview Survey
NIDDK	National Institute of Diabetes and Digestive and Kidney Diseases
NIH	National Institutes of Health
NIOSH	National Institute for Occupational Safety and Health
NIPS	noninvasive prenatal screening
NKF	National Kidney Foundation
NORC	National Opinion Research Center at the University of Chicago
OMB	Office of Management and Budget
ONC	Office of the National Coordinator for Health Information Technology
OR	odds ratio
OSHA	Occupational Safety and Health Administration
PC	psychological consultant
PCOS	polycystic ovarian syndrome
PF	pulmonary fibrosis
PFT	pulmonary function test
PPC	primary peritoneal carcinoma
PrEP	pre-exposure prophylaxis

POMS   Program Operations Manual System
PTSD   posttraumatic stress disorder

SDOH   social determinants of health
SGM   sexual and gender minority
SHADAC   State Health Access Data Assistance Center
SIM   State Innovation Model
SMR   standardized mortality ratio
SIR   standardized incidence ratio
SOC   *Standards of Care* (WPATH)
SOGI   sexual orientation and gender identity
SSA   Social Security Administration
SSDI   Social Security Disability Insurance
SSI   Supplemental Security Income

TGD   transgender and gender diverse

UCSF   University of California, San Francisco
UDS   Uniform Data System

VA   U.S. Department of Veterans Affairs
VHA   Veterans Health Administration
VST   variation in sex traits
VTE   venous thromboembolism

WHO   World Health Organization
WPATH   World Professional Association for Transgender Health

YRBS   Youth Risk Behavior Survey

Summary[1]

With limited resources to provide income support to Americans with chronic disease and disability, the criteria used in the Social Security Administration's (SSA's) disability determination process need to operationalize its definition of disability as validly as possible, consistent with the best scientific evidence. Over the years, SSA has asked the National Academies of Sciences, Engineering, and Medicine (the National Academies) to convene experts to offer conclusions about how current medical guidelines, scientific research, and clinical practices can inform SSA's processes for determining the distribution of disability benefits. This report responds to a request from SSA for the National Academies to convene a committee of experts to evaluate how contemporary conceptions of sex and gender in medicine and current clinical guidelines may impact certain of SSA's adult and childhood Listing of Impairments (Listings) that use sex-specific diagnostic criteria or address conditions traditionally associated with only one sex. These Listings include respiratory disorders, chronic kidney disease, childhood growth failure, cancers of the reproductive system, and certain gynecological conditions related to HIV infection. The conclusions drawn by this committee are intended to offer guidance to SSA on how best to serve applicants for disability benefits who are transgender and gender diverse or have variations in sex traits.

"Transgender and gender diverse" (TGD) is an umbrella term the committee uses throughout this document to refer to people whose gender

---

[1] This summary does not include references. Citations to support the text and conclusions herein are provided in the respective chapters of the report.

identity differs from what is typically associated with their sex recorded at birth. It is estimated that approximately 0.6 percent (nearly 1.64 million people) over age 13 in the United States identify as TGD. The committee uses the term "variations in sex traits" (VSTs) to refer to people born with a variety of genetic, anatomical, and hormonal variations that affect the genitourinary tract and reproduction systems; people with VSTs may have a sex and/or gender identity that differs from their sex recorded at birth. Estimates of the percentage of the population born with VSTs vary from 0.05 to 1.7 percent.

While only a small portion of disability applicants are likely to be TGD or have VSTs, adjudicating their applications appropriately is important. Numerous studies demonstrate that TGD people and people with VSTs experience stigma attached to their nonconformity in sex and/or gender identity and expression, which can result in cascading and consequential patterns of discrimination in health care settings. These considerable challenges and inequalities lead to delayed preventive screenings, late detection of chronic disease, and poor health outcomes. A growing body of data consistently demonstrates that TGD people experience a greater burden of poor physical health, mental health, and health-related quality of life compared with their cisgender counterparts. TGD people also experience a greater burden of disability overall, and TGD people with disabilities are more likely than cisgender people with disabilities to report an unmet need, such as the inability to obtain prescription medications or to see a health provider when needed. Research is lacking on disability among people with VSTs, but available data suggest that they experience greater morbidity from chronic disease compared with the general population, and some VST diagnoses may cause lifelong chronic health concerns.

SSA does not offer gender-affirming treatment or care (or health care services of any kind). However, it does receive applications for disability benefits that come from TGD applicants or applicants with VSTs. It is not known how many TGD people or people with VSTs currently receive disability benefits from SSA or how many have applied and been denied. However, given that TGD people and people with VSTs may experience a greater burden of disability overall relative to the general population, SSA requested this study to ensure that its disability determination process provides an accurate and clear assessment of function among these and all populations that may apply.

STUDY APPROACH

To carry out this study, the National Academies empaneled an ad hoc committee of 15 experts in the areas of endocrinology, gender and sexual development, gender-affirming care and treatment, the health of persons with VSTs, clinical psychology, pediatrics and adolescent medicine, pulmonology, nephrology, oncology, data collection, health policy, disability policy, and health disparities.

The committee held five meetings between May 2023 and February 2024. These meetings included two public sessions during which the committee heard presentations by experts in the field on appropriate evaluation criteria for TGD people with chronic kidney disease; breaking the gender–cancer association; gender identity–related data collection and care decision making within the Veterans Health Administration; appropriate evaluation criteria for TGD people with chronic respiratory disease; and collection of gender identity data in electronic health records (EHRs). Finally, in a third public session, the committee listened to three patient–provider panels that examined the lived experience of chronic disease and disability among TGD people and people with VSTs. In addition, the committee and National Academies staff conducted an extensive review of the literature.

OVERALL CONCLUSIONS

The committee formulated thirteen overall conclusions in seven categories: (1) collection of data on sex and gender identity, (2) variability of documentation for TGD people and people with VSTs in medical records, (3) Listings with sex-specific diagnostic criteria, (4) chest binders and considerations for pulmonary function tests, (5) alternative growth failure measurements, (6) inclusive language in Listings, and (7) guidance for adjudicators on assessing disability for TGD applicants and applicants with VSTs. In accordance with its statement of task, the committee offers conclusions, but not recommendations. Conclusions presented below are based on best available data. The committee acknowledges that clinical decisions need to be made—and are being made—even when evolving scientific data are limited, and that SSA needs a reasonable approach for adjudicating claims for TGD applicants and applicants with VSTs. The conclusions presented here represent the consensus of committee members based on their clinical expertise and professional judgment.

Collection of Data on Sex and Gender Identity

Recent advances in EHRs and health information technology provide opportunities to increase the visibility of TGD patients and patients with VSTs through the routine collection of sexual orientation and gender identity (SOGI) data. SOGI data collection—which allows for health care providers and patients to record sexual orientation, gender identity, sex recorded at birth, information about VSTs, and similar information within individual patient charts—is a key strategy for reducing the many health disparities faced by TGD people and people with VSTs. For TGD patients and patients with VSTs, robust SOGI data collection can enhance meaningful dialogue during clinical encounters, promote appropriate preventive screenings based on anatomy, reduce unequal and discriminatory health care practices, and foster respectful and patient-centered long-term care. Furthermore, comprehensive SOGI data collection enables accurate interpretation of common sex-specific measurements that are important for disability evaluations. Yet despite the importance of collecting these data and the capacity for medical records to facilitate that process, SOGI data collection and documentation by health care providers remains highly variable. Medical records therefore cannot be relied upon to capture accurately all patients with TGD or VST identity or lived experience.

> *Conclusion 1. Medical records alone may fail to identify the gender diversity of TGD applicants or appropriately capture biological characteristics relevant to applicants with VSTs. SSA application forms do not ask applicants about gender identity or sex recorded at birth. Because these patient characteristics matter for disability determination, the committee concludes giving applicants the option to enter their own gender identity and sex recorded at birth information when submitting a disability application would enable a more accurate assessment.*

This approach would help fill the gaps that result when health care providers and institutions do not collect the patient data that SSA may need to adjudicate accurately the applications for disability benefits of TGD people and people with VSTs. Best practices include allowing people to enter gender identity separately from sex recorded at birth, offering a range of appropriate response options and providing a free-text response option, such as "I use something else." It is also important to include either separate questions about VSTs or free-text options that allow people with VSTs to share their individual experience. SSA forms give prompts to applicants to "explain in remarks" additional details about various questions on the application (e.g., citizenship status, military service), and similar prompts could be appropriate for applicants to describe additional information related to gender identity or sex recorded at birth. SSA might also benefit from including such optional questions in its National Beneficiary Survey to help it better understand the lived experience of those people it serves who are TGD or have VSTs. It is important to provide information to applicants and survey respondents on why these questions are being asked and how these data may impact disability determinations. In addition, best practices call upon health care providers and institutions to consistently refer to patients by their correct name (i.e., their chosen and presently used name) and pronouns in all records. SSA could conduct a review of its processes to ensure they meet this standard.

Variability of Documentation for Transgender and Gender Diverse People and People with Variations in Sex Traits in Medical Records

Gender-affirming care comprises an array of services for TGD people that may include medical, surgical, mental health, and nonmedical care. There is no "one size fits all" approach to gender-affirming care: health care services provided to TGD people may differ based on when the care was provided (both historically and across the lifespan), differences in access to care, and tailoring of care to the needs of individual patients. Likewise, appropriate care and treatment for people with VSTs is highly variable and condition and patient specific. Medical records specific to care for chronic conditions may not fully describe gender-affirming care or care related to VSTs. In addition, some TGD people and people with VSTs do not seek or are not able to access medical intervention, so one should not assume that TGD or VST identity or lived experience confers any particular type or amount of care.

Conclusion 2. There is considerable observed variability in gender-affirming care across the country for TGD people. This variability may impact documentation in medical records submitted to SSA for disability applications. The committee concludes that SSA would best serve TGD applicants by communicating to them that medical records related to gender-affirming care are likely relevant to certain disability determinations.

Having a sufficiently complete medical record of gender-affirming care is important for disability evaluations, as understanding the nature of any such care (along with its timing and duration) may be important to improve understanding of functional assessment and eligibility for disability benefits.

Conclusion 3. Individuals with VSTs are a heterogeneous group that includes persons with genetic, anatomical, and hormonal variations and/or variations in genitourinary system development affecting the genitourinary tract and reproduction system. The diverse VST diagnoses may differ as to the extent and type of impact they have on chronic disease and disability. Hence, care and treatment for these diagnoses is variable and patient specific, and medical records that merely list a VST diagnosis may fail to provide sufficient historical information for evaluating the need for disability benefits. The committee concludes that SSA would best serve applicants with VSTs by communicating to them that medical records related to VST care may be relevant to disability applications and their submission is greatly encouraged whenever possible.

Some people with VSTs experience lifelong and ongoing disability, whereas others experience sporadic severe health crises (e.g., experiencing sudden needs for lengthy hospitalization followed by periods of stability) or mental health and/or neurodiversity disabilities associated with VST-related stressors. To provide thorough disability adjudication, SSA needs to have medical records that sufficiently document care related to the management of VSTs. Given that a VST diagnosis is often made during early childhood and adolescence, records from many years ago may be relevant to the adjudication process; however, the committee acknowledges that old records may be very difficult to obtain, and an undue burden should not be placed on applicants to locate such records.

Listings with Sex-Specific Diagnostic Criteria

Listings for respiratory disease, childhood growth failure, and chronic kidney disease include sex-specific diagnostic criteria. Clinicians interpreting tests and measurements for these conditions must select an appropriate reference sex—male or female—to predict lung function, growth failure, or kidney function, respectively. For many applicants for disability benefits, sex recorded at birth is the appropriate reference sex. However, selecting the reference sex for TGD people or people with VSTs is often difficult, and it is not always clear which sex is the most appropriate to use.

Errors in the selection of reference sex may happen for a number of reasons, including incorrect sex recorded in the patient chart (especially when the medical record does not ask for gender identity separately from sex recorded at birth), failure to ask patients about VSTs, failure to ask patients about relevant gender-affirming care (e.g., timing of any hormone therapy), biases held by providers that negatively influence patient care, and the absence of guidelines for interpreting relevant tests and measurements for TGD patients and patients with VSTs. Moreover, even when medical records contain a complete and accurate accounting of patient sex and gender identity characteristics such that providers are aware they are assessing TGD patients or patients with VSTs, providers may lack training and experience in caring for these patients and may not know how or when TGD or VST lived experience impacts patient care and clinical decision making. Thus, providers may have to make difficult or arbitrary judgment calls about which reference sex is most appropriate for a given patient at a given time.

Gender-affirming hormone therapy (GAHT) further complicates this picture. In the case of pulmonary function, some research suggests that "hormonal sex at puberty"—the hormone that was predominant during puberty (estrogen or testosterone) and that influenced the shape and size of the thoracic cavity—may be a more accurate metric for choosing a reference sex for a pulmonary function test for individuals who initiated pubertal delay and began GAHT during puberty. For this portion of the population, affirmed gender—not sex recorded at birth—may be the more appropriate reference sex for this test. Similarly, some researchers propose, for the purposes of calculating body mass index (BMI), continuing to use the growth chart corresponding to sex recorded at birth during pubertal delay but switching to the affirmed-sex growth chart once GAHT has been initiated. In the case of assessing chronic kidney disease, the receipt of GAHT at any time (not just during puberty) is an important consideration for assessing kidney function, but conclusions cannot be drawn regarding the accuracy of either the male or female gender-based estimating equations for estimated glomerular filtration rate (eGFR) in populations receiving GAHT. To aid in clinical decision making for patients receiving GAHT, it may be appropriate for providers to interpret lung function, adolescent growth, and kidney function in comparison with both reference sex ranges ("dual calculations") or use measurements that are independent of sex, when available. However, these approaches to patient care have yet to be prospectively validated for clinical use. Where people with VSTs take GAHT, the above approaches may be appropriate; however, research is limited on the impact of GAHT in populations with VSTs. The committee notes that people with VSTs take hormone therapy for a multitude of reasons beyond gender-affirming care and care is extremely individualized; the impact of various hormone therapies on sex-specific measurements is unknown.

> *Conclusion 4. Sex recorded at birth may be the appropriate reference sex to use for some—but not all—TGD applicants and applicants with VSTs who apply for disability benefits by submitting medical records with sex-specific measurements of pulmonary function (i.e., spirometry and diffusion capacity of the lungs for carbon monoxide [DLCO] measurements), growth failure (i.e., weight-for-length and BMI-for-age measurements), or kidney function (i.e., estimated glomerular filtration rate [eGFR]). However, SSA's disability criteria use the term "gender" in reference to pulmonary function and growth failure measurements, which may incorrectly indicate that "gender identity" is the determining factor in the interpretation of these measurements.*

SSA might consider changing the language in the respiratory disorder Listings[2] and Listings related to childhood growth failure[3] to replace the word "gender" with "sex recorded at birth." Making this change would

---

[2] Listing of Impairments 3.02, 3.03, 3.04, 103.02, and 103.04.

[3] Listing of Impairments 105.08B, as applied across 100.05, 103.06, 104.02, 105.08, 106.08, and 114.11(I).

allow for clearer assessments for some TGD applicants and some applicants with VSTs. Using the phrase "sex recorded at birth" rather than simply "sex" clarifies that sex as recorded at birth is the important patient characteristic for these specific assessments, not "sex" as may be recorded on other administrative records (e.g., driver's license, passport). The current SSA Listings for chronic kidney disease[4] do not use gender- or sex-specific language, and language changes are not necessary. The committee stresses that even though sex recorded at birth is important for the assessments listed here, this does not negate the importance of gender identity for disability applicants in general or for other types of disability assessments. In addition, the committee acknowledges that for some people with VSTs, sex assignment at birth (which becomes the sex recorded on birth certificates and medical records) may not be straightforward and can change after the initial determination.

> *Conclusion 5. Sex recorded at birth may* not *be the appropriate reference sex for assessing pulmonary function or growth failure for some TGD people or people with VSTs, particularly for those who began pubertal delay and GAHT during puberty. While considerable research is needed to determine best approaches, the committee concludes that SSA would best serve applicants who receive GAHT by using the lowest value recorded (e.g., lower percentile for BMI-for-age and weight-for-length/lower spirometry or DLCO reading) to determine the presence of disability.*

Some providers use "dual calculations" (e.g., interpreting spirometry using both male and female reference ranges) to enhance decision making for patients receiving GAHT, but use of this approach is not universal, and most assessments are likely to use whatever sex is listed in the medical record (even if this information is inaccurate). Medical records may also contain calculations from both charts because providers were mistaken or lacked training on which chart to use. Given these challenges, the committee concludes that when a disability applicant's medical record contains calculations from both reference ranges, SSA will best serve applicants who receive GAHT by using the *lowest recorded value* to determine disability under respiratory and childhood growth failure Listings.

> *Conclusion 6. Medical records submitted to SSA may provide an inaccurate estimation of kidney function in people who receive GAHT. The committee concludes that where medical records contain eGFR measurements based on both the male and female coefficients, SSA would best serve applicants who receive GAHT by using measured GFR (when available) or the lowest eGFR value recorded to determine the presence of disability.*

---

[4] Listing of Impairments 6.05A3 and 106.05C.

Comprehensive data are lacking regarding the bias introduced by using binary sex coefficients in eGFR calculations for TGD people and people with VSTs, and clear conclusions cannot be drawn regarding the accuracy of either the male or female sex-based estimating equations for eGFR in populations receiving GAHT. Until further research clarifies the influence of GAHT on biomarkers that are important for calculating eGFR and determining kidney function, existing eGFR measurements for people who receive GAHT may be inaccurate and may overestimate kidney function. Given these challenges, SSA might consider using the *lowest eGFR value recorded* in the medical record for applicants receiving GAHT to determine disability under chronic kidney disease Listings.

Conclusion 7. In order to improve access to an accurate interpretation of pulmonary function, kidney function, or growth percentile, SSA may offer a consultative exam to TGD applicants and applicants with VSTs where SSA sees evidence in the medical record that measurements were or may have been calculated using an incorrect reference sex or where dual calculations were not provided but may be appropriate.

In such cases, it may be beneficial, where clinically appropriate, to order a test that does not contain sex-specific criteria (e.g., pulse oximetry for evaluation of cystic fibrosis) or that offers more precise measurement of function (e.g., measured GFR to assess kidney function). Where more specific tests are not available or clinically appropriate, SSA could instruct the consultative examiner to interpret results using both male and female reference ranges. This approach would ensure fairness for TGD people and people with VSTs who have lacked access to providers trained to interpret their results thoughtfully and with specific consideration of individual patient histories (e.g., duration and timing of GAHT). It is essential that individual applicants always have the choice of whether to submit to a consultative examination without any detriment to their application if declined.

Chest Binders and Considerations for Pulmonary Function Tests

Chest binders are a common gender-affirming practice for transgender men and other TGD individuals. Some people with VSTs also use chest binders. Chest binding is not merely an elective activity to enhance appearance, but an essential daily practice for reducing chest dysphoria (distress from unwanted breast development) and improving mental health outcomes. While minimal research exists on the impact of chest binders on pulmonary function, some patients may wear a chest binder during administration of a pulmonary function test (PFT). The committee strongly believes providers should not require TGD people to remove chest binders prior to undergoing a PFT.

Conclusion 8. Evidence that an individual applying for disability benefits wore a chest binder during a PFT should not disadvantage their application.

As many people who bind do so daily and for extended periods of time (often exceeding 10 hours each day), SSA needs to be aware that when a chest binder has been removed for the purposes of undergoing a PFT, that measurement of lung function may not reflect daily lived experience. The medical record may not indicate whether a chest binder was worn during a PFT, but when the medical record contains different PFT values, SSA needs to be aware that those differences could be attributable to the fact that the patient wore a binder during one test but not another. For this reason, the committee concludes that SSA would best serve TGD applicants and applicants with VSTs by using the lowest recorded PFT value to determine disability under respiratory disorder Listings.

Alternative Growth Failure Measurements

Literature and guidelines call for the use of alternative measures of body composition along with BMI-for-age, given concerns about the utility and accuracy of BMI-for-age as the sole measure. BMI-for-age may be an especially poor measure for identifying growth failure in children, as it is not considered a reliable indicator for children below the third percentile of weight. In addition, because BMI does not differentiate between lean body mass and body fat, it may not adequately measure elements of body composition that matter for children who are experiencing growth failure related to underlying chronic disease.

Conclusion 9. Studies clearly show that for many children, BMI is a suboptimal measure for identifying growth failure. BMI can be particularly inaccurate in identifying growth failure in TGD adolescents receiving GAHT, which may affect linear growth and fat distribution.

In these adolescents, linear growth velocity may be a better indicator of growth failure. Similarly, a large-percentage weight loss strongly indicates malnutrition that places an individual at very high risk for growth failure. SSA might consider including alternative measures across various childhood growth failure Listings, as well as changing the window of time during which measurements must be taken. This approach might provide for more accurate assessment of not just TGD youth but all pediatric populations applying for disability benefits.

Inclusive Language in Listings

Increasingly, national organizations are moving away from using gendered language that restricts cancers and gynecological conditions to one's gender or sex recorded at birth. Simple updates to language—for example, changing "women with cervical cancer" to "people with cervical cancer"—serve to include all populations that may have or may be at risk of developing these conditions, regardless of gender identity or sex recorded at birth.

Conclusion 10. National organizations, such as the American Cancer Society and the American Society of Clinical Oncology, have begun to call for a more gender-inclusive approach to cancer screening, treatment, and care, whereby cancer terms reflect the organ in which they arise instead of being tied to gender. SSA might best serve disability applicants by removing gendered language from its cancer Listings.

The current SSA Listings for cancers of the prostate gland, testicles, and penis[5] exemplify this approach and are consistent with how the field is shifting toward inclusiveness in cancer language. SSA might consider changing the Listing for "Cancers of the female genital tract"[6] to "Cancers of the uterus, uterine cervix, vulva, vagina, fallopian tubes, and ovaries," which would align this Listing with organs rather than gender. Such a change would clarify that this Listing can apply to anyone who can meet the SSA criteria, regardless of their sex recorded at birth or gender identity. Similarly, SSA might consider removing the differentiation of women versus men within criteria under primary peritoneal carcinoma[7] and instead base this condition on the histopathology. This approach recognizes that primary peritoneal mesothelioma can occur in all people regardless of the presence or absence of ovaries, while primary peritoneal adenocarcinoma is almost exclusively diagnosed in people born with ovaries.

Conclusion 11. Using more inclusive language in Listings would help achieve appropriate disability adjudication for TGD people and people with VSTs living with HIV. The committee concludes that SSA might best serve applicants with HIV by removing sex-specific language from its HIV disability criteria.

---

[5] Listing of Impairments 13.24, 13.25, and 13.26.
[6] Listing of Impairments 13.23.
[7] Listing of Impairments 13.00K7.

SSA might consider changing the Listing category from "HIV infection manifestations specific to women"[8] to "Gynecologic manifestations of HIV," to make this Listing inclusive of and appropriate for all people with HIV who exhibit these medical conditions. Such an inclusive approach promotes equitable care by recognizing that gendered representations in HIV screening and treatment may misidentify patient care needs.

Guidance for Adjudicators on Assessing Disability for Transgender and Gender Diverse Applicants and Applicants with Variations in Sex Traits

Similar to health care providers who make difficult choices about appropriate chronic disease management for TGD patients and patients with VSTs, experts involved in the disability determination process must determine how TGD or VST lived experience may impact various disability applications (if at all) and whether additional information is needed to aid in accurate adjudication. In addition, these experts must understand how the multiple social determinants of health that disproportionately impact TGD applicants and applicants with VSTs intersect with chronic disease and disability.

> *Conclusion 12. Given the complexities of the disability determination process for some TGD applicants and some applicants with VSTs, experts involved in the disability adjudication process may need guidance on how aspects of gender-affirming care or other aspects of health, treatment, and care impact disability determinations. SSA might consider supporting adjudicators in these complex disability determinations by delivering national-level trainings and consultive services.*

Guidance to adjudicators can take many forms, including (1) training on the intersection of disability with TGD/VST lived experience; (2) access to national- or regional-level medical and mental health experts who can consult on disability applications submitted by TGD applicants and applicants with VSTs (the Veteran Health Administration's e-consult might serve as a model); (3) clear statements within the Program Operations Manual System that medical records related to gender-affirming care and care for people with VSTs may be relevant for accurate disability evaluation; and (4) communications to applicants that medical records related to gender-affirming care and care for VSTs may be relevant to certain disability applications and that it may be appropriate to use the "remarks" section on disability applications to describe how TGD or VST lived experience has impacted their health or opportunity to receive appropriate care for their

---

[8] Listing of Impairments 14.00F7.

impairment(s). Consistent training and guidance across the 54 Disability Determination Services offices is important, as geographic variability or lack of local expertise may mean that individual offices are not equipped to deliver trainings or provide consultation on these topics.

> *Conclusion 13. Multilevel obstacles to optimal health occur across the life course of TGD people and people with VSTs. These barriers contribute to a greater burden of co-occurring physical and mental health conditions and poorer overall health outcomes compared with the general population. SSA might consider supporting adjudicators in making determinations for TGD applicants and applicants with VSTs by including in guidance and trainings content on the structural disadvantages faced by these populations and how they may impact disability.*

While many applicants for disability benefits experience challenges with their health, TGD applicants and applicants with VSTs face significant and well-described structural disadvantages, including intrapersonal factors (internalized transphobia due to stigma and stress), interpersonal factors (e.g., lack of access to knowledgeable providers, exposure to discriminatory and suboptimal health care, consequences of implicit bias), and structural factors (e.g., lack of access to health insurance, inequitable access to employment opportunities). In addition, TGD people and people with VSTs are members of multiple diverse communities and may experience concomitant barriers to optimal health due to additional dimensions (e.g., race, ethnicity, age, socioeconomic status, and other domains) that influence their experiences with health care and the social drivers of health.

Thus, TGD people and people with VSTs may have systematically experienced delayed preventive screenings, late detection of chronic disease (and the predisposing conditions that contribute to chronic disease), and inadequate care to address chronic health concerns. These barriers coalesce, leading to poorer self-care, inadequate management of chronic disease, and poorer quality of life. These factors may ultimately result in delayed and/or inadequate care for multiple impairments that form the basis of a disability application. It is essential that disability adjudicators remain attuned to the structural and sociocontextual factors that shape the applications of TGD people and people with VSTs. For example, adjudicators might receive guidance and training to consider, as part of a disability evaluation, potential stigmatizing language found in medical records that signals suboptimal care delivery.

1

Introduction

The U.S. Census Bureau (2022) estimates that 44 million Americans (13.4 percent of the U.S. population) have a disability. However, only about one-third of these Americans (15.1 million as of December 2022[1]) meet the rigorous medical and other criteria for receiving disability benefits from the Social Security Administration (SSA). Despite a more limited definition of disability, SSA's programs are an important safety net for all Americans, given that "a young person starting a career today has a roughly 1-in-3 chance of dying or qualifying for [disability] before reaching Social Security's full retirement age" (CBPP, 2023, p. 1). SSA disability programs are especially significant for severely disabled Americans, as chronic illness can have devastating economic consequences for those unable to work because of their condition(s) and health needs.

Given the limited resources for providing income support to Americans with chronic disease and disability, the criteria used in SSA's disability determination process need to operationalize its definition of disability as validly as possible, consistent with the best scientific evidence. Over the years, SSA has sought to bring greater accuracy to its disability criteria by updating its Listing of Impairments (Listings) (medical criteria that apply to the evaluation of disability) to recognize advances in medical technology and alternative medical criteria that are more appropriate to disability evaluation for certain populations. In June 2023, for example, SSA revised

---

[1] As of December 2022, 8.8 million people received disability benefits from the Social Security Disability Insurance program, and 6.3 million received Supplemental Security Income benefits, qualifying for this program as a result of meeting disability criteria (SSA, 2023a,b).

its medical criteria for evaluating chronic liver disease by adding another type of measurement (serum sodium levels), which research shows offers a clearer assessment for individuals with certain liver conditions (SSA, 2023c). Likewise, in 2016 SSA added measurement of CD4 count to its HIV Listings to allow for clearer assessment for certain populations with HIV, and in 2022 it proposed revising its criteria for measuring congenital heart disease to recognize advances in medical technology that allow for more accurate measurement (SSA, 2016, 2022).

Over the years, SSA has asked the National Academies of Sciences, Engineering, and Medicine (the National Academies) to convene experts for the purpose of studying various aspects of its disability criteria and offering conclusions as to how it could update or modify its Listings or other policies to reflect current medical guidelines, findings of scientific research, and clinical practices relevant for persons with severe chronic disease. This report responds to a request from SSA for the National Academies to convene an ad hoc committee of experts to evaluate how modern conceptions of sex and gender in medicine and current clinical guidelines may impact certain of SSA's adult and childhood disability Listings that use sex-specific diagnostic criteria or address conditions traditionally associated with only one sex. Conclusions drawn by this committee (and presented in Chapter 14 of this report) represent an attempt to add clarity and accuracy to SSA's disability criteria for all disabled Americans, but in particular, and as requested by SSA, for Americans who meet disability criteria and also are transgender or gender diverse (TGD) or have variations in sex traits (VSTs). In addition, the materials presented in this report are intended to aid SSA in creating resources for training disability adjudicators in several areas, including on how sex and gender identity impact disability determinations and how to best understand the medical records it receives from TGD applicants and applicants with VSTs—including the sex and gender identity data contained therein, the descriptions of care and treatment specific to these populations, and common co-occurring conditions that contribute to impairment—so that SSA may appropriately adjudicate these disability applications.

TRANSGENDER AND GENDER DIVERSE PEOPLE AND PEOPLE WITH VARIATIONS IN SEX TRAITS: BACKGROUND, PREVALENCE, AND DISABILITY EXPERIENCE

"Transgender and gender diverse" is an umbrella term the committee uses throughout this document to refer to people whose gender identity differs from what is typically associated with their sex recorded at birth. The committee uses the term "variations in sex traits" to refer to people born with a variety of genetic, anatomical, and hormonal variations that affect the genitourinary tract and reproduction systems; people with VSTs may have a sex and/or gender identity that differs from their sex recorded at birth. A wide range of terminology is used to refer to sex and gender identity and to TGD people and people with VSTs, as elaborated in Chapter 2.

Population Size

Transgender and Gender Diverse People

According to a 2022 analysis of data from the Centers for Disease Control and Prevention's Behavior Risk Factor Surveillance System (BRFSS) and Youth Risk Behavior Survey (YRBS), nearly 1.64 million people over age 13 in the United States identify as transgender (Herman et al., 2022). This analysis, conducted by the Williams Institute at the University of California, Los Angeles, estimates that 0.5 percent of U.S. adults (about 1.3 million) and 1.4 percent of U.S. youth ages 13–17 (about 300,000) identify as transgender (Herman et al., 2022). While these figures represent the best available data on estimates of the TGD population in the United States, they may be an undercount, as questions about gender identity were, at the time of the study, included in the YRBS in only 15 states. Still, these figures show that a growing proportion of the younger population identifies as TGD. A 2022 survey by the Pew Research Center echoes these findings, showing that adults under age 30 (5.1 percent) are more likely than older adults (1.6 percent of those ages 30–49 and 0.3 percent of those ages 50 and older) to be TGD (Brown, 2022).

People with Variations in Sex Traits

Estimates of the percentage of the population born with VSTs vary between 0.05 and 1.7 percent, depending on the definition used for VST (e.g., restricting the definition to include only ambiguous genitalia or taking a broader approach to include other differences in characteristics or reproductive anatomy) and the type of study conducted (medical or general population study) (Blackless et al., 2000; Fausto-Sterling, 2000; Hughes et al., 2007). Overall, the statistics for the occurrence of VST are possibly inaccurate, given the difficulty of accessing knowledgeable medical providers and variability in documentation.

Disability Experience among Transgender and Gender Diverse People and People with Variations in Sex Traits

A growing body of data consistently demonstrates that TGD people experience a greater burden of poor physical health, mental health, and health-related quality of life compared with their cisgender counterparts

(Fredriksen Goldsen et al., 2022). TGD people also experience a greater burden of disability overall, and TGD people with disabilities are more likely than cisgender people with disabilities to report an unmet need, such as the inability to obtain a needed prescription medication or to see a doctor when needed (Downing and Przedworski, 2018; Fredriksen Goldsen et al., 2022; Mulcahy et al., 2022). These findings have been echoed in multiple studies, including a study using nationally representative data from the BRFSS which found that TGD people have a greater probability of reporting a disability compared with their cisgender peers (Smith-Johnson, 2022). In this study, TGD adults were found to have a "27 percent chance of having at least one disability at age 20 and a 39 percent chance of disability at age 55, nearly twice the rate of cisgender counterparts" (Smith-Johnson, 2022, p. 1470). Likewise, a 2015 study by the National Center for Transgender Equality found that 39 percent of transgender survey respondents (n = 28,000) reported one or multiple disabilities, compared with 15 percent of the general U.S. population (James et al., 2016). That survey also found that transgender respondents were almost four times as likely as the general population to report difficulty in conducting basic activities of daily living (including visiting a doctor's office or going shopping), and six times as likely to report having serious difficulty concentrating, remembering, or making decisions because of a physical, mental, or emotional condition (James et al., 2016).

These studies examine disability overall and not necessarily disability in the SSA context, as federal law requires a very strict definition of disability within SSA programs (as described in Box 1-1).[2] However, TGD populations served by SSA may also experience greater disability: Dragon and colleagues (2017) showed that 71 percent of TGD Medicare beneficiaries were entitled to disability benefits and had more disabilities overall compared with their non-TGD counterparts. Notably, in this study, a greater proportion of TGD Medicare beneficiaries were younger than age 65, identified as Black, and had chronic conditions (including chronic obstructive pulmonary disease [COPD] and depression), as well as additional potentially disabling pain and neurologic conditions, compared with non-TGD beneficiaries (Dragon et al., 2017).

While research is lacking on disability among people with VSTs, the available data suggest that, compared with the general population, they

---

[2] BRFSS surveys ask a set of six questions related to disability; answering "yes" to one or more of these questions means a respondent is considered to have a disability: (1) "Are you deaf or do you have serious difficulty hearing?" (2) "Are you blind or do you have serious difficulty seeing, even when wearing glasses?" (3) "Because of a physical, mental, or emotional condition, do you have serious difficulty concentrating, remembering, or making decisions?" (4) "Do you have serious difficulty walking or climbing stairs?" (5) "Do you have difficulty dressing or bathing?" (6) "Because of a physical, mental, or emotional condition, do you have difficulty doing errands alone such as visiting a doctor's office or shopping?" (CDC, 2018).

experience greater morbidity from chronic disease, including some of the specific chronic conditions examined in this report, and experience a range of chronic care needs, as described in Chapter 7 (Bojesen et al., 2006; Gaston et al., 2021; Romejko et al., 2022).

In addition, and of importance in considering SSA's work-related disability criteria, social stigma, gender dysphoria, and other mental health concerns may interfere with the educational trajectory of TGD/VST youth (Budge et al., 2020; Hatchel et al., 2019; Johns et al., 2021), and TGD people at any age may face significant employment discrimination (Davidson, 2016; Kattari et al., 2016). Education and employment are predictors of more positive health outcomes and healthy aging (McDowell et al., 2019), so challenges in these areas increase vulnerability to poor health outcomes.

SOCIAL SECURITY ADMINISTRATION: DISABILITY DETERMINATIONS

To understand the committee's charge and the scope of this report, it is first helpful to understand the basics of SSA disability determinations. SSA administers benefits for disabled Americans through two programs: (1) the Supplemental Security Income (SSI) Program for adults and children (under age 18) who meet disability criteria and qualify based on limited income and resources[3]; and (2) the Social Security Disability Insurance (SSDI) Program for disabled workers who have worked for a sufficient period of time to qualify for SSDI benefits (in other words, people who are "insured" under the Social Security Act because they have contributed to the Social Security trust fund by paying taxes on their earnings over time). SSDI covers certain disabled dependents as well. A person with both limited income/ resources and a work history can qualify for both SSI and SSDI.

To receive disability benefits (SSDI or SSI) from SSA, an individual must meet the statutory definition of disability, which, for adults, is the "inability to engage in any substantial gainful activity by reason of any medically determinable physical or mental impairment which can be expected to result in death or which has lasted or can be expected to last for a continuous period of not less than 12 months."[4] SSA considers a medically determinable physical or mental impairment to be an impairment that results from anatomical, physiological, or psychological abnormalities that can be shown by medically acceptable clinical and laboratory diagnostic techniques. A child under age 18 is considered disabled if he or she "has a medically determinable physical or mental impairment, which results in

---

[3] "Income" includes wages, Social Security benefits, and pensions, and "resources" are things of value an applicant may own, such as a second vehicle or money in a bank account (SSA, 2024).

[4] 42 U.S.C. § 1382c(a)(3)(A) (2004).

marked and severe functional limitations, and which can be expected to result in death or which has lasted or can be expected to last for a continuous period of not less than 12 months."[5] SSA's definition of a "medically determinable physical or mental impairment" is the same for adults and children. A finding of disability in both adults and children depends on the severity of functional limitations arising from the applicant's impairment or combination of impairments.

SSA evaluates eligibility for both SSI and SSDI for adult applicants through a five-step sequential evaluation process, described in Box 1-1. The evaluation process is modified for child applicants, as described below.

BOX 1-1
SSA Disability Determinations:
Five-Step Sequential Evaluation Process

The Social Security Administration (SSA) engages in a five-step sequential evaluation process to determine adult eligibility for Supplemental Security Income (SSI) and Social Security Disability Insurance (SSDI) programs. The five steps are as follows:

Step 1: SSA considers the disability applicant's current work activity. If the applicant is currently engaged in what SSA considers to be "substantial gainful activity," the applicant is not eligible for disability benefits under either SSI or SSDI and the process ends here, regardless of the applicant's medical condition. In 2024, the threshold income—the most a person can earn and still be eligible for disability benefits—is $1,550 a month ($18,600 per year) for people who are not blind ($2,590 per month for blind applicants).

Step 2: SSA considers the medical severity of the applicant's impairment(s) and whether their impairment meets the duration requirement. Under 20 C.F.R. § 404.1509, unless an applicant's impairment is expected to result in death, the impairment "must have lasted or must be expected to last for a continuous period of at least 12 months." If an applicant cannot provide sufficient documentation that their impairment(s) meets the duration requirement, the disability application will be denied.

Step 3: SSA considers the medical severity of the applicant's impairment(s) and whether they have an impairment(s) that "meets" or "medically equals" one of the categories in the

continued

---

[5] 42 U.S.C. § 1382c(a)(3)(C)(i) (2004).

For children, SSA determines at step 3 whether the impairment(s) meets, medically equals (is equivalent in severity to), or functionally equals (i.e., the impairment[s] results in functional limitations equivalent in severity to) the criteria in SSA's Child Listings.[6] If a child's impairment or combination of impairments "does not meet or medically equal any listing, [SSA] will decide whether it results in limitations that functionally equal the listings."[7] Functional equivalence refers to functionally equaling the Listings: SSA's technique for determining functional equivalence is a "whole child" approach that "accounts for all of the effects of a child's impairments singly and in combination—the interactive and cumulative effects of the impairments—because it starts with a consideration of actual functioning in all settings" (SSA, 2009).

---

regulations called the Listing of Impairments (the Listings). For adults, the Listings describe, for each of the major body systems, impairments SSA considers to be severe enough to prevent a person from engaging in any gainful activity, regardless of his or her age, education, or work experience, and serve as a "screen-in" step. If SSA finds that the applicant's impairment meets or medically equals a Listing, then the application is accepted and benefits are awarded (and the analysis does not proceed to steps 4 and 5). Applicants proceed to step 4 when their impairment is severe but does not meet or medically equal any Listing within the Listing of Impairments.

Step 4: SSA assesses the applicant's "residual functional capacity" and past relevant work. Residual functional capacity is the maximum level of physical or mental performance that the applicant can achieve given the functional limitations resulting from their medical impairment(s). If an applicant has the capacity to engage in some portion of their past relevant work, the application will be denied.

Step 5: SSA determines whether the applicant can perform any work in the national economy on the basis of the assessment of residual functional capacity and the applicant's age, education, and work experience. If the applicant can make an adjustment to perform other work, SSA will deny the disability application. Otherwise, the application will be approved and disability benefits awarded.

SOURCES: 20 C.F.R. § 404.1520 (2012); SSA, 2024.

---

[6] 20 C.F.R. §§ 416.926, 416.926a.
[7] 20 C.F.R. § 416.926a.

STUDY CHARGE AND SCOPE

SSA requested that the National Academies convene an ad hoc committee of experts to evaluate how modern conceptions of sex and gender in medicine and current clinical guidelines may impact certain of SSA's adult and childhood disability Listings that use sex-specific diagnostic criteria or address conditions traditionally associated with only one sex. In addition, SSA asked for a description of the current collection and use of sex and gender identity data in clinical practice and across the health care system; an examination of the impact of gender-affirming hormone therapy on physiological sex differences; and a discussion of how common therapies, treatment, and care used in practice today for TGD people and people with VSTs may impact disability evaluation. This report responds to these requests. The statement of task provided by SSA is displayed in Box 1-2.

Social Security Disability Applicants Who Are Transgender and Gender Diverse or Have Variations in Sex Traits

Although the statement of task asks the committee to review gender-affirming care and other treatments for TGD people and people with VSTs, it should be noted that SSA itself does not offer gender-affirming treatment or care (or health care services of any kind). Furthermore, SSA does not stand in a position to determine what gender-affirming treatment and care should be, or how these health care services should be financed through public or private insurance. SSA is a federal agency distinct from the Department of Health and Human Services (HHS). The policy decisions made by HHS (or federal or state programs that receive HHS funding) regarding gender-affirming care do not impact decision making at SSA, just as SSA's policy decisions on disability criteria do not impact care for chronic diseases within HHS-funded programs.

While SSA does not determine what appropriate care for TGD people and people with VSTs should be, it does receive applications for disability benefits that may come from these populations. SSA does not currently ask its applicants questions around gender identity, sex recorded at birth, or other matters that might be related to the lived experience of TGD people or people with VSTs; therefore, this committee cannot know how many TGD people or people with VSTs currently receive disability benefits from SSA or how many have applied for benefits and been denied. However, given research presented above on chronic disease and disability experienced by TGD people and people with VSTs, these populations may make up a larger portion of SSA's population than of the general population.

On the other hand, as examined in Chapter 3, TGD people and people with VSTs encounter considerable challenges and inequities in their ability

---

BOX 1-2
Statement of Task

An ad hoc committee of the National Academies of Sciences, Engineering, and Medicine will review the latest published research and medical guidelines addressing the current status of sex-specific medical diagnosis, evaluation, and treatment of individuals who are transgender or who are undergoing gender-affirming procedures. Based on the available evidence, the committee's report will strive to

1. Describe the current clinical conceptions of sex and gender accepted by the medical community, including
   a. How sex and gender are medically defined and the preferred nomenclature for transgender individuals, those who have undergone some amount of gender-affirming therapy, treatments, or care, and others with intersex sex traits, expression, or identity;
   b. The recognized categories of individuals with intersex sex traits, expression, or identity, and to the extent possible, identify
      i. Each category's prevalence in the American public;
      ii. How does the medical community handle decisions involving intersex, transgender, and transitioning patients and what are the particular impacts each trait, expression, or identity has on medical evaluation and care; and
      iii. Any trends or potential changes in how physiological sex differences are conceptualized, measured, or accounted for in the provision of medical care and what is driving these trends;
   c. How and when sex and gender identification information is collected and used in the clinical practice of medicine; and
   d. How other large, national health organizations, besides the Social Security Administration (SSA), collect sex and gender information, and whether and how they use that information to make health care decisions (e.g., Veterans Health Administration, Medicaid, health management organizations).
2. Identify the usual physiological differences between the male and female sex and describe what is known about
   a. How differences between the sexes are measured and change in quantity or quality over the course of development, puberty, and growth;
   b. Exceptions to these usual differences, their prevalence, and what can cause them;

continued

BOX 1-2 Continued

    c. The specific effect hormonal or other gender-affirming therapies, treatments, or care (or similar therapies used for other reasons) have on expected physiological sex differences such as height and weight, including how those differences change based on the onset, duration, or intensity of the employed therapy, treatment, or care; and

    d. The diagnostic or evaluative testing that may be impacted by sex differences or sex transition and how to account for that impact.

3. Describe the gender-affirming therapies, treatments, and care utilized most commonly today to aid in sex affirmation and detail for each

    a. The method of action and expected physiological effect;

    b. Prerequisite testing or treatment before the therapy, treatment, or care is prescribed;

    c. Ways of categorizing the therapies, treatments, and care;

    d. The general course of treatment, specific impacts, and potential side effects from the therapy, treatment, or care, including how progress is measured and indicators that would lead to cessation of the therapy, treatment, or care; and

    e. Common comorbid impairments for those seeking, undergoing, or under the effects of the therapy, treatment, or care.

4. For the criteria in the listing of impairments that currently consider an individual's gender[a] describe the evidence related to

    a. If these criteria were changed to vary based upon an individual's birth sex, or, alternatively, to vary based upon an individual's affirmed sex after gender-affirming therapy, treatment, or care, rather than their gender, would the criteria appropriately measure the severity of the underlying medical concept?

    b. Based on the current criteria, could sex assigned at birth or affirmed sex (or some other categorization) be used to measure the severity of the underlying medical concept as a medically appropriate indicator of severity?

    c. What guidelines are available to maintain the specificity of these criteria for persons who have undergone some type and amount of gender-affirming therapy, treatment, or care or who have an intersex sex expression, trait, or identity?

    d. Are there alternative tests, evaluations, or laboratory values that would offer similar insight into functional capability as what is revealed by the current criteria?

    e. If and how other large, national health organizations, besides SSA, assess the impairments associated with these criteria and determine eligibility for individuals who have undergone some type and amount of gender-affirming therapy,

BOX 1-2 Continued

treatment, or care or who have an intersex sex expression, trait, or identity, to the extent applicable?

   f. If there are alternative tests that would offer similar insight into functional capability, could an individual's sex assigned at birth or affirmed sex (or some other categorization) be applied to appropriately assess medical severity for each of those tests?

5. For the criteria or Listings in the Listing of Impairments that currently consider conditions generally associated with only one sex, what is known about[b]

   a. How does the medical community diagnose and what terminology is appropriate to evaluate the considered conditions when they affect an individual that has undergone some type and amount of gender-affirming therapy, treatment, or care or who has an intersex sex expression, trait, or identity?

   b. Which of SSA's existing Listing criteria could be most appropriately used to evaluate these conditions in individuals affected by some type and amount of gender-affirming therapy, treatment, or care or who have an intersex sex expression, trait, or identity?

   c. What are the circumstances under which an individual with a different sex assigned at birth could appropriately be evaluated under the criteria?

   d. What, if any, changes to the current criteria would be necessary for them to serve as medically appropriate indicators of severity for claimants outside of the generally associated sex?

   e. Are there any screening recommendations or guidelines related to the considered conditions specific to individuals who have undergone some type and amount of gender-affirming therapy, treatment, or care or who have an intersex sex expression, trait, or identity?

   f. Do other large, national health organizations, besides SSA, assess these impairments and determine eligibility for individuals who have undergone some type and amount of gender-affirming therapy, treatment, or care or who have an intersex sex expression, trait, or identity?

The report will include findings and conclusions but not recommendations.

---

[a]*Adult Listings with different criteria for males and females include 3.02, 3.03, 3.04, and 6.05. Child Listings with different criteria for males and females include 103.02, 103.04, 105.08, and 106.05. Listings that refer to male and female growth charts under Listing 105.08B include 100.05, 104.02, 106.08, and 114.11(I).*

[b]*Listings considering conditions generally associated with only one sex include 13.23, 13.24, 13.25, 13.26, and 14.11(I).*

to access quality health care services, and experience a disproportion-ate burden of structural barriers, including discrimination, violence, and stigmatizing experiences, inside and outside of health care interactions (Bockting et al., 2013; Brown and Jones, 2016; Caceres et al., 2020; Feldman et al., 2021; Grant et al., 2011; Haghighat et al., 2023; Jackson et al., 2008; Maragh-Bass et al., 2017; Poteat et al., 2013, 2016; Seelman et al., 2017). These well-established structural barriers and inequities may mean that fewer TGD people and people with VSTs have the support they need from providers to submit an application for disability benefits to SSA.

Regardless of their actual numbers among populations applying for and receiving disability benefits from SSA, logic dictates that at least some applicants for SSA benefits will have TGD or VST lived experience. SSA developed the committee's statement of task with these applicants in mind in effort to ensure that its disability criteria provide an accurate and clear assessment of function for these and all populations that may apply.

Disability Listings Included in the Statement of Task

While questions around sex assigned at birth and gender identity are important to diagnosis, treatment, health disparities, and morbidity for many chronic diseases, SSA asked the committee to examine how these concepts impact a few specific conditions within SSA's disability criteria as described under the Listing of Impairments. Imbedded within the statement of task are several adult and childhood disability Listings that refer to an applicant's sex or gender by using sex-specific diagnostic criteria. These Listings (Box 1-3) comprise adult and childhood respiratory disorders, adult and childhood chronic kidney disease, and various childhood Listings related to growth failure.

SSA also asked the committee to review those disability Listings that are traditionally associated with one sex, comprising several cancers of the reproductive system and criteria for assessing human immunodeficiency virus (HIV) infection in women (Box 1-4).

The committee acknowledges that many chronic diseases vary by sex beyond those listed in Boxes 1-3 and 1-4. Sex differences in disease prevalence, presentation, manifestation, incidence, diagnosis, response to treatment, long-term effects, and disability are common in nearly every major chronic disease, including cardiovascular disease, stroke, Alzheimer's disease, diabetes, mental health conditions, and autoimmune disorders (Mauvais-Jarvis et al., 2020). While these sex differences may matter for chronic disease and disability among TGD people and people with VSTs, the committee did not endeavor to review all disability Listings to determine whether and how those differences may impact these populations. Rather, the committee was tasked with examining only those chronic diseases that

---

BOX 1-3
SSA Disability Listings with Sex-Specific Diagnostic Criteria

Respiratory Disorders (Adult and Childhood)
    3.00 Respiratory Disorders—Adult[a]:
        3.02: Chronic respiratory disorders due to any cause except CF
        [cystic fibrosis]
        3.03: Asthma
        3.04: Cystic fibrosis
    103.00 Respiratory Disorders—Childhood[b]:
        103.02: Chronic respiratory disorders due to any cause except CF
        103.04: Cystic fibrosis
Chronic Kidney Disease (Adult and Childhood)
    6.00 Genitourinary Disorders—Adult[c]
        6.05: Chronic kidney disease
    106.00 Genitourinary Disorders—Childhood[d]
        106.05: Chronic kidney disease
Growth Failure (Childhood)[e]
    100.05 Failure to thrive in children from birth to attainment of age 3
    103.06 Growth failure due to any chronic respiratory disorder
    104.02 Chronic heart failure
    105.08 Growth failure due to any digestive disorder
    106.08 Growth failure due to any chronic renal disease
    114.11(I) Human immunodeficiency virus (HIV) infection; immune sup-
        pression and growth failure

SOURCES:[1]
[a] https://www.ssa.gov/disability/professionals/bluebook/3.00-Respiratory-Adult.htm (accessed March 11, 2024)
[b] https://www.ssa.gov/disability/professionals/bluebook/103.00-Respiratory-Childhood.htm (accessed March 11, 2024)
[c] https://www.ssa.gov/disability/professionals/bluebook/6.00-Genitourinary-Adult.htm (accessed March 11, 2024)
[d] https://www.ssa.gov/disability/professionals/bluebook/106.00-Genitourinary-Childhood.htm (accessed March 11, 2024)
[e] https://www.ssa.gov/disability/professionals/bluebook/100.00-GrowthImpairment-Childhood.htm (accessed March 11, 2024)

---

[1]All sources accessed March 11, 2024.

have sex-specific diagnostic criteria (outlined in Box 1-3) or are traditionally associated with one sex (outlined in Box 1-4). From the perspective of how SSA evaluates disability under its Listings, sex differences in other chronic conditions do not have a sex or gender component, and therefore are not within the purview of this study.

BOX 1-4
SSA Disability Listings Traditionally Associated with One Sex

Cancers of the Reproductive System (Adult)[a]
    13.00 Cancer—Adult
    13.23: Cancers of the female genital tract—carcinoma or sarcoma
    13.24: Prostate gland—carcinoma
    13.25: Testicles
    13.26: Penis
HIV Infection Manifestations Specific to Women (Adult)[b]
    14.00 Immune System Disorders—Adult
    14.11(I): HIV [human immunodeficiency virus] infection manifestations
    specific to women

SOURCES:[1]
[a] https://www.ssa.gov/disability/professionals/bluebook/13.00-Neoplastic Diseases-Malignant-Adult.htm (accessed March 11, 2024)
[b] https://www.ssa.gov/disability/professionals/bluebook/14.00-Immune-Adult.htm (accessed March 11, 2024)

---

[1]All sources accessed March 11, 2024.

Take, for example, cardiovascular disease. Ischemic heart disease (IHD)—heart problems caused by narrowed heart arteries, which can lead to heart attack—is the leading cause of morbidity and mortality in women in the United States (Aggarwal et al., 2018). Recognizing and understanding the sex-specific pathophysiology of cardiovascular disease has resulted in improved clinical outcomes for women. Compared with men, women have different risk factors for developing IHD, often exhibit different symptoms of IHD, show pathophysiologic differences, and may require different or additional diagnostic imaging to fully determine the extent and severity of their condition (Aggarwal et al., 2018; Mieres et al., 2014). Sex hormones have been shown to impact IHD as well (e.g., the negative impact of estrogen loss during menopause), and research suggests that estrogen administration increases the risk of cardiovascular events in transgender women (Iqbal and Zaidi, 2009; Masumori and Nakatsuka, 2023; Wellons et al., 2012). Despite the importance of considering sex and gender identity in IHD for appropriate diagnosis and treatment, however, the diagnostic tools[8]

---

[8] While there is evidence to suggest sex differences in common diagnostic tools that measure cardiac function, current guidelines do not use gender-specific diagnostic criteria (Kligfield et al., 2007; Tomaszewski et al., 2019).

commonly used to measure cardiac function are not sex specific, meaning test results are not interpreted differently for males and females (Kligfield et al., 2007). Therefore, criteria for determining disability under SSA Listing 4.04, Ischemic heart disease, do not include any sex-specific diagnostic tests or other criteria (SSA, 2008). For this reason, SSA did not include IHD or other cardiovascular conditions within the purview of this committee.

Some disability Listings, however, use sex-specific diagnostic criteria (outlined in Box 1-3 and presented in detail in Chapters 8, 9, and 10), and these criteria can be challenging to put into practice when determining disability for TGD applicants and applicants with VSTs. For example, spirometry is a common test for measuring lung function. SSA evaluation criteria include the use of spirometry measurements as part of evaluating respiratory disorders under adult Listing 3.00 and childhood Listing 103.00. Current clinical guidelines from the European Respiratory Society/American Thoracic Society advise that spirometry be calculated based on age, height, and sex, meaning "biological sex" (Graham et al., 2019; Stanojevic et al., 2022). Clinicians interpreting spirometry for TGD people and people with VSTs must select an appropriate reference sex—male or female—when using spirometry results to predict lung function. This can be a challenge, as sex is not always an easy question to answer for many people with VSTs. For TGD people who undergo pubertal delay and/or receive gender-affirming hormone treatment during puberty (a critical phase in lung development), affirmed gender—not sex recorded at birth—may be the more appropriate reference sex for interpreting spirometry. Chapter 8 of this report reviews respiratory disease Listings in greater depth and considers what the current science and guidelines may mean for evaluating disability among TGD people and people with VSTs.

Similar questions arise in evaluating the various growth failure categories listed in Box 1-3, as these disability listings all utilize the weight-for-length table for children from birth to attainment of age 2 years and the body mass index (BMI) table for children from age 2 to attainment of age 18, both of which are dependent on sex for determining growth as it relates to disability; these conditions are discussed in Chapter 9. Likewise, sex and gender identity are important when considering estimated glomerular filtration rate (eGFR), a common measurement of kidney function, that is calculated based on the patient's age, sex, and creatinine/cystatin C; chronic kidney disease is discussed in Chapter 10.

Regarding SSA disability Listings traditionally associated with one sex, SSA included in the statement of task reproductive cancers and HIV manifestations specific to women, as outlined in Box 1-4. The committee acknowledges that certain other conditions may be more common in one sex or the other, or present for one sex in specific ways that matter for disability. For example, some common chronic conditions—such as autoimmune diseases and depression—occur at substantially higher rates in women than in men (Temkin et al., 2023). However, none of these conditions are female specific. For example, while males may constitute only 20 percent of the population affected by autoimmune diseases, they may still suffer from disability related to such diseases, and SSA's criteria do not limit autoimmune disease Listings to female applicants (Nussinovitch and Shoenfeld, 2012). This report addresses (in Chapters 11 and 12) the question of whether any of the SSA categories traditionally associated with one sex should remain reserved for just one sex; however, reproductive cancers and HIV manifestations specific to women are the only disability Listings that have criteria limited to (or potentially limited to) one sex.

The committee acknowledges that mental health conditions are of significant concern for TGD people and people with VSTs. While this report does not examine disability Listings related to any mental health condition, the committee describes these important issues throughout this report as these conditions may impact care, quality of life, and disability.

SSA Disability Evaluation Processes Included in the Statement of Task

It should be noted that none of the sex-specific measures outlined above determine, on their own, whether an applicant will receive disability benefits. SSA disability criteria under these Listings require that applicants submit additional medical evidence to document the severity of their condition and show the extent of their impairment in support of their disability application. In the case of adult respiratory disorders, for example, applicants may submit, in addition to results of pulmonary function tests, results of imaging tests and other laboratory tests, descriptions of prescribed treatment and the patient's response to treatment, documentation of recurrent hospitalizations, and other documentation included under Listing 3.00, Respiratory Disorders—Adult. Likewise, people with reproductive cancers provide medical evidence in support of their disability application that may include documentation of their treatment history, response to anticancer therapy, cancer recurrence, evidence of metastasis, or other documentation listed under Listing 13.00, Cancer—Adult or under any specific cancer listing.

Furthermore, medical evidence to document impairment under the Listings is just one type of information applicants are required to submit to prove eligibility for disability benefits from SSA. Applicants must document that they are financially eligible for the SSA program to which they are applying and that they are, as a result of their disability, unable to engage in "substantial gainful activity." As presented in Box 1-1, if an applicant has a severe impairment but does not meet or medically equal any of the Listings, the sequential process assesses whether the applicant's physical or mental residual functional capacity allows them to perform past relevant work (step 4) or whether the applicant can adjust to other work in the national economy (step 5).

The statement of task asks the committee to focus on medical criteria within SSA's Listing of Impairments; therefore, this report focuses on aspects of the disability determination process related to assessing medical impairment under SSA's Listings. However, the committee notes that the functional capacity–related questions within SSA's process are important for TGD applicants and applicants with VSTs, as they are for all disability applicants. As this report highlights, assessing disability for TGD people and people with VSTs is not easily done within the rubric of the Listings, especially where questions of sex and gender identity arise. Where an applicant cannot meet or medically equal a Listing—especially where the complexities raised by sex and gender identity make it challenging to meet Listing criteria—the evaluation of functional capacity becomes a critical component of determining disability for TGD applicants and applicants with VSTs. Certainly, TGD or VST identity or lived experience will factor into the assessment of functional capacity, but the report does not focus on these areas as they are outside of the statement of task and areas of expertise among committee members. However, information provided in this report may support understanding of evaluating functional capacity within disability determination.

STUDY APPROACH

The committee empaneled by the National Academies to conduct this study consisted of 15 members with expertise in the areas of endocrinology, gender and sexual development, gender-affirming care and treatment, the health of persons with variations in sex traits, clinical psychology, pediatrics and adolescent medicine, pulmonology, nephrology, oncology, data collection, health policy, disability policy, and health disparities (see Appendix B for biographical sketches of the committee members).

The committee held five meetings between May 2023 and February 2024, which included four public sessions. At the first public session, SSA reviewed the statement of task with the committee and provided more specifics on its objectives for the study. At the second public session, the committee heard presentations on (1) sex differences in kidney disease, the impact of gender-affirming care, and appropriate evaluation criteria for TGD people with chronic kidney disease, and (2) recent efforts to break the gender–cancer association in preventive screenings and quality measurement. In the third public session, the committee heard presentations on (1) collection of gender identity data and care decision making within the Veterans Health Administration; (2) respiratory disease among TGD people and the selection of an appropriate reference sex for pulmonary function tests for TGD patients; and (3) collection of sexual orientation and gender identity data in electronic health records. Finally, in the fourth public session, the committee listened to three patient–provider panels that addressed (1) VSTs and implications for disability; (2) chronic lung disease and chronic kidney disease in TGD people and implications for disability; and (3) cancer treatment and care for TGD people and implications for disability. (See Appendix A for the public session agendas.)

In addition, the committee conducted an extensive review of the literature pertaining to (1) care and treatment for chronic disease in TGD people and people with VSTs; (2) current guidelines pertaining to reproductive cancers, HIV, and the sex-specific measurements commonly used to measure pulmonary function, kidney function, and childhood growth; and (3) collection and reporting of sex and gender identity data within clinical practice and across the health care system. Committee members and project staff identified additional literature and information using traditional academic research methods and online searches throughout the course of the study. The committee's work was further informed by previous reports of the National Academies related to disability and the health of LGBTQ+ populations, which are referenced throughout the report.

ORGANIZATION OF THE REPORT

Given the length and complexity of the statement of task, the committee divided this report into three parts.

Part I: Sex and Gender Data Collection and Clinical Practice

Here, the report examines modern definitions of sex and gender and how medical records document sex, gender, and other important data on the experiences of TGD people and people with VSTs in medical settings. Chapter 2 reviews contemporary understandings of sex and gender in clinical practice and implications for the work of SSA. This chapter includes definitions of key concepts and terms important for understanding sex and gender within the context of clinical medicine. Chapter 3 describes how and when sex and gender information is collected and used in clinical practice of medicine; the committee describes the substantial benefits to the collection of sexual orientation and gender identity (SOGI) data and the significant biases and structural barriers that prevent robust SOGI data collection in health care settings, including unequal and discriminatory care delivery experienced by TGD people and people with VSTs. Chapter 4 provides an overview of SOGI data collection across the health care system. A common thread across the chapters in Part I is the recognition that medical records from various providers form the bulk of the information gathered and received by SSA as it makes disability determinations. Given that individuals applying for disability benefits from SSA access health insurance in different ways and access care from different types of providers, it is important to understand how the SOGI data collection that takes place—or does not take place—in health care institutions and across various sectors of the health care system impacts the quality of SOGI data available in medical records received by SSA.

Part II: Affirming Treatment and Care for Transgender and Gender Diverse People and People with Variations in Sex Traits

Affirming care and treatment for TGD people and people with VSTs is a broad and variable area of clinical care. While there are guidelines in existence that put forward the highest standard of care, the committee acknowledges that outdated treatment and care practices may still be in common use today. In addition, there is no "one size fits all" approach to care, and care is often variable and patient specific. Some TGD people and people with VSTs do not seek or are not able to access medical intervention, and TGD or VST identity or lived experience does not confer any particular type or amount care. Chapter 5 focuses on the range of gender-affirming care practices, including gender-affirming hormone therapy and surgeries, that may be documented in medical records provided to SSA. Chapter 6 builds on this knowledge by describing various co-occurring conditions that may have a disproportionate impact on TGD populations. Chapter 7 examines the numerous categories that may fall under VSTs and appropriate care for these populations.

Part III: Sex, Gender, and Disability Determinations

With an understanding of the collection of sex and gender data in clinical practice (Part I) and a foundation of care and treatment for TGD people and people with VSTs (Part II), the final part of the report examines the specific disability Listings within the statement of task and responds to SSA's questions about whether changes in disability criteria may be warranted to assess these conditions accurately for TGD people and people with VSTs within current guidelines and standards of care. Chapter 8 reviews adult and childhood respiratory disorder Listings, including asthma, COPD, and cystic fibrosis. Here, the committee reviews the sex-specific pulmonary function tests included in the disability criteria (including spirometry and diffusing capacity of the lungs for carbon monoxide [DLCO] tests), assessing whether these tests are appropriate for measuring pulmonary function among TGD and VST populations or whether there are alternative measurements that may be more appropriate. Chapter 9 examines the pediatric weight-for-length table and BMI-for-age table, both of which are gendered and may have implications for appropriate measurement for childhood disability applicants who are TGD or who have VSTs. Chapter 10 reviews adult and childhood kidney disease and looks at eGFR—a common test of kidney function that has sex-specific criteria—considering whether eGFR is appropriate for measuring kidney function among TGD and VST populations or whether alternative measurements may be more appropriate. Chapter 11 focuses on reproductive cancers, including "cancers of the female genital tract" (which includes cancers of the uterus, uterine cervix, vulva, vagina, fallopian tubes, and ovaries) and cancers of the prostate gland, testicles, and penis; here, the committee reviews current guidelines that recommend screening based on organs rather than gender identity or sex recorded at birth and evaluates whether the language SSA uses to describe reproductive cancers could be updated to be more inclusive of TGD people and people with VSTs. Chapter 12 addresses the gender-specific language under the disability Listing "HIV infection manifestations specific to women," and, similar to the analysis of reproductive cancers in Chapter 11, considers whether language under this Listing could be worded differently to capture data on TGD people and people with VSTs more accurately. Finally, in Chapter 13 the committee gives an overview of the various types of experts who inform SSA disability determinations at different stages in the process, and draws conclusions about where, within its current policies and processes, SSA might think about opportunities for ensuring that these experts have the information and tools they need to make appropriate disability determinations for TGD applicants and applicants with VSTs.

Conclusions

While the committee presents key points at the end of each chapter, Chapter 14 provides the committee's overall conclusions for the study.

Appendix C

The report contains one substantive appendix, Appendix C, exploring sex differences in physiology and disease pathophysiology, the impact of gender-affirming hormone therapy on physiological health, and the affect exogenous hormones may have on common diagnostic or evaluative tests. Appendix C covers the following topic areas: bone health and body composition, cardiovascular system, immune system, metabolism, gastrointestinal system, nervous system, pulmonary system, renal system, integumentary system, fertility, and sexual function.

REFERENCES

Aggarwal, N. R., H. N. Patel, L. S. Mehta, R. M. Sanghani, G. P. Lundberg, S. J. Lewis, M. A. Mendelson, M. J. Wood, A. S. Volgman, and J. H. Mieres. 2018. Sex differences in ischemic heart disease. *Circulation: Cardiovascular Quality and Outcomes* 11(2):E004437.

Blackless, M., A. Charuvastra, A. Derryck, A. Fausto-Sterling, K. Lauzanne, and E. Lee. 2000. How sexually dimorphic are we? Review and synthesis. *American Journal of Human Biology* 12(2):151–166.

Bockting, W. O., M. H. Miner, R. E. Swinburne Romine, A. Hamilton, and E. Coleman. 2013. Stigma, mental health, and resilience in an online sample of the US transgender population. *American Journal of Public Health* 103(5):943–951.

Bojesen, A., S. Juul, N. H. Birkebaek, and C. H. Gravholt. 2006. Morbidity in Klinefelter syndrome: A Danish register study based on hospital discharge diagnoses. *Journal of Clinical Endocrinology & Metabolism* 91(4):1254–1260.

Brown, A. 2022. *About 5% of young adults in the U.S. say their gender is different from their sex assigned at birth.* https://www.pewresearch.org/short-reads/2022/06/07/about-5-of-young-adults-in-the-u-s-say-their-gender-is-different-from-their-sex-assigned-at-birth/ (accessed March 2024).

Brown, G. R., and K. T. Jones. 2016. Mental health and medical health disparities in 5135 transgender veterans receiving healthcare in the Veterans Health Administration: A case-control study. *LGBT Health* 3(2):122–131.

Budge, S. L., S. Domínguez, Jr., and A. E. Goldberg. 2020. Minority stress in nonbinary students in higher education: The role of campus climate and belongingness. *Psychology of Sexual Orientation and Gender Diversity* 7(2):222–229.

Caceres, B. A., K. B. Jackman, D. Edmondson, and W. O. Bockting. 2020. Assessing gender identity differences in cardiovascular disease in US adults: An analysis of data from the 2014–2017 BRFSS. *Journal of Behavioral Medicine* 43(2):329–338.

CBPP (Center on Budget and Policy Priorities). 2023. *Chart book: Social security disability insurance.* https://www.cbpp.org/research/social-security/social-security-disability-insurance-0 (accessed March 2024).

CDC (Centers for Disease Control and Prevention). 2018. *A data users' guide to the disability questions included in the Behavioral Risk Factor Surveillance System.* https://www.cdc.gov/brfss/data_documentation/pdf/BRFSS_Data_Users_Guide_on_Disability_Questions_2018-508.pdf (accessed May 2024).

Davidson, S. 2016. Gender inequality: Nonbinary transgender people in the workplace. *Cogent Social Sciences* 2(1):1236511.

Downing, J. M., and J. M. Przedworski. 2018. Health of transgender adults in the U.S., 2014–2016. *American Journal of Preventive Medicine* 55(3):336–344.

Dragon, C. N., P. Guerino, E. Ewald, and A. M. Laffan. 2017. Transgender Medicare beneficiaries and chronic conditions: Exploring fee-for-service claims data. *LGBT Health* 4(6):404–411.

Fausto-Sterling, A. 2000. *Sexing the body: Gender politics and the construction of sexuality.* New York: Basic Books.

Feldman, J. L., W. E. Luhur, J. L. Herman, T. Poteat, and I. H. Meyer. 2021. Health and health care access in the US transgender population health (TransPop) survey. *Andrology* 9(6):1707–1718.

Fredriksen Goldsen, K. I., M. Romanelli, C. P. Hoy-Ellis, and H. Jung. 2022. Health, economic and social disparities among transgender women, transgender men and transgender nonbinary adults: Results from a population-based study. *Preventive Medicine* 156:106988.

Gaston, B., N. Marozkina, D. C. Newcomb, N. Sharifi, and J. Zein. 2021. Asthma risk among individuals with androgen receptor deficiency. *JAMA Pediatrics* 175(7):743–745.

Graham, B. L., I. Steenbruggen, M. R. Miller, I. Z. Barjaktarevic, B. G. Cooper, G. L. Hall, T. S. Hallstrand, D. A. Kaminsky, K. McCarthy, M. C. McCormack, C. E. Oropez, M. Rosenfeld, S. Stanojevic, M. P. Swanney, and B. R. Thompson. 2019. Standardization of spirometry 2019 update. An official American Thoracic Society and European Respiratory Society technical statement. *American Journal of Respiratory and Critical Care Medicine* 200(8):E70–E88.

Grant J. M., L. A. Mottet, J. Tanis, J. Harrison, J. L. Herman, and M. Keisling. 2011. *Injustice at every turn: A report of the national transgender discrimination survey*. Washington, DC: National Center for Transgender Equality and National Gay and Lesbian Task Force.

Haghighat, D., T. Berro, L. Torrey Sosa, K. Horowitz, B. Brown-King, and K. I. Zayhowski. 2023. Intersex people's perspectives on affirming healthcare practices: A qualitative study. *Social Science & Medicine* 329:116047.

Hatchel, T., A. Valido, K. T. De Pedro, Y. Huang, and D. L. Espelage. 2019. Minority stress among transgender adolescents: The role of peer victimization, school belonging, and ethnicity. *Journal of Child and Family Studies* 28(9):2467–2476.

Herman, J. L., A. R. Flores, and K. K. O'Neill. 2022. *How many adults and youth identify as transgender in the United States?* Los Angeles, CA: UCLA School of Law, Williams Institute.

Hughes, I. A., C. Nihoul-Fekete, B. Thomas, and P. T. Cohen-Kettenis. 2007. Consequences of the ESPE/ LWPES guidelines for diagnosis and treatment of disorders of sex development. *Best Practice & Research Clinical Endocrinology & Metabolism* 21:351–365.

Iqbal, J., and M. Zaidi. 2009. Understanding estrogen action during menopause. *Endocrinology* 150(8):3443–3445.

Jackson, N. C., M. J. Johnson, and R. Roberts. 2008. The potential impact of discrimination fears of older gays, lesbians, bisexuals and transgender individuals living in small-to moderate-sized cities on long-term health care. *Journal of Homosexuality* 54(3): 325–339.

James, S. E., J. L. Herman, S. Rankin, M. Keisling, L. Mottet, and M. Anafi. 2016. *The report of the 2015 U.S. Transgender survey*. Washington, DC: National Center for Transgender Equality.

Johns, M. M., A. Zamantakis, J. Andrzejewski, L. Boyce, C. N. Rasberry, and P. E. Jayne. 2021. Minority stress, coping, and transgender youth in schools-results from the resilience and transgender youth study. *Journal of School Health* 91(11):883–893.

Kattari, S. K., D. L. Whitfield, N. E. Walls, L. Langenderfer-Magruder, and D. Ramos. 2016. Policing gender through housing and employment discrimination: Comparison of discrimination experiences of transgender and cisgender LGBQ individuals. *Journal of the Society for Social Work and Research* 7(3):427–447.

Kligfield, P., L. S. Gettes, J. J. Bailey, R. Childers, B. J. Deal, E. W. Hancock, G. van Herpen, J. A. Kors, P. Macfarlane, D. M. Mirvis, O. Pahlm, P. Rautaharju, G. S. Wagner, M. Josephson, J. W. Mason, P. Okin, B. Surawicz, and H. Wellens. 2007. Recommendations for the standardization and interpretation of the electrocardiogram: Part I: The electrocardiogram and its technology: A scientific statement from the American Heart Association Electrocardiography and Arrhythmias Committee, Council on Clinical Cardiology; the American College of Cardiology Foundation; and the Heart Rhythm Society: Endorsed by the International Society for Computerized Electrocardiology. *Circulation* 115(10): 1306–1324.

Maragh-Bass, A. C., M. Torain, R. Adler, E. Schneider, A. Ranjit, L. M. Kodadek, R. Shields, D. German, C. Snyder, S. Peterson, J. Schuur, B. Lau, and A. H. Haider. 2017. Risks, benefits, and importance of collecting sexual orientation and gender identity data in healthcare settings: A multi-method analysis of patient and provider perspectives. *LGBT Health* 4(2):141–152.

Masumori, N., and M. Nakatsuka. 2023. Cardiovascular risk in transgender people with gender-affirming hormone treatment. *Circulation Reports* 5(4):105–113.

Mauvais-Jarvis, F., N. Bairey Merz, P. J. Barnes, R. D. Brinton, J. J. Carrero, D. L. DeMeo, G. J. De Vries, C. N. Epperson, R. Govindan, S. L. Klein, A. Lonardo, P. M. Maki, L. D. McCullough, V. Regitz-Zagrosek, J. G. Regensteiner, J. B. Rubin, K. Sandberg, and A. Suzuki. 2020. Sex and gender: Modifiers of health, disease, and medicine. *Lancet* 396(10250):565–582.

McDowell, M. J., J. M. W. Hughto, and S. L. Reisner. 2019. Risk and protective factors for mental health morbidity in a community sample of female-to-male trans-masculine adults. *BMC Psychiatry* 19(1):16.

Mieres, J. H., M. Gulati, N. Bairey Merz, D. S. Berman, T. C. Gerber, S. N. Hayes, C. M. Kramer, J. K. Min, L. K. Newby, J. V. Nixon, M. B. Srichai, P. A. Pellikka, R. F. Redberg, N. K. Wenger, L. J. Shaw, and on behalf of the American Heart Association Cardiac Imaging Committee of the Council on Clinical Cardiology and the Cardiovascular Imaging and Intervention Committee of the Council on Cardiovascular Radiology and Intervention. 2014. Role of noninvasive testing in the clinical evaluation of women with suspected ischemic heart disease: A consensus statement from the American Heart Association. *Circulation* 130(4):350–379.

Mulcahy, A., C. G. G. Streed, A. M. Wallisch, K. Batza, N. Kurth, J. P. P. Hall, and D. J. McMaughan. 2022. Gender identity, disability, and unmet healthcare needs among disabled people living in the community in the United States. *International Journal of Environmental Research and Public Health* 19(5):2588.

Nussinovitch, U., and Y. Shoenfeld. 2012. The role of gender and organ specific autoimmunity. *Autoimmunity Reviews* 11(6–7):A377–A385.

Poteat, T., D. German, and D. Kerrigan. 2013. Managing uncertainty: A grounded theory of stigma in transgender health care encounters. *Social Science & Medicine* 84:22–29.

Poteat, T., D. German, and C. Flynn. 2016. The conflation of gender and sex: Gaps and opportunities in HIV data among transgender women and MSM. *Global Public Health* 11(7–8):835–848.

Romejko, K., A. Rymarz, H. Sadownik, and S. Niemczyk. 2022. Testosterone deficiency as one of the major endocrine disorders in chronic kidney disease. *Nutrients* 14(16):3438.

Seelman, K. L., S. R. Young, M. Tesene, L. R. Alvarez-Hernandez, and L. Kattari. 2017. A comparison of health disparities among transgender adults in Colorado (USA) by race and income. *International Journal of Transgender Health* 18(2):199–214.

Smith-Johnson, M. 2022. Transgender adults have higher rates of disability than their cisgender counterparts. *Health Affairs* 41(10):1470–1476.

SSA (Social Security Administration). 2008. *Disability evaluation under Social Security (blue book-October 2008)*. https://www.ssa.gov/disability/professionals/bluebook/4.00-Cardiovascular-Adult.htm (accessed March 14, 2024).

SSA. 2009. *SSR 09-1p: Title XVI: Determining childhood disability under the functional equivalence rule - the "whole child" approach.* Woodlawn, MD: SSA. https://www.ssa.gov/OP_Home/rulings/ssi/02/SSR2009-01-ssi-02.html#fn4 (accessed October 10, 2023).

SSA. 2016. Revised medical criteria for evaluating human immunodeficiency virus (HIV) infection and for evaluating functional limitations in immune system disorders. Final rule. *Federal Register* 81(232):86915–86928.

SSA. 2022. Revised medical criteria for evaluating cardiovascular disorders. *Federal Register* 87(124):38838–38867.

SSA. 2023a. Table 5.A1—All beneficiaries: Number and average monthly benefit, by type of benefit and sex, December 2022. *Annual Statistical Supplement:*5.1. https://www.ssa.gov/policy/docs/statcomps/supplement/2023/5a.pdf (accessed March 12, 2024).

SSA. 2023b. Table 7.E4—Number and percentage distribution of recipients of federally administered payments with and without representative payees, by eligibility category and age, December 2022. *Annual Statistical Supplement:*7.26. https://www.ssa.gov/policy/docs/statcomps/supplement/2023/7e.pdf (accessed March 12, 2024).

SSA. 2023c. Revised medical criteria for evaluating digestive disorders and skin disorders. *Federal Register* 88(11):37704–37747.

SSA. 2024. *Disability benefits: How you qualify.* https://www.ssa.gov/benefits/disability/qualify.html (accessed March 12, 2024).

Stanojevic, S., D. A. Kaminsky, M. R. Miller, B. Thompson, A. Aliverti, I. Barjaktarevic, B. G. Cooper, B. Culver, E. Derom, G. L. Hall, T. S. Hallstrand, J. D. Leuppi, N. MacIntyre, M. McCormack, M. Rosenfeld, and E. R. Swenson. 2022. ERS/ATS technical standard on interpretive strategies for routine lung function tests. *European Respiratory Journal* 60(1):2101499.

Temkin, S. M., E. Barr, H. Moore, J. P. Caviston, J. G. Regensteiner, and J. A. Clayton. 2023. Chronic conditions in women: The development of a National Institutes of Health framework. *BMC Women's Health* 23(1):162.

Tomaszewski, M., W. Topyła, B. G. Kijewski, P. Miotła, and P. Waciński. 2019. Does gender influence the outcome of ischemic heart disease? *Przeglad Menopauzalny* 18(1):51–56.

U.S. Census Bureau. 2022. *American Community Survey. S1810 disability characteristics.* https://data.census.gov/table?q=disability (accessed March 12, 2024).

Wellons, M., P. Ouyang, P. J. Schreiner, D. M. Herrington, and D. Vaidya. 2012. Early menopause predicts future coronary heart disease and stroke: The multi-ethnic study of atherosclerosis. *Menopause* 19(10):1081–1087.

Part I

Sex and Gender Data Collection and Clinical Practice

The primary information the Social Security Administration (SSA) has at its disposal for adjudicating disability applications is the applicant's medical record. Therefore, part of understanding disability for transgender and gender diverse (TGD) people and people with variations in sex traits (VSTs) is understanding how information related to sex and gender identity becomes part of the medical record. The data collection related to these important patient characteristics that takes place—or does not take place— across clinical practice and within various sectors of the health care system impacts the quality of information contained in medical records received by SSA, influencing its ability to adjudicate disability applications from TGD people and people with VSTs appropriately.

In response to questions in the statement of task, the three chapters that form this part of the report focus on current and evolving practices for collecting sex and gender data across the health care system. Beginning with Chapter 2, the committee provides background on the medical definitions of sex and gender, which serve as the basis of self-identification, sex-specific medical evaluations, sex-specific disease risks, and appropriate therapeutic interventions, all of which may be relevant for disability evaluation. Here, the committee offers definitions of key concepts and terms important for understanding sex and gender within the context of clinical medicine and medical records. Next, Chapter 3 examines the substantial benefits of collecting sexual orientation and gender identity (SOGI) data, along with the significant biases and structural barriers that prevent robust SOGI data collection within health care settings. Chapter 4 provides an overview of SOGI data collection across the health care system, examining the fact that while certain components of the system collect SOGI data for the populations they serve, few federal- or state-level policies are in place that require health care providers or health insurers to record information about patient gender identity or sex recorded at birth, both considered key to documenting the health care experiences of TGD people and people with VSTs. Given that individuals applying for disability benefits from SSA access care from different types of providers and access health insurance in different ways, recognizing these challenges at all levels in the health care system is important to understanding the gaps in SOGI data seen in medical records, including those submitted to SSA as part of disability determinations.

2

Clinical Conceptions of Sex and Gender

This committee was tasked with examining contemporary under-standings of sex and gender as applied in clinical practice and implications for the work of the Social Security Administration (SSA). To accomplish this task, the committee determined that an essential first step would be to provide background on the medical definitions of sex and gender, which serve as the basis of self-identification, sex-specific medical evaluations, sex-specific disease risks, and appropriate therapeutic interventions, particularly as relevant for disability evaluation. Elsewhere in this report, the committee describes how and when sex and gender data are collected and used in the clinical practice of medicine as reflected in the health record, whether electronic or historically documented on paper (refer to Chapter 3 for a detailed discussion of these topics). The committee strongly believes that these complexities are relevant for how certain conditions are diagnosed; how laboratory results are derived and interpreted; and, in the case of applicants for SSA disability benefits who are transgender and gender diverse (TGD) or have variations in sex traits (VSTs), how disability determinations are made. Unfortunately, some terms are used interchangeably and others have multiple definitions, likely creating hurdles in this process.

What follows are the range of terminologies currently accepted by the medical community, which can serve as a reference point for SSA. In the tables below, the committee presents a main term (a term that is more commonly used in clinical settings today) along with its definition, as well as a range of alternative, similar, and synonymous terms. The committee presents terms and definitions organized in the following categories:

- Sex and gender definitions
- Gender identity terms
- Terms for individuals with variations in sex traits
- Sexual orientation terms
- Legal and administrative terms
- Diagnosis, care, and treatment terms

As the body of possible terminology that may be used in referring to sex and gender is substantial, the committee developed six guiding principles to inform and focus this work. Following the presentation of terms, the committee offers a discussion of these guiding principles—including a discussion of why terminology presented centers on those terms commonly used in the clinical practice of medicine (as opposed to terminology in common usage in various social contexts) and why the committee chose to include some terminology and language that may be considered outdated or offensive. The committee intends for the discussion of these guiding principles to further inform understanding of how various terminology related to sex and gender is relevant for disability determinations.

SEX AND GENDER DEFINITIONS

Table 2-1 presents definitions of sex and gender and related terms as commonly used in clinical practice and within medical records. While these definitions attempt to define and clarify concepts, the committee calls to SSA's attention that terms related to sex and gender are commonly conflated or used interchangeably within medical records and different clinicians and patients may use the same word to mean different things.

GENDER IDENTITY TERMS

Table 2-2 offers common gender identity terms that may be found in medical records, including some outdated terms that may still be in use by certain providers or communities. Where used appropriately within the medical record, these terms may describe people with TGD identity. The committee recognizes that TGD people may define their gender identity in numerous ways. For the purposes of this report, whenever the term "transgender and gender diverse" or "TGD" is used, the committee intends for it to encompass all of the alternative terms listed under the definition of "transgender and gender diverse" in Table 2-2.

TABLE 2-1 Sex and Gender Terms Commonly Found in Medical Records

Term	Definition	Alternative Term(s)
Sex	The biological components, including anatomical and physiological traits, largely related to sexual reproduction. Not all components align for all people.	• Biological sex
Gender	A multidimensional construct that links language with social and cultural expectations about status, characteristics, and behavior that are supposedly associated with sex traits.	
Male	A term identifying individuals who are typically capable of producing sperm for fertilizing ova. Males typically have XY chromosomes. Not everyone who is male has all the traits (e.g., chromosomes, hormone prevalence, external and internal anatomy) that are typically defined as male.	• Male sex • Man • Boy
Female	A term identifying individuals who typically have ovaries and produce eggs. Females typically have XX chromosomes. Not everyone who is female has all the traits (e.g., chromosomes, hormone prevalence, external and internal anatomy) that are typically defined as female.	• Female sex • Woman • Girl
Sex recorded at birth	The sex recorded on the original birth certificate (based on appearance of external genitals observed at birth by physical exam).	• Sex assigned at birth • Sex designated at birth • Birth sex • Assigned female at birth • Assigned male at birth
Sex of rearing	The sex assigned to a child at birth, most often based on the appearance of the child's external genital anatomy. Traditionally, sex of rearing is assigned as "male" or "female," although in some geographic regions, there is the option of "X." Assigned sex of rearing becomes the sex recorded on birth certificates and medical records. When a child is born with atypical genitalia, there may be a delay in assigning sex of rearing until the child's condition or diagnosis is better understood. Through a shared decision-making process between a multidisciplinary care team and the child's parents/guardians/caregivers, the goal is to select a sex of rearing that has the greatest likelihood of matching gender identity in adulthood.	• Sex assignment at birth • Gender of rearing • Assigned sex of rearing • Assigned gender of rearing

continued

TABLE 2-1 Continued

Term	Definition	Alternative Term(s)
Gender marker	Designation of "male" (M) "female" (F) or other (X) on a document, including on the original birth certificate. Depending on the document, this marker may represent an individual's sex recorded at birth or gender identity and a designation of "X," where present on records, may be defined in different ways.	• Sex marker
Gender identity	Used by individuals to label themselves and their internal sense of themselves. One's gender identity can be the same as or different from one's sex recorded at birth.	• Affirmed gender • Gender
Gender expression	One's mannerisms and appearance—including through behavior, clothing, body characteristics, or voice—that are, in a given culture, associated with masculinity or femininity.	
Gender attribution	The process through which others assign a gender to a person, with or without knowledge of that person's sex recorded at birth or gender identity.	

TERMS FOR INDIVIDUALS WITH VARIATIONS IN SEX TRAITS

For the purposes of this report, whenever the term "variations in sex traits"[1] or "VSTs" is used, the committee intends for it to encompass all of the alternative terms listed in Table 2-3, along with the diagnostic terms listed in Table 2-6 and other specific conditions described in detail in Chapter 7. Table 2-3 offers a definition of VSTs along with several alternative terms that may be common in clinical use or preferable to certain communities. The committee acknowledges that the umbrella of VSTs encompasses a great diversity of conditions, traits, and variations, all of which may not be included in this table. In addition, sexual orientation

---

[1] The committee uses the term "variations in sex traits" (VSTs) for this report to describe individuals with variations in development of the reproductive system (sex determination and sex development). The term "differences of sex development" (DSD) is commonly used in medical records and in the medical literature. However, some patients and clinicians consider the term DSD to be inaccurate and distasteful. "Intersex" is another commonly used term, but some individuals take issue with the notion that their reproductive anatomy falls between the binary and question this terminology. "Variations in sex traits," therefore, is intended to encompass all variations in reproductive tract development while being attentive to patient lived experience. However, the committee acknowledges that stakeholders have different and varied opinions on appropriate terminology and, like other terminology in this report, terminology is likely to evolve over time.

TABLE 2-2 Gender Identity Terms Commonly Found in Medical Records

Term	Definition	Alternative Term(s)
Transgender and gender diverse (TGD)	Umbrella term for people whose gender identity differs from what is typically associated with their sex recorded at birth. Not all transgender individuals seek treatment by health care providers.	• Transgender • Gender diverse • Trans • Transsexual • Transmasuline • Transfeminine • Transgender man/male • Trans man/male • Transgender woman/female • Trans woman/female • Male-to-female • Female-to-male • Gender nonconforming • Gender nonbinary • Nonbinary • Gender incongruent • Genderqueer • Gender fluid • Gender creative • Gender expansive • Gender independent • Intergender • Ambigender • Noncisgender • Agender • Bigender • Neutrois
Gender fluid	Describes a person whose gender identity is not fixed. A person who is gender fluid may feel like a mix of more than one gender, but may feel more aligned with a certain gender some of the time, another gender at other times, both genders sometimes, and sometimes no gender at all.	• Gender fluidity
Gender expansive	Describes a person with a wider, more flexible range of gender identity and/or expression than is typically associated with the binary gender system. Often used as an umbrella term when referring to people still exploring the possibilities of their gender expression and/or gender identity.	• Gender diverse
Agender	Describes a person who identifies as having no gender, or who does not experience gender as a primary identity component.	

continued

TABLE 2-2 Continued

Term	Definition	Alternative Term(s)
Two-Spirit	Describes a person who embodies both a masculine and a feminine spirit. This is a culture-specific term used among some Native American, American Indian, and First Nations people to describe their gender and/or spiritual identity (this term may also describe sexual orientation).	
Cisgender	Describes a person whose sex and gender identities match the sex recorded at birth.	• Nontransgender
Pronouns	The self-defined words to be used when others refer to a person in lieu of their name. Examples include "he/him/his/himself," "she/her/hers/herself," and "they/them/theirs/themselves."	

and gender identity (SOGI) data collection within electronic health records (EHRs) does not typically include VST categories, so VSTs may be indicated by various diagnostic codes (see Table 2-6). However, these codes do not represent every known VST or every VST community. There are more than 30 medical terms for specific combinations of VSTs, and every person with a VST is unique.

Table 2-3 includes terms found in medical records; some terms, including "hermaphrodite" and "pseudohermaphrodite," are now considered harmful and pejorative, and should be avoided today.

TABLE 2-3 Terms Related to Variations in Sex Traits Commonly Found in Medical Records

Term	Definition	Alternative Term(s)
Variations in sex traits (VSTs)	People with VSTs are born with a variety of differences in their sex traits and reproductive anatomy. The diversity of these variations is evident in the physical differences in external genitalia, chromosome composition, gonadal differentiation, internal sex organs, hormone production, hormone response, and/or development of secondary sex traits. This can be labeled as "phenotypic heterogeneity."	• Intersex • Intersex variations • Differences of sex development (DSD) (also known as disorders of sex development) • Variations of sex characteristics • Ambiguous genitalia • Congenital variations of sex characteristics • Intersexuality • Hermaphrodite • Pseudohermaphrodite • Hermaphroditism • Pseudohermaphroditism

SEXUAL ORIENTATION TERMS

Along with terms related to gender identity, sexual orientation terms are frequently included in SOGI data fields within EHR systems. As described below in the discussion of guiding principles, terms related to sexual orientation are often used interchangeably with gender identity terms. Therefore, the committee believes it is helpful to define and clarify these constructs separately. Table 2-4 presents various sexual orientation terms commonly found in medical records.

TABLE 2-4 Sexual Orientation Terms Commonly Found in Medical Records

Term	Definition	Alternative Term(s)
Sexual orientation	An individual's identity, attraction, behavior and emotional attachment to another person. Gender identity and sexual orientation are not the same.	• Sexual identity • Sexuality
Straight	Sexually oriented only toward people of a different, usually binary, sex.	• Heterosexual
Lesbian	A woman who is emotionally, romantically, and/or sexually attracted to other women. Women and nonbinary people may use this term to describe themselves.	• Women who have sex with women (WSW)
Gay	A person who is emotionally, romantically, and/ or sexually attracted to members of the same sex or gender. Men, women, and nonbinary people may use this term to describe themselves.	• Homosexual • Men who have sex with men (MSM)
Bisexual	A person emotionally, romantically, or sexually attracted to more than one sex, gender, or gender identity, though not necessarily simultaneously, in the same way, or to the same degree.	• Pansexual
Asexual	A person who may have little interest in having sex, even though they desire emotionally intimate relationships. Asexuality exists on a spectrum and people may identify somewhere between sexual and asexual.	• Ace • Aces • Queerplatonic • Demisexual • Grey-A
Sexual and gender minority (SGM)	An umbrella term that encompasses a diverse array of sexual orientations and gender identities, including lesbian, gay, bisexual, and transgender (LGBT), as well as queer/questioning, intersex, and others.	• Sexual and gender minoritized • Sexual and gender diverse
LGBTQ+	An acronym for "lesbian, gay, bisexual, transgender, and queer" with a "+" sign to recognize the limitless sexual orientations and gender identities.	• LGBTQI • LGBTQIA • LGBTQIA+ • LGBTQIA2+
Two-Spirit	Describes a person who embodies both a masculine and a feminine spirit. This is a culture-specific term used among some Native American, American Indian, and First Nations people to describe their sexual orientation (this term may also describe gender and/or spiritual identity).	

TABLE 2-5 Administrative Terms Commonly Found in
Medical Records

Term	Definition	Alternative Term(s)
Administrative sex or gender	One's gender as recorded on an identity document (e.g., passport, driver's license, birth certificate).	• Legal gender • Legal sex • Recorded gender • Recorded sex

LEGAL AND ADMINISTRATIVE TERMS

Although often assumed to be concordant with clinical terms, administrative terminology is often designated for business purposes, such as insurance billing. This type of information is commonly collected during patient registration rather than in the process of clinical care. Patients may not have the opportunity to update this information as frequently as other records, since modification typically requires legal documentation. Also, patients may be embarrassed, frightened, intimidated, or just uncomfortable about sharing their sex and gender identity with the person collecting this information. Within legal and administrative records, sex and gender may be delineated interchangeably and may not align with the patient's gender identity. Table 2-5 presents legal and administrative terms commonly found in medical records.

DIAGNOSIS, CARE, AND TREATMENT TERMS

Beyond terms related to patient identity and characteristics, other terms related to diagnosis, care, or treatment that may be present in the medical record are relevant for TGD people and people with VSTs. These terms may be present within diagnostic codes or within clinical notes that describe patient care and, importantly, may provide a tool for identifying these populations in the medical record where SOGI data are incomplete or unreliable.

Table 2-6 presents commonly used care and treatment terms and corresponding codes from the International Classification of Diseases and Related Health Problems (10th revision) (ICD-10). The language of diagnostic codes may be used in the medical record despite any patient or provider terminology preferences. For people with VSTs, the wide range of variations is commonly classified into three major categories by the patient's karyotype: sex chromosomes DSD [difference of sex development], 46,XY DSD, and 46,XX DSD (Hughes et al., 2006). These classifications are presented in Table 2-6, as this classification structure may be present in medical records.

TABLE 2-6 Terms Commonly Found in Medical Records That May Relate to Care and Treatment for TGD People and People with VSTs, Along with Corresponding ICD-10 Codes

Term	Definition	Alternative Term(s)
Gender dysphoria	Distress experienced by some people whose gender identity does not correspond with their sex recorded at birth. The *Diagnostic and Statistical Manual of Mental Disorders* (DSM-5-TR) includes gender dysphoria as a diagnosis for people whose distress is clinically significant or impairs social, occupational, or other important areas of functioning. The degree and severity of gender dysphoria are highly variable among TGD people.	• Gender incongruence *Related ICD-10 codes:* • F64 Gender identity disorders • F64.0 Transsexualism • F64.1 Dual role transvestism • F64.2 Gender identity disorder of childhood • F64.8 Other gender identity disorders • F64.9 Gender identity disorder, unspecified • Z87.890 Personal history of sex reassignment
Gender transition	The process by which some people strive to align their outward appearance more closely with their internal experience of their gender. Some people socially transition, whereby they might begin dressing, using names and pronouns, and/or being socially recognized as another gender. Others undergo physical transitions in which they modify their bodies through medical interventions.	• Transition • Medical transition • Transitioning • Gender affirmation • Gender confirmation • Social transition • Legal transition
Gender-affirming hormone treatment and surgery	Medical/surgical interventions performed to align appearance with gender identity.	• Gender-confirming hormone treatment and surgery • Medical transition • Hormone therapy • Hormone replacement therapy • Bottom surgery • Top surgery
Retransition	A process through which a person discontinues some or all aspects of gender affirmation. Refers to the stopping, reversal, or other change to transitioning, which could be social (gender presentation, pronouns), medical (hormone therapy), surgical, or legal.	• Detransition • Gender evolution

continued

TABLE 2-6 Continued

Term	Definition	Alternative Term(s)
Sex Chromosome DSD	A category of VSTs that includes any condition in which there is an atypical number/arrangement of the sex chromosomes. For example, Turner syndrome (45,X) is a condition that occurs when a child is born with only 45 chromosomes because one of the sex chromosomes (an X chromosome) is missing. The sex chromosome DSD category also includes Klinefelter syndrome (47,XXY), 45,X/46,XY gonadal dysgenesis, and chimeric 46,XX/46,XY individuals.	*Related ICD-10 codes:* • Q96.0–Q96.9 Turner syndrome and variants • Q97.0–Q97.9 Other sex chromosome abnormalities, female phenotype, not elsewhere classified • Q98.0, Q98.1 • Q98.2, Q98.4 Klinefelter syndrome and variants • Q98.5–Q98.9 Other sex chromosome abnormalities, male phenotype, not elsewhere classified • Q99.0 Chimera 46, XX/46, XY
46,XY DSD	Children born with XY chromosomes (46,XY) usually develop typical male sex characteristics. However, some children born with one X and one Y chromosome have underdeveloped gonads or cannot produce or respond to sex hormones to develop the typical male physical characteristics. Individuals with 46,XY DSD encompass the greatest diversity in diagnoses. This category includes individuals with genetic variants involved in testicular differentiation, androgen biosynthesis, and androgen action. Common VSTs in this category include androgen insensitivity syndrome, 46,XY gonadal dysgenesis, 5-alpha reductase deficiency, penoscrotal hypospadias, and persistent Müllerian duct syndrome.	*Related ICD-10 codes:* • E34.50 Androgen insensitivity syndrome, unspecified • E34.51 Complete androgen insensitivity syndrome • E34.52 Partial androgen insensitivity syndrome • Q53.2 Undescended testicle, bilateral • Q54.2 Hypospadias, penoscrotal • Q54.3 Hypospadias, perineal • Q55.00 Absence and aplasia of testis • Q55.01 Anorchia • Q56.1 Male pseudoherma phroditism, not elsewhere classified • Q97.3 Female with 46,XY karyotype

TABLE 2-6 Continued

Term	Definition	Alternative Term(s)
46,XX DSD	Children born with two X chromosomes (46,XX) usually develop typical female physical sex characteristics. However, some children born with two X chromosomes were exposed before birth to excess male sex hormones that led to genitals that appear atypical. Individuals with 46,XX DSD may have aberrant ovarian development and typical female external genitalia at birth; they typically present during the adolescent years with delayed onset of female puberty. Another frequent cause of 46,XX DSD is classic congenital adrenal hyperplasia, a group of autosomal recessive disorders associated with impaired adrenal cortisol biosynthesis. The most common form is 21-hydroxylase deficiency due to deleterious variants in the 21-hydroxylase (*CYP21A2*) gene.	*Related ICD-10 codes:* • Q52.0 Congenital absence of vagina • Q52.1 Doubling of vagina • Q56.2 Female pseudoherma phroditism, not elsewhere classified • Q98.3 Other male with 46,XX karyotype • E25.00 Salt-losing congenital adrenal hyperplasia • E25.01 Congenital adrenal hyperplasia
Anatomical inventory	A structured form that tracks the presence or absence of a patient's reproductive organs, as well as any surgical history relevant to those organs. The inventory can be integrated into the electronic health record and can help guide preventive health screenings and postsurgical care plans.	• Anatomy inventory • Organ inventory

NOTE: There are many more ICD-10 codes related to various VST diagnosis. A full list of these codes is presented in Chapter 3. DSD = difference of sex development; ICD = International Classification of Diseases and Related Health Problems (10th revision); TGD = transgender and gender diverse; VST = variation in sex traits.
SOURCES: CDC, 2024; Kohva et al., 2018.

GUIDING PRINCIPLES

The body of terminology that may be used in referring to sex and gender identity and TGD populations and populations with VSTs is substantial. Hence, the committee developed six guiding principles to inform and focus terminology and its definitions.

(1) Terms commonly used in the clinical practice of medicine are most relevant to SSA for determining gender identity and other relevant biology of disability applicants. Medical records, clinician reports, and test results are a primary source of information used by SSA to determine disability status. Therefore, in considering which commonly used terms to bring forward to SSA, it is important to ground those terms in the context of the sources of information available to SSA (e.g., the medical record). Accordingly, this

chapter does not include sex and gender identity terms that are more likely to be used in a social or political context, or definitions and concepts that may be considered aspirational (what terminology should look like in an ideal world). Rather, the focus here is on terminology likely to be found in medical records today and definitions of those terms used currently in clinical practice.

(2) Most contemporary electronic health records (EHRs) contain fields to capture sexual orientation and gender identity (SOGI) data, although mandates to collect these data are not widely in place. Most EHR systems in the United States have the capacity to record SOGI data as the result of a federal requirement for EHR developers and vendors to enable patients and providers to record SOGI data in the EHR (HHS, 2015). As described in detail in Chapter 3, however, while EHRs may have data fields with which to capture SOGI data, there is no mandate for providers or health care institutions to collect these data, and there are many systemic barriers to such data collection. As a result, health care providers and systems routinely fail to collect and record SOGI data (Goldhammer et al., 2018, 2022; Liu et al., 2023; May et al., 2023).

When available and used, SOGI data collected in medical records may provide SSA with important data to inform decision making for TGD applicants and applicants with VSTs. At this time, however, given incomplete data collection, SOGI data cannot be used as a sole reference point in disability determinations. Despite these limitations, the committee expects the collection of SOGI data in medical records to continue to expand and evolve over time. For this reason, the committee sought to capture and provide examples of SOGI terminology in current use within medical records.

(3) Diagnostic codes may have limited utility in helping SSA understand the sex and gender of disability applicants. For some applicants, however, diagnostic codes provide indicators of sex and gender that may not be captured elsewhere. The ICD, a health care classification system of diagnostic codes for diseases, diagnoses, and procedures, provides a uniform way of collecting and maintaining patient data. These codes are imbedded within EHRs and used by health care systems to document patient care and seek insurance reimbursement. Several ICD-10 codes relate to gender dysphoria and VSTs; Chapter 3 describes these ICD-10 codes in detail, along with the coming reconceptualization and reorganization of diagnostic codes under ICD-11 and codes related to social determinants of health.

While the committee notes that ICD codes may not always be used or may be used incorrectly, they may serve to document patient characteristics, particularly where the SOGI data captured in EHRs do not include sufficient categories to identify TGD people or people with VSTs. For this reason, the committee sought to capture relevant ICD codes in current use in the definitions presented in this chapter.

(4) Given the limitations in data collection using fields and diagnostic codes imbedded in medical records, clinical notes may capture additional dimensions of patient identity, experience, and care. Narrative clinical notes can serve as an important source of patient health information, including SOGI data and information related to health care and therapeutic interventions for TGD people and people with VSTs, capturing additional dimensions related to patient identity, experience, and care that provide important context for any disability application. Recognizing that expression of gender identity may be fluid, malleable, and inconsistent over time, review of the medical record can clarify an individual person's trajectory with respect to gender identity and any gender-affirming care sought over time. Indeed, where health care providers do not utilize SOGI data collection fields within the medical record or do not categorize care using current ICD diagnostic codes, clinical notes may be the *only* source of information indicating gender identity, gender-affirming care, or VSTs.

Although SSA views an applicant's record and need for disability benefits at a specific moment in time, for certain conditions—as described in chapters of this report related to pulmonary function (chapter 8), growth failure (chapter 9), and kidney function (chapter 10)—it is important to understand whether a person utilized gender-affirming hormone therapy, and, if so, whether they utilized this care during puberty or in adulthood. These details may impact clinical interpretation of key measurements that indicate disability; therefore, understanding this care trajectory is important for disability adjudication. Similarly, it is important to know sex recorded at birth for certain measurements utilized in SSA's Listing of Impairments, and narrative clinical notes may illuminate the unique trajectory an applicant with a VST has had with determining their sex (e.g., that sex was assigned incorrectly at birth, and, therefore, sex as recorded in birth records is incorrect). Such details are not captured in standard SOGI data collection fields within the medical record. Therefore, the committee determined that it is important to define for SSA additional terms beyond the basic SOGI demographic fields or diagnostic codes found in medical records.

(5) Given that gender identity and sexual orientation can sometimes be conflated or used interchangeably in clinical settings, it is also important to define terms related to sexual orientation. The statement of task does not specifically ask for definitions and terms related to sexual orientation. However, the committee finds that it should not leave sexual orientation terminology and definitions out of this report because, in clinical settings, gender and sexual identities can often be conflated, confused, or misconstrued. Patients may be assumed to be TGD when they do not fit into stereotypical gender roles, and clinicians may document patients as TGD when they may instead define themselves as gay or lesbian. The opposite may also be true, with health care providers believing a TGD person is

actually a cisgender person who is gay or lesbian. Defining certain terms related to sexual orientations should enable SSA to separate and clarify these concepts.

(6) Health care providers and patients use a wide range of terminology, and it is important for SSA to understand that range, along with the fluidity of terms over time. By their nature, narrative, free-text clinical descriptions are not uniform, and the language and descriptions found within medical records will vary greatly, as not all health care providers use the same terminology, and not all patients use the same language when describing themselves or their experiences. Choice of terminology can vary with age, nationality, sex recorded at birth, life experiences, and educational attainment (Carrier et al., 2020; Michaels et al., 2017; Panfil, 2020; Sloboda et al., 2018; Suen et al., 2020; Walker, 2020). Medical records also may contain outdated terminology and language that was previously utilized and now considered to be pejorative and disparaging. Older medical records may still be relevant to a disability adjudication, particularly for people with VSTs, despite containing outdated language that is considered offensive by today's standards. For these reasons, the committee believes it is important to present a wide range of possible gender identity terms and diagnostic categories so that SSA can search for this helpful information in medical records or elsewhere on disability application forms. Hence, the tables presented above offer alternative, similar, and synonymous terms—that may include some outdated terms—with the intent of capturing the range of nomenclature that could be present in medical records received by SSA.

The committee anticipates that terms presented here will change over time, as language and popular culture evolve. Terms once common may become outdated; terms once offensive may become preferred. New terms come into the lexicon and eventually become conventional in clinical care. The committee acknowledges and emphasizes to SSA this fluidity of terminology.

SUMMARY OF KEY POINTS

This chapter offers a range of terms and definitions that may be present in medical records and relevant for people with TGD or VST lived experience or identity. Disability adjudicators may need to become aware of these many terms for appropriate understanding of the characteristics of disability applicants. Further chapters in this report describe in greater depth why these concepts may matter for disability evaluation.

Although they are the primary source of information for SSA, medical records may not accurately reflect the current status of a disability applicant's gender identity and/or other biology. The committee acknowledges the reality of what medical records contain, where SOGI information may be sparse or inaccurate or difficult to ascertain within clinical notes.

While most EHRs have capabilities to collect SOGI data, many institutions do not activate the SOGI fields and do not collect these data. And even when these fields are "turned on," patients may have difficulty responding to questions as asked, or the fields may not allow for adequate responses. Within written portions of the medical record, health care providers may conflate or confuse sex recorded at birth, gender identity, anatomy, and sexual orientation in a patient's medical history or fail to record these data entirely. Furthermore, even where medical records contain some level of SOGI data, these data may not be accurate for a particular patient at a particular point in time, as patients may come to understand their sex or gender identity as different from that previously recorded in the medical record (or previously recorded in disability applications). For these many reasons, the medical record may not accurately reflect the current status of a disability applicant's sex or gender identity.

REFERENCES

Carrier, L., J. Dame, and J. Lane. 2020. Two-Spirit identity and Indigenous conceptualization of gender and sexuality: Implications for nursing practice. *Creative Nursing* 26(2):96–100. https://doi.org/10.1891/CRNR-D-19-00091.

CDC (Centers for Disease Control and Prevention). 2024. *National Center for Health Statistics ICD-10-CM, FY2024.* https://icd10cmtool.cdc.gov/?fy=FY2024 (accessed March 12, 2024)

Goldhammer, H., C. Grasso, S. L. Katz-Wise, K. Thomson, A. R. Gordon, and A. S. Keuroghlian. 2022. Pediatric sexual orientation and gender identity data collection in the electronic health record. *Journal of American Medical Informatics Association* 29(7):1303–1309. https://doi.org/10.1093/jamia/ocac048.

Goldhammer, H., E. D. Maston, and L. A. Kissock. 2018. National findings from an LGBT healthcare organizational needs assessment. *LGBT Health* 5(8):461–468. https://doi.org/10.1089/lgbt.2018.0118.

HHS (U.S. Department of Health and Human Services). 2015. 2015 Edition health information technology (health IT) certification criteria, 2015 edition base electronic health record (EHR) definition, and ONC health IT certification program modifications. *Federal Register* 80(200):62602–62759. https://www.govinfo.gov/content/pkg/FR-2015-10-16/pdf/2015-25597.pdf (accessed March 11, 2024).

Hughes, I. A., C. Houk, S. F. Ahmed, and P. A. Lee. 2006. Consensus statement on management of intersex disorders. *Archives of Disease in Childhood* 91(7):554–563. https://doi.org/10.1136/adc.2006.098319.

Kohva, E., P. J. Miettinen, S. Taskinen, M. Hero, A. Tarkkanen, and T. Raivio. 2018. Disorders of sex development: Timing of diagnosis and management in a single large tertiary center. *Endocrine Connections* 7(4):595–603. https://doi.org/10.1530/EC-18-0070.

Liu, M., D. King, K. H. Mayer, C. Grasso, and A. Keuroghlian. 2023. Sexual orientation and gender identity data completeness at U.S. federally qualified health centers, 2020 and 2021. *American Journal of Public Health* 113(8):883–892. https://doi.org/10.2105/AJPH.2023.307323.

May, J. T., J. Myers, D. Noonan, E. McConnell, and M. P. Cary, Jr. 2023. A call to action to improve the completeness of older adult sexual and gender minority data in electronic health records. *Journal of the American Medical Informatics Association* 30(10): 1725–1729. https://doi.org/10.1093/jamia/ocad130.

Michaels, S., C. Milesi, M. Stern, M. H. Viox, H. Morrison, P. Guerino, C. N. Dragon, and S. C. Haffer. 2017. Improving measures of sexual and gender identity in English and Spanish to identify LGBT older adults in surveys. *LGBT Health* 4(6):412–418. https://doi.org/10.1089/lgbt.2016.0168.

Panfil, V. R. 2020. "Nobody don't really know what that mean": Understandings of "queer" among urban LGBTQ young people of color. *Journal of Homosexuality* 67(12):1713–1735. https://doi.org/10.1080/00918369.2019.1613855.

Sloboda, A., A. Mustafa, and J. Schober. 2018. An approach to discussing personal and social identity terminology with patients. *Clinical Anatomy* 31(2):136–139. https://doi.org/10.1002/ca.23022.

Suen, L. W., M. R. Lunn, K. Katuzny, S. Finn, L. Duncan, J. Sevelius, A. Flentje, M. R. Capriotti, M. E. Lubensky, C. Hunt, S. Weber, K. Bibbins-Domingo, and J. Obedin-Maliver. 2020. What sexual and gender minority people want researchers to know about sexual orientation and gender identity questions: A qualitative study. *Archives of Sexual Behavior* 49(7):2301–2318. https://doi.org/10.1007/s10508-020-01810-y.

Walker, A. 2020. "I'm not like that, so am I gay?" The use of queer-spectrum identity labels among minor-attracted people. *Journal of Homosexuality* 67(12):1736–1759. https://doi.org/10.1080/00918369.2019.1613856.

3

Data on Sexual Orientation and Gender Identity: Collection and Use in the Clinical Practice of Medicine

Recent advances in electronic health records (EHRs) and health information technology provide opportunities to increase the visibility of transgender and gender diverse (TGD) patients and patients with variations in sex traits (VSTs) through the collection of sexual orientation and gender identity (SOGI) patient data. SOGI data collection—whereby health care providers and patients can record sexual orientation, gender identity, legal sex, sex recorded at birth, and similar information in individual patient charts—is a key strategy for reducing the many health disparities faced by LGBTQ+ populations. For patients who are TGD or have VSTs, data collection that involves asking for a patient's gender identity and sex recorded at birth can enhance meaningful dialogue during clinical encounters, aid in clinical decision making, promote appropriate preventive screenings, reduce inequitable and discriminatory health care practices, and foster respectful and patient-centered long-term care.

In recent years, new federal policies—including mandates for certified EHR systems to have the capacity to record SOGI demographic data—have been major drivers of the expansion of SOGI demographic data collection among EHR vendors and across the health care system. Yet despite the importance of collecting SOGI data and the capacity for EHRs to do so, uptake of the collection and documentation of SOGI data by health care systems and providers is suboptimal. The persistent lack of routine data collection on sexual orientation, gender identity, and variations in sex traits is a substantial roadblock to the health and well-being of sexual and gender minorities.

This chapter examines the importance of collecting SOGI data within health care settings, best practices for collecting these data, structural barriers to collecting these data, and the future of SOGI data collection within medical records. Given that one of the important reasons for collecting SOGI data in medical records is to help combat discriminatory health care provided to sexual and gender minorities, the chapter begins with an examination of the uneven health care delivery experienced by TGD people and people with VSTs.

UNEQUAL CARE DELIVERY IMPACTING TRANSGENDER AND GENDER DIVERSE PEOPLE AND PEOPLE WITH VARIATIONS IN SEX TRAITS

Sex and gender bias and discrimination in health care—unequal treatment by providers for patients who are TGD or have VSTs—is a well-documented experience. Numerous studies demonstrate that TGD people experience cascading patterns of discriminatory experiences in health care, ranging from providers having limited clinical understanding of transgender health to overt refusals of care. These studies, spanning decades and care settings (including primary care, mental health care, subspecialty care, and social service settings), show how discriminatory care practices adversely affect access to and quality of health care, leading to poor physical and mental health outcomes among TGD people (Jackson et al., 2008; Maragh-Bass et al., 2017a; Poteat et al., 2013; Seelman et al., 2017). People with VSTs experience similar marginalization and discrimination in their health care, due largely to the stigma of not conforming to providers' binary views of sex (Crocetti et al., 2021; Haghighat et al., 2023). According to a 2020 survey from the Center for American Progress, people with VSTs, compared with LGBTQ+ people who do not have VSTs, experience higher rates of stigma and discrimination (69 percent vs. 35 percent) and are more likely to avoid going to the doctor or engaging in other behavior that could expose them to discriminatory treatment (Medina and Mahowald, 2021).

In a second survey from the Center for American Progress, conducted in 2022, 21 percent of transgender and nonbinary respondents (including 28 percent of transgender and nonbinary respondents of color) reported that a health care provider had refused to provide reproductive or sexual health services because of their gender identity (Medina and Mahowald, 2021). More than half (55 percent) of respondents with VSTs reported refusal of care because of their sex characteristics. These experiences were notably more prevalent among TGD individuals and individuals with VSTs who also had a disability. This finding echoes those of previous studies that show higher rates of discrimination against TGD individuals with disabilities (Kattari et al., 2017, 2020). While these studies use a broader definition of disability than SSA's, they still indicate the discrimination faced by TGD/VST populations with serious chronic health needs. Racially minoritized TGD people also experience higher rates of discrimination in health care settings (Gonzales and Henning-Smith, 2017; Grant et al., 2011; Kattari et al., 2015).

Panelist Perspective

"I have also had asthma my whole life, which, out of all the things is the last thing I thought being trans would impact my care for. But sure enough, I was denied an appointment this year to get an inhaler prescription renewed. Solely because [at] the health care facility that I had been to for 6 years, my doctor retired this summer, and they decided they would no longer accept transgender patients for anything. And this was particularly traumatizing since my mother died last year from an asthma attack during a brief lapse in insurance coverage."

—Statement from patient–provider panel,
presented to the committee on December 1, 2023.

The downstream impacts of this discrimination include patients with TGD or VST lived experience postponing or avoiding needed medical care because of medical providers' disrespect or overt discrimination and the fear of such mistreatment repeating itself in future clinical encounters (Feldman et al., 2021; MacDougall et al., 2023; Romanelli and Lindsey, 2020; Streed et al., 2017; White Hughto et al., 2015). In the 2015 U.S. Transgender Survey, 33 percent of transgender respondents reported having had negative experiences with health care providers, and 23 percent reported avoiding necessary medical care for fear of being mistreated as a transgender person (James et al., 2016). These findings are consistent with those of a review by Jaffee and colleagues (2016), which found that nearly one-third (30.8 percent) of transgender people delayed or did not seek medical treatment because of discrimination (Jaffee et al., 2016). Repeated incidents of discrimination in health care settings may also contribute to coping-motivated substance abuse, and even suicide (Glick et al., 2020; Kidd et al., 2018; Romanelli et al., 2018; Zollweg et al., 2023).

Panelist Perspective

"I walk into a clinic and I'm immediately—*immediately*—either deadnamed,[a] or somebody uses the wrong pronouns. And these are the things where you walk into a room, and you're like you can't even use a correct pronoun? How am I supposed to trust you with my medical care, with the most vulnerable aspects of my life and my identity when you can't even level with me and treat me with respect as a human being?"

—Statement from patient–provider panel, presented to the committee on November 30, 2023.

---

[a]"Deadnaming" refers to when a person is called by the name they were given at birth instead of their chosen and presently used name (Lieurance et al., 2021).

TGD people also face other forms of structural stigma that impact their ability to receive quality health care, including "societal-level conditions, cultural norms, and institutional policies that constrain the opportunities, resources, and wellbeing of the stigmatized" (Hatzenbuehler, 2014; Price et al., 2024). For TGD people, this stigma may result in a lack of legal protections, as well as discriminatory laws, policies, and/or attitudes. For instance, growing and evolving restrictions on access to gender-affirming medical care have a negative impact on the physical and mental health of TGD people (Abreu et al., 2022; Hughes et al., 2021; Poteat and Simmons, 2022; Velasco et al., 2022).

BENEFITS OF SOGI DATA COLLECTION

Traditionally, data on sex and gender collected by health care providers and institutions place patients into one of two categories based on "administrative sex": male or female (Hines et al., 2023). The constrained selection of either "male" or "female" within medical encounters imposes the idea of a societal "norm" whereby everyone falls neatly into one of two categories. However, this binary categorization does not reflect the reality of sex and gender variations, and so can render TGD people and people with VSTs invisible and leave them with the sense that they are non-normative and, perhaps, unwelcome. When medical records and clinical encounters do not provide the opportunity for patients to describe important characteristics about their identity, or body and experiences— for example, to state their gender as different from their sex recorded at birth, to declare a gender identity that does not conform to expectations based on sex recorded at birth, or to describe variations in sex traits—patients cannot receive the culturally responsive, patient-centered services they need.

While many structural factors contribute to discriminatory health care, one important way providers, health systems, and social programs can combat discrimination and advance equity is through the collection of SOGI data in medical records. Giving TGD patients and patients with VSTs the ability to disclose SOGI data to health care providers can be enormously beneficial to these patient populations as it provides clinicians and staff with more accurate information and has the potential to make the health care environment more welcoming—and, in turn, opens the door to a more trusting patient–provider relationship. In short, SOGI data collection can promote inclusivity, increase patient comfort with providers, reduce misgendering, reduce health care avoidance, and enhance the patient experience (Hines et al., 2023; Kronk et al., 2022; Streed et al., 2020).

SOGI data collection arms providers with critical data they need to inform decision making for vulnerable patients at all levels of care: from preventive screening to chronic disease management. Without knowing a patient's gender identity and sex recorded at birth, for example, a provider may not flag that a transgender man who retains a cervix should be offered cervical cancer screening. Likewise, without asking about VSTs, a health care provider may not appreciate important health conditions that may disproportionately affect a patient, such as chronic pain or infertility. Asking patients about their gender identity and sex recorded at birth thus allows providers to get to know their patients and allows them to offer the patient-centered services TGD people and people with VSTs need and deserve (National LGBTQIA+ Health Education Center, 2022). Additionally, when SOGI data collection includes asking about pronoun(s) and name(s), providers can engage in respectful conversations with their patients, all of which enriches the patient–provider relationship, improves care delivery, and enhances patient satisfaction (Streed et al., 2020).

SOGI documentation has specific advantages within pediatric primary care practices. When pediatricians have these data for their patients, they can make more informed decisions, offer referrals for psychosocial support, and encourage gender identity acceptance among family members and caregivers (Goldhammer et al., 2022).

Outside of clinical care, SOGI data collection is an indispensable tool for helping researchers, policy makers, and advocates understand and address challenges facing communities that are diverse with respect to sexual orientation and gender identity (NASEM, 2022). Chapter 4 of this report looks at SOGI data collection in federal surveys and recent strides toward improving such data collection across federal agencies.

Patient Attitudes toward SOGI Data Collection

Research shows that most patients endorse the collection of SOGI data in medical records. One survey of a racially diverse group of patients (N = 301, including 15.6 percent of the respondents identifying as transgender) across four community health centers found that most understood the importance of answering SOGI questions and were willing to answer them in a health care setting (Cahill et al., 2014). The two-step question asked in the study ("What is your current gender identity?" and "What sex were you assigned at birth on your original birth certificate?") was widely understood by survey respondents, and 86 percent reported willingness to answer the gender identity portion of the question, while 84 percent reported willingness to answer the sex recorded at birth portion. Respondents of all ages endorsed the importance of asking SOGI questions, with transgender and cisgender respondents reporting similar comfort levels with the collection of gender identity data (Cahill et al., 2014). Another study of the attitudes of heterosexual and cisgender patients toward SOGI data (N = 491) found that 97 percent believed SOGI data collection to be an acceptable part of routine clinical intake forms (Rullo et al., 2018). Other surveys have found similarly high patient willingness to complete SOGI data collection within EHRs (Bjarnadottir et al., 2017; Maragh-Bass et al., 2017a; Ruben et al., 2017).

Beyond questions on gender identity and sex recorded at birth, TGD patients may prefer to have additional identification documented in their EHRs. For example, one survey of transgender youth (aged 12–26 years, N = 204) found that 79 percent wished to have their preferred name and pronouns documented in the EHR, these details being critical to cultivating a respectful and affirming interaction between provider and patient (Sequeira et al., 2020). When providers refer to patients by their correct name (i.e., their chosen and presently used name) and pronouns, this is an added step in ensuring that patients feel seen, heard, and respected in their identities.

However, other research describes the possible negative implications of SOGI data disclosure in health care settings. For example, in a qualitative study of 30 transgender adults, participants reported that disclosing transgender status resulted in increased stigma and poorer care (e.g., participants were not misgendered *until* they disclosed receipt of gender-affirming hormone therapy; providers began asking stigmatizing questions only after learning of TGD status) (Alpert et al., 2023). Participants in this study reported feeling reticent about sharing SOGI data to avoid such negative clinical encounters. Other studies have reported a similar phenomenon: for example, studies show patients may receive invasive questioning when gender identity is disclosed or providers may misattribute medical concerns as being a result of the patient's gender identity or gender-affirming care, leading to reduced access to needed health care interventions (Wall et al., 2023).

The decision to provide SOGI data is often complicated, but research shows TGD patients are more likely to disclose where they perceive the information is directly relevant to their health concern, they are told why SOGI collection is needed, and providers give assurances of confidentiality (Maragh-Bass et al., 2017b). In addition, TGD people report a greater willingness to disclose SOGI data where there are a wide range of response options that allow for more accurate reflection of identities and experiences (Puckett et al., 2020).

SOGI DATA COLLECTION: BEST PRACTICES

Given its many benefits to patients, health equity, and clinical care, best practices call for the collection of SOGI data in medical records. The National Academy of Medicine (NASEM, 2022), The Joint Commission (2011), the National Science and Technology Council (NSTC, 2023), and Healthy People 2030 (OASH, n.d.), among others, have all called for the collection of SOGI data in routine patient care.

For data collection related to gender identity, researchers and advocates call for a two-step gender identity question, like that posed in the study referenced above (Cahill et al., 2014), to identify transgender and nonbinary people in health care settings (Kronk et al., 2022; NASEM, 2022; National LGBTQIA+ Health Education Center, 2022; Thompson, 2021). The two-step gender identity question is a pair of questions asked in sequence, one asking about current gender identity and the other about sex recorded at birth (sometimes referred to as "sex assigned at birth"). Table 3-1 provides three examples of the two-step question.

While gender identity information can be obtained with a one-step question (e.g., by asking "Are you male, female, or transgender?" or "Do you consider yourself transgender?"), some transgender people describe their gender identity as either "male" or "female," so the one-step question does not always identify people with transgender lived experience (Schilt and Bratter, 2015; Tate et al., 2013). Furthermore, listing various gender identities—transgender woman, transgender male, transfeminine, transmasculine, etc.—in a one-step question may not comport with terminology preferred by the individual, and can enforce a level of distinction between transgender and cisgender individuals that is unnecessary and can feel alienating for TGD people (Kronk et al., 2022).

The two-step question method is considered a better proxy for gender- and/or sex-related information than any one-step question alone (Kronk et al., 2022; NASEM, 2022). With the two-step method, when a patient

TABLE 3-1 Examples of a Two-Step Question on Gender Identity and Sex Recorded at Birth

Question 1	Q1 Response Options	Question 2	Q2 Response Options	Source
What sex were you assigned at birth, on your original birth certificate?	☐ Female ☐ Male ☐ Don't know ☐ Prefer not to answer	What is your current gender? [Mark only one]	☐ Female ☐ Male ☐ Transgender ☐ [If respondent is American Indian/Alaska Native] Two Spirit ☐ I use a different term: [free text] ☐ Don't know ☐ Prefer not to answer	NASEM, 2022
What is your current gender identity?	☐ Female/woman/girl ☐ Male/man/boy ☐ Nonbinary, genderqueer, or not exclusively female or male ☐ Transgender female/woman/girl ☐ Transgender male/man/boy ☐ Another gender: [free text] ☐ Don't know ☐ Prefer not to answer	What sex were you assigned at birth, on your original birth certificate? (Check one.)	☐ Female ☐ Male ☐ X/Another sex: [free text] ☐ Don't know ☐ Prefer not to answer	National LGBTQIA+ Health Education Center, 2022
What is your gender identity? *Choose all that apply.*	☐ Female; Woman; Girl ☐ Male; Man; Boy ☐ Nonbinary ☐ Questioning; Exploring ☐ Prefer not to respond; Prefer not to disclose ☐ Gender identity not listed (please specify): [free text]	What is your assigned gender at birth, meaning the gender marker which appears on your original birth certificate? *Choose one.*	☐ Female ('F') ☐ Male ('M') ☐ X ☐ Unsure ☐ Prefer not to respond; Prefer not to disclose ☐ Assigned gender at birth not listed (please specify): [free text]	Kronk et al., 2022

NOTE: Although some literature states that best practices are to ask the gender identity question first before the sex recorded at birth question, the questions presented above are presented in the order they appear within these sources.
SOURCES: Kronk et al., 2022; NASEM, 2022; National LGBTQIA+ Health Education Center, 2022.

selects, for example, "female" as gender identity and "male" as sex recorded at birth, health care providers can understand that the patient is transgender without the patient having to specifically select "transgender" on health forms. Researchers estimate that without a two-step question for gender identity, roughly one-quarter of transgender patients would not be clinically visible (Dubin et al., 2022). The two-step approach also helps count cisgender patient populations accurately because it allows for separate counts of cisgender men and cisgender women (NASEM, 2022). Importantly, because the two-step method allows for more accurate recording of sex and gender identity compared with the traditional "administrative sex" categories of male/female, providers can use these data to inform appropriate clinical decision making. For example, the Veterans Health Administration's (VHA's) EHR system uses data on sex recorded at birth to guide health screenings (e.g., cervical cancer screening for transgender men) and to help determine laboratory ranges and medication dosing (VHA, 2022).

Best practices call for medical records to offer enough categories so individuals do not have to select an "other" category; the inclusion of terms—for example, "X" as a response under sex recorded at birth or "nonbinary" as a category for gender identity—communicates to patients that they are included and welcome (Kronk et al., 2022; Puckett et al., 2020). In addition, providing a free-text response option, such as "I use something else," allows individuals to use their own terminology to accurately reflect their identity and experience. Health care organizations may also prefer to modify response options to better fit the populations they serve. For example, for an organization that serves a large number of American Indians/Alaska Natives, it may be appropriate to include "Two-Spirit" as an option for gender identity (NASEM, 2022; National LGBTQIA+ Health Education Center, 2022), as the Indian Health Service does on its patient intake forms (IHS, 2023). Another example would be to include the terms "raerae" or "māhū" when serving a Polynesian community, as these are culturally specific terms that recognize a third gender (Ford and Coleman, 2023). Many cultures and regions have culturally specific terminology, which points to the importance of including free-text options so individuals have the autonomy to identify themselves accurately.

Occasionally, medical records may include variations in sex traits—sometimes using the term "intersex" or "differences of sex development"—under the gender identity or sex recorded at birth question. However, people with VSTs have a range of gender identities, just like the general population; thus, some people with VSTs may consider their gender to be "intersex," whereas others identify as female, male, nonbinary, or a different gender. In addition, as the process of assigning gender at birth can be highly complex for many people born with VSTs, individuals may have a sex recorded on their birth certificate that differs from their current sex and/or gender

TABLE 3-2 Examples of Questions That Ask Patients About Variations in Sex Traits

Question Example:	Response Options:
Have you ever been diagnosed by a medical doctor or other health professional with any variations in sex traits (this is sometimes called an intersex condition or a difference of sex development), or were you born with (or developed naturally in puberty) genitals, reproductive organs, or chromosomal patterns that do not fit standard definitions of male or female?	☐ Yes ☐ No ☐ Don't know ☐ Prefer not to answer
Were you born with any variations in your physical sex characteristics (this is sometimes called being intersex or having a variation in sex trait or difference of sex development)?	☐ Yes ☐ No ☐ Don't know ☐ Prefer not to answer
Have you ever been diagnosed by a medical doctor as having any variations in sex traits (this is sometimes called an intersex condition or a difference of sex development)?	☐ Yes ☐ No ☐ Don't know ☐ Prefer not to answer

SOURCE: Adapted from NASEM, 2022.

identity. For these reasons, instead of listing "intersex" along with other categories in the two-step question, it may be better to capture identifications related to VSTs through free-text response options, such as "another sex, please specify" or "another gender, please specify" (Kronk et al., 2022).

Providers may also record VSTs by using a separate question. Table 3-2 offers examples of questions that ask about patients' VSTs.

Best practices also call for medical records to record patient name[1] and pronoun-related information, to update this information regularly as part of routine practice, and to use algorithms to automatically populate provider notes with a person's selected pronouns (Alpert et al., 2023; Goldhammer et al., 2022; Kronk et al., 2022). Kronk and colleagues (2022) offer a comprehensive example of pronoun selection within the medical record, as shown in Box 3-1.

Finally, best practices call for all gender identity data to be modifiable by patients without the consent of their provider (Kronk et al., 2022). If EHR systems or institutional policies allow only providers or office staff to change these data, patients may be put in the uncomfortable position of having to out themselves to individuals they do not know or trust, and, where providers have not had appropriate education in caring for TGD patients and patients with VSTs, it can lead to the entry of incorrect or transphobic information in the EHR (Kronk et al., 2022). Finally, as the

---

[1] Allowing patients to record their chosen and presently used name helps avoid the distress TGD people or people with VSTs may feel when referred to by a former name ("dead name").

BOX 3-1
Examples of Pronoun Selection Within the Medical Record

What pronouns do you use? Choose all that apply.

- ☐ he/him/his/himself
- ☐ she/her/hers/herself
- ☐ they/them/theirs/themself
- ☐ xe/xem/xyr/xyrs/xemself
- ☐ e/em/eir/eirs/eirself
- ☐ unsure; questioning; exploring
- ☐ I use all/any pronouns
- ☐ none; I avoid pronouns; I use only my name
- ☐ I use different pronouns in different contexts
- ☐ prefer not to respond; prefer not to disclose
- ☐ pronouns/option not listed (please specify): [free text]

SOURCE: Kronk et al., 2022.

---

decision to provide SOGI data may be complicated (given privacy concerns or dynamics of the patient–provider relationship, as explored below), best practices call for patients to have the ability to choose whether to disclose SOGI data and provide consent on how their SOGI data might be used.

BARRIERS TO SOGI DATA COLLECTION

Despite established best practices and documentation of patients' willingness to answer SOGI questions, significant gaps in SOGI data collection remain across the U.S. health care system. Research has identified several systemic barriers—including lack of requirements to record and report SOGI data, provider misconceptions, lack of provider education/training, institutional barriers, and privacy concerns—that prevent the U.S. health care system from achieving the many benefits ascribed to SOGI data collection. This section examines these barriers.

Lack of Federal Requirements

One significant barrier to SOGI data collection in the United States is the fact that there are few requirements for the collection and reporting of SOGI demographic data.

Increasingly, more federal health care programs are encouraging SOGI data collection, most often by including data fields for gender identity and sex recorded at birth in program enrollment forms. Yet with the exception of a mandate from the Health Resources and Services Administration (HRSA) for federally qualified health centers (FQHCs) to collect and report SOGI data for patients, SOGI data collection within federal health care programs is optional, meaning that patients do not have to answer these questions and providers do not have to ask them. Chapter 4 examines the current state of SOGI data collection policies across the federal health care system, describing these and other ongoing SOGI data collection efforts in detail. As described in Chapter 4, most federal efforts to advance SOGI data collection are only recently under way or are still in the proposal state. While SSA (n.d.) does not ask about gender identity or sex recorded at birth or other SOGI data on applications for disability benefits or in beneficiary surveys, it does allow people to change their sex identification on their Social Security records. SSA does not require people to support a change in sex identification with any medical or legal evidence, but sex identification must be either male or female.[2]

Providers who work outside of federal health care programs and facilities are increasingly able to collect and record SOGI data, but there are no federal requirements for them to do so. Since 2018, the Centers for Medicare & Medicaid Services (CMS) and the Office of the National Coordinator for Health Information Technology (2023) have required EHR developers and vendors to allow patients and providers to record SOGI data in EHRs as part of certification under the Meaningful Use incentive program (HHS, 2015). Meaningful Use certification does not require providers or health care institutions to collect SOGI data; it requires only that certified EHR technologies have the ability (i.e., the data fields) to record these data. In addition, certification requirements do not specify which SOGI data questions should be in place or what response options should be available to patients. As a result, there is great variability in whether providers turn on SOGI data capabilities in EHRs and if so, what questions they ask patients.

Indeed, without requirements in place, health care providers and systems routinely fail to collect and record SOGI data. A survey of more than 6,000 staff members and leaders across 18 health care organizations revealed that more than half of clinicians (55.4 percent) "rarely or never"

---

[2] SSA (n.d.) states: "Currently, our record systems require a sex designation of female or male, and cannot accommodate a non-binary or unspecified sex designation, such as X. We are examining ways to address this in the future." SSA disability application forms contain a free-text "remarks" space for applicants to include additional details about any aspect of their disability application. Applicants could use the remarks section of the application form to provide details about gender identity or sex recorded at birth, but the committee does not know how frequently applicants enter such information.

engaged patients in discussion about sexual orientation, and almost two-thirds (71.9 percent) failed to engage in discussions about gender identity (Goldhammer et al., 2018). A survey of 153,827 older adults discharged from one hospital showed that 67.6 percent of records were missing data on sexual orientation, and 63 percent of records lacked data on gender identity (May et al., 2023). Where reporting is mandated, levels of SOGI data collection are higher, although persistent gaps remain: a review of data from 1,297 FQHCs serving more than 30 million patients revealed that, 6 years after HRSA mandated SOGI data collection and reporting, sexual orientation data were missing from 29.1 percent of patient records and gender identity data from 24 percent (Liu et al., 2023). It is unclear whether these gaps exist because providers are not asking the questions or patients are unwilling to disclose. However, previous research has found similar gaps in data collection among FQHCs, although SOGI data collection at FQHCs has increased substantially since 2016 (the year reporting requirements began) (Grasso et al., 2019; McDowell et al., 2022).

Even institutions that are otherwise recognized as providing quality care to LGBTQ+ patients find it difficult to adapt to recording SOGI data in EHRs. In an analysis of Rush University Medical Center—recognized by the Human Rights Campaign's Health Equality Index as being a national leader in the care of LGBTQ+ patients—researchers found that only one-quarter of patient records included gender identity data (Thompson et al., 2021). Likewise, a review of charts at New York University Langone Health (an urban quaternary care academic hospital system that provides gender-affirming surgery and pediatric gender-affirming care, has a child and adolescent mental health gender clinic, and conducts staff training in SOGI data collection) revealed that almost two-thirds of transgender patients (63.05 percent) had no SOGI demographic data attached to their record that would identify them as a gender minority (Dubin et al., 2022).

Provider Misconceptions

Another factor contributing to insufficient SOGI data collection is providers' frequent misconception that their patients do not want to answer SOGI questions. Research finds that patients and providers have discordant views on the appropriateness of SOGI questions in clinical settings: the majority of patients are willing to provide SOGI information, but the majority of providers assume that SOGI questions will make their patients feel uncomfortable or that patients will find these questions offensive (Callahan et al., 2015; Goldhammer et al., 2018; Haider et al., 2017; Maragh-Bass et al., 2017a; Mullins et al., 2020). Providers may also assume that SOGI data are relevant only to certain populations—for example, patients who report sexual health complaints—and not medically relevant to other patient encounters, believing that quality clinical care can be delivered to the majority of patients on the basis of administrative sex (Goldhammer et al., 2018; Kodadek et al., 2019; McClure et al., 2022; Newsom et al., 2022). Providers may also assume that gender identity is static and may not understand the importance of asking SOGI questions over time (Davison et al., 2021).

Even where providers understand the need for documenting patient SOGI in theory, they may prioritize other inquiries they deem more relevant to clinical decision making, such as those relevant to patients' behaviors and experiences rather than to their sexual orientation or gender identity (Dichter et al., 2018). In a qualitative study entailing in-depth individual interviews of health care providers, providers stated that one reason they do not prioritize SOGI data collection is that understanding whether their patient has a sex recorded at birth that is different from their gender identity is clinically necessary information only in certain circumstances (Dichter et al., 2018). While this may be true, it points to another misconception among providers—that clinical decision making is the only reason for collecting SOGI data. This view disregards other important benefits of obtaining and documenting these data, such as building an inclusive and affirming environment for patients.

Lack of Provider Education and Training

Provider misconceptions indicate a lack of education and training in the importance of SOGI data for clinical use and patient care. Providers often lack formal education focused on populations for whom SOGI data are particularly important. Indeed, conventional medical curricula do not include adequate education on treatment and care for TGD people (Haymer, 2014; Jelinek et al., 2020; Safer et al., 2016). One study of 176 undergraduate medical schools in the United States and Canada demonstrated a median time of 5 hours of dedicated content related to sexual and gender minorities across the full curriculum (Obedin-Maliver et al., 2011). Where such content was offered, few schools presented information beyond sexual history, and only 11 of the 176 (8.3 percent; 95 percent confidence interval 3.6–13.0 percent) taught all 16 topics identified by the authors as critical features of LGBT experiences that affect health (Obedin-Maliver et al., 2011). Another study estimates that medical school students receive approximately 18.3 minutes of education about transgender health and related care (Kronk et al., 2022). Studies show similar deficiencies in transgender health training among medical residency programs, with one study finding that 60 percent of residency programs surveyed lacked any clinical rotation in which residents directly worked with transgender patients (Kopel et al., 2023). Nursing students lack access to such training as well: one study estimates that baccalaureate nursing programs dedicate only 2.12 hours of curriculum time to LGBT-related content, and there is no estimation of how much of this content is related specifically to transgender health care (Lim et al., 2015).

Panelist Perspective

"The reason that most adult providers don't provide care for inter-sex folks is because they're just not trained in providing that care. The current model in medical education is that people will get like one or two lectures in general during medical school, and it's usually about a specific condition. . . . We've conceptualized this in medicine for so long as a pediatric problem that is corrected during childhood, and then has no implications for adulthood. So, we have the vast majority of adult health care providers—though they are interacting with patients with VST [variations in sex traits] on a daily basis—[who] have no training, no framework, no skills to be able to provide that care."

—Statement from patient–provider panel,
presented to the committee on November 30, 2023.

Multiple studies examining self-perceived knowledge among health care professionals have demonstrated inadequate knowledge of health issues impacting TGD people (Dubin et al., 2018; Lelutiu-Weinberger et al., 2016; McPhail et al., 2016; Morris et al., 2019; Pratt-Chapman et al., 2022). Without training, providers feel uncertain and ambivalent during clinical encounters with transgender patients; feel less familiar with transgender patient health needs as compared with those of lesbian, gay, and bisexual patients; and have low confidence in their ability to discuss patient gender identity properly (Goldhammer et al., 2018; Morris et al., 2019; Poteat et al., 2013).

Insufficient training also reduces health care providers' literacy in these topics. Providers report that they lack the appropriate language for engaging in SOGI discussions with their patients (Goldhammer et al., 2018; Mullins et al., 2020; Thompson et al., 2021). Providers may also lack a firm understanding of foundational concepts: one study found that 20 percent of nursing students believe sex and gender are synonymous (Sherman et al., 2021; Strong and Folse, 2015).

TGD patients have voiced concern regarding their clinicians' level of knowledge about transgender care. In a study of 27,715 TGD respondents, for example, 5,612 individuals (23.8 percent) reported the need to teach their clinician about transgender people (Miller et al., 2023). TGD respondents who had to educate their provider about their health care needs had higher odds of reporting fair or poor health (versus good or excellent health) and higher odds of severe psychological distress compared with individuals who did not have to do so (Miller et al., 2023). Similar concerns exist regarding the transition of people with VSTs to adult care providers, who may have limited experience with the diversity and special needs of people with VSTs (Nowotny and Reisch, 2023).

Panelist Perspective

"An example of me experiencing a discriminatory event was when I was inpatient at my hospital for a lung collapse and an orderly . . . was bringing me from X-ray to my room, and . . . he either said my dead name or misgendered me, and I corrected him, and he kind of flipped out . . . saying, 'you people, you know, can't just give us a break. Why, you need so much, or you think you're special,' or something like that. And he didn't use any kind of explicitly transphobic language. But it was very clear that he was talking to me as a trans person, or at least nonbinary. So that was shocking, and I was really, really scared by that. . . . [T]he first time I didn't report it, which is crazy. . . . I guess I was too scared. But then he brought me somewhere again . . . and I didn't say anything to him, and he pretended like nothing had ever happened."

—Statement from patient–provider panel,
presented to the committee on November 30, 2023.

The lack of training and support in these areas leads to significant missed opportunities for collecting SOGI data within clinical encounters. But despite these barriers, several studies describe promising models for educating health care providers about transgender health, including those focused at the undergraduate and graduate medical education levels and continuing medical education (Dubin et al., 2018; Ruprecht et al., 2023). Health care institutions must also be responsible for providing SOGI training: to be effective, these trainings need to encompass the full scope of individuals engaged in health care delivery—including administrative staff and others engaged in the process of collecting and updating accurate and affirming SOGI data (Dimant et al., 2019; Dubin et al., 2018; Lelutiu-Weinberger et al., 2016; Pratt-Chapman et al., 2022; Reisner et al., 2016).

Geographic Variability and Variability among Provider Types

As might be expected, SOGI data collection varies with geography. One study of FQHCs found that those located in municipalities that implement sexual and gender minority nondiscrimination laws collect more complete SOGI data for patients relative to those located in municipalities that lack these provisions (Almazan et al., 2021). Another study of community oncology practices found that providers were more likely to ask patients about their SOGI if their clinic was located in a western region of the United States or in a region with higher proportions of sexual and gender minority–identifying individuals (Cathcart-Rake et al., 2019).

Variation is seen among professional disciplines as well. While SOGI records are incomplete in many clinical settings, patient records in home health care settings are particularly so, with one study reporting that only 0.17 percent of records (35 of 20,447 records) contained documentation of the patient's sexual orientation or gender identity (Bjarnadottir et al., 2019). Among comprehensive cancer centers, only 14 percent regularly collected sexual orientation data, and only 19 percent regularly collected gender identity data (Wheldon et al., 2018). In general, gender identity data may not be well documented outside of clinics that specialize in gender-affirming care (Sequeira et al., 2020), and these differences point to specific training needs for different provider types and for outreach to providers who work in regions where SOGI data collection is low.

Institutional Barriers

Even assuming providers have the training and competency to obtain SOGI data from their patients appropriately, obstacles within health care institutions may impede data collection. For example, health care settings may lack an established clinical workflow (e.g., who asks for SOGI data and when), standardized intake forms, or supportive institutional policies and guidelines, all of which hinder the collection of SOGI data (Dunne et al., 2017; Goldberg et al., 2018; Wheldon et al., 2018).

The design of the EHR system itself may inhibit SOGI data collection. For example, while the VHA has collected self-identified gender identity data through administrative systems since 2018, the system was not initially set up to link these data to patient EHRs, meaning that VHA providers could not see these important demographic data during clinic visits (GAO, 2020). Even though VHA providers can now find gender identity information in the EHR's "patient inquiry box," for privacy reasons, this information is not on the "banner" at the top of the patient's record, which may make it difficult for VHA providers to find (Matza and McConnell, 2023). The VHA example shows that even where health care systems and institutions want to collect SOGI data, it can take time to design an appropriate EHR format and to iron out compatibility issues and workflow processes between systems.

Another design challenge surfaces when the EHR platform does not contain a sufficient range of appropriate choices—for example, when the EHR lacks gender options for nonbinary patients or a free-text box in which patients can describe their identity if it differs from available response options—patients may be unable to disclose their SOGI information accurately and may not respond to these questions (Dunne et al., 2017). In addition, institutions may deploy EHR platforms that use outdated or potentially offensive terms or define key terms inconsistently, all of which hinders data collection (Baker et al., 2023b).

Privacy Concerns

The collection and maintenance of SOGI data poses the risk that gender identity status, presence of a VST, or other intimate personal information about an individual will be shared without their informed consent. Unwanted disclosure of SOGI data can pose both immediate harms (e.g., disclosure of SOGI data to a hostile family member who could pose immediate safety risks) and ongoing harms, such as differential treatment by health care providers or office staff (Alpert et al., 2023; Wall et al., 2023; Wood et al., 2022). Caution with disclosing SOGI information is justified considering the stigma often faced by TGD people and people with VSTs in health and social services contexts where SOGI data are collected. However, the committee did not uncover research examining the extent to which privacy concerns reduce the likelihood of TGD adults or adults with VSTs disclosing SOGI data within medical records.

The acute privacy concerns for TGD adolescents make SOGI data collection particularly challenging in pediatric settings. Adolescents face a risk of unwanted disclosure of SOGI to parents/guardians, who have access to their medical records. Given this, pediatric providers may have corresponding worries that they cannot sufficiently protect a pediatric patient's privacy (Carlson et al., 2021; Goldhammer et al., 2022). In addition, the 21st Century Cures Act prevents health care providers from blocking guardians' access to medical records and any sensitive information therein (Carlson et al., 2021). This dynamic may explain why few adolescents and adolescent medicine providers report asking their adolescent patients their SOGI data. A 2020 survey of transgender youth (aged 12–26 years, N = 204) found that only 9 percent were always or often asked about their preferred pronouns outside of specialty gender centers (Sequeira et al., 2020). In a recent survey of pediatric residents, only 20 percent reported asking their patients "often" about gender pronouns (Jelinek et al., 2020). More sophisticated EHR systems are in development that may allow adolescent patients to set controls and permissions with respect to the visibility of their data or may allow clinicians to view data different from what is accessible to guardians via a patient portal (Vance and Mesheriakova, 2017). Until such systems become accessible, SOGI data collection in adolescent populations will remain a challenge.

ICD-10 CODES AND OTHER DATA

Where SOGI data are not well documented—either because of the failure of providers or institutions to collect such data or because EHR platforms are not designed with an appropriate two-step question—researchers and institutions can use codes in the International Classification of Diseases and Related Health Problems (ICD) to identify TGD patients and patients with VSTs.

The ICD is a health care classification system developed by the World Health Organization (WHO) that provides a system of diagnostic codes for categorizing diseases, diagnoses, and procedures. Because ICD codes provide a uniform way of collecting and maintaining patient data, they are imbedded in EHRs and used by health care systems to document patient care and seek insurance reimbursement.

Several codes in the 10th edition of the ICD (ICD-10) relate to care for TGD people (Box 3-2) and people with VSTs (Box 3-3). The committee notes that the ICD-10 codes originally became available in 1999 and contain several out-of-date and pejorative terms (CDC, 2023).

BOX 3-2
ICD-10 Codes Related to Care for Transgender and Gender Diverse People

CHAPTER 5: Mental, Behavioral and Neurodevelopmental Disorders (F01–F99)
F64 Gender identity disorders
- F64.0 Transsexualism
- F64.1 Dual role transvestism
- F64.2 Gender identity disorder of childhood
- F64.8 Other gender identity disorders
- F64.9 Gender identity disorder, unspecified

CHAPTER 21: Factors Influencing Health Status and Contact with Health Services (Z00–Z99)
Z87.89 Personal history of other specified conditions
- Z87.890 Personal history of sex reassignment

SOURCE: CDC, 2024.

BOX 3-3
**ICD-10 Codes Related to Care for People with
Variations in Sex Traits**

**CHAPTER 4: Endocrine, Nutritional and Metabolic Diseases
(E00–E89)**
E25 Adrenogenital disorders
- E25.00 Salt-losing congenital adrenal hyperplasia
- E25.01 Congenital adrenal hyperplasia
- E25.8 Other adrenogenital disorders
- E25.9 Adrenogenital disorder, unspecified

E34.5 Androgen insensitivity syndrome
- E34.50 Androgen insensitivity syndrome, unspecified
- E34.51 Complete androgen insensitivity syndrome
- E34.52 Partial androgen insensitivity syndrome

**CHAPTER 17: Congenital Malformations, Deformations and
Chromosomal Abnormalities (Q00–Q99)**
Q52 Other congenital malformations of female genitalia
- Q52.0 Congenital absence of vagina
- Q52.1 Doubling of vagina

Q53 Undescended and ectopic testicle
- Q53.2 Undescended testicle, bilateral

Q54 Hypospadias
- Q54.2 Hypospadias, penoscrotal
- Q54.3 Hypospadias, perineal

Q55 Other congenital malformations of male genital organs
- Q55.00 Absence and aplasia of testis
- Q55.01 Anorchia

Q56 Indeterminate sex and pseudohermaphroditism
- Q56.0 Hermaphroditism, not elsewhere classified
- Q56.1 Male pseudohermaphroditism, not elsewhere classified
- Q56.2 Female pseudohermaphroditism, not elsewhere classified
- Q56.3 Pseudohermaphroditism, unspecified
- Q56.4 Indeterminate sex, unspecified

BOX 3-3 Continued

Q96 Turner's syndrome
- Q96.0 Karyotype 45, X
- Q96.1 Karyotype 46, X iso (Xq)
- Q96.2 Karyotype 46, X with abnormal sex chromosome, except iso (Xq)
- Q96.3 Mosaicism, 45, X/46, XX or XY
- Q96.4 Mosaicism, 45, X/other cell line(s) with abnormal sex chromosome
- Q96.8 Other variants of Turner's syndrome
- Q96.9 Turner's syndrome, unspecified

Q97 Other sex chromosome abnormalities, female phenotype, not elsewhere classified
- Q97.0 Karyotype 47, XXX
- Q97.1 Female with more than three X chromosomes
- Q97.2 Mosaicism, lines with various numbers of X chromosomes
- Q97.3 Female with 46, XY karyotype
- Q97.8 Other specified sex chromosome abnormalities, female phenotype
- Q97.9 Sex chromosome abnormality, female phenotype, unspecified

Q98 Other sex chromosome abnormalities, male phenotype, not elsewhere classified
- Q98.0 Klinefelter syndrome karyotype 47, XXY
- Q98.1 Klinefelter syndrome, male with more than two X chromosomes
- Q98.3 Other male with 46, XX karyotype
- Q98.4 Klinefelter syndrome, unspecified
- Q98.5 Karyotype 47, XYY
- Q98.6 Male with structurally abnormal sex chromosome
- Q98.7 Male with sex chromosome mosaicism
- Q98.8 Other specified sex chromosome abnormalities, male phenotype
- Q98.9 Sex chromosome abnormality, male phenotype, unspecified

continued

BOX 3-3 Continued

Q99 Other chromosome abnormalities, not elsewhere classified
- Q99.0 Chimera 46, XX/46, XY
- Q99.1 46, XX true hermaphrodite
- Q99.2 Fragile X chromosome
- Q99.8 Other specified chromosome abnormalities
- Q99.9 Chromosomal abnormality, unspecified

NOTE: A number of other ICD-10 codes may be relevant for people with VSTs, including E25.9 Adrenogenital disorder, unspecified; Q43.7 Persistent cloaca; Q53.0 Ectopic testis; Q53.1 Undescended testicle, unilateral; Q53.9 Undescended testicle, unspecified; Q54.0 Hypospadias, balanic; Q54.1 Hypospadias, penile; Q54.4 Congenital chordee; Q54.8 Other hypospadias; Q54.9 Hypospadias, unspecified; Q55.1 Hypoplasia of testis and scrotum; Q55.20 Retractile testis; Q55.28 Unspecified congenital malformations of testis and scrotum; Q55.6 Other congenital malformations of penis; Q55.8 Other specified congenital malformations of male genital organs; Q55.9 Congenital malformation of male genital organ, unspecified; Q52.2 Congenital rectovaginal fistula; Q52.3 Imperforate hymen; Q52.4 Other congenital malformations of vagina; Q52.5 Fusion of labia; Q52.8 Other specified congenital malformations of female genitalia; Q52.9 Congenital malformation of female genitalia, unspecified; Q64.1 Exstrophy of urinary bladder; Z79.890 Hormone replacement therapy; E29.1 Hyprogondaism; E34.9 Endocrine disorder, unspecified.

SOURCE: CDC, 2024.

Using ICD Codes to Identify TGD Patients and Patients with VSTs

Because ICD codes may be present where other gender-identifying information is not, these codes have proved useful to researchers in identifying medical records of TGD patients. For example, research conducted at an urban quaternary care hospital specializing in gender-affirming care found that ICD-10 codes were more reliable than patient demographic data for identifying TGD patient medical records—identifying 63.05 percent versus only 14.49 percent of TGD patients, respectively (a combination of ICD-10 codes and demographic data identified the remaining 22.36) (Dubin et al., 2022). Other studies have found similar rates of TGD patient identification using ICD codes (Jasuja et al., 2020).

In the case of people with VSTs, ICD codes may be particularly important, as SOGI demographic categories in medical records typically do not include questions or response options that would document this identity. ICD codes corresponding to different VST diagnoses (see Box 3-3) may therefore be the only indication in medical records of patients with VSTs. These codes are helpful for tracking patients, especially as many

VSTs are rare. For example, researchers recently developed an algorithm of diagnostic codes and other data for identifying patients with Turner syndrome, a rare condition affecting about 1 in 2,000 live female births (Huang et al., 2023).

The committee notes that ICD codes do not represent every known VST or every population with VSTs. There are more than 30 medical terms for specific combinations of VSTs, and all people with VSTs are unique.

ICD-10 "Z Codes" Documenting Social Determinants of Health in the Medical Record

Beyond documenting specific clinical diagnoses, ICD-10 codes can document various factors that influence health. An extensive body of scientific evidence demonstrates that sociocontextual factors—outside of individual patient interactions with clinicians and health care systems—have a significant influence on individual- and population-level health (Chaiyachati et al., 2016; Chen et al., 2020; Hatef et al., 2019). Known as the social determinants of health (SDOH), these sociocontextual factors can be categorized into multiple domains, including (1) economic stability, (2) education access and quality, (3) neighborhood and built environmental factors, (4) social and community contextual factors, and (5) health care access and quality (OASH, n.d.). SDOH are key factors influencing long-term functional status and quality of life; they are modifiable and so have been identified as points of intervention for health systems and policies designed to improve health equity (Adler et al., 2016; Brown et al., 2019; Stonington et al., 2018; Warnecke et al., 2008; Weir et al., 2020). ICD-10 "Z codes" ranging from Z55 to Z65 capture these factors (CMS, 2021, 2023; Maksut et al., 2021) (see Box 3-4).

CMS, the National Academies, and other groups have encouraged use of these Z codes to advance health equity and reduce health disparities, and EHR vendors and health systems have increasingly added fields designed to promote the capture of SDOH data in structured formats (CMS, 2023; Wang et al., 2021). Some health systems have leveraged these codes to identify social needs and provide context-specific resources to enhance care for people with substantial health-related needs (Bensken et al., 2022; Wang et al., 2021).

Z codes enable health care providers to identify and appropriately document social factors impacting a patient's health, and they can enhance the capture of unequal care and SDOH impacting TGD individuals. Importantly for SSA, Z codes may help identify factors outside of specific health care interactions that delay care or contribute to poorer outcomes among TGD people with SSA-designated disabilities. These considerations are especially important in light of the well-established disproportionate

---

BOX 3-4
ICD-10 "Z Codes" Related to Social Determinants of Health

Z55 – Problems related to education and literacy
- Z55.5 – Less than a high school diploma
- Z55.6 – Problems related to health literacy

Z56 – Problems related to employment and unemployment
Z57 – Occupational exposure to risk factors
Z58 – Problems related to physical environment
- Z58.6 – Inadequate drinking-water supply
- Z58.8 – Other problems related to physical environment
- Z58.81 – Basic services unavailable in physical environment
- Z58.89 – Other problems related to physical environment

Z59 – Problems related to housing and economic circumstances
- Z59.0 – Homelessness
- Z59.00 – Homelessness unspecified
- Z59.01 – Sheltered homelessness
- Z59.02 – Unsheltered homelessness
- Z59.1 – Inadequate Housing
- Z59.10 – Inadequate housing, unspecified
- Z59.11 – Inadequate housing environmental temperature
- Z59.12 – Inadequate housing utilities
- Z59.19 – Other inadequate housing
- Z59.4 – Lack of adequate food
- Z59.41 – Food insecurity
- Z59.48 – Other specified lack of adequate food
- Z59.8 – Other problems related to housing and economic circumstances
- Z59.81 – Housing instability, housed
- Z59.811 – Housing instability, housed, with risk of homelessness
- Z59.812 – Housing instability, housed, homelessness in past 12 months
- Z59.819 – Housing instability, housed unspecified
- Z59.82 – Transportation insecurity
- Z59.86 – Financial insecurity
- Z59.87 – Material hardship due to limited financial resources, not elsewhere classified
- Z59.89 – Other problems related to housing and economic circumstances

Z60 – Problems related to social environment

BOX 3-4 Continued

Z62 – Problems related to upbringing
- Z62.2 – Upbringing away from parents
- Z62.23 – Child in custody of non-parental relative
- Z62.24 – Child in custody of non-relative guardian
- Z62.8 – Other specified problems related to upbringing
- Z62.81 – Personal history of abuse in childhood
- Z62.814 – Personal history of child financial abuse
- Z62.815 – Personal history of intimate partner abuse in childhood
- Z62.82 – Parent-child conflict
- Z62.823 – Parent-step child conflict
- Z62.83 – Non-parental relative or guardian-child conflict
- Z62.831 – Non-parental relative-child conflict
- Z62.832 – Non-relative guardian-child conflict
- Z62.833 – Group home staff-child conflict
- Z62.89 – Other specified problems related to upbringing
- Z62.892 – Runaway [from current living environment]

Z63 – Other problems related to primary support group, including family circumstances
Z64 – Problems related to certain psychosocial circumstance
Z65 – Problems related to other psychosocial circumstances

SOURCE: CDC, 2024.

---

burden of health-harming SDOH among TGD people across the life course, resulting from limited or no protection from discrimination, marginalization, and other key stressors, as well as inequitable access to a range of health-promoting conditions (Blosnich et al., 2017; Braveman and Gottlieb, 2014; Glick et al., 2020; Marcus et al., 2024; NASEM, 2019, 2020; Scheim et al., 2022). Examples include high rates of unemployment, violence, and homelessness that disproportionately impact TGD people (Glick et al., 2020; Henderson et al., 2022; Kuhns et al., 2021; Scheer and Poteat, 2021). For example, in a study examining the prevalence of health-harming SDOH among transgender U.S. veterans using data collected from 1997 to 2014 at the VHA, violence, housing instability, and housing strain were highly prevalent among TGD people and significantly associated with multiple medical conditions, including hepatitis C, mood disorders, and posttraumatic stress disorder (Blosnich et al., 2017).

Using Z codes, providers can capture these aspects of their patients' lives, and Z codes in the medical record may indicate the broader context impacting health and health behaviors among TGD people and people with VSTs applying for disability benefits from SSA. For example, nonadherence to medication can be considered in the context of an individual's financial means, transportation availability, and ability to access basic services within their physical environment (e.g., available mental health infrastructure, access to specialty providers). It should be noted, however, that despite their promise, Z codes are not widely used by providers. One review of Z code utilization among Medicare beneficiaries estimates that less than 2 percent of patients have Z codes documented in their medical record (Maksut et al., 2021).

Pharmacy Data and Natural Language Processing

In addition to identifying TGD patients through the use of ICD codes, researchers and health care entities use search algorithms that include pharmacy data to track the provision of gender-affirming hormones or natural language processing to track key words (such as "transgender" or "gender dysphoria") within free-text clinical notes as alternative means of ascertaining TGD patients where SOGI data are incomplete (Ehrenfeld et al., 2019; Hines et al., 2023; Hua et al., 2023; Huang et al., 2023; Quinn et al., 2017; Streed et al., 2023; Xie et al., 2021). ICD-10 codes, SOGI data fields, pharmacy data, and clinical notes all have strengths and weaknesses for identifying TGD patients, but used in combination, they can provide more complete documentation (Jasuja et al., 2020). One study of patients at an academic medical center combined data from EHR SOGI fields, ICD-10 codes related to gender dysphoria, and pharmacy data on prescriptions for estradiol and testosterone; using this approach, researchers identified more than 99 percent of the total TGD population (Hines et al., 2023).

Using natural language processing algorithms may also be useful for correcting information where SOGI data collection is inaccurate. One study comparing the accuracy of SOGI data fields versus a keyword search or ICD code found that a small number of cisgender patients had been identified as possibly transgender by their gender identity selections within SOGI data fields. For these patients, keywords within free-text clinical notes helped clarify patient identity where SOGI data collection produced inaccuracies (Foer et al., 2020).

Documenting TGD patients via ICD codes can help health systems understand disparities experienced by the patients they serve. For example, a recent study used ICD-10 codes and prescription data to find a cohort of Medicaid-enrolled TGD people living with HIV, finding that they had lower viral suppression rates (76 percent) than cisgender women (80.4 percent) and cisgender men (83.3 percent); however, that study found higher viral suppression rates among TGD people who had gender-affirming surgery than among the cisgender population (Rodriguez-Hart et al., 2023). An examination of medical records at one university health system (which included diagnostic codes, recorded sex, and clinical narrative text that indicated gender identity and sex) found a chronic kidney disease prevalence of 36 percent among transgender patients, substantially higher than would be expected relative to cisgender data (Eckenrode et al., 2022). By examining ICD-10 codes and specific key words in free-text clinical notes within three Kaiser Permanente health plan regions, researchers uncovered a higher frequency of certain adverse events for TGD people, leading to a follow-up study on diabetes incidence among TGD patients (Islam et al., 2022; Quinn et al., 2017). The VHA has also used ICD codes to identify TGD veterans within its system, revealing numerous health disparities for them compared with cisgender veterans, including higher rates of suicidality, housing instability, and substance use (Blosnich et al., 2013, 2018; Fletcher et al., 2022).

Limitations of ICD Data

While these examples show the potential value of ICD codes and similar data for health systems' documentation of health disparities among TGD patients, researchers caution that these data may not be reliable in all circumstances. For one thing, not every TGD person will seek gender-affirming services that generate an ICD code or utilize gender-affirming hormone therapies that generate pharmacy data (Hines et al., 2023). Chapters 5–7 of this report describe the multiple and varied gender-affirming services available for TGD people and people with VSTs, many of which do not correspond to an ICD code. In addition, ICD-10 codes related to care for TGD people may be used less frequently outside of specialty gender care clinics (Dubin et al., 2022). Use of these codes may also fail to count individuals who are unable to access gender-affirming interventions, which may result in disproportionately undercounting those of lower socioeconomic status who are not connected to health plans that cover gender-affirming services or cannot pay for these services out of pocket (Kronk et al., 2022). ICD-10 codes have also been seen as pathologizing, as codes related to care for TGD people fall underneath a mental health diagnostic code (Wesp et al., 2019). Some providers may refrain from using these codes for this reason.

In addition, the consistent and accurate reporting of SDOH Z codes has been inadequate to date, in part because of providers' lack of knowledge of SDOH and limited time to spend with patients uncovering underlying needs. Current Z coding in TGD/VST patient charts also is likely to be poorly reflective of the actual burden of social needs (Chang et al., 2024; Jacobs, 2021; Kostelanetz et al., 2022; Truong et al., 2020; Yang et al., 2022).

While identifying TGD people or people with VSTs through ICD codes, pharmacy data, or other such information has benefits for research, the committee notes that individual patients may object to their medical records being examined in this way. While the research presented above examines this type of data in the aggregate to better understand health disparities in a way that may improve services, there is a risk that organizations could use these data to identify individual TGD patients or patients with VSTs who would not have chosen to report such identities or experiences. For these reasons, rather than relying on ICD-10 codes, health care settings can seek to improve SOGI data collection to capture all patients with TGD or VST identity or lived experience (Dubin et al., 2022), while offering patients the autonomy to select for themselves how they want to be identified in medical records.

Panelist Perspective

"One of the big problems, though, is that there is a huge number of ICD codes that are used to refer to folks with VST. I think folks who have tried to study [and] have tried to take a big data approach to understanding the health of folks with VST have really struggled actually to capture everybody in a health care system or in CMS data—for example, by ICD codes, because there's just so much heterogeneity in how individual physicians will code when they're seeing an individual patient."

—Statement from patient–provider panel,
presented to the committee on November 30, 2023.

NOTES: CMS = Centers for Medicare & Medicaid Services; ICD = International Classification of Diseases and Related Health Problems; VST = variations in sex traits.

FUTURE OF SOGI DATA COLLECTION WITHIN ELECTRONIC HEALTH RECORDS

Where SOGI data collection is in place, there remains significant variability in how these data are collected and how they are used in clinical practice. Despite a deep body of research on the benefits of SOGI data and best practices for collecting these data appropriately, the health care system has been slow to adopt these practices. Efforts are under way that may address some of these challenges. This section explores the recent update of the ICD classification system that may better capture TGD people and people with VSTs in the medical record, as well as other data collection tools—such as the "anatomical inventory" and "sex for clinical use" data field—that are aimed at advancing and expanding SOGI data collection in ways that support patient-centered clinical decision making.

ICD-11

WHO (n.d.-b) recently updated the ICD classification system to incorporate advances in science, medicine, disease treatment, and prevention, with the goal of enabling more precise and more detailed data recording and collection. Effective January 1, 2022, the International Classification of Diseases and Related Health Problems, 11th edition (ICD-11), reconceptualizes and reorganizes diagnostic codes related to TGD health to "reflect modern understanding of sexual health and gender identity" (WHO, n.d.-a). Box 3-5 lists the revised ICD-11 codes under the new term "gender incongruence," along with the language used by the ICD to describe each category.

ICD-11 replaces outdated terms such as "transsexualism" with "gender incongruence" and removes the pathologizing label of "disorder." The new edition locates "gender incongruence" categories, organizationally, within a new chapter titled "Conditions Related to Sexual Health." In previous versions of the ICD, the "gender identity disorder" category was placed in the chapter on "Mental, Behavioral or Neurodevelopmental Disorders" (see Box 3-2). By reconceptualizing gender incongruence under sexual health, the ICD recognizes that it is inappropriate to classify TGD identity as a mental health disorder, as the mental health component leading to distress or functional limitation for some TGD people is not linked to gender identity itself but to the experience of violence and discrimination (Baleige et al., 2022; Robles et al., 2022). This reclassification may help reduce the social stigma associated with TGD identity and the perception that some TGD people have disorders or sicknesses that should be cured.

However, this new classification is not without limitations: organizing categories of gender identity under sexual health can incorrectly leave the impression that these are sexual health problems (Giordano, 2023). This concern aside, the move away from mental health classification may have practical implications for care, as it may mean more coverage of gender-affirming care by insurance companies, and thus more accurate coding by providers who see TGD people. In general, it is often more difficult for patients to receive coverage for mental health–related claims, such as those under the ICD-10 (F64 and Q56.3) gender identity disorder classification (CSE, 2019), than for medical claims. In these cases, providers may get creative with the codes they use to record patient care, meaning that ICD-10 codes may not accurately record TGD treatment and care. With gender incongruence now classified within a sexual health framework,

---

BOX 3-5
Revised ICD-11 Codes for Gender Incongruence

CHAPTER 17: Conditions Related to Sexual Health

Gender Incongruence: Gender incongruence is characterised by a marked and persistent incongruence between an individual's experienced gender and the assigned sex. Gender variant behaviour and preferences alone are not a basis for assigning the diagnoses in this group.

HA60 – Gender incongruence of adolescence and adulthood: Gender Incongruence of Adolescence and Adulthood is characterised by a marked and persistent incongruence between an individual´s experienced gender and the assigned sex, which often leads to a desire to 'transition', in order to live and be accepted as a person of the experienced gender, through hormonal treatment, surgery or other health care services to make the individual´s body align, as much as desired and to the extent possible, with the experienced gender. The diagnosis cannot be assigned prior the onset of puberty. Gender variant behaviour and preferences alone are not a basis for assigning the diagnosis.

HA61 – Gender incongruence of childhood: Gender incongruence of childhood is characterised by a marked incongruence between an individual's experienced/expressed gender and the assigned sex in pre-pubertal children. It includes a strong desire to be a different gender than the assigned sex; a strong dislike on the child's part of his or her sexual anatomy or anticipated secondary sex characteristics and/or a strong desire for the primary and/or anticipated secondary sex characteristics that match the experienced gender; and make-believe or fantasy play, toys, games, or activities and playmates that are typical of the experienced gender rather than the assigned sex. The incongruence must have persisted for about 2 years. Gender variant behaviour and preferences alone are not a basis for assigning the diagnosis.

HA6Z – Gender incongruence, unspecified: This category is an 'unspecified' residual category.

SOURCE: WHO, 2024.

ICD-11 may enable providers to code accurately, which could serve to increase the presence of such ICD codes within medical records; however, this approach may have drawbacks, where coding under a sexual health framework may not capture all patient circumstances.

ICD-11 also reorganizes and updates WHO's classification related to VSTs. Box 3-6 lists the revised ICD-11 codes, which fall into two main groupings: (1) "Adrenogenital disorders" in Chapter 17: Conditions Related

BOX 3-6
Revised ICD-11 Codes for Variations in Sex Traits

CHAPTER 17: Conditions related to sexual health

5A71 – Adrenogenital disorders: Disorders of the reproductive system resulting from pathologic androgen production secondary to abnormalities in cortisol and/or aldosterone production

- *5A71.0 – 46,XX disorders of sex development induced by androgens of fetal origin.* This refers to 46,XX disorders of sex development induced by any natural or synthetic compound, usually a steroid hormone, that stimulates or controls the development and maintenance of male characteristics in vertebrates by binding to androgen receptors, of fetal origin.

- *5A71.00 – Glucocorticoid resistance.* Glucocorticoid resistance is a rare genetic endocrine condition characterised by generalised, partial, target tissue resistance to glucocorticoids. The clinical spectrum of the condition is broad, ranging from asymptomatic to severe cases of hyperandrogenism, fatigue and/or mineralocorticoid excess.

- *5A71.01 – Congenital adrenal hyperplasia.* Congenital adrenal hyperplasia (CAH) refers to a group of conditions associated with either complete (classical form) or partial (non-classical) anomalies in the biosynthesis of adrenal hormones. The condition is characterised by insufficient production of cortisol, or of aldosterone (classical form with salt wasting), associated with overproduction of adrenal androgens. In the classical form, metabolic decompensation (dehydration with hyponatraemia, hyperkalaemia and acidosis associated with mineralocorticoid deficiency, and hypoglycaemia associated with glucocorticoid deficiency) may be life-threatening from the neonatal period onwards. Genital variations may be noted at birth in affected females. Chronic hyperandrogenism may lead to accelerated growth during childhood, but advanced bone maturation may lead to a deficit in final height. Adults tend to be overweight and metabolic disturbances, bone anomalies and fertility problems may also be present. Non-classical forms are associated with later onset, during the peri- or post-pubertal period, and manifest with signs of hyperandrogenism (acne, hirsutism, menstrual problems and infertility).

- *5A71.0Y – Other specified 46,XX disorders of sex development induced by androgens of fetal origin.* This category is an 'other specified' residual category.

continued

BOX 3-6 Continued

- 5A71.*0Z* – *46,XX disorders of sex development induced by androgens of fetal origin, unspecified.* This category is an 'unspecified' residual category.
- *5A71.1 – 46,XX disorders of sex development induced by androgens of maternal origin.* This refers to 46,XX disorders of sex development induced by any natural or synthetic compound, usually a steroid hormone, that stimulates or controls the development and maintenance of male characteristics in vertebrates by binding to androgen receptors, of maternal origin.
- *5A71.Y – Other specified adrenogenital disorders.* This category is an 'other specified' residual category
- *5A71.Z – Adrenogenital disorders, unspecified.* This category is an 'unspecified' residual category

CHAPTER 20: Developmental Abnormalities

LD2A – Malformative disorders of sex development: Any condition caused by failure of the genitals to correctly develop during the antenatal period.

- *LD2A.0 – Ovotesticular disorder of sex development:* Ovotesticular disorder of sex development, formerly called true hermaphroditism, is a rare cause of genital ambiguity characterised by the presence of ovarian and testicular tissue in an individual, leading to development of both male and female structures.
- *LD2A.1 – 46,XY gonadal dysgenesis.* This is any congenital developmental disorder of the reproductive system characterised by a progressive loss of primordial germ cells on the developing gonads of an embryo.
- *LD2A.2 – Testicular agenesis.* (No description provided)
- *LD2A.3 – 46,XY disorder of sex development due to a defect in testosterone metabolism* (No description provided)
- *LD2A.4 – 46,XY disorder of sex development due to androgen resistance.* Androgen insensitivity syndrome (AIS) is a disorder of sex development (DSD) characterised by the presence of female external genitalia, ambiguous genitalia or variable defects in virilization in a 46,XY individual with absent or partial responsiveness to age-appropriate levels of androgens. It comprises two clinical subgroups: complete AIS (CAIS) and partial AIS (PAIS).
- *LD56 – Chimaera 46, XX, 46, XY.* A disease caused by XX and XY embryonic fusion or the distinct loss event of a sex chromosome from a XXY embryo early in development. This results in

---

BOX 3-6 Continued

a subset of cells in the body having a XX karyotype, while other cells demonstrate a XY karyotype. This disease may present with abnormal genital development.
  - LD56.0 – Androgenetic chimaera
  - LD56.1 – Gynogenetic chimaera
  - LD56.Y – Other specified chimaera 46, XX, 46, XY
  - LD56.Z – Chimaera 46, XX, 46, XY, unspecified
- *LD2A.Y – Other specified malformative disorders of sex development.* This category is an 'other specified' residual category
- *LD2A.Z – Malformative disorders of sex development, unspecified.* This category is an 'unspecified' residual category

SOURCE: WHO, 2024.

---

to Sexual Health, and (2) "Malformative disorders of sex development" in Chapter 20: Developmental Abnormalities. While ICD-11 removes outdated terms such as "hermaphroditism" and "pseudohermaphroditism" and expands the categories of VSTs, ICD-11 has been criticized for using the language "disorders of sex development," which may inaccurately pathologize VSTs as "disorders" (Carpenter, 2018). Previous studies have demonstrated that this nomenclature is offensive and distressing to patients and may cause individuals to avoid seeking health care (Johnson et al., 2017). In addition, placing certain VST categories in the sexual health chapter does not have the same effect of reducing social stigma as the gender incongruence codes, as these variations were not previously classified under mental health categories in ICD-10 (rather, they were included in a chapter on endocrine diseases).

Finally, ICD-11 reorganizes Z codes related to SDOH under a new heading, "Factors Influencing Health Status." ICD-11 includes additional codes related to SDOH (e.g., including "insufficient insurance coverage," coded as QE30), but it omits others that are present in ICD-10 (e.g., "personal history of abuse in childhood") (Handerer et al., 2021).

ICD-11 is in the process of being adopted by WHO member countries, but it may take several years for its successful rollout in the United States, given the challenge of cross-walking the more than 70,000 current ICD-10 codes to corresponding ICD-11 codes and updating every ICD-dependent process, including billing and reimbursement systems, quality measurement, and data reporting systems within the U.S. health care system (Feinstein et al., 2023). Still, to the extent that the reclassification of TGD health-related diagnoses encourages providers to use these diagnostic codes to document care and treatment, ICD-11 could become a more dependable way to document TGD patient care within medical records. And to the extent that expanded ICD-11 codes for VSTs bring more accurate recording of patient treatment and experience, these codes, too, may be useful for health systems and researchers seeking to better understand the many experiences of people with VSTs.

However, ICD-11 codes alone are unlikely to be a way to identify all TGD patients and patients with VSTs, as some populations will remain undercounted. Similar to the problems with ICD-10, not every health experience can be coded under this new framework, and the ICD-11 reorganization does nothing to improve access to gender-affirming care and treatment for populations that are currently unable to access them.

Anatomical Inventory

While EHR data collection that asks for a person's gender identity and sex recorded at birth may enable clinicians to address patients in a respectful manner and offer culturally responsive and individually tailored care, such data collection does not tell clinicians about their patients' anatomy. TGD patients and patients with VSTs may have features of their anatomy that do not match traditional expectations based on gender identity or sex recorded at birth. While some TGD people undergo medical and surgical interventions to affirm their gender identity—including genital surgery, hysterectomy, or breast augmentation—others do not. Even if clinicians are aware that their patients are TGD, they cannot know the organs their patients have without asking.

Likewise, people with VSTs may have organs that do not match their gender identity or sex recorded at birth. For example, individuals born with androgen insensitivity syndrome (AIS) present physically as female, are usually recorded female at birth, and typically identify with a female gender identify (Hines et al., 2003). However, because they are born with XY chromosomes, they have internal, undescended testes and do not have a uterus. Some people with AIS will have their testes surgically removed; others will not. If clinicians make assumptions about organs based on gender identity and sex recorded at birth, they may miss an important opportunity to discuss cancer risk with patients with AIS.

There have been recent efforts to encourage clinicians to ensure that an anatomical inventory of their patients has been completed, either by the patient or as part of the standard practice of taking a medical history (Grasso et al., 2021). This may also be referred to as an "organ inventory." The goal of an anatomical inventory is to document and track the presence or absence of sexual/reproductive organs within the patient's EHR along with any surgeries related to those organs. Such inventories have obvious advantages for TGD patients and patients with VSTs, but they are important for all patients. A clinician may be unaware, for example, that a cisgender female patient has had a hysterectomy (removal of the uterus) as treatment for endometriosis, or that a cisgender male patient has had an orchiectomy (removal of the testicles) as part of treatment for prostate cancer. With an accurate understanding of patient anatomy together with data on gender identity and sex recorded at birth, clinicians can offer appropriate preventive health screenings, chronic disease management, and long-term care that are tailored to the needs of every patient.

Today, some EHR vendors include a standardized anatomical inventory template within their platform; other EHR vendors permit health care organizations to customize their own anatomical inventory template (Grasso et al., 2021). Yet while EHR capabilities may be present, anatomical inventories are not yet used in common practice.

There have been some efforts to bring the anatomical inventory into wider use. In 2022, for example, the Oregon Health Authority issued draft SOGI data collection recommendations that, in addition to questions on gender identity and sex recorded at birth, include an anatomic inventory (OEI, 2023). As part of "best practice recommendations to assure quality medical care," the draft recommendations call on health care providers to ask patients about their anatomy using the question presented in Box 3-7 (OEI, 2023, Appendix A).

BOX 3-7
Oregon Health Authority: Draft Recommendations for Anatomic Inventory Question

YOUR BODY
Are you (Check all that apply):
- ☐ A person with breasts
- ☐ A person with a cervix
- ☐ A person with ovaries
- ☐ A person with a uterus
- ☐ A person with a vagina
- ☐ A person with a penis
- ☐ A person with a prostate
- ☐ A person with testes
- ☐ A person with intersex genitalia
- ☐ A person who had genital reassignment surgery
- ☐ Don't know
- ☐ I don't know what this question is asking
- ☐ I don't want to say

As anatomical inventories become more commonplace, thought leaders suggest that anatomical inventory data should correspond to ICD codes to enhance the accuracy and tracking of quality-of-care measures (Grasso et al., 2021).

Sex for Clinical Use

The Health Level Seven International Gender Harmony Model is a conceptual model produced through a collaborative, international effort that aims to improve the standardization of SOGI data collection by specifying gender-inclusive standards that can be used by health care providers and health systems (McClure et al., 2022). EHR developers can look to the Gender Harmony Model for updated terminology that is both clinically useful and culturally appropriate (Baker et al., 2023a).

The intent of the model is to push the system to advance the collection of information that will aid in the provision of affirmative and quality person-centered care. Many aspects of the Gender Harmony Model match best practices in SOGI data collection described throughout this chapter. One additional element of this model is the concept of "sex for clinical use," or the idea that "a given patient can have one sex for routine clinical care, but another sex for reproductive care or cancer screenings or for certain clinical assessments where sex-based assessments may be necessary (e.g., kidney function tests and lung function tests)" (McClure et al., 2022).

The concept of sex for clinical use is not used regularly within the U.S. health care system, and providers do not commonly collect the data elements required—such as an anatomical inventory, measurement of hormone levels, or chromosomal analysis—for this type of clinical patient care to become a reality. However, the Gender Harmony Model demonstrates the possibility of data that could be collected and serves as an aspiration for providers and institutions to move toward collecting these data elements.

SUMMARY OF KEY POINTS

SOGI data collection is enormously beneficial to patients because it promotes patient trust and comfort with providers, reduces health care avoidance among TGD people and people with VSTs, and enhances the patient experience by helping providers make informed and patient-centered clinical decisions about treatment and care. However, this chapter has documented the varied and complex challenges involved in bringing widespread and meaningful SOGI data collection to the U.S. health care system. While efforts are under way to advance and expand SOGI data collection, these model efforts are not part of current practice, and many providers and institutions across the health care system may not record or collect adequate or accurate SOGI data for the patients they serve. While people can change their gender identity on their Social Security records, SSA does not ask about sex recorded at birth or gender identity or other SOGI data on applications for disability benefits.

As medical records alone may fail to identify the gender diversity of TGD applicants or appropriately capture biological characteristics relevant to applicants with VSTs, giving applicants the option to enter their own sex and gender identity information when submitting a disability application to SSA would enable a more accurate understanding of applicant characteristics and, ultimately, more accurate assessment of disability. Asking SOGI questions of applicants up front allows applicants to choose how to report their identity to SSA (rather than having adjudicators piece together their identity through other information in the medical record). However, it is important that applicants always have the option to keep SOGI data private from SSA.

REFERENCES

Abreu, R. L., J. P. Sostre, K. A. Gonzalez, G. M. Lockett, E. Matsuno, and D. V. Mosley. 2022. Impact of gender-affirming care bans on transgender and gender diverse youth: Parental figures' perspective. *Journal of Family Psychology* 36(5):643–652. https://doi.org/10.1037/fam0000987.

Adler, N. E., M. M. Glymour, and J. Fielding. 2016. Addressing social determinants of health and health inequalities. *JAMA* 316(16):1641–1642. https://doi.org/10.1001/jama.2016.14058.

Almazan, A. N., D. King, C. Grasso, S. Cahill, M. Lattanner, M. L. Hatzenbuehler, and A. S. Keuroghlian. 2021. Sexual orientation and gender identity data collection at U.S. health centers: Impact of city-level structural stigma in 2018. *American Journal of Public Health* 111(11):2059–2063. https://doi.org/10.2105/AJPH.2021.306414.

Alpert, A. B., J. E. Mehringer, S. J. Orta, T. Hernandez, E. F. Redwood, L. Rivers, C. Manzano, R. Ruddick, S. Adams, J. Sevelius, E. Belanger, D. Operario, and J. J. Griggs. 2023. Transgender people's experiences sharing information with clinicians: A focus group-based qualitative study. *Annals of Family Medicine* 21(5):408–415. https://doi.org/10.1007/s11606-022-07671-6.

Baker, K., D. Compton, E. Fechter-Leggett, C. Grasso, and C. Kronk. 2023a. Will clinical standards not be part of the choir? Harmonization between the HL7 gender harmony project model and the NASEM measuring sex, gender identity, and sexual orientation report in the United States. *Journal of the American Medical Informatics Association* 30(1):83–93. https://doi.org/10.1093/jamia/ocac205.

Baker, K. E., E. Sarkodie, J. Kwait, C. Medina, A. Radix, and R. Flynn. 2023b. Advancing sexual and gender minority population health using electronic health record data. *American Journal of Public Health* 113(12):1287–1289. https://doi.org/10.2105/AJPH.2023.307467.

Baleige, A., M. de la Cheneliere, C. Dassonneville, and M. J. Martin. 2022. Following ICD-11, rebuilding mental health care for transgender persons: Leads from field experimentations in Lille, France. *Transgender Health* 7(1):1–6. https://doi.org/10.1089/trgh.2020.0143.

Bensken, W. P., P. M. Alberti, K. C. Stange, M. Sajatovic, and S. M. Koroukian. 2022. ICD-10 Z-code health-related social needs and increased healthcare utilization. *American Journal of Preventive Medicine* 62(4):E232–E241. https://doi.org/10.1016/j.amepre.2021.10.004.

Blosnich, J., G. R. Brown, J. C. Shipherd, M. Kauth, R. I. Piegari, and R. M. Bossarte. 2013. Prevalence of gender identity disorder and suicide risk among transgender veterans utilizing Veterans Health Administration care. *American Journal of Public Health* 103(10):E27–E32. https://doi.org/10.2105/AJPH.2013.301507.

Blosnich, J. R., M. C. Marsiglio, M. E. Dichter, S. Gao, A. J. Gordon, J. C. Shipherd, M. R. Kauth, G. R. Brown, and M. J. Fine. 2017. Impact of social determinants of health on medical conditions among transgender veterans. *American Journal of Preventive Medicine* 52(4):491–498. https://doi.org/10.1016/j.amepre.2016.12.019.

Blosnich, J., J. Cashy, A. J. Gordon, J. C. Shipherd, M. Kauth, G. Brown, and M. J. Fine. 2018. Using clinician text notes in electronic medical record data to validate transgender-related diagnosis codes. *Journal of the American Medical Informatics Association* 25(7):905–908. https://doi.org/10.1093/jamia/ocy022.

Bjarnadottir, R. I., W. Bockting, and D. W. Dowding. 2017. Patient perspectives on answering questions about sexual orientation and gender identity: An integrative review. *Journal of Clinical Nursing* 26(13–14):1814–1833. https://doi.org/10.1111/jocn.13612.

Bjarnadottir, R. I., W. Bockting, S. Yoon, and D. W. Dowding. 2019. Nurse documentation of sexual orientation and gender identity in home healthcare. *Computers, Informatics, Nursing* 37(4):213–221. https://doi.org/10.1097/CIN.0000000000000492.

Braveman, P., and L. Gottlieb. 2014. The social determinants of health: It's time to consider the causes of the causes. *Public Health Reports* 129 (Suppl 2):19–31. https://doi.org/10.1177/00333549141291S206

Brown, A. F., G. X. Ma, J. Miranda, E. Eng, D. Castille, T. Brockie, P. Jones, C. O. Airhihenbuwa, T. Farhat, L. Zhu, and C. Trinh-Shevrin. 2019. Structural interventions to reduce and eliminate health disparities. *American Journal of Public Health* 109(S1):S72–S78. https://doi.org/10.2105/AJPH.2018.304844.

Cahill, S., R. Singal, C. Grasso, D. King, K. Mayer, K. Baker, and H. Makadon. 2014. Do ask, do tell: High levels of acceptability by patients of routine collection of sexual orientation and gender identity data in four diverse American community health centers. *PLoS ONE* 9(9):E107104. https://doi.org/10.1371/journal.pone.0107104.

Callahan, E. J., N. Sitkin, H. Ton, W. S. Eidson-Ton, J. Weckstein, and D. Latimore. 2015. Introducing sexual orientation and gender identity into the electronic health record: One academic health center's experience. *Academic Medicine* 90(2):154–160. https://doi.org/10.1097/ACM.0000000000000467

Carlson, J., R. Goldstein, K. Hoover, and N. Tyson. 2021. NASPAG/SAHM statement: The 21st Century Cures Act and adolescent confidentiality. *Journal of Adolescent Health* 68(2):426–428. https://doi.org/10.1016/j.jadohealth.2020.10.020.

Carpenter, M. 2018. Intersex variations, human rights, and the international classification of diseases. *Health and Human Rights* 20(2):205–214.

Cathcart-Rake, E. J., T. Zemla, A. Jatoi, K. E. Weaver, H. Neuman, A. E. Kazak, R. Carlos, L. Gansauer, J. M. Unger, N. M. Pajewski, and C. Kamen. 2019. Acquisition of sexual orientation and gender identity data among NCI Community Oncology Research Program practice groups. *Cancer* 125(8):1313–1318. https://doi.org/10.1002/cncr.31925.

CDC (Centers for Disease Control and Prevention). 2023. *International Classification of Diseases, Tenth Revision, Clinical Modification (ICD-10-CM)*. https://www.cdc.gov/nchs/icd/icd-10-cm.htm#:~:text=The%20ICD%2D10%20is%20used,as%20of%20January%201%2C%201999 (accessed April 3, 2024).

CDC. 2024. *National Center for Health Statistics–ICD-10-CM*. https://icd10cmtool.cdc.gov/?fy=FY2024&query=Q99 (accessed April 3, 2024).

Chaiyachati, K. H., D. T. Grande, and J. Aysola. 2016. Health systems tackling social determinants of health: Promises, pitfalls, and opportunities of current policies. *American Journal of Managed Care* 22(11):E393–E394.

Chang, J. E., N. Smith, Z. Lindenfeld, and W. B. Weeks. 2024. Hospital use of common Z-codes for Medicare fee-for-service beneficiaries, 2017–2021. *Health Affairs Scholar* 2(1). https://doi.org/10.1093/haschl/qxad086.

Chen, M., X. Tan, and R. Padman. 2020. Social determinants of health in electronic health records and their impact on analysis and risk prediction: A systematic review. *Journal of the American Medical Informatics Association* 27(11):1764–1773. https://doi.org/10.1093/jamia/ocaa143.

CMS (Centers for Medicare & Medicaid Services). 2021. *Utilization of Z codes for social determinants of health among Medicare fee-for-service beneficiaries, 2019. Data Highlight No. 24.* Rockville, MD: Office of Minority Health. https://www.cms.gov/files/document/z-codes-data-highlight.pdf (accessed March 14, 2024).

CMS. 2023. *Using Z codes: The social determinants of health (SDOH) data journey to better outcomes.* Rockville, MD: Office of Minority Health. https://www.cms.gov/files/document/zcodes-infographic.pdf (accessed March 14, 2024).

Crocetti, D., S. Monro, V. Vecchietti, and T. Yeadon-Lee. 2021. Towards an agency-based model of intersex, variations of sex characteristics (VSC) and DSD/DSD health. *Culture, Health, & Sexuality* 23(4):500–515. https://doi.org/10.1080/13691058.2020.1825815.

CSE (Campaign for Southern Equality). 2019. *Insurance coding alternatives for trans healthcare.* https://southernequality.org/wp-content/uploads/2019/03/InsuranceCoding.pdf (accessed May 3, 2023).

Davison, K., R. Queen, F. Lau, and M. Antonio. 2021. Culturally competent gender, sex, and sexual orientation information practices and electronic health records: Rapid review. *JMIR Medical Informatics* 9(2):E25467. https://doi.org/10.2196/25467.

Dichter, M. E., S. N. Ogden, and K. L. Scheffey. 2018. Provider perspectives on the application of patient sexual orientation and gender identity in clinical care: A qualitative study. *Journal of General Internal Medicine* 33(8):1359–1365. https://doi.org/10.1007/s11606-018-4489-4.

Dimant, O. E., T. E. Cook, R. E. Greene, and A. E. Radix. 2019. Experiences of transgender and gender nonbinary medical students and physicians. *Transgender Health* 4(1):209–216. https://doi.org/10.1089/trgh.2019.0021.

Dubin, S. N., I. T. Nolan, C. G. Streed, Jr., R. E. Greene, A. E. Radix, and S. D. Morrison. 2018. Transgender health care: Improving medical students' and residents' training and awareness. *Advances in Medical Education and Practice* 9(9):377–391. https://doi.org/10.2147/amep.s147183.

Dubin, S., T. Cook, A. Liss, G. Doty, K. Moore, R. Greene, A. Radix, and A. Janssen. 2022. Comparing electronic health record domains' utility to identify transgender patients. *Transgender Health* 7(1):78–84. https://doi.org/10.1089/trgh.2020.0069.

Dunne, M. J., L. A. Raynor, E. K. Cottrell, and W. J. A. Pinnock. 2017. Interviews with patients and providers on transgender and gender nonconforming health data collection in the electronic health record. *Transgender Health* 2(1):1–7. https://doi.org/10.1089/trgh.2016.0041.

Eckenrode, H. E., O. M. Gutierrez, G. Osis, A. Agarwal, and L. M. Curtis. 2022. Kidney disease prevalence in transgender individuals. *Clinical Journal of the American Society of Nephrology* 17(2):280–282. https://doi.org/10.2215/cjn.04660421.

Ehrenfeld, J. M., K. G. Gottlieb, L. B. Beach, S. E. Monahan, and D. Fabbri. 2019. Development of a natural language processing algorithm to identify and evaluate transgender patients in electronic health record systems. *Ethnicity & Disease* 29(Suppl 2):441–450. https://doi.org/10.18865/ed.29.S2.441.

Feinstein, J., P. Gill, and B. Anderson. 2023. Preparing for International Classification of Diseases, 11th Revision (ICD-11) in the U.S. health care system. *JAMA Health Forum* 4(7):E232253. https://doi.org/10.1001/jamahealthforum.2023.2253.

Feldman, J. L., W. E. Luhur, J. L. Herman, T. Poteat, and I. H. Meyer. 2021. Health and health care access in the U.S. transgender population health (TransPop) survey. *Andrology* 9(6):1707–1718. https://doi.org/10.1111/andr.13052.

Fletcher, O. V., J. A. Chen, J. van Draanen, M. C. Frost, A. D. Rubinsky, J. R. Blosnich, and E. C. Williams. 2022. Prevalence of social and economic stressors among transgender veterans with alcohol and other drug use disorders. *SSM-Population Health* 19:101153. https://doi.org/10.1016/j.ssmph.2022.101153.

Foer, D., D. M. Rubins, A. Almazan, K. Chan, D. W. Bates, and O. R. Hamnvik. 2020. Challenges with accuracy of gender fields in identifying transgender patients in electronic health records. *Journal of General Internal Medicine* 35(12):3724–3725. https://doi.org/10.1007/s11606-019-05567-6.

Ford, J. V., and E. Coleman. 2023. Gender diversity, gender liminality in French Polynesia. *International Journal of Transgender Health* 1–17. https://doi.org/10.1080/26895269.2023.2291128.

GAO (U.S. Government Accountability Office). 2020. VA health care: Better data needed to assess the health outcomes of lesbian, gay, bisexual, and transgender veterans. GAO-21-69. https://www.gao.gov/assets/gao-21-69.pdf (accessed March 14, 2024).

Giordano, S. 2023. Gender incongruence as a condition related to sexual health. In *Children and gender: Ethical issues in clinical management of transgender and gender diverse youth, from early years to late adolescence.* Oxford University Press eBooks. Pp. 55–C54P37. https://doi.org/10.1093/oso/9780192895400.003.0004.

Glick, J. L., A. Lopez, M. Pollock, and K. P. Theall. 2020. Housing insecurity and intersecting social determinants of health among transgender people in the USA: A targeted ethnography. *International Journal of Transgender Health* 21(3):337–349. https://doi.org/10.1080%2F26895269.2020.1780661.

Goldberg, J. E., L. Moy, and A. B. Rosenkrantz. 2018. Assessing transgender patient care and gender inclusivity of breast imaging facilities across the United States. *Journal of the American College of Radiology* 15(8):1164–1172. https://doi.org/10.1016/j.jacr.2018.05.007.

Goldhammer, H., C. Grasso, S. L. Katz-Wise, K. Thomson, A. R. Gordon, and A. S. Keuroghlian. 2022. Pediatric sexual orientation and gender identity data collection in the electronic health record. *Journal of the American Medical Informatics Association* 29(7): 1303–1309. https://doi.org/10.1093/jamia/ocac048.

Goldhammer, H., E.D. Maston, L.A. Kissock, J.A. Davis, and A.S. Keuroghlian. 2018. National findings from an LGBT healthcare organizational needs assessment. *LGBT Health.* 5(8):461–468. doi: 10.1089/lgbt.2018.0118.

Gonzales, G., and C. Henning-Smith. 2017. Barriers to care among transgender and gender nonconforming adults. *Milbank Quarterly* 95(4):726–748. https://doi.org/10.1111/1468-0009.12297.

Grant, J. M., L. A. Mottet, J. Tanis, J. Harrison, J. L. Herman, and M. Keisling. 2011. *Injustice at every turn: A report of the National Transgender Discrimination Survey.* Washington, DC: National Center for Transgender Equality and National Gay and Lesbian Task Force.

Grasso, C., H. Goldhammer, D. Funk, D. King, S. L. Reisner, K. H. Mayer, and A. S. Keuroghlian. 2019. Required sexual orientation and gender identity reporting by U.S. health centers: First-year data. *American Journal of Public Health* 109(8):1111–1118. https://doi.org/10.2105/AJPH.2019.305130.

Grasso, C., H. Goldhammer, J. Thompson, and A. S. Keuroghlian. 2021. Optimizing gender-affirming medical care through anatomical inventories, clinical decision support, and population health management in electronic health record systems. *Journal of the American Medical Informatics Association* 28(11):2531–2535. https://doi.org/10.1093/jamia/ocab080.

Haghighat, D., T. Berro, L. Torrey Sosa, K. Horowitz, B. Brown-King, and K. Zayhowski. 2023. Intersex people's perspectives on affirming healthcare practices: A qualitative study. *Social Science & Medicine* 329:116047. https://doi.org/10.1016/j.socscimed.2023.116047.

Haider, A. H., E. B. Schneider, L. M. Kodadek, R. R. Adler, A. Ranjit, M. Torain, R. Y. Shields, C. Snyder, J. D. Schuur, L. Vail, D. German, S. Peterson, and B. D. Lau. 2017. Emergency department query for patient-centered approaches to sexual orientation and gender identity: The equality study. *JAMA Internal Medicine* 177(6):819–828. https://doi.org/10.1001/jamainternmed.2017.0906

Handerer, F., P. Kinderman, and S. Tai. 2021. The need for improved coding to document the social determinants of health. *Lancet Psychiatry* 8(8):653. https://doi.org/10.1016/s2215-0366(21)00208-x

Hatef, E., H. Kharrazi, K. Nelson, P. Sylling, X. Ma, E. C. Lasser, K. M. Searle, Z. Predmore, A. J. Batten, I. Curtis, S. Fihn, and J. P. Weiner. 2019. The association between neighborhood socioeconomic and housing characteristics with hospitalization: Results of a national study of veterans. *Journal of the American Board of Family Medicine* 32(6):890–903. https://doi.org/10.3122/jabfm.2019.06.190138.

Hatzenbuehler, M. L. 2014. Structural stigma and the health of lesbian, gay, and bisexual populations. *Current Directions in Psychological Science* 23(2):127–132. https://doi.org/10.1177/0963721414523775.

Haymer, M. 2014. *Transgender patients: Prejudice and training needs among trainees in 6 U.S. emergency medicine residency programs.* Presentation at the 142nd American Public Health Association Annual Meeting and Exposition, New Orleans, LA.

Henderson, E. R., J. T. Goldbach, and J. R. Blosnich. 2022. Social determinants of sexual and gender minority mental health. *Current Treatment Options in Psychiatry* 9(3):229–245. http://dx.doi.org/10.1007/s40501-022-00269-z.

HHS (U.S. Department of Health and Human Services). 2015. 2015 edition health information technology (health IT) certification criteria, 2015 edition base electronic health record (EHR) definition, and ONC health IT certification program modifications. *Federal Register* 80(200):62602–62759. https://www.govinfo.gov/content/pkg/FR-2015-10-16/pdf/2015-25597.pdf (accessed March 14, 2024).

Hines, M., S. F. Ahmed, and I. A. Hughes. 2003. Psychological outcomes and gender-related development in complete androgen insensitivity syndrome. *Archives of Sexual Behavior* 32(2):93–101. https://doi.org/10.1023/a:1022492106974.

Hines, N. G., D. N. Greene, K. L. Imborek, and M. D. Krasowski. 2023. Patterns of gender identity data within electronic health record databases can be used as a tool for identifying and estimating the prevalence of gender-expansive people. *JAMIA Open* 6(2):OOAD42. https://doi.org/10.1093/jamiaopen/ooad042.

Hua, Y., L. Wang, V. Nguyen, M. Rieu-Werden, A. McDowell, D. W. Bates, D. Foer, and L. Zhou. 2023. A deep learning approach for transgender and gender diverse patient identification in electronic health records. *Journal of Biomedical Informatics* 147:104507. https://doi.org/10.1016/j.jbi.2023.104507.

Huang, S. D., V. Bamba, S. Bothwell, P. Y. Fechner, A. Furniss, C. Ikomi, L. Nahata, N. J. Nokoff, L. Pyle, H. Seyoum, and S. M. Davis. 2023. Development and validation of a computable phenotype for Turner syndrome utilizing electronic health records from a national pediatric network. *American Journal of Medical Genetics Part A* 194(4):E63496. https://doi.org/10.1002/ajmg.a.63495.

Hughes, L. D., K. M. Kidd, K. E. Gamarel, D. Operario, and N. Dowshen. 2021. "These laws will be devastating": Provider perspectives on legislation banning gender-affirming care for transgender adolescents. *Journal of Adolescent Health* 69(6):976–982. https://doi.org/10.1016/j.jadohealth.2021.08.020.

IHS (Indian Health Service). 2023. Data capture of sexual orientation and gender identity information. *Indian Health Service Circular* (23-02). Rockville, MD: Department of Health and Human Services. https://www.ihs.gov/ihm/circulars/2023/data-capture-of-sexual-orientation-and-gender-identity-information/ (accessed March 13, 2024).

Islam, N., R. Nash, Q. Zhang, L. Panagiotakopoulos, T. Daley, S. Bhasin, D. Getahun, J. Sonya Haw, C. McCracken, M. J. Silverberg, V. Tangpricha, S. Vupputuri, and M. Goodman. 2022. Is there a link between hormone use and diabetes incidence in transgender people? Data from the STRONG cohort. *Journal of Clinical Endocrinology & Metabolism* 107(4):E1549–E1557. https://doi.org/10.1210/clinem/dgab832.

Jackson, N. C., M. J. Johnson, and R. Roberts. 2008. The potential impact of discrimination fears of older gays, lesbians, bisexuals and transgender individuals living in small- to moderate-sized cities on long-term health care. *Journal of Homosexuality* 54(3):325–339. https://doi.org/10.1080/00918360801982298.

Jacobs, Z. G. 2021. Codifying social determinants of health: A gap in the ICD-10-CM. *Journal of General Internal Medicine* 36(10):3205–3207. https://doi.org/10.1007/s11606-021-06742-4.

Jaffee, K. D., D. A. Shires, and D. Stroumsa. 2016. Discrimination and delayed health care among transgender women and men: Implications for improving medical education and health care delivery. *Medical Care* 54(11):1010–1016. https://doi.org/10.1097/mlr.0000000000000583.

James, S. E., J. L. Herman, S. Rankin, M. Keisling, L. Mottet, and M. Anafi. 2016. *The report of the 2015 U.S. Transgender survey*. Washington, DC: National Center for Transgender Equality. https://transequality.org/sites/default/files/docs/usts/USTS-Full-Report-Dec17.pdf (accessed March 14, 2024).

Jasuja, G. K., A. de Groot, E. K. Quinn, O. Ameli, J. M. W. Hughto, M. Dunbar, M. Deutsch, C. G. Streed, M. K. Paasche-Orlow, H. L. Wolfe, and A. J. Rose. 2020. Beyond gender identity disorder diagnoses codes an examination of additional methods to identify transgender individuals in administrative databases. *Medical Care* 58(10):903–911. https://doi.org/10.1097/mlr.0000000000001362.

Jelinek, S., F. Toor, K. Becker, K. Smith, B. Schindel, N. Puoplo, C. Hebert, B. Winik, N. Mann, L. Ambler, C. Birbiglia, A. Stengel, L. N. Hodo, C. Tenore, and C. Katz. 2020. Building inclusive healthcare for LGBTQ+ youth: Improving the collection and utilization of patients' sexual orientation and gender identity (SOGI) information, preferred names and gender pronouns in a pediatric clinic. *Journal of Scientific Innovation in Medicine* 3(3). https://doi.org/10.29024/jsim.76.

Johnson, E., I. Rosoklija, and C. Finlayson. 2017. Attitudes towards "disorders of sex development" nomenclature among affected individuals. *Journal of Pediatric Urology* 13(6):608. E601–E608. https://doi.org/10.1016/j.jpurol.2017.03.035.

The Joint Commission. 2011. *Advancing effective communication, cultural competence, and patient- and family-centered care for the lesbian, gay, bisexual, and transgender (LGBT) community: A field guide*. Oak Brook, IL: The Joint Commission. https://www.jointcommission.org/-/media/tjc/documents/resources/patient-safety-topics/health-equity/lgbtfield-guide_web_linked_verpdf.pdf?db=web&hash=FD725DC02CFE6E4F21A35EBD839BBE97&hash=FD725DC02CFE6E4F21A35EBD839BBE97 (accessed March 14, 2024).

Kattari, S. K., N. E. Walls, D. L. Whitfield, and L. Langenderfer-Magruder. 2015. Racial and ethnic differences in experiences of discrimination in accessing health services among transgender people in the United States. *International Journal of Transgenderism* 16(2):68–79. https://doi.org/10.1080/15532739.2015.1064336.

Kattari, S. K., N. E. Walls, and S. R. Speer. 2017. Differences in experiences of discrimination in accessing social services among transgender/gender nonconforming individuals by (dis)ability. *Journal of Social Work in Disability & Rehabilitation* 16(2):116–140. https://doi.org/10.1080/1536710x.2017.1299661.

Kattari, S. K., M. Bakko, H. K. Hecht, and M. K. Kinney. 2020. Intersecting experiences of healthcare denials among transgender and nonbinary patients. *American Journal of Preventive Medicine* 58(4):506–513. https://doi.org/10.1016/j.amepre.2019.11.014.

Kidd, J. D., K. B. Jackman, M. Wolff, C. B. Veldhuis, and T. L. Hughes. 2018. Risk and protective factors for substance use among sexual and gender minority youth: A scoping review. *Current Addiction Reports* 5(2):158–173. https://doi.org/10.1007/s40429-018-0196-9.

Kodadek, L. M., S. Peterson, R. Y. Shields, D. German, A. Ranjit, C. Snyder, E. Schneider, B. D. Lau, and A. H. Haider. 2019. Collecting sexual orientation and gender identity information in the emergency department: The divide between patient and provider perspectives. *Emergency Medicine Journal* 36(3):136–141. https://doi.org/10.1136/emermed-2018-207669.

Kopel, J., N. Beck, M. H. Almekdash, and S. Varma. 2023. Trends in transgender healthcare curricula in graduate medical education. *Proceedings (Baylor University Medical Center)* 36(5):620–626. https://doi.org/10.1080/08998280.2023.2228140.

Kostelanetz, S., M. Pettapiece-Phillips, J. Weems, T. Spalding, C. Roumie, C. H. Wilkins, and S. Kripalani. 2022. Health care professionals' perspectives on universal screening of social determinants of health: A mixed-methods study. *Population Health Management* 25(3):367–374. https://doi.org/10.1089/pop.2021.0176.

Kronk, C. A., A. R. Everhart, F. Ashley, H. M. Thompson, T. E. Schall, T. G. Goetz, L. Hiatt, Z. Derrick, R. Queen, A. Ram, E. M. Guthman, O. M. Danforth, E. Lett, E. Potter, S. E. D. Sun, Z. Marshall, and R. Karnoski. 2022. Transgender data collection in the electronic health record: Current concepts and issues. *Journal of the American Medical Informatics Association* 29(2):271–284. https://doi.org/10.1093/jamia/ocab136.

Kuhns, L. M., J. Hereth, R. Garofalo, M. Hidalgo, A. K. Johnson, R. Schnall, S. L. Reisner, M. Belzer, and M. J. Mimiaga. 2021. A uniquely targeted, mobile app-based HIV prevention intervention for young transgender women: Adaptation and usability study. *Journal of Medical Internet Research* 23(3):e21839. https://doi.org/0.2196/21839.

Lelutiu-Weinberger, C., P. Pollard-Thomas, W. Pagano, N. Levitt, E. I. Lopez, S. A. Golub, and A. E. Radix. 2016. Implementation and evaluation of a pilot training to improve transgender competency among medical staff in an urban clinic. *Transgender Health* 1(1):45–53. https://doi.org/10.1089/trgh.2015.0009.

Lieurance, D., S. Kuebbing, M. A. McCary, and M. A. Nuñez. 2021. Words matter: How to increase gender and LGBTQIA + inclusivity at *Biological Invasions*. *Biological Invasions* 24:341–344. https://doi.org/10.1007/s10530-021-02665-7.

Lim, F., M. J. Johnson, and M. J. Eliason. 2015. A national survey of faculty knowledge, experience, and readiness for teaching lesbian, gay, bisexual, and transgender health in baccalaureate nursing programs. *Nursing Education Perspectives* 36:144–152. https://doi.org/10.5480/14-1355

Liu, M., D. King, K. H. Mayer, C. Grasso, and A. S. Keuroghlian. 2023. Sexual orientation and gender identity data completeness at U.S. Federally Qualified Health Centers, 2020 and 2021. *American Journal of Public Health* 113(8):883–892. https://doi.org/10.2105/AJPH.2023.307323.

MacDougall, H., C. Henning-Smith, G. Gonzales, and A. Ott. 2023. Access to health care for transgender and gender-diverse adults in urban and rural areas in the United States. *Medical Care Research and Review* 81(1):68–77. https://doi.org/10.1177/10775587231191649.

Maksut, J. L., C. Hodge, C. D. Van, A. Razmi, and M. T. Khau. 2021. Utilization of Z codes for social determinants of health among Medicare fee-for-service beneficiaries, 2019. *Data Highlight* 24. Baltimore, MD: Centers for Medicare and Medicaid Services, Office of Minority Health.

Maragh-Bass, A. C., M. Torain, R. Adler, E. Schneider, A. Ranjit, L. M. Kodadek, R. Shields, D. German, C. Snyder, S. Peterson, J. Schuur, B. Lau, and A. H. Haider. 2017a. Risks, benefits, and importance of collecting sexual orientation and gender identity data in healthcare settings: A multi-method analysis of patient and provider perspectives. *LGBT Health* 4(2):141–152. https://doi.org/10.1089/lgbt.2016.0107.

Maragh-Bass, A. C., M. Torain, R. Adler, A. Ranjit, E. Schneider, R. Y. Shields, L. M. Kodadek, C. F. Snyder, D. German, S. Peterson, J. Schuur, B. D. Lau, and A. H. Haider. 2017b. Is it okay to ask: Transgender patient perspectives on sexual orientation and gender identity collection in healthcare. *Academic Emergency Medicine* 24(6):655–667. https://doi.org/10.1111/acem.13182.

Marcus, R., L. Trujillo, E. Olansky, S. Cha, R. B. Hershow, A. R. Baugher, C. Sionean, and K. Lee. 2024. Transgender women experiencing homelessness—national HIV behavioral surveillance among transgender women, seven urban areas, United States, 2019–2020. In collaboration with the National HIV Behavioral Surveillance Among Transgender Women Study Group. *Morbidity and Mortality Weekly Report* 73(1):40–50. https://doi.org/10.15585/mmwr.su7301a5.

Matza, L., and L. McConnell, A. 2023. *Veterans Health Administration: LGBTQ+ health program.* Presentation to the National Academies of Science, Engineering & Medicine, Washington, DC.

May, J. T., J. Myers, D. Noonan, E. McConnell, and M. P. Cary. 2023. A call to action to improve the completeness of older adult sexual and gender minority data in electronic health records. *Journal of the American Medical Informatics Association* 30(10):1725–1729. https://doi.org/10.1093/jamia/ocad130.

McClure, R. C., C. L. Macumber, C. Kronk, C. Grasso, R. J. Horn, R. Queen, S. Posnack, and K. Davison. 2022. Gender harmony: Improved standards to support affirmative care of gender-marginalized people through inclusive gender and sex representation. *Journal of the American Medical Informatics* 29(2):354–363. https://doi.org/10.1093/jamia/ocab196.

McDowell, A., C. Myong, D. Tevis, and V. Fung. 2022. Sexual orientation and gender identity data reporting among U.S. Health centers. *American Journal of Preventive Medicine* 62(6):e325–e332. https://doi.org/10.1016/j.amepre.2021.12.017.

McPhail, D., M. Rountree-James, and I. Whetter. 2016. Addressing gaps in physician knowledge regarding transgender health and healthcare through medical education. *Canadian Medical Education Journal* 7(2):E70–E78.

Medina, C., and L. Mahowald. 2021. *Key issues facing people with intersex traits.* Developed by the Center for American Progress. https://www.americanprogress.org/article/key-issues-facing-people-intersex-traits/ (accessed March 13, 2024).

Miller, G. H., G. Marquez-Velarde, A. R. Mills, S. M. Hernandez, L. E. Brown, M. Mustafa, and J. E. Shircliff. 2023. Patients' perceived level of clinician knowledge of transgender health care, self-rated health, and psychological distress among transgender adults. *JAMA Network Open* 6(5):E2315083. https://doi.org/10.1001%2Fjamanetworkopen.2023.15083.

Morris, M., R. L. Cooper, A. Ramesh, M. Tabatabai, T. A. Arcury, M. Shinn, W. Im, P. Juarez, and P. Matthews-Juarez. 2019. Training to reduce LGBTQ-related bias among medical, nursing, and dental students and providers: A systematic review. *BMC Medical Education* 19(1):325. https://doi.org/10.1186%2Fs12909-019-1727-3.

Mullins, M. A., P. A. Matthews, J. J. Plascak, T. A. Hastert, L. K. Ko, M. S. Gray, and Y. Molina. 2020. Why aren't sexual orientation and gender identity being measured and what role do cancer researchers play? *Cancer Epidemiology, Biomarkers & Prevention* 29(9):1837–1839. https://doi.org/10.1158/1055-9965.epi-20-0540.

NASEM (National Academies of Sciences, Engineering, and Medicine). 2019. *Integrating social care into the delivery of health care: Moving upstream to improve the nation's health.* Washington, DC: The National Academies Press.

NASEM. 2020. *Understanding the well-being of LGBTQI+ populations.* Edited by C. J. Patterson, M.-J. Sepúlveda, and J. White. Washington, DC: The National Academies Press.

NASEM. 2022. *Measuring sex, gender identity, and sexual orientation.* Edited by N. Bates, M. Chin, and T. Becker. Washington, DC: The National Academies Press.

National LGBTQIA+ Health Education Center. 2022. *Ready, set, go! Guidelines and tips for collecting patient data on sexual orientation and gender identity (SOGI) – 2022 update.* Developed by the U.S. Health Resources and Services Administration (HRSA). https://www.lgbtqiahealtheducation.org/publication/ready-set-go-a-guide-for-collecting-data-on-sexual-orientation-and-gender-identity-2022-update/ (accessed March 14, 2024).

Newsom, K. D., G. Carter, and J. J. Hille. 2022. Assessing whether medical students consistently ask patients about sexual orientation and gender identity as a function of year in training. *LGBT Health* 9(2):142–147. https://doi.org/10.1089/lgbt.2021.0109.

Nowotny, H. F., and N. Reisch. 2023. Challenges waiting for an adult with DSD. *Hormone Research in Paediatrics* 96(2):207–221. https://doi.org/10.1159/000527433.

NSTC (National Science and Technology Council). 2023. *Federal evidence agenda on LGBTQI+ equity*. https://www.whitehouse.gov/wp-content/uploads/2023/01/Federal-Evidence-Agenda-on-LGBTQI-Equity.pdf (accessed May 3, 2024).

OASH (Office of the Assistant Secretary for Health). n.d. *Healthy people 2030: LGBT*. Developed by the Department of Health and Human Services (HHS). https://health.gov/healthypeople/objectives-and-data/browse-objectives/lgbt (accessed February 21, 2024).

Obedin-Maliver, J., E. S. Goldsmith, L. Stewart, W. White, E. Tran, S. Brenman, M. Wells, D. M. Fetterman, G. Garcia, and M. R. Lunn. 2011. Lesbian, gay, bisexual, and transgender-related content in undergraduate medical education. *JAMA* 306(9):971–977. https://doi.org/10.1001/jama.2011.1255.

OEI (Office of Equity and Inclusion). 2023. *OHA SOGI draft data collection recommendations*. Developed by the Oregon Health Authority. https://www.oregon.gov/oha/EI/REALD%20Documents/DRAFT-SOGI-Recommendations.pdf (accessed March 14, 2024).

Office of the National Coordinator for Health Information Technology. 2023. *2023 interoperability standards advisory*. Developed by the Department of Health and Human Services. https://www.healthit.gov/sites/isa/files/inline-files/2023%20Reference%20Edition_ISA_508.pdf (accessed February 29, 2024).

Poteat, T., and A. Simmons. 2022. Intersectional structural stigma, community priorities, and opportunities for transgender health equity: Findings from TRANSforming the Carolinas. *Journal of Law, Medicine & Ethics* 50(3):443–455. https://doi.org/10.1017/jme.2022.86.

Poteat, T., D. German, and D. Kerrigan. 2013. Managing uncertainty: A grounded theory of stigma in transgender health care encounters. *Social Science & Medicine* 84:22–29. https://doi.org/10.1016/j.socscimed.2013.02.019.

Pratt-Chapman, M. L., K. Eckstrand, A. Robinson, L. B. Beach, C. Kamen, A. S. Keuroghlian, S. Cook, A. Radix, M. P. Bidell, D. Bruner, and L. Margolies. 2022. Developing standards for cultural competency training for health care providers to care for lesbian, gay, bisexual, transgender, queer, intersex, and asexual persons: Consensus recommendations from a national panel. *LGBT Health* 9(5):340–347. https://doi.org/10.1089/lgbt.2021.0464.

Price, M. A., N. L. Hollinsaid, S. McKetta, E. J. Mellen, and M. Rakhilin. 2024. Structural transphobia is associated with psychological distress and suicidality in a large national sample of transgender adults. *Social Psychiatry & Psychiatric Epidemiology* 59(2):285–294. https://doi.org/10.1007/s00127-023-02482-4.

Puckett, J. A., N. C. Brown, T. Dunn, B. Mustanski, and M. E. Newcomb. 2020. Perspectives from transgender and gender diverse people on how to ask about gender. *LGBT Health* 7(6):305–311. https://doi.org/10.1089/lgbt.2019.0295.

Quinn, V. P., R. Nash, E. Hunkeler, R. Contreras, L. Cromwell, T. A. Becerra-Culqui, D. Getahun, S. Giammattei, T. L. Lash, A. Millman, B. Robinson, D. Roblin, M. J. Silverberg, J. Slovis, V. Tangpricha, D. Tolsma, C. Valentine, K. Ward, S. Winter, and M. Goodman. 2017. Cohort profile: Study of transition, outcomes and gender (STRONG) to assess health status of transgender people. *BMJ Open* 7(12):E018121. https://doi.org/10.1136/bmjopen-2017-018121.

Reisner, S. L., T. Poteat, J. Keatley, M. Cabral, T. Mothopeng, E. Dunham, C. E. Holland, R. Max, and S. D. Baral. 2016. Global health burden and needs of transgender populations: A review. *Lancet* 388(10042):412–436. https://doi.org/10.1016/s0140-6736(16)00684-x.

Robles, R., J. Keeley, H. Vega-Ramírez, J. Cruz-Islas, V. Rodríguez-Pérez, P. Sharan, S. Purnima, R. Rao, M. I. Rodrigues-Lobato, B. Soll, F. Askevis-Leherpeux, J. L. Roelandt, M. Campbell, G. Grobler, D. J. Stein, B. Khoury, J. E. Khoury, A. Fresán, M. E. Medina-Mora, and G. M. Reed. 2022. Validity of categories related to gender identity in ICD-11 and DSM-5 among transgender individuals who seek gender-affirming medical procedures. *International Journal of Clinical and Health Psychology* 22(1):100281. https://doi.org/10.1016/j.ijchp.2021.100281.

Rodriguez-Hart, C., G. Zhao, Z. Goldstein, A. Radix, and L. Torian. 2023. An exploratory study to describe transgender people with HIV who accessed Medicaid and their viral suppression over time in New York City, 2013–2017. *Transgender Health* 8(5):429–436. https://doi.org/10.1089/trgh.2021.0195.

Romanelli, M., and M. A. Lindsey. 2020. Patterns of healthcare discrimination among transgender help-seekers. *American Journal of Preventive Medicine* 58(4):E123–E131. https://doi.org/10.1016/j.amepre.2019.11.002.

Romanelli, M., W. Lu, and M. A. Lindsey. 2018. Examining mechanisms and moderators of the relationship between discriminatory health care encounters and attempted suicide among U.S. transgender help-seekers. *Administration and Policy in Mental Health* 45(6):831–849. https://doi.org/10.1007/s10488-018-0868-8.

Ruben, M. A., J. R. Blosnich, M. E. Dichter, L. Luscri, and J. C. Shipherd. 2017. Will veterans answer sexual orientation and gender identity questions? *Medical Care* 55(Suppl 9 Suppl 2): S85–S89. https://doi.org/10.1097/mlr.0000000000000744.

Rullo, J. E., J. L. Foxen, J. M. Griffin, J. R. Geske, C. A. Gonzalez, S. S. Faubion, and M. van Ryn. 2018. Patient acceptance of sexual orientation and gender identity questions on intake forms in outpatient clinics: A pragmatic randomized multisite trial. *Health Services Research* 53(5):3790–3808. https://doi.org/10.1111/1475-6773.12843.

Ruprecht, K., W. Dunlop, E. Wah, C. Phillips, and S. Martin. 2023. 'A human face and voice': Transgender patient-educator and medical student perspectives on gender-diversity teaching. *BMC Medical Education* 23(1):621. https://doi.org/10.1186/s12909-023-04591-9.

Safer, J. D., E. Coleman, J. Feldman, R. Garofalo, W. Hembree, A. Radix, and J. Sevelius. 2016. Barriers to healthcare for transgender individuals. *Current Opinion in Endocrinology, Diabetes, and Obesity* 23(2):168–171. https://doi.org/10.1097/med.0000000000000227.

Scheer, J. R., and V. P. Poteat. 2021. Trauma-informed care and health among LGBTQ intimate partner violence survivors. *Journal of Interpersonal Violence* 36(13-14):6670–6692. https://doi.org/10.1177/0886260518820688.

Scheim, A. I., K. E. Baker, A. J. Restar, and R. L. Sell. 2022. Health and health care among transgender adults in the United States annual review of public health. *Annual Review of Public Health* 43:503–523. https://doi.org/10.1146/annurev-publhealth-052620-100313.

Schilt, K., and J. Bratter. 2015. From multiracial to transgender? Assessing attitudes toward expanding gender options on the U.S. census. *Transgender Studies Quarterly* 2(1):77–100. https://doi.org/10.1215/23289252-2848895.

Seelman, K. L., M. J. P. Colón-Diaz, R. H. LeCroix, M. Xavier-Brier, L. Kattari. 2017. Transgender noninclusive healthcare and delaying care because of fear: Connections to general health and mental health among transgender adults. *Transgender Health* 2(1):17–28. https://doi.org/10.1089/trgh.2016.0024.

Sequeira, G. M., K. Kidd, R. W. S. Coulter, E. Miller, R. Garofalo, and K. N. Ray. 2020. Affirming transgender youths' names and pronouns in the electronic medical record. *JAMA Pediatrics* 174(5):501–503. https://doi.org/10.1001/jamapediatrics.2019.6071.

Sherman, A. D. F., A. McDowell, K. D. Clark, M. Balthazar, M. Klepper, and K. Bower. 2021. Transgender and gender diverse health education for future nurses: Students' knowledge and attitudes. *Nurse Education Today* 97:104690. https://doi.org/10.1016/j.nedt.2020.104690.

SSA (Social Security Administration). n.d. *Gender identity: How do I change the sex identification on my Social Security record?* https://www.ssa.gov/people/lgbtq/gender-identity.html#:~:text=How%20do%20I%20change%20the,sometimes%20citizenship%20or%20immigration%20status (accessed May 17, 2024).

Stonington, S. D., S. M. Holmes, H. Hansen, J. A. Greene, K. A. Wailoo, D. Malina, S. Morrissey, P. E. Farmer, and M. G. Marmot. 2018. Case studies in social medicine—attending to structural forces in clinical practice. *The New England Journal of Medicine* 379(20):1958–1961. https://doi.org/10.1056/nejmms1814262.

Streed, C. G., E. P. McCarthy, and J. S. Haas. 2017. Association between gender minority status and self-reported physical and mental health in the United States. *JAMA Internal Medicine* 177(8):1210–1212. https://doi.org/10.1001/jamainternmed.2017.1460.

Streed, C. G., C. Grasso, S. L. Reisner, and K. H. Mayer. 2020. Sexual orientation and gender identity data collection: Clinical and public health importance. *American Journal of Public Health* 110(7):991–993. https://doi.org/10.2105%2FAJPH.2020.305722.

Streed, C. G., D. King, C. Grasso, S. L. Reisner, K. H. Mayer, G. K. Jasuja, T. Poteat, M. Mukherjee, A. Shapira-Daniels, H. Cabral, V. Tangpricha, M. K. Paasche-Orlow, and E. J. Benjamin. 2023. Validation of an administrative algorithm for transgender and gender diverse persons against self-report data in electronic health records. *Journal of the American Medical Informatics Association* 30(6):1047–1055. https://doi.org/10.1093/jamia/ocad039.

Strong, K. L., and V. N. Folse. 2015. Assessing undergraduate nursing students' knowledge, attitudes, and cultural competence in caring for lesbian, gay, bisexual, and transgender patients. *The Journal of Nursing Education* 54(1):45–49. https://doi.org/10.3928/01484834-20141224-07.

Tate, C. C., J. N. Ledbetter, and C. P. Youssef. 2013. A two-question method for assessing gender categories in the social and medical sciences. *Journal of Sex Research* 50(8):767–776. https://doi.org/10.1080/00224499.2012.690110.

Thompson, H. M. 2021. Stakeholder experiences with gender identity data capture in electronic health records: Implementation effectiveness and a visibility paradox. *Health Education & Behavior* 48(1):93–101. https://doi.org/10.1177/1090198120963102.

Thompson, H. M., C. A. Kronk, K. Feasley, P. Pachwicewicz, and N. S. Karnik. 2021. Implementation of gender identity and assigned sex at birth data collection in electronic health records: Where are we now? *International Journal of Environmental Research and Public Health* 18(12):6599. https://doi.org/10.3390/ijerph18126599.

Truong, H. P., A. A. Luke, G. Hammond, R. K. Wadhera, M. Reidhead, and K. E. Joynt Maddox. 2020. Utilization of social determinants of health ICD-10 Z-codes among hospitalized patients in the United States, 2016-2017. *Medical Care* 58(12):1037–1043. https://doi.org/10.1097/mlr.0000000000001418.

Vance, S. R., Jr., and V. V. Mesheriakova. 2017. Documentation of gender identity in an adolescent and young adult clinic. *Journal of Adolescent Health* 60(3):350–352. https://doi.org/10.1016/j.jadohealth.2016.10.018.

Velasco, R. A. F., K. Slusser, and H. Coats. 2022. Stigma and healthcare access among transgender and gender-diverse people: A qualitative meta-synthesis. *Journal of Advanced Nursing* 78(10):3083–3100. https://doi.org/10.1111/jan.15323.

VHA (Veterans Health Administration). 2022. *Provider fact sheet on birth sex and gender identity.* Developed by the Department of Veterans Affairs. https://www.patientcare.va.gov/LGBT/docs/2022/Birth-Sex-Gender-Identity-FactSheet-for-Providers-2022.pdf (accessed March 14, 2024).

Wall, C. S. J., A. J. Patev, and E. G. Benotsch. 2023. Trans broken arm syndrome: A mixed-methods exploration of gender-related medical misattribution and invasive questioning. *Social Science & Medicine* 320:115748. https://doi.org/10.1016/j.socscimed.2023.115748.

Wang, M., M. S. Pantell, L. M. Gottlieb, and J. Adler-Milstein. 2021. Documentation and review of social determinants of health data in the EHR: Measures and associated insights. *Journal of the American Medical Informatics Association* 28(12):2608–2616. https://doi.org/10.1093/jamia/ocab194.

Warnecke, R. B., A. Oh, N. Breen, S. Gehlert, E. Paskett, K. L. Tucker, N. Lurie, T. Rebbeck, J. Goodwin, J. Flack, S. Srinivasan, J. Kerner, S. Heurtin-Roberts, R. Abeles, F. L. Tyson, G. Patmios, and R. A. Hiatt. 2008. Approaching health disparities from a population perspective: The National Institutes of Health Centers for Population Health and Health Disparities. *American Journal of Public Health* 98(9):1608–1615. https://doi.org/10.2105/ajph.2006.102525.

Weir, R. C., M. Proser, M. Jester, V. Li, C. M. Hood-Ronick, and D. Gurewich. 2020. Collecting social determinants of health data in the clinical setting: Findings from national PRAPARE implementation. *Journal of Health Care for the Poor & Underserved* 31(2):1018–1035. https://doi.org/10.1353/hpu.2020.0075.

Wesp, L. M., L. H. Malcoe, A. Elliott, and T. Poteat. 2019. Intersectionality research for transgender health justice: A theory-driven conceptual framework for structural analysis of transgender health inequities. *Transgender Health* 4(1):287–296. https://doi.org/10.1089/trgh.2019.0039.

Wheldon, C. W., M. B. Schabath, J. Hudson, M. Bowman Curci, P. A. Kanetsky, S. T. Vadaparampil, V. N. Simmons, J. A. Sanchez, S. K. Sutton, and G. P. Quinn. 2018. Culturally competent care for sexual and gender minority patients at National Cancer Institute-Designated Comprehensive Cancer Centers. *LGBT Health* 5(3):203–211. https://doi.org/10.1089/lgbt.2017.0217.

White Hughto, J. M., S. L. Reisner, and M. J. Mimiaga. 2015. Characteristics of transgender residents of Massachusetts cities with high HIV prevalence. *American Journal of Public Health* 105(12):E14–18. https://doi.org/10.2105/ajph.2015.302877.

WHO (World Health Organization). n.d.-a. *Gender incongruence and transgender health in the ICD.* https://www.who.int/standards/classifications/frequently-asked-questions/gender-incongruence-and-transgender-health-in-the-icd (accessed March 14, 2024).

WHO n.d.-b. *ICD-11 implementation.* https://www.who.int/standards/classifications/frequently-asked-questions/icd-11-implementation#:~:text=When%20will%20ICD%2D11%20come,be%20reported%20in%20ICD%2D11 (accessed March 14, 2024).

WHO. 2024. *ICD-11 for mortality and morbidity statistics: Gender incongruence.* https://icd.who.int/browse/2024-01/mms/en#344733949 (accessed March 26, 2024).

Wood, C., K. Ringrose, C. Gutierrez, A. Stepanovich, and C. Colson, 2022. *The role of data protection in safeguarding sexual orientation and gender identity information.* Developed by LGBT Tech and The Future of Privacy Forum. https://fpf.org/wp-content/uploads/2022/06/FPF-SOGI-Report-R2-singles-1.pdf (accessed May 16, 2024).

Xie, F., D. Getahun, V. P. Quinn, T. M. Im, R. Contreras, M. J. Silverberg, T. C. Baird, R. Nash, L. Cromwell, D. Roblin, T. Hoffman, and M. Goodman. 2021. An automated algorithm using free-text clinical notes to improve identification of transgender people. *Informatics for Health & Social Care* 46(1):18–28. https://doi.org/10.1080/17538157.2020.1828890.

Yang, X., B. Yelton, S. Chen, J. Zhang, B. A. Olatosi, S. Qiao, X. Li, and D. B. Friedman. 2022. Examining social determinants of health during a pandemic: Clinical application of Z codes before and during COVID-19. *Frontiers in Public Health* 10:888459. https://doi.org/10.3389/fpubh.2022.888459.

Zollweg, S. S., J. A. Belloir, L. A. Drabble, B. Everett, J. Y. Taylor, and T. L. Hughes. 2023. Structural stigma and alcohol use among sexual and gender minority adults: A systematic review. *Drug and Alcohol Dependence Reports* 8:100185. https://doi.org/10.1016/j.dadr.2023.100185.

4

Data on Sex and Gender Identity: Collection Across the U.S. Health Care System

Individuals applying for disability benefits from the Social Security Administration (SSA) access health insurance in different ways and access care from different types of providers. Therefore, it is important to understand how the collection of data on sexual orientation and gender identity (SOGI) that takes place—or does not—within various sectors of the health care system impacts the quality of SOGI data that will be present in medical records received by SSA. SSA can also learn from those parts of the health care system that are beginning to embrace the importance of SOGI data by moving toward policies that encourage payers and providers to document these data, and in some cases, use this information for clinical decision making. The health care system is evolving with respect to SOGI data collection, and it may be useful for SSA to understand current practices and upcoming changes so it can evaluate whether and how it may need to update its own internal data collection policies to fill the gaps when SOGI data collection in other sectors falls short.

Chapter 3 of this report examines the substantial benefits of SOGI data collection, along with the significant biases and structural barriers that prevent robust SOGI data collection in health care settings. A key barrier discussed in Chapter 3 is the fact the United States does not have federal standards or mandates for the collection and reporting of SOGI data. While certain components of the health care system collect SOGI data for the populations they serve, few federal-level policies are in place that require health care providers or health insurers to record information about patient gender identity or sex recorded at birth, both considered key data points for documenting the health care experience of transgender and gender diverse (TGD) people and people with variations in sex traits (VSTs). Currently, application forms for SSA disability programs do not ask applicants about gender identity, sex recorded at birth, or other SOGI data.[1]

This chapter provides an overview of SOGI data collection policies across the health care system, starting with a discussion of recent efforts to increase the collection of these data among public and private health insurers, including Medicaid, Medicare, TRICARE, and private health plans. Next, the chapter examines what SOGI data collection looks like within various federal-level health care delivery systems—including federally qualified health centers (FQHCs), the Veterans Health Administration (VHA), and the Indian Health Service (IHS)—and reviews state-level efforts to encourage and incentivize providers to collect these data. Finally, the chapter describes SOGI data collection within federal surveys and other population-level data collection tools.

SOGI DATA COLLECTION AND HEALTH INSURERS: MEDICAID, MEDICARE, TRICARE, AND PRIVATE HEALTH INSURERS

Increasingly, health insurers are collecting SOGI data from individuals who apply for or enroll in various health insurance programs. In 2022, the Biden administration issued Executive Order 14075, *Advancing Equality for Lesbian, Gay, Bisexual, Transgender, Queer, and Intersex Individuals.*[2] Among other priorities, it calls on federal agencies to "advance the responsible and effective collection and use of data on sexual orientation, gender identity, and sex characteristics."[3] Stemming from this directive, in 2023 the U.S. Department of Health and Human Services (HHS, 2023) developed the SOGI Data Action Plan, a roadmap for federal agencies' development of agency-specific SOGI data collection policies. Among other activities, the plan calls on HHS programs and divisions to add SOGI data elements to existing surveys and forms and, where possible, to remove binary gender and sex data measures and replace them with tested and inclusive gender identity data measures. The plan does not put forward specific SOGI questions and response options, but promotes the two-step question

---

[1] SSA disability application forms contain a free-text "remarks" space for applicants to include additional details about any aspect of their disability application. Applicants could use the remarks section of the application form to provide details about gender identity or sex recorded at birth, but the committee does not know how frequently applicants enter such information.

[2] Executive Office of the President. 2022. Exec. Order No. 14,075, 87 *Federal Register* 37189-37195 (June 15, 2022).

[3] Executive Office of the President. 2022. Exec. Order No. 14,075, 87 *Federal Register* 37194 (June 15, 2022).

methodology (i.e., inclusion of separate questions on gender identity and sex recorded at birth, as described in Chapter 3) and stresses the importance of including items on "sex characteristics."

The Centers for Medicare & Medicaid Services (CMS) has responded to HHS's SOGI Data Action Plan by implementing changes to enrollment forms to allow CMS to collect these data at the point of enrollment in Medicaid and the Children's Health Insurance Program (CHIP); CMS is in the process of examining how to incorporate SOGI data collection into Medicare. This section explores these changes, as well as programs at the federal and state levels designed to incentivize providers who seek Medicaid and Medicare reimbursement to record SOGI data during patient encounters. This section also explores similar efforts under way among private health insurers.

Medicaid

Medicaid is an important source of health insurance coverage for many individuals who apply for and receive disability benefits from SSA. Some applicants for disability benefits may already be covered by Medicaid at the time they apply, while others may gain Medicaid coverage after they qualify for disability benefits, either because they fall into a categorical Medicaid category, as is the case for many Supplemental Security Income (SSI) recipients, or because they meet Medicaid income eligibility criteria as they await Medicare enrollment, as is the case for many Social Security Disability Insurance (SSDI) recipients. (For background information on Medicare and Medicaid coverage for SSI and SSDI recipients, refer to the discussion in Box 4-1.)

Medicaid may be especially important for sexual and gender minorities with disabilities. A 2022 KFF survey of people aged 18–64 examined access to insurance coverage, finding that a greater portion of LGBT+ people receive Medicaid compared with their non-LGBT+ counterparts (21 vs. 16 percent) (Dawson et al., 2023). The survey also found that a higher portion of LGBT+ respondents had a "disability or chronic disease preventing full participation in work, school, housework or other activities" compared with non-LGBT+ respondents (25 vs. 16 percent).[4] Among LGBT+ people, those with Medicaid had much higher rates of disability compared with LGBT+ people with private insurance coverage (45 vs. 15 percent). These significant health concerns do not occur in a vacuum: as described in Chapters 5 and 7, TGD people and people with VSTs experience multilevel stigma and structural factors that may put them at greater risk for disease, with reduced ability to seek the services they need for optimal care and management.

---

[4] The KFF survey's definition of disability was "chronic disease preventing full participation in work, school, housework, or other activities."

How the Medicaid program collects and records SOGI data impacts the quality of the information on which SSA can rely for making appropriate disability determinations for Medicaid-enrolled applicants for whom questions on gender identity and sex recorded at birth are important. This section describes the current state of SOGI data collection among providers that serve people with Medicaid coverage and the delivery systems and organizations that manage their care. The section begins with an analysis of the state- and federal-level Medicaid policies for collecting SOGI data, including a description of the changes to policy at CMS that promote SOGI data collection within the Medicaid system.

Medicaid and SOGI Data Collection: CMS's Model Application

On November 1, 2023, CMS (2023a) issued an informational bulletin putting forward a new model application for enrollment in Medicaid and CHIP. This model application includes, for the first time, optional questions about gender identity, sex recorded at birth and sexual orientation. Accurate and quality SOGI data are critical to advancing health equity within the Medicaid program, and this new data collection policy has the potential to provide CMS and state Medicaid programs with a more accurate depiction of the needs, health outcomes, and disparities experienced by their enrollees based on sex, gender identity, and other related characteristics. CMS recommends that the new SOGI questions be asked of all Medicaid and CHIP applicants aged 12 and older.

CMS's model application uses the two-step question methodology, asking about sex recorded at birth (using the phrase "sex assigned at birth") and gender identity separately. This approach, detailed in Table 4-1, generally follows best practices in the field that call on health insurers and providers to collect SOGI data using this methodology (Chapter 3 of this report discusses the two-step question, along with other best practices for SOGI data collection). The model application does not include a separate question about VSTs, but free-text responses may prompt applicants to disclose this information. In communications about its model approach, CMS (2023b) states the importance of including free-text responses so consumers can enter their own preferred terms or describe characteristics about their identity that are not otherwise captured in response options.

Prior to the introduction of these new SOGI data fields, CMS's model application required applicants to respond to a single binary "sex" question with "male" and "female" responses. The updated model application retains the binary sex question, and this question remains the only *required* question. The new sex recorded at birth and gender identity questions are *optional*, and Medicaid/CHIP applicants may skip these questions during enrollment with no impact on eligibility determination.

TABLE 4-1 Questions on Sex Recorded at Birth and Gender Identity in Federal Health Insurance Programs

Program	Question 1	Q1 Response Options	Question 2	Q2 Response Options	Data Collection Requirements
Medicaid/Children's Health Insurance Program, 2023	**What was [First Name]'s sex assigned at birth?** *You can find this on an original birth certificate or similar document. (optional, single select)*	☐ Female ☐ Male ☐ A sex that's not listed: [free text] ☐ Not sure ☐ Prefer not to answer	**What's [First Name]'s gender identity?** *(optional, single select)*	☐ Female ☐ Male ☐ Transgender female ☐ Transgender male ☐ A gender identity that's not listed: [free text] ☐ Not sure ☐ Prefer not to answer	Optional for states to adopt the model application; Optional for Medicaid applicants to answer questions on sexual orientation and gender identity (SOGI)
Medicare Advantage (MA) & Medicare Part D Plans (proposed, 2025)	**What sex were you assigned at birth?** *(this information may be found on your original birth certificate)*	☐ Male ☐ Female ☐ Other: [free text] ☐ Don't know ☐ I choose not to answer	**What is your current gender?**	☐ Female ☐ Male ☐ Transgender female ☐ Transgender male ☐ I use a different term: [free text] ☐ Don't know ☐ I choose not to answer	Proposed for inclusion on forms in calendar year 2025. Optional for MA and Part D enrollees to answer these questions
Medicare Part A and Part B	**Not Collected**	N/A	**Not Collected**	N/A	Not included in the recent update proposed by the Centers for Medicare & Medicaid Services (CMS)
TRICARE	**Not collected**	N/A	**Not collected**	N/A	Prohibited

NOTES: While many of the federal programs listed above ask questions about sexual orientation, these questions and responses are not listed here. The table presents SOGI data questions in the order they are asked (or proposed to be asked) by CMS—i.e., that a question related to sex recorded at birth is asked first, followed by a question about gender identity. As described in Chapter 3, it is considered best practice to order the questions in the reverse order: ask first about gender identity then about sex recorded at birth (Deutsch et al., 2013).

CMS's model application—and the updated SOGI questions therein—represent an enormous improvement in SOGI data collection within the Medicaid and CHIP programs. CMS (2023a) encourages all states to adopt the model application, but CMS policy does not require them to do so. States may elect to add some SOGI questions but not others, or to use different language/wording or response options. States may also continue to use current applications without change. The only requirement set by CMS is that SOGI data collection must be optional; states may not require Medicaid/CHIP applicants to answer any SOGI questions other than the required binary sex question.

Where states use the model application, it will help create uniformity and ensure that data collection serves to improve consumer experience by allowing people to attest to their gender identity and sex in a way that reflects their lived experience. CMS (2023a) states that it will use the new SOGI questions to "improve demographic data collection to identify disparities in access to care and, ultimately, to support appropriate and equitable health care" (p. 1). CMS is targeting 2025 to begin receiving SOGI data submissions in the Transformed Medicaid Statistical Information System.

Current SOGI Data Collection within Medicaid

Given the recency of CMS's guidance on SOGI data collection, no data are available on how many states will adopt the model SOGI data questions. However, a recent review of SOGI data collection across state Medicaid programs demonstrates the considerable variability in and lack of SOGI data collection overall that this new CMS model application is designed to address.

In August 2023, the State Health Access Data Assistance Center (SHADAC) reviewed paper Medicaid applications for all 50 states and the District of Columbia, along with 44 online Medicaid applications (Zylla and Lukanen, 2024). SHADAC's survey found that the majority of state Medicaid program applications (41 paper and 42 online applications) provided only binary "male" and "female" response options to any questions asked about sex or gender. SHADAC found that while some paper applications allowed for a write-in option (where applicants could indicate something other than male or female under either sex or gender), only a handful of states provided more than "male" and "female" checkboxes as responses on their paper or online applications. In addition, the review found that questions about sex and gender could be confused or conflated on Medicaid applications or omitted altogether. Table 4-2 provides a few examples of SOGI questions uncovered by SHADAC's state Medicaid review, showing the variability in questions and response options.

As shown in Table 4-2, prior to the new model application, Oregon was the only state to use a two-step methodology for asking applicants about sex recorded at birth (using the phrase "sex assigned at birth") and gender

TABLE 4-2 Examples of SOGI Questions from Various State Medicaid Applications (as of August 2023)

State	Question(s) with Response Categories	
Maine	Gender: ☐ Female ☐ Male ☐ Non-binary	
New York	Gender identity (optional) ☐ Female ☐ Male ☐ Non-Binary / Non-Conforming ☐ X ☐ Transgender ☐ Different Identity. Describe your identity (optional): [free text]	
Oregon	For data matching purposes, what was your sex assigned at birth? ☐ Male ☐ Female	Gender Identity: ☐ Male ☐ Female ☐ Trans Male (FTM) ☐ Trans Female (MTF) ☐ Gender Non-Binary / Two Spirit ☐ Not listed ☐ Decline to answer ☐ Other: [free text]
California	What is [person's name]'s Sex? ☐ Female ☐ Male ☐ Transgender: Female to Male ☐ Transgender: Male to Female	

SOURCE: Zylla and Lukanen, 2024.

identity, although Oregon's approach does not currently offer options beyond male and female for the sex recorded at birth question. Washington State is reportedly in the process of exploring options for adding a gender identity question (Washington State Health Care Authority, 2024[5]); the state already asks a mandatory question about each applicant's "sex assigned at birth" (responses: male or female) (Washington State Health Care Authority, 2022a).

---

[5] Washington State Health Care Authority has stated that it intends to align with other state programs and policies that ask a mandatory question about sex assigned at birth and an optional gender identity question. It reportedly uses the mandatory sex assigned at birth field to coordinate benefit coverage (e.g., uterine cancer screenings are covered only for those who were assigned female sex at birth, and prostate exams are covered only for those who were assigned male sex at birth) (Washington State Health Care Authority, 2024).

Medicare

As described in Box 4-1, Medicare is an important source of health insurance coverage for individuals who qualify for SSA disability benefits under the SSDI program. In contrast with Medicaid, individuals seeking benefits under the SSDI program are not likely to be covered through Medicare when they submit a disability application to SSA. However, SSDI recipients are likely to be covered by Medicare by the time of their first continuing disability review (CDR),[6] and having accurate and up-to-date SOGI information during the CDR may be important. After all, SOGI data are not static. In the interim between the initial disability determination and first CDR (or between one CDR and another), SSDI beneficiaries may have undergone some amount of gender-affirming treatment or care, while others may have learned they have a VST, and still others may have had no specific change in their personal understanding of their own sex traits and gender identity but are now ready to disclose such information to health care providers or insurers. Therefore, whether and how the Medicare program and the providers who serve Medicare-enrolled populations collect and record SOGI data may impact the quality of information on which SSA can rely for making appropriate CDR determinations, especially those for which questions around gender identity and sex recorded at birth are important.

CMS currently does not collect any SOGI data to identify and track TGD Medicare beneficiaries or beneficiaries with VSTs. As noted above, however, CMS is in the process of examining how to incorporate SOGI data collection into Medicare. In 2022, CMS (2022b) issued a framework for health equity that included, among other priorities, collecting, reporting, and analyzing data on "gender identity, sex, [and] sexual orientation" (p. 10). Building on these efforts, CMS (2023e) is currently engaged in a rulemaking process to update enrollment forms for individuals enrolling in Medicare Advantage (MA or Part C) plans and Medicare Prescription Drug (Part D) plans. On September 29, 2023, CMS (2023c) released a proposed model enrollment form for MA and Part D plans that includes a sex assigned at birth question and a gender identity question, in addition to questions about sexual orientation, race, and ethnicity. CMS has proposed that these enrollment form changes would go into effect for calendar year 2025. However, the agency is in the process of collecting public comments from interested stakeholders and has not issued a final rule.

---

[6] Any person who receives disability benefits must have their medical conditions reviewed periodically through a process called continuing disability review (CDR). How often the CDR takes place depends on the nature of the disability and whether a condition is likely to improve. A review by SSA (n.d.) typically occurs every 3 years but could take place as soon as 6–18 months after the most recent disability determination (for conditions that are expected to improve), or as long as 7 years later (where medical improvement is not expected).

BOX 4-1
Medicare and Medicaid Coverage for
Supplemental Security Income (SSI) and
Social Security Disability Insurance (SSDI) Recipients

As described in Chapter 1, the Social Security Administration administers benefits for disabled Americans through two programs:

(I) The **Supplemental Security Income (SSI) program** for adults and children (under age 18) who meet disability criteria and qualify based on limited income and assets. Some individuals over age 65 are eligible for SSI without a disability if they have very low income, but the vast majority of SSI beneficiaries (approximately 85 percent) are eligible because of a qualifying disability.

(II) The **Social Security Disability Insurance (SSDI) program** for disabled workers who have worked for a sufficient period of time to qualify for SSDI benefits (in other words, people who are "insured" under the Social Security Act because they have contributed to the Social Security trust fund by paying taxes on their earnings over time). SSDI covers certain disabled dependents as well. Unlike SSI, SSDI has no income or asset limits for eligibility.

A person with both limited income/resources and a work history can qualify for both SSI and SSDI.

Whether they qualify through SSI or SSDI, SSA uses the same medical criteria to determine whether applicants meet disability criteria (described in Chapter 1). However, the programs have different implications for public insurance coverage, with most SSI recipients becoming eligible for Medicaid and most SSDI recipients becoming eligible for Medicare.

Supplemental Security Income (SSI) Program

Medicaid and SSI. Medicaid serves as primary insurer for many SSI recipients, but Medicaid eligibility is not guaranteed. In most states, once individuals qualify for SSI, they automatically qualify for Medicaid without having to file a separate Medicaid application with the state. In these states, SSI recipients are categorically eligible for Medicaid, and Medicaid eligibility starts the same month as SSI eligibility. Other states require a separate Medicaid application,[a] but Medicaid eligibility levels are generally high enough that SSI recipients are eligible for the program. Because beneficiaries typically have no other source of income, more than half of SSI recipients receive the maximum monthly SSI benefit; in 2024 this was $943 per month for an individual (or $11,316 annually),[b] which is well below the income threshold for Medicaid in most states.[c] However, because states are allowed to set their own Medicaid eligibility requirements, several states set Medicaid eligibility below 50 percent of the federal poverty line for certain populations (e.g., low-income parents).[d] In these states, SSI recipients are not guaranteed to qualify for Medicaid.

Continued

Given strict income limits set by SSA, many applicants may already be on Medicaid when they apply for SSI disability benefits. SSI is reserved for low-income populations, and SSA uses a set of criteria to determine what income and other resources "count" for purposes of eligibility in each program. In general, the most a person can earn and still be eligible for SSI disability benefits is $1,550 a month in 2024 ($18,600 per year). This is below the income threshold for Medicaid in most states.[c]

Medicare and SSI. SSI recipients do not automatically qualify for Medicare and will qualify only if they fall into one of the Medicare eligibility categories. Medicare is the federal health insurance program for Americans over age 65, but younger people with certain disabilities— permanent kidney failure, or amyotrophic lateral sclerosis (ALS)—can also qualify for Medicare. SSI recipients with other types of disabilities are generally not eligible for Medicare until they turn 65, unless they separately qualify for SSDI (as detailed below). States may pay Medicare premiums for SSI recipients who qualify for Medicaid (see the section below on dual eligibles).

Social Security Disability Insurance (SSDI) Program

Medicare and SSDI. Individuals who qualify for SSDI benefits automatically become eligible for Medicare Part A (inpatient hospital insurance) after a 24-month waiting period. The waiting period is waived for persons with ALS. Once enrolled in Medicare, SSDI recipients can obtain other Medicare coverage, such as Medicare Part B (which includes doctors' visits, outpatient care, home health care, and certain preventive services) and Medicare Part D (prescription drug coverage) if they select these options and pay a monthly premium. For individuals with limited resources, their state may cover Medicare premiums and other out-of-pocket medical expenses (see the section below on dual eligibles).

Medicaid and SSDI. Some SSDI recipients may be eligible for Medicaid while awaiting Medicare coverage. If SSDI recipients are unable to work because of their disability and they have no other source of income, their SSDI benefit becomes their primary source of income. The average monthly SSDI benefit in January 2024 was $1,395.33 (or $16,743.96 annually). This is below the income threshold for Medicaid in most states,[c] but Medicaid coverage is not guaranteed in states that set very low income thresholds. SSDI recipients who have additional income that puts them above Medicaid thresholds may still qualify for Medicaid if they have high medical bills. Some states have "spend down" programs that allow individuals to deduct certain medical expenses from income to reduce their income below the Medicaid ceiling.

Dual Eligibles. Even once SSDI recipients become Medicare eligible (after the 24-month waiting period), some may still qualify for Medicaid if they continue to meet state Medicaid eligibility criteria. These individuals are known as "dual eligibles." For dual eligibles, Medicare becomes their primary insurance, but Medicaid may cover additional care that is not covered or only partially covered under Medicare, such as wheelchairs and home- and community-based services (services that help people with disabilities live in their homes and communities). Medicaid may also cover Medicare premiums and, in some cases, other out-of-pocket medical expenses, such as deductibles, copayments, and coinsurance.

----

[a] *Some states and territories require a separate Medicaid application but use SSI eligibility criteria for Medicaid eligibility (Alaska, Idaho, Kansas, Nebraska, Nevada, Northern Mariana Islands, Oregon, Utah); other states use their own Medicaid eligibility criteria for Medicaid, which may be different from SSI eligibility criteria (Connecticut, Hawaii, Illinois, Minnesota, Missouri, New Hampshire, North Dakota, Oklahoma, Virginia).*

[b] *SSA reduces these benefit amounts for beneficiaries who have other sources of income, and the average monthly SSI benefit for adults aged 18–64 in January 2024 was $723.10 (or $8,677.20 annually).*

[c] *As of February 7, 2024, 41 states (including the District of Columbia) expanded their Medicaid programs to cover nearly all adults with incomes up to 138 percent of the federal poverty line ($20,783 for an individual in 2024). In these states, most SSI recipients will qualify for Medicaid. Many SSDI recipients will qualify as well.*

[d] *The federal poverty line is $15,060 per year for individuals in 2024. Where states have not elected to expand their Medicaid program to 138 percent of the federal poverty line, these states retain very low eligibility levels for parents and have no coverage pathway for adults without dependent children (who are not elderly or receiving SSI).*

SOURCES: Center on Budget & Policy Priorities, 2023a,b; CMS, 2022a, 2024a; HHS, 2024; KFF, 2023a, 2024a; SSA 2024a,b,c,d,e,f,g.

Table 4-1 displays CMS's proposed sex recorded at birth and gender identity questions for MA and Part D plans. The proposed model form contains the minimum amount of information required to process Medicare enrollment in MA and Part D plans, but CMS gives plan administrators flexibility to modify the language and content of the enrollment form. This means that going forward, CMS is not proposing to require standardized SOGI data collection across Medicare plans; public commenters have noted this problem and have urged CMS to work with other HHS agencies to adopt standardized measures (National Health Law Program, 2023). Notably, the proposed Medicare questions/responses are similar to, but not the same as, the newly adopted Medicaid/CHIP questions and responses, and both sets of SOGI data options are again different from the SOGI data collected by other components of the health care system (as discussed below and displayed in Tables 4-1 and 4-3).

Public commenters have also urged CMS to add SOGI demographic fields to the Medicare Part B application, and have requested that CMS's data collection efforts include identifying populations with VSTs and other demographic characteristics, such as preferred language and disability status (National Health Law Program, 2023). CMS has not indicated whether or when it will move toward wider adoption of SOGI data collection across all Medicare programs or whether it will adopt a wider range of demographic questions. Still, the proposed MA and Part D enrollment questions are a major step forward toward meeting the goals of CMS's health equity framework for many Medicare beneficiaries.[7]

TRICARE

TRICARE is the U.S. Department of Defense (DoD) health care insurance program for active-duty service members and their families (including National Guard and Reserve members and their family members, retirees and retiree family members, survivors, and certain former spouses). Service members who separate from service because of a service-connected injury or illness may become eligible for Social Security disability benefits (and therefore, Medicare or Medicaid coverage), but may also retain TRICARE benefits, depending on their circumstances (TRICARE, 2023).

Although LGBTQ+ individuals may now serve openly in the military, DoD (2021) policy and practice have prohibited the collection of SOGI data from military personnel, stating:

> Gender identity is a personal and private matter. DoD Components, including the Military Departments and Services, require written approval from the USD (P&R) to collect transgender and transgender related data or publicly release such data. (p. 17)

Given this policy, TRICARE has not moved to adopt SOGI data collection on its enrollment forms and has not set expectations for TRICARE plan administrators to collect these data.

---

[7] More than half of the Medicare-enrolled population is enrolled in an MA plan, and about three-quarters are enrolled in a Part D plan (CMS, 2021).

Private Health Insurers

Private health insurance is a significant source of coverage for TGD people—a 2022 KFF survey found that 59 percent of LGBT+ respondents aged 18–64 were covered by a private health insurance plan (Dawson et al., 2023). Whether any federal SOGI data requirements apply to individual private health plans depends on whether the plan is sold through state marketplaces or through the employer-sponsored market.

Qualified Health Plans Operating through State Marketplaces

Under the Affordable Care Act (ACA), consumers may purchase private health insurance policies, known as "qualified health plans," that meet certain ACA-mandated standards (including a group of essential health benefits and limits on out-of-pocket expenses). States are required to have a single, streamlined application for people to apply for Medicaid/CHIP coverage or financial assistance (e.g., tax credits or cost-sharing reductions that reduce insurance costs) to purchase qualified health plans sold on state health insurance marketplaces (also known as exchanges).[8] States can use the CMS-developed model application or an approved alternative to determine eligibility for these programs. CMS's model application (and the SOGI questions therein, as described above) is effective immediately in the 32 state marketplaces that use the Federally Facilitated Marketplace (FFM) platform (CMS, 2023a).

Nineteen states (including the District of Columbia) operate their own state-based marketplace platforms[9]; the remaining states use the FFM either fully or just for select functions (application processing and certain eligibility and enrollment activities). States that operate their own health insurance marketplaces do so with the goal of saving money and gaining more control and authority over marketplace functions. Consumers in these states apply for and enroll in coverage through separate marketplace websites maintained by the states. As states operating their own marketplaces use state-specific enrollment forms that may differ from federal forms, they will not automatically incorporate CMS's new SOGI questions (although CMS guidance encourages states to adopt the model application).

In states that utilize the FFM and enrollment forms on HealthCare.gov, consumers applying for qualified health plans will use CMS's new model

---

[8] Patient Protection and Affordable Care Act, 42 U.S.C. §§ 18083, 1396w–3 (2010).

[9] The following states operate their own state-based marketplaces, and therefore, will not automatically utilize the SOGI questions on CMS's model application: California, Colorado, Connecticut, District of Columbia, Idaho, Kentucky, Maine, Maryland, Massachusetts, Minnesota, Nevada, New Jersey, New Mexico, New York, Pennsylvania, Rhode Island, Vermont, Virginia, and Washington (KFF, 2024b).

application forms (outlined above), including the SOGI data questions displayed in Table 4-1.[10] Despite CMS's new enrollment forms, however, FFM participation may not guarantee SOGI data collection. Through a process called "direct enrollment," the federal government allows health plan issuers and third-party web brokers operating in states that use the FFM to enroll consumers directly from their own websites instead of requiring them to use HealthCare.gov (CMS, 2023d).[11] Whether a consumer enters the process through HealthCare.gov or via a direct enrollment website is often a matter of chance, and the direct enrollment pathway raises several concerns for consumers, as these websites have been found to offer health plans that do not comply with ACA standards and may not direct consumers toward Medicaid or other subsidies to which they are entitled (Straw, 2019). In the case of CMS's model application form, it is unclear whether direct enrollment entities will adopt this new form or the SOGI data collection therein, meaning that SOGI data collection may vary depending on which website a consumer stumbles onto when enrolling in marketplace coverage.

Employer-Sponsored Health Plans

Employer-sponsored health plans are offered to employees and their dependents as a benefit of employment. These plans currently provide some level of health care coverage for approximately 153 million Americans (KFF, 2023b). While the ACA includes certain requirements for employer-sponsored health plans (including requirements on cost and benefits and a mandate for companies with 50 or more employees to offer health insurance coverage for employees), the law did not change the way health plans are sold, and employees who access these plans continue to enroll through their employers as they did prior to the ACA (in other words, they do not enroll through HealthCare.gov or a state-run marketplace). Therefore, CMS's model application form is not applicable to health plans that are sold through the employer-sponsored market, nor are other recent HHS initiatives aimed at improving data collection.

Increasingly, health plans operating in the employer-sponsored market are taking note of the importance of SOGI data collection. The National

---

[10] While states may participate in the FFM, this does not mean that the SOGI data collected are automatically generated into state Medicaid applications as applications may be processed separately. As described above, states must elect to adopt CMS's model application for use in their Medicaid program.

[11] In some cases, consumers applying through a direct enrollment entity are directed to HealthCare.gov to fill out an eligibility application and then redirected back to the direct enrollment entity to compare health plans and enroll in coverage. In other cases, the direct enrollment entity conducts the full application and enrollment process without directing consumers to HealthCare.gov at any point in the process.

Association of Insurance Commissioners (NAIC, 2021)[12] issued a set of principles for data collection in December 2021, calling on health insurers to systematically collect a series of voluntarily reported enrollee data, including data on sex recorded at birth, gender identity, and sexual orientation. NAIC advises health insurance companies to follow best practices in data collection and ensure that data collection is always voluntary for plan enrollees (e.g., by ensuring that there is always a "prefer not to answer" option for each question). NAIC also cautions that such demographic data should be used only to analyze health disparities and inequities and never for benefit determinations (as prohibited by law).

When NAIC drafted these principles, it received numerous comments from interested industry organizations. Judging from these comments, the employer-sponsored health insurance industry as a whole appears supportive of SOGI data collection at the point of health plan enrollment, but some organizations have expressed concerns. For example, America's Health Insurance Plans (AHIP, 2021a), an advocacy organization for health insurance providers, agrees that it is important for health plans to collect SOGI data systematically but cautions that sometimes these questions may be "extremely uncomfortable" for consumers to answer (especially where the questions are not developed through a consumer-driven process) and should be collected only in a trusted patient–provider relationship. AHIP (2021b) states further that employers may be reluctant to update enrollment forms and ask employees to provide this information, and that the health insurance industry should work with other components of the health care system to develop stakeholder-driven demographic data standards. Other leaders have also stressed the need for industry-wide standards for SOGI data collection (BCBSA, 2022).

Even without health care system–wide standards in place, NAIC's (2021) final principles for data collection cite the National Academies' 2022 consensus study *Measuring Sex, Gender Identity, and Sexual Orientation* as a guide to SOGI data collection, stating:

> When asking about sex, it is recommended to use a "two-step" approach. Respondents should be asked what sex they were assigned at birth or what sex is indicated on their birth certificate, and should also be asked how they describe their current gender identity. When describing current gender identity, respondents should be allowed to 'check all that apply' or fill in their own descriptor. (p. 7)

It is unclear how many employer-sponsored health plans currently collect SOGI data and how many employers require employees to report

---

[12] NAIC is a standards-setting organization governed by the chief insurance regulators from all 50 states, the District of Columbia, and five U.S. territories.

such data at the point of plan enrollment. This committee did not uncover any research studies examining this question. However, a few health plans have made statements about their approach to SOGI data collection:

- *Blue Cross Blue Shield Association* (BCBSA, 2022)—a national federation of 35 Blue Cross Blue Shield plans—published a report on the use of data to reduce health disparities, describing the changes that need to be made across the health care system to make robust collection of SOGI data a reality. BCBSA's report is not a statement about what its plans are doing in terms of SOGI data collection, but a call to action for the industry to address the challenges in the system, including the lack of standard data sets for the collection of SOGI data. In addition, BCBSA is working with the National Minority Quality Forum to advance the standardization of SOGI data collection across the industry (Houston, 2023).
- *Kaiser Permanente* has been a leader in establishing systems of care geared toward transgender health. In 2017, Kaiser stated that all Kaiser Permanente regions are updating electronic health records (EHRs) to "allow for gender markers to indicate what primary care prompts should go with a patient's record" as a means of improving care coordination (Seto, 2017). In 2017, Kaiser Permanente Mid-Atlantic States (KPMAS, 2018) announced a new EHR form that collects SOGI data and ensures that appropriate prompts based on anatomy for cancer screening are documented in a transgender registry. As of 2018, KPMAS's EHR had 460 patients documented in a transgender registry, 164 (35 percent) of whom had an organ inventory completed (an organ inventory is also termed "anatomical inventory"; the importance of these inventories for TGD people and people with VSTs is discussed in Chapter 3).
- *Optum Health* announced in 2023 plans to build a "disparities analytics dashboard" to capture SOGI and other data important for documenting health equity among its members (Optum, 2023; Raths, 2023).

SOGI DATA COLLECTION WITHIN FEDERAL HEALTH SYSTEMS

In addition to operating public health insurance programs, the federal government operates three major systems of health care: (1) federally qualified health centers (FQHCs), (2) the Veteran's Health Administration (VHA), and (3) the Indian Health Service (IHS). This section examines the SOGI data collection in place within these systems.

Federally Qualified Health Centers Funded by the Health Resources and Services Administration

FQHCs are safety net health care providers that deliver primary care in underserved communities regardless of insurance status or ability to pay. FQHCs are funded by the Health Resources and Services Administration (HRSA), and in 2022 delivered comprehensive primary and preventive health care to more than 30.5 million of the most vulnerable Americans, including nearly 1.4 million people experiencing homelessness; more than 395,000 veterans; and 24.2 million people who were either uninsured or covered by Medicaid or Medicare (HRSA, 2024b), including an estimated 1 in 5 Medicaid enrollees (Cole et al., 2021).[13] HRSA (2024a) estimates that 90 percent of the patients served by FQHCs are at or below 200 percent of the federal poverty line. Given that TGD populations can experience disproportionately higher rates of poverty and lower rates of insurance coverage (Crissman et al., 2017; Dickey et al., 2016), they may benefit from access to FQHCs (Grasso et al., 2019).

To enhance care and equity among the populations it serves, including TGD patients, HRSA mandates that FQHCs collect and report SOGI data for all patients. Unlike other providers and health systems that may or may not utilize SOGI data collection capabilities within EHRs, FQHCs must report aggregate SOGI data for patients aged 18 and older as part of standard reporting of demographic data to the U.S. Bureau of Primary Health Care under the Uniform Data System (UDS) (HRSA, 2016).[14] Under these requirements, FQHCs must collect and report data on sex recorded at birth (using the term "sex assigned at birth") and gender identity. Table 4-3 illustrates the questions and response options required by HRSA under the UDS (HRSA, 2023).

HRSA's SOGI reporting requirements—in place since 2016—are the only federal mandate requiring SOGI data collection in any U.S. health care setting. Yet despite this mandate, HRSA has faced challenges in getting FQHCs to comply with SOGI data reporting; these challenges are described in Chapter 3 of this report.

---

[13] Medicaid and Medicare beneficiaries may receive care and services from FQHCs. In these circumstances, SOGI data collection and reporting take place in accordance with HRSA requirements, even if Medicare and Medicaid providers elsewhere are not required to collect and report SOGI data. The same is true for people eligible for VHA or IHS programs who access care within an FQHC.

[14] HRSA's UDS captures a range of data on patient characteristics, services provided, and health outcomes across HRSA's 1,400 health centers. Currently, HRSA (2024b) requires reporting of patient data in the aggregate, but through a recent UDS modernization initiative, certain FQHCs are now able to submit deidentified patient-level data to HRSA.

TABLE 4-3 Sex Assigned at Birth and Gender Identity Questions Within Federal Health Care Delivery Systems

Program	Question 1	Q1 Response Options	Question 2	Q2 Response Options	Data Collection Requirements
Health Resources and Services Administration, Bureau of Primary Health Care, 2023	Sex Assigned at Birth	☐ Male ☐ Female	Gender Identity	☐ Male ☐ Female ☐ Transgender Man/ Transgender Male/ Transmasculine ☐ Transgender Woman/ Transgender Female/ Transfeminine ☐ Other ☐ Chose not to disclose ☐ Unknown	Mandatory
Department of Veterans Affairs, 2021	Birth Sex	☐ Male ☐ Female	Self-Identified Gender Identity	☐ Male ☐ Female ☐ Transmale[a]/Transman/ Female-to-Male ☐ Transfemale/Transwoman/ Male-to-Female ☐ Choose not to answer	Optional

TABLE 4-3 Continued

Program	Question 1	Q1 Response Options	Question 2	Q2 Response Options	Data Collection Requirements
Indian Health Service, 2023	**Birth Sex:** *sex assigned at birth*	□ Female □ Male □ Intersex □ Other	**Gender Identity** (optional)	□ Female □ Male □ Two Spirit □ Transgender Male □ Transgender Female □ Non-Binary □ Genderqueer □ Gender Expansive □ Gender Diverse □ Don't know □ Decline to answer □ Other: [free text]	Optional
	Legal Sex: *if different from birth sex*	□ Female □ Male □ Other			

[a] The committee notes the use of the "transwoman" and "transman" (one word), as opposed to "trans woman," "trans man," "transgender woman" and "transgender man" (two words), can be seen as offensive.
NOTE: While many of the federal programs listed in this table ask questions about sexual orientation, these questions and responses are not listed here. The table presents sexual orientation and gender identity data questions in the order they are asked—i.e., that a question related to sex recorded at birth is asked first, followed by a question about gender identity. As described in Chapter 3, it is considered best practice to order the questions in the reverse order: ask first about gender identity then about sex recorded at birth (Deutsch et al., 2013).

Veterans Health Administration

VHA is an integrated health care system providing health care services to more than 9 million veterans (VA, 2023). VHA is not a health insurer but a health care system; eligible populations may have other types of health insurance coverage (such as Medicare, Medicaid, TRICARE, or a private insurance plan).[15]

To better serve TGD veterans and veterans with VSTs, VHA (2018) issued a national directive in 2011 that established policies for delivering affirming and respectful health care services to all people enrolled in the Department of Veterans Affairs (VA) health care system. This directive represented a significant advance in care for thousands of veterans: the VHA estimates that as of July 2023, its system served 28,659 TGD veterans (Matza and McConnell, 2023), and researchers estimate that TGD people are at least two to three times more likely to have served in the U.S. armed forces compared with cisgender people (Gates and Herman, 2014). The VHA serves many disabled veterans, some of whom may also be eligible for SSA programs,[16] so SOGI data collection within the VHA is important for veterans applying for disability benefits.

Since 2018, the VHA has also had a directive in place for the collection of data on sex recorded at birth and gender identity (termed by within the VHA system as "birth sex" and "self-identified gender," respectfully) (VHA, 2018). Table 4-3 displays the SOGI questions and response options used by the VHA. Unlike FQHCs, which are required by HRSA to collect and report SOGI data, the VHA system relies on veterans to self-report their sex and gender identity when applying for health benefits and when checking in for health care at a VHA facility. The VHA estimates that, currently, 25 percent

---

[15] Retired service members may be eligible for both TRICARE and Department of Veterans Affairs (VA) benefits. Service members who separate from service because of a service-connected injury or illness may become eligible for VA benefits but also retain certain TRICARE benefits depending on the nature of their illness or injury. In addition, all VHA facilities are TRICARE network providers, and TRICARE beneficiaries may access care through VHA providers. Finally, retired service members who qualify for SSDI (and as a result, Medicare) may retain TRICARE and/or VA benefits. Given the connections between these programs, SOGI data collection for retired service members may depend on whether an individual seeks care from VHA providers or from providers that seek reimbursement through TRICARE or Medicare (VA, 2021, 2022).

[16] Many veterans are disabled. According to the Bureau of Labor Statistics, as of August 2022, 4.9 million veterans (27 percent of all veterans) had a service-connected disability. When veterans can show that they have a disability condition that was incurred or aggravated by military service, they are entitled to disability compensation provided by the VA. Veterans may be separately eligible for SSA disability programs or for both SSA and VA disability programs if they meet criteria for each. SSA gives processing priority to disability claims of veterans. The VA and SSA work cooperatively in these cases, with the VA sharing the medical evidence it has used to make its own disability decisions with SSA (BLS, 2023; SSA, 2021).

of veteran enrollee records contain gender identity information (Matza and McConnell, 2023).

While other components of the federal health care system may collect SOGI data at enrollment or patient encounters, VHA stands above others with requirements in place to use collected SOGI data to aid in clinical decision making. Within the VHA EHR system, clinical reminders are cued to "birth sex," so TGD veterans receive appropriate preventive screening specific to their sex recorded at birth (VHA, 2018). In addition, the VHA system automatically uses sex recorded at birth data to determine appropriate laboratory ranges for certain conditions and doses for medication (along with data on height, weight, and age) (VHA, 2022).

Prior to 2018, when the singular demographic field of "sex" within the VHA records system represented both birth sex and gender identity, some veterans chose to change their birth sex information to better align with their gender identity. Now that the system captures birth sex and gender identity separately in a two-step question, VHA has had to contend with the fact that some "birth sex" records in their system do not align with the patient's actual sex recorded at birth (Burgess et al., 2019). VHA (2022) does not have a policy to automatically change these records back but encourages providers to engage veterans in discussion about how information in the birth sex field may impact their care and why it is important for the birth sex field to be consistent with sex recorded at birth.

The VHA is currently working to better capture and expand veterans' SOGI data by deploying new EHR systems that capture pronouns and administrative sex data in addition to birth sex and gender identity (Matza and McConnell, 2023). These data collection policies follow prior directives for all VHA providers to offer affirming care to TGD veterans and veterans with VSTs (Wolfe et al., 2023).

Indian Health Service

IHS, an agency within HHS, is responsible for providing comprehensive health services to approximately 2.6 million American Indians and Alaska Natives (AI/ANs) in 37 states. IHS either operates health facilities directly or funds tribes to operate health facilities themselves.[17]

AI/AN people who seek care within the IHS system are not required to have health insurance. Many AI/AN populations meet eligibility requirements for Medicaid and CHIP, and since Medicaid/CHIP coverage provides access to other providers or services beyond what is available through IHS alone, AI/AN populations may seek these coverage options (CMS, n.d.-a).

---

[17] Sometimes, tribes may operate a health facility that qualifies as an FQHC. In these cases, the IHS facility must meet HRSA requirements for SOGI data collection and reporting.

In 2019, IHS launched an initiative to train staff in the collection of voluntary SOGI data to help IHS "identify the health care needs and address the disparities of our Two Spirit, lesbian, gay, bisexual, transgender, and queer patients" (Haverkate, 2022). In June 2023, IHS created a standard for the capture of structured SOGI data within IHS patient medical records (Haverkate, 2023). Its standard registration intake form contains fields for birth sex, legal sex, gender identity, preferred name, pronouns, and sexual orientation. However, IHS policy does not require IHS providers to collect and report SOGI data or to use the standard intake form. As with VHA policy, patients receiving services within the IHS are allowed to provide SOGI data voluntarily for capture in their EHRs (IHS, 2023). Table 4-3 displays questions on sex recorded at birth and gender identity on the IHS standard intake form.

AI/AN people may be eligible for SSA disability programs if they meet eligibility requirements; overall, these populations experience chronic disease and related morbidity at a higher rate compared with other groups (Goins et al., 2007; Siordia et al., 2017). The Centers for Disease Control and Prevention (CDC, 2008) found that AI/AN people are 50.3 percent more likely to have a disability compared with the national average. Although the CDC estimate comes from the 2006 Behavioral Risk Factor Surveillance System surveys that use a broader definition of disability[18] than would meet SSA requirements, these data are nonetheless an indicator of need within AI/AN populations.

SOGI DATA COLLECTION AMONG PROVIDERS AND HEALTH CARE DELIVERY SYSTEMS: STATE-LEVEL REQUIREMENTS AND INCENTIVES

As detailed in Chapter 3, while EHRs are required to have data fields that allow end users to record SOGI information, the federal government does not require providers and health care systems to use these data fields.[19]

---

[18] The 2006 Behavioral Risk Factor Surveillance System used a definition of disability consistent with Healthy People 2010, asking respondents: "Are you limited in any way in any activities because of physical, mental, or emotional problems?" and "Do you now have any health problem that requires you to use special equipment, such as a cane, a wheelchair, a special bed, or a special telephone?" Participants who responded "yes" to either question were classified as having a disability.

[19] CMS's Meaningful Use program incentivizes providers and health care systems to modernize data collection through EHRs. In 2015, CMS and the Office of the National Coordinator for Health Information Technology (ONC) added a requirement that EHRs certified under Stage 3 of the Meaningful Use program allow users to record SOGI data. Effective January 1, 2018, these requirements apply to EHR developers and vendors and health institutions and to practices that are using EHR systems as part of their participation in the Meaningful Use incentive program. Meaningful Use certification does not require providers or health care institutions to collect SOGI data; it requires only that certified EHR technologies have the ability (i.e., the data fields) to record such data (ONC and HHS, 2015).

Although some providers work in systems (e.g., VHA or an FQHC) that require or encourage SOGI reporting, many providers routinely fail to collect SOGI data, and the many barriers to SOGI data collection described in Chapter 3 are persistent problems. New efforts by CMS to collect SOGI data within its programs do not address these system-wide challenges.

CMS's new model marketplace application—where adopted by states—changes SOGI data collection only at the point of application for Medicaid, CHIP, or a qualified health plan purchased through the state marketplace. The model application does not require providers who seek reimbursement from Medicaid/CHIP to collect or record SOGI data for their patients. Similarly, the questions proposed by CMS for inclusion in Medicare's enrollment forms are applicable only for the collection of data at the point of enrollment; this proposed policy does not require providers who offer services for Medicare beneficiaries to collect or report SOGI data. Finally, neither model application impacts SOGI data collection within the employer-sponsored health insurance market or the providers who seek reimbursement from these insurers.

The collection of SOGI data at the point of enrollment is useful in helping public and private health insurers understand the populations they serve, but these efforts may not change what SOGI data are recorded in any given individual's medical record. There are, however, a few current and former state-level efforts to require or incentivize providers and payers to collect and report SOGI data, as described below.

Oregon Health Authority: Proposed SOGI Reporting Requirements

Legislation in Oregon passed in 2021 requires the Oregon Health Authority to build a data collection system for SOGI data reporting and to create a grant program to help community partners and community-based organizations serving underrepresented communities collect and report these data (OEI, n.d.). As part of this effort, the Oregon Health Authority issued draft SOGI data collection recommendations in 2023 (OEI, 2023). Table 4-4 outlines Oregon's proposed approach and the robust SOGI demographic questions recommended for inclusion. In addition, the draft recommendations put forward additional questions providers may ask of patients as part of ensuring quality medical care. These include a series of questions about gender-affirming care—for example, *Are you currently taking gender-affirming hormones and/or hormone blockers? If Yes, when did you start? What is your current dose and frequency?*—and best practices for taking a patient's anatomical inventory (Oregon's anatomical inventory questions are discussed in Chapter 3 of this report). The Oregon Health Authority plans to have its SOGI data collection system active "no sooner than" late 2024, and once the system is active, providers and insurers will be asked to submit SOGI data annually (OEI, n.d.). Patients will also have direct access to the system to update their SOGI information.

TABLE 4-4 Oregon Health Authority: Draft SOGI Data Collection Recommendations

---

Please describe your gender in any way you prefer: [free text]

What is your gender? (check all that apply)
- ☐ Girl, Woman
- ☐ Boy, Man
- ☐ Non-binary
- ☐ Agender/No gender
- ☐ Questioning
- ☐ Not listed. Please specify: [free text]
- ☐ Don't know
- ☐ I don't know what this question is asking
- ☐ I don't want to answer

Are you transgender?
- ☐ Yes
- ☐ No
- ☐ Questioning
- ☐ Don't know
- ☐ I don't know what this question is asking
- ☐ I don't want to answer

What pronouns do you want us to use? (select all that apply)
- ☐ They/Them
- ☐ She/Her
- ☐ He/Him
- ☐ No pronouns, use my name
- ☐ Don't know
- ☐ Not listed. Please specify: [free text]
- ☐ I don't know what this question is asking
- ☐ I don't want to answer

Sex- It is anticipated that if you need to ask about sex (not gender) you will probably just need to ask 1 or 2 of the questions below – depending on WHY you need this information.

When you were born what sex was assigned to you? (Pick one)
- ☐ Male
- ☐ Female
- ☐ Intersex
- ☐ Unspecified
- ☐ Not listed. Please specify: [free text]
- ☐ Don't know
- ☐ I don't know what this question is asking
- ☐ I don't want to answer

What is your current legal sex in your state? (Pick one) (OR simply: What is your current sex?)
- ☐ Male
- ☐ Female
- ☐ X
- ☐ Intersex
- ☐ Non-binary
- ☐ Unspecified
- ☐ Don't know
- ☐ Not listed. Please specify: [free text]
- ☐ I don't know what this question is asking

NOTES: The Oregon Health Authority recommends including questions about sexual orientation, but these questions and responses are not listed here. The gender identity questions are recommended for inclusion in every setting, whereas the sex assigned at birth and pronouns questions are recommended for social services and eligibility systems.
SOURCE: OEI, 2023.

Incentives for Providers and Payers to Collect SOGI Data: Massachusetts and Oregon

State Medicaid programs use payment models to incentivize improved collection of health equity data (Ubri et al., 2023). Massachusetts, for example, is using innovative payment models to provide incentives for providers to collect and report SOGI data. MassHealth's Section 1115 Demonstration Waiver[20] financially incentivizes Accountable Care Organizations (ACOs)[21] and ACO-participating hospitals to provide complete SOGI data starting in fiscal year 2023. The 1115 waiver application states that gender identity will be among the data collected by ACOs in Massachusetts but does not specify further what SOGI data will be collected (CMS, 2024b).

Oregon is planning a similar initiative. According to a 2023 survey of state Medicaid agencies and Medicaid Managed Care Organizations (MCOs)[22] conducted by the National Opinion Research Center (NORC) at the University of Chicago, the Oregon Health Authority is exploring ways to incentivize hospitals and other providers participating in Coordinated Care Organizations within the state to report SOGI data (Ubri et al., 2023). NORC reports that Medicaid leaders in other states are beginning to recognize the importance of collecting SOGI data to better understand the experiences and needs of enrollees. Overall, however, states are much further along with incentivizing data collection on race, ethnicity, language, and disability, and few MCOs collect SOGI data (Ubri et al., 2023).

Building SOGI Data Collection Capacity among Providers: Connecticut

From 2015 to 2020, the state of Connecticut received federal funding through a State Innovation Model (SIM) grant to test reforms to health care payment and service delivery models within the state. Connecticut's SIM focused in part on health equity and was aimed at building capacity at participating FQHCs and patient-centered medical homes to collect SOGI data (Connecticut Office of Health Strategy, 2020). Although the SIM grant has ended, the Connecticut Office of Health Strategy reports that all health care entities participating in the SIM developed infrastructure and workflows for collecting SOGI data and most began to document these data in their EHR systems.

---

[20] Medicaid 1115 demonstration waivers allow the Secretary of Health and Human Services to "waive" certain provisions of Medicaid law to give states additional flexibility to design and improve their Medicaid or CHIP programs. Massachusetts has received a waiver from CMS to use an innovative service delivery system model (the ACO), with the goal of improving care, increasing efficiency, and reducing costs.

[21] ACOs are a delivery system model designed to improve care coordination and delivery by holding providers financially accountable for the health of the patient population they serve. More than 80 percent of eligible MassHealth members are covered by ACOs in the state (MassHealth, 2022).

[22] States design and administer their own Medicaid programs within federal rules. Many states elect to administer Medicaid through contracts with MCOs, which accept a per member, per month fee from the state to organize care delivery and manage cost and quality. MCOs are the dominant delivery system for Medicaid enrollees, and 72 percent of Medicaid beneficiaries are enrolled in an MCO (Hinton and Raphel, 2023).

TABLE 4-5 Gender Identity Question Included in Washington State's Comprehensive Hospital Abstract Reporting System

---

Patient's gender identity shall be identified by the patient and reported using one or more of the following options. If the patient self-identifies more than one gender, each gender shall be reported.

(a) Male;	(j) Gender fluid;
(b) Female;	(k) Bigender;
(c) Man or Masculine/Masc;	(l) Agender;
(d) Woman or Feminine/Femme;	(m) Demigirl;
(e) Trans* or transgender;	(n) Demiboy;
(f) Cis or cisgender;	(o) Gender not listed above, please specify;
(g) Genderqueer;	(p) Patient declined to respond; or
(h) Nonbinary;	(q) Unknown
(i) Two spirit;	

SOURCE: Washington State Health Care Authority, 2022b.

Hospital Requirements for SOGI Reporting: Washington State

In 2021, Washington state became the first in the United States to require hospitals to collect and submit detailed patient self-identified demographic data, including race, ethnicity, language, disabilities, sexual orientation, and gender identity (Strong, 2022). Hospitals in the state had to comply with these new rules by January 1, 2023, and had to report on patient sex recorded at birth and gender identity to the state's Comprehensive Hospital Abstract Reporting System database (Washington State Health Care Authority, 2022b). The 17 response options for gender identity are listed in Table 4-5. While reporting demographic information to the Department of Health is mandatory for hospitals, patient participation is voluntary.

FEDERAL SURVEYS AND SOGI DATA COLLECTION

Federal surveys play a vital role in generating the data needed by government agencies to understand the demographics of the American public in support of evidence-based policy making. Measuring sexual and gender minority populations within federal surveys improves understanding of these populations, helping the public health and health care systems identify and track health disparities among TGD people and people with VSTs, and design and monitor strategies for reducing these disparities.

In July 2021, for example, the U.S. Census Bureau began including questions on sex assigned at birth, current gender identity, and sexual orientation in the Household Pulse Survey (HPS) (Anderson et al., 2021). National HPS data from 2021 and 2022 show that LGBT respondents reported experiencing greater anxiety and depression compared with non-LGBT respondents (Marlay et al., 2022). Examining HPS data specific to California, the California Budget and Policy Center found that about 6 in 10 LGBTQ+ Californians in households with annual incomes of less than $50,000 experienced poor mental health, compared with only 4 in 10 non-LGBTQ+ Californians in that same income category (Kitson and Ramos-Yamamoto, 2022). Given this high rate of poor mental health among low-income LGBTQ+ adults in California, the California Budget and Policy Center made recommendations for state policy makers to bolster the state's mental health workforce in order to reduce disparities for LGBTQ+ adults (e.g., by ensuring that behavioral health care providers serving people with Medi-Cal receive LGBTQ+-affirming training). These data points are coming at an important juncture for California, as the state legislature recently funded new initiatives for providing training on inclusive care for TGD people and people with VSTs within continuing medical education curricula (Coursolle, 2023), and as California's governor is looking to modernize the state's mental health system in an effort to better prioritize residents with the most severe mental health needs (Office of Governor Gavin Newsom, 2023).

California's use of HPS data is just one example of how, armed with SOGI data, policy makers can quickly target funding and policies to better serve TGD people and people with VSTs. Increasingly, other federal surveys are collecting and reporting SOGI data, and because of data collection on gender identity, federal surveys now can examine tobacco use (CMS, n.d.-b.), educational experiences (NCES, 2023), and patterns of violence against TGD people (Truman and Morgan, 2022). Coupling SOGI data with other measures—for example, many federal surveys collect data on disability status (CDC, 2020)—can help researchers and policy makers understand and describe how the intersectionality of various identities impacts health and well-being.

However, not every federal survey includes the gender identity questions necessary to fully explore health and disparities among TGD people and people with VSTs. In 2022, the National Academies examined the state of SOGI data collection across 47 federal surveys and other data systems, identifying 24 federal surveys that include one or more SOGI data questions (NASEM, 2022). As in other areas of SOGI data collection, terms and response options vary widely across federal surveys. In addition, fewer federal surveys collect any data on gender identity, and only 12 of the surveys examined in the National Academies report collect gender identity data using a two-step question methodology (NASEM, 2022). Furthermore, where surveys include a question on sex recorded at birth, most include only male and female as response options and do not allow free-text responses that would enable respondents to indicate VSTs.

The variability in SOGI data collection overall and gender identity data in particular stems from the fact that federal law does not require federal surveys to collect any SOGI data beyond asking about "biological sex" (male/female).[23] However, federal surveys are increasingly asking SOGI questions beyond what is required by law, prompted in part by a January 2023 White House Office of Management and Budget (OMB) report outlining best practices for the collection of self-reported SOGI data in federal statistical surveys, including using a two-step methodology for collecting data on sex recorded at birth and gender identity (Office of the Chief Statistician of the United States, 2023). Building on recommendations from the OMB report, the Census Bureau is in the process of testing SOGI questions to be included in the American Community Survey (ACS).[24] In addition, beginning in 2023, the National Survey on Drug Use and Health (an annual survey sponsored by the Substance Abuse and Mental Health Services Administration) asked respondents about their sex assigned at birth and their gender identity (SAMHSA, 2023).

Increased and expanded SOGI data collection will greatly enhance documentation of the experience of TGD people and may also provide opportunities to document people with VSTs.

Federal Surveys, SOGI Data, and SSA

Federal surveys, by their nature, are at the population level and cannot supplement information about any particular SSA disability applicant. However, data collected from various federal surveys may help SSA

---

[23] Federal surveys are not required to collect SOGI data. While Section 4302 of the ACA contains provisions to strengthen federal data collection by requiring that all national federal data collection efforts collect information on race, ethnicity, sex, primary language, and disability status, current minimum data collection standards published by HHS in 2011 define the category of sex only as "biological sex." HHS considered sexual orientation and gender identity to be concepts separate from biological sex and did not address them within the 2011 standards. However, the 2011 standards are just the minimum data collection requirements, and ACA § 4302 allows for federal surveys to collect additional data beyond what is described in the law (ASPE, 2011).

[24] Agency Information Collection Activities; Submission to the Office of Management and Budget (OMB) for Review and Approval; Comment Request; American Community Survey Methods Panel: 2024 Sexual Orientation and Gender Identity Test, 88 Fed. Reg. 64404–64407 (September 19, 2023). While the ACS is not a health care survey, it is still an important tool for advancing health care equity. In April 2023, for example, researchers in the U.S. Census Bureau linked ACS data with Medicaid data, which helped identify gaps in estimates about health disparities. Including SOGI data in the ACS adds an important demographic layer to this information (Limburg, 2023).

understand important characteristics of the populations who are likely to apply for and benefit from SSI/SSDI. For example, where federal surveys ask about both SOGI data and health insurance coverage—the Census Bureau Household Pulse Survey, for example, includes questions on health insurance (NCHS, 2023)—this may help illuminate access to health care coverage for TGD people and people with VSTs where there are gaps in SOGI data collection across Medicare, Medicaid, state exchanges, and private insurers. As this data collection evolves and improves, it may help SSA better understand the populations applying for disability benefits, particularly those who access insurance through Medicaid.

Currently, the National Beneficiary Survey administered by SSA asks only a question about biological sex (response options: male or female) (McDonald et al., 2021). While other federal surveys may provide useful data points for SSA, only the National Beneficiary Survey is geared toward the populations that receive SSI and SSDI. Including questions about sex recorded at birth and gender identity in this survey would enable SSA to better understand the experience of populations it serves who are TGD or have VSTs.

SUMMARY OF KEY POINTS

SOGI data collection is increasing across the U.S. health care system through promising enrollment policies within Medicaid and Medicare, focused efforts within private health plans and health systems, innovative state-level incentives to providers and payers, and expanded survey instruments. However, many of these initiatives are only just emerging, and almost all efforts to collect and report these data are optional or voluntary, with the exception of the HRSA mandate for FQHCs to collect SOGI data from their patients and new efforts in Oregon and Washington to require providers to submit SOGI data. As described in Chapter 3, optional reporting requirements have not produced robust SOGI data collection, and there are significant gaps in data collection even where collection and reporting of SOGI data are mandatory. Thus it could still be a long time before robust or even adequate SOGI data collection occurs across the system.

While this committee expects that SOGI data collection will continue to evolve, the health care system today is far from achieving the goals of SOGI data collection in ways that can support care for TGD people and people with VSTs. For this reason, SSA may best serve TGD applicants and applicants with VSTs by conducting its own SOGI data collection at the point of application. This approach would help fill the gaps where health care providers, insurers, and institutions are not yet collecting the patient data that SSA may need to fairly adjudicate disability applications from TGD people and people with VSTs. Asking SOGI questions of applicants up front allows applicants to choose how to report their identity to SSA (rather than having adjudicators piece together their identity through other information in the medical record). SSA disability application forms give prompts to applicants to "explain in remarks" additional details about various questions on the application (e.g., citizenship status, military service), and similar prompts could be included alongside SOGI data questions to invite applicants to describe additional information related to gender identity, sex recorded at birth, or other SOGI data. However, it is important that applicants always have the option to keep SOGI data private from SSA.

SSA could also consider whether to include SOGI questions in its National Beneficiary Survey. While other federal surveys increasingly ask SOGI questions, these survey instruments are not geared toward the specific populations served by SSA; the inclusion of SOGI data in the National Beneficiary Survey could therefore help SSA better understand the experience of the sexual and gender minority populations it serves.

REFERENCES

AHIP (America's Health Insurance Plans). 2021a. *AHIP comments-Draft principles for data collection.* Washington, DC. https://content.naic.org/sites/default/files/call_materials/AHIP%20Comments_0.pdf (accessed March 13, 2024).

AHIP. 2021b. *NAIC special (EX) committee on race and insurance 2021 charges.* Washington, DC. https://content.naic.org/sites/default/files/inline-files/America%27s%20Health%20Insurance%20Plans.pdf (accessed March 13, 2024).

Anderson, L., T. File, J. Marshall, K. McElrath, and Z. Scherer. 2021. *Census bureau survey explores sexual orientation and gender identity.* Suitland, MD: United States Census Bureau. https://www.census.gov/library/stories/2021/11/census-bureau-survey-explores-sexual-orientation-and-gender-identity.html (accessed March 13, 2024).

ASPE (Office of the Assistant Secretary for Planning and Evaluation). 2011. *HHS implementation guidance on data collection standards for race, ethnicity, sex, primary language, and disability status.* Washington, DC: Department of Health and Human Services. https://aspe.hhs.gov/reports/hhs-implementation-guidance-data-collection-standards-race-ethnicity-sex-primary-language-disability-0 (accessed April 2, 2024).

BCBSA (Blue Cross Blue Shield Association). 2022. *The ethical and transparent use of data to reduce health disparities.* Chicago, IL. https://www.bcbs.com/sites/default/files/healthequity/REL/HE_REL_Data_Paper.pdf (accessed March 13, 2024).

BLS (Bureau of Labor Statistics). 2023. *Employment situation of veterans-2022. USDL-23-0537.* Washington, DC: U.S. Department of Labor. https://www.bls.gov/news.release/pdf/vet.pdf (accessed March 13, 2024).

Burgess, C., M. Kauth, C. Klemt, H. Shanawani, and J. C. Shipherd. 2019. Evolving sex and gender in electronic health records. *Federal Practitioner* 36(6):271–277.

Center on Budget & Policy Priorities. 2023a. *Policy basics: Social Security disability insurance.* Washington, DC. https://www.cbpp.org/research/retirement-security/policy-basics-social-security-disability-insurance (accessed March 13, 2024).

Center on Budget & Policy Priorities. 2023b. *Policy basics: Supplemental security income.* Washington, DC. https://www.cbpp.org/research/social-security/policy-basics-introduction-to-supplemental-security-income (accessed March 13, 2024).

CDC (Centers for Disease Control and Prevention). 2008. Racial/ethnic disparities in self-rated health status among adults with and without disabilities—United States, 2004–2006. *Morbidity and Mortality Weekly Report* 57(39):1069–1073.

CDC. 2020. *Disability and health promotion: Disability datasets.* https://www.cdc.gov/ncbddd/disabilityandhealth/datasets.html (accessed March 13, 2024).

CMS (Centers for Medicare & Medicaid Services). n.d.-a. *Medicaid & CHIP for American Indians and Alaska natives.* https://www.healthcare.gov/american-indians-alaska-natives/medicaid-chip/ (accessed March 13, 2024).

CMS. n.d.-b. *Population Assessment of Tobacco and Health (PATH): Years survey included sexual and gender minority (SGM)-related questions, 2013-present.* https://www.cms.gov/files/document/sgm-clearinghouse-path-updated.pdf (accessed March 13, 2024).

CMS. 2021. *CMS program statistics.* https://data.cms.gov/collection/cms-program-statistics (accessed March 13, 2024).

CMS. 2022a. *Beneficiaries dually eligible for Medicare & Medicaid.* https://www.cms.gov/outreach-and-education/medicare-learning-network-mln/mlnproducts/downloads/medicare_beneficiaries_dual_eligibles_at_a_glance.pdf (accessed March 13, 2024).

CMS. 2022b. *CMS framework for health equity 2022–2032.* https://www.cms.gov/files/document/cms-framework-health-equity.pdf (accessed March 13, 2024).

CMS. 2023a. *CMCS informational bulletin: Guidance on adding sexual orientation and gender identity questions to state Medicaid and CHIP applications for health coverage.* https://www.medicaid.gov/sites/default/files/2023-11/cib11092023.pdf (accessed March 12, 2024).

CMS. 2023b. *New sexual orientation and gender identity (SOGI) questions on the marketplace application.* https://www.cms.gov/files/document/sogi-questions-marketplace-application.pdf (accessed March 12, 2024).

CMS. 2023c. *Model Medicare Advantage and Medicare prescription drug plan individual enrollment request: CMS-10718.* https://www.cms.gov/regulations-and-guidancelegislationpaperworkreductionactof1995pra-listing/cms-10718 (accessed March 13, 2024).

CMS. 2023d. *Direct enrollment and enhanced direct enrollment.* Developed by the Center for Consumer Information & Insurance Oversight. https://www.cms.gov/marketplace/agents-brokers/direct-enrollment-partners (accessed March 13, 2024).

CMS. 2023e. Agency information collection activities: Proposed collection; Comment request. *Federal Register* 88:67298–67299 (September 29, 2023).

CMS. 2024a. *People with disabilities: Supplementary Security Income (SSI) disability & Medicaid coverage.* https://www.healthcare.gov/people-with-disabilities/ssi-and-medicaid/ (accessed March 13, 2024).

CMS. 2024b. *CMS amendment approval: MassHealth Medicaid and Children's Health Insurance Plan (CHIP) section 1115 demonstration.* https://www.medicaid.gov/medicaid/section-1115-demonstrations/downloads/ma-masshealth-ca-04192024.pdf (accessed May 7, 2024).

Cole, M. B., J-H. Kim, T. W. Levengood, and A. N. Trivedi. 2021. Association of Medicaid expansion with 5-year changes in hypertension and diabetes outcomes at federally qualified health centers. *JAMA Health Forum* 2(9):E212375. https://doi.org/10.1001/jamahealthforum.2021.2375

Connecticut Office of Health Strategy. 2020. *The state of Connecticut state innovation model final & annual report.* Hartford, CT. https://portal.ct.gov/-/media/OHS/SIM/WorkStream-Updates/Final-AY4-Annual-Report_SIM_Master.pdf (accessed March 13, 2024).

Coursolle, A. 2023. *NHeLP welcomes the TGI Inclusive Care Act in California.* Washington, DC: National Health Law Program. https://healthlaw.org/nhelp-welcomes-the-tgi-inclusive-care-act-in-california/ (accessed March 13, 2024).

Crissman, H. P., M. B. Berger, L. F. Graham, and V. K. Dalton. 2017. Transgender demographics: A household probability sample of U.S. adults, 2014. *American Journal of Public Health* 107(2):213–215. https://doi.org/10.2105/ajph.2016.303571.

Dawson, L., M. Long, and B. Frederiksen. 2023. *LGBT+ people's health status and access to care*. San Francisco, CA: Keiser Family Foundation. https://www.kff.org/report-section/lgbt-peoples-health-status-and-access-to-care-issue-brief/ (accessed March 12, 2024).

Deutsch, M. B., J. Green, J. Keatley, G. Mayer, J. Hastings, A. M. Hall, R. Allison, O. Blumer, S. Brown, M. K. Cody, K. Fennie, G. Moscoe, R. St Claire, M. River Stone, A. Wilson, and C. Wolf-Gould. 2013. Electronic medical records and the transgender patient: Recommendations from the World Professional Association for Transgender Health EMR Working Group. *Journal of the American Medical Informatics Association* 20(4):700–703. https://doi.org/10.1136/amiajnl-2012-001472.

Dickey, L. M., S. L. Budge, S. L. Katz-Wise, and M. V. Garza. 2016. Health disparities in the transgender community: Exploring differences in insurance coverage. *Psychology of Sexual Orientation and Gender Diversity* 3(3):275–282. https://doi.org/10.1037/sgd0000169.

DoD (U.S. Department of Defense). 2021. *DoD instruction 1300.28: In-service transition for transgender service members*. Arlington, VA. https://www.esd.whs.mil/Portals/54/Documents/DD/issuances/dodi/130028p.pdf (accessed March 13, 2024).

Gates, J., and J. L. Herman. 2014. *Transgender military service in the United States*. Los Angeles, CA: UCLA School of Law, Williams Institute. https://williamsinstitute.law.ucla.edu/publications/trans-military-service-us/ (accessed March 13, 2024).

Goins, R. T., M. Moss, D. Buchwald, and J. M. Guralnik. 2007. Disability among older American Indians and Alaska Natives: An analysis of the 2000 census public use microdata sample. *Gerontologist* 47(5):690–696. https://doi.org/10.1093/geront/47.5.690.

Grasso, C., H. Goldhammer, D. Funk, D. King, S. L. Reisner, K. H. Mayer, and A. S. Keuroghlian. 2019. Required sexual orientation and gender identity reporting by U.S. health centers: First-year data. *American Journal of Public Health* 109(8):1111–1118. https://doi.org/10.2105/AJPH.2019.305130.

Haverkate, R. 2022. *IHS encourages the inclusion of sexual orientation and gender identity in electronic health records*. Rockville, MD: Indian Health Service, U.S. Department of Health and Human Services. https://www.ihs.gov/newsroom/ihs-blog/june-2022-blogs/ihs-encourages-the-inclusion-of-sexual-orientation-and-gender-identity-in-electronic-health-records/ (accessed March 13, 2024).

Haverkate, R. 2023. *IHS includes sexual orientation and gender identity in electronic health records*. Rockville, MD: Indian Health Service, U.S. Department of Health and Human Services. https://www.ihs.gov/newsroom/ihs-blog/june-2023-blogs/ihs-includes-sexual-orientation-and-gender-identity-in-electronic-health-records/ (accessed March 13, 2024).

HHS (U.S. Department of Health and Human Services). 2023. *Sexual orientation and gender identity (SOGI) data action plan*. Washington, DC. https://www.hhs.gov/sites/default/files/hhs-sogi-data-action-plan.pdf (accessed March 12, 2024).

HHS. 2024. Annual update of the HHS poverty guidelines. *Federal Register* 89:2961–2963. https://www.govinfo.gov/content/pkg/FR-2024-01-17/pdf/2024-00796.pdf (accessed March 13, 2024).

Hinton, E., and J. Raphel. 2023. *10 things to know about Medicaid managed care*. San Francisco, CA: KFF. https://www.kff.org/medicaid/issue-brief/10-things-to-know-about-medicaid-managed-care/ (accessed March 13, 2024).

Houston, C. 2023. *New data collection recommendations to address health disparities*. Chicago, IL: Blue Cross Blue Shield Association. https://www.bcbs.com/the-health-of-america/healthequity/new-data-collection-recommendations-address-health-disparities/ (accessed March 13, 2024).

HRSA (Health Resources and Services Administration). 2016. *Program assistance letter: Approved uniform data system changes for calendar year 2016.* North Bethesda, MD. https://bphc.hrsa.gov/sites/default/files/bphc/data-reporting/program-assistance-letter-2016-02.pdf (accessed March 13, 2024).

HRSA. 2023. *Uniform data system: 2023 manual, health center data reporting requirements.* North Bethesda, MD. https://bphc.hrsa.gov/sites/default/files/bphc/data-reporting/2023-uds-manual.pdf (accessed March 13, 2024).

HRSA. 2024a. *Health center program: Impact and growth.* North Bethesda, MD. https://bphc.hrsa.gov/about-health-centers/health-center-program-impact-growth (accessed March 13, 2024).

HRSA. 2024b. *Uniform Data System (UDS) Modernization Initiative.* https://bphc.hrsa.gov/data-reporting/uds-training-and-technical-assistance/uniform-data-system-uds-modernization-initiative (accessed May 7, 2024).

IHS (Indian Health Service). 2023. Data capture of sexual orientation and gender identity information. *Indian Health Service Circular* (23-02). Rockville, MD: Department of Health and Human Services. https://www.ihs.gov/ihm/circulars/2023/data-capture-of-sexual-orientation-and-gender-identity-information/ (accessed March 13, 2024).

KFF. 2023a. *2023 Employer health benefits survey.* San Francisco, CA. https://www.kff.org/report-section/ehbs-2023-survey-design-and-methods/ (accessed March 13, 2024).

KFF. 2023b. *State health facts: Medicaid income eligibility limits for adults as a percent of the federal poverty level.* San Francisco, CA. https://www.kff.org/affordable-care-act/state-indicator/medicaid-income-eligibility-limits-for-adults-as-a-percent-of-the-federal-poverty-level/?currentTimeframe=0&selectedDistributions=other-adults-for-an-individual&sortModel=%7B%22colId%22:%22Location%22,%22sort%22:%22asc%22%7D (accessed March 13, 2024).

KFF. 2024a. *Status of state Medicaid expansion decisions: Interactive map.* San Francisco, CA. https://www.kff.org/medicaid/issue-brief/status-of-state-medicaid-expansion-decisions-interactive-map/ (accessed March 13, 2024).

KFF. 2024b. *State health insurance marketplace types, 2024.* San Francisco, CA. https://www.kff.org/health-reform/state-indicator/state-health-insurance-marketplace-types/?currentTimeframe=0&sortModel=%7B%22colId%22:%22Location%22,%22sort%22:%22asc%22%7D (accessed March 13, 2024).

Kitson, K., and A. Ramos-Yamamoto. 2022. *State leaders should prioritize LGBT+ Californians' mental health.* Sacramento, CA: California Budget & Policy Center. https://calbudgetcenter.org/resources/state-leaders-should-prioritize-lgbtq-californians-mental-health (accessed March 13, 2024).

KPMAS (Kaiser Permanente Mid-Atlantic States). 2018. *New KPHC smartform helps provide culturally appropriate care for transgender patients.* Rockville, MD. https://kpproud-midatlantic.kaiserpermanente.org/new-kphc-smartform-helps-provide-culturally-appropriate-care-transgender-patients/ (accessed March 13, 2024).

Limburg, A. 2023. *New research links Medicaid and Census Bureau data to improve study of racial/ethnic health disparities.* Suitland, MD: U.S. Census Bureau. https://www.census.gov/library/stories/2023/04/missing-medicaid-data-on-race-ethnicity-may-bias-health-research.html (accessed March 13, 2024).

Marlay, M., T. File, and Z. Scherer. 2022. *Mental health struggles higher among LGBT adults than non-LGBT adults in all age groups.* Suitland, MD: U.S. Census Bureau. https://www.census.gov/library/stories/2022/12/lgbt-adults-report-anxiety-depression-at-all-ages.html (accessed March 13, 2024).

MassHealth. 2022. *Comprehensive quality strategy.* Quincy, MA. https://www.mass.gov/doc/masshealth-2022-comprehensive-quality-strategy-2/download (accessed March 13, 2024).

Matza, L., and A. McConnell. 2023. *Gender identity data collection & care decision-making within the Veterans Health Administration.* Washington, DC: Presentation to the National Academies of Science, Engineering & Medicine's Consensus Committee on Sex and Gender Identification and Implications for Disability Evaluation.

McDonald, K., A. Wec, R. Callahan, J. Markesich, B. Mory, and E. Grau. 2021. *National beneficiary survey-general waves round 7: Public use file codebook final report.* Washington, DC: Mathematica. https://www.ssa.gov/disabilityresearch/documents/NBSR7_PUFCodebook_Final_508C.pdf (accessed May 3, 2024).

NAIC (National Association of Insurance Commissioners). 2021. *Special committee on race and insurance–Workstream 5 (health) principles for data collection.* Washington, DC. https://content.naic.org/sites/default/files/inline-files/Principles%20for%20Data%20Collection%20-%20Final%20-%20Dec%202021.docx (accessed March 13, 2024).

NASEM (National Academies of Sciences, Engineering, and Medicine). 2022. *Measuring sex, gender identity, and sexual orientation.* Edited by N. Bates, M. Chin, and T. Becker. Washington, DC: The National Academies Press.

National Health Law Program. 2023. *Comment on CMS-2023-0161-0001.* Washington, DC: Centers for Medicare & Medicaid Services. https://www.regulations.gov/comment/CMS-2023-0161-0007 (accessed March 13, 2024).

NCES (National Center for Education Statistics). 2023. *NCES celebrates LGBTQ+ pride month.* Washington, DC: Institute of Education Sciences. https://nces.ed.gov/blogs/nces/post/nces-celebrates-lgbtq-pride-month (accessed March 13, 2024).

NCHS (National Center for Health Statistics). 2023. *Health insurance coverage: Household pulse survey, 2020-2023.* Atlanta, GA: Centers for Disease Control and Prevention. https://www.cdc.gov/nchs/covid19/pulse/health-insurance-coverage.htm (accessed March 13, 2024).

OEI (Office of Equity and Inclusion). n.d. *Using REALD and SOGI to identify and address health inequities.* Salem, OR: Oregon Health Authority. https://www.oregon.gov/oha/ei/pages/demographics.aspx (accessed March 13, 2024).

OEI. 2023. *OHA SOGI draft data collection recommendations.* Salem, OR: Oregon Health Authority. https://www.oregon.gov/oha/EI/REALD%20Documents/DRAFT-SOGI-Recommendations.pdf (accessed March 13, 2024).

Office of Governor Gavin Newsom. 2023. *Governor Newsom puts historic mental health transformation on March 2024 ballot.* https://www.gov.ca.gov/2023/10/12/governor-newsom-puts-historic-mental-health-transformation-on-march-2024-ballot/ (accessed March 13, 2024).

Office of the Chief Statistician of the United States. 2023. *Recommendations on the best practices for the collection of sexual orientation and gender identity data on federal statistical surveys.* https://www.whitehouse.gov/wp-content/uploads/2023/01/SOGI-Best-Practices.pdf (accessed March 13, 2024).

ONC (Office of the National Coordinator for Health Information Technology) and HHS (Department of Health and Human Services). 2015. 2015 Edition health information technology (Health IT) certification criteria, 2015 edition base electronic health record (EHR) definition, and ONC health IT certification program modifications. *Federal Register* 80(200):62602–62759. https://www.govinfo.gov/content/pkg/FR-2015-10-16/pdf/2015-25597.pdf (October 16, 2015).

Optum. 2023. *Health equity pillar.* Eden Prairie, MN. https://www.optum.com/content/dam/o4-dam/resources/pdfs/white-papers/OPA-Health-Equity-1-pager.pdf (accessed March 13, 2024).

Raths, D. 2023. *Humana, Optum Health execs describe building health equity infrastructure.* Healthcare Innovation. https://www.hcinnovationgroup.com/population-health-management/health-equity/article/53080313/humana-optum-health-execs-describe-building-health-equity-infrastructure (accessed March 13, 2024).

SAMHSA (Substance Abuse and Mental Health Services Administration). 2023. *Lesbian, gay, and bisexual behavioral health: Results from the 2021 and 2022 national surveys on drug use and health*. Rockville, MD: Department of Health and Human Services. https://www. samhsa.gov/data/sites/default/files/reports/rpt41899/2022NSDUHLGBBrief061623.pdf (accessed March 13, 2024).

Seto, B. 2017. *A coordinated transgender person care pathway*. Permanente Medicine. https:// permanente.org/coordinated-transgender-person-care-pathway/ (accessed March 13, 2024).

Siordia, C., R. A. Bell, and S. L. Haileselassie. 2017. Prevalence and risk for negative disability outcomes between American Indians-Alaskan Natives and other race-ethnic groups in the southwestern United States. *Journal of Racial & Ethnic Health Disparities* 4(2):195–200. https://doi.org/10.1007/s40615-016-0218-z

Social Security Administration. n.d. *Disability Benefits, Your Continuing Eligibility*. Baltimore, MD. https://www.ssa.gov/benefits/disability/work.html (accessed March 13, 2024).

SSA (Social Security Administration). 2021. *Social security disability and veterans affairs disability—How do they compare? Publication No. 64-125*. Baltimore, MD. https://www. ssa.gov/pubs/EN-64-125.pdf (accessed March 13, 2024).

SSA. 2024a. *A guide to supplemental security insurance (SSI) for groups and organizations. Publication No. 05-11015*. Baltimore, MD. https://www.ssa.gov/pubs/EN-05-11015.pdf (accessed March 13, 2024).

SSA. 2024b. *Disability benefits: How you qualify*. https://www.ssa.gov/benefits/disability/ qualify.html (accessed March 13, 2024).

SSA. 2024c. *Medicare. Publication No. 05-10043*. Baltimore, MD. https://www.ssa.gov/pubs/ EN-05-10043.pdf (accessed March 13, 2024).

SSA. 2024d. *Monthly statistical snapshot, January 2024*. Baltimore, MD. https://www.ssa.gov/ policy/docs/quickfacts/stat_snapshot/2024-02.pdf (accessed March 13, 2024).

SSA. 2024e. *Program operations manual system (POMS)*. http://policy.ssa.gov/poms.nsf/ lnx/0501715010 (accessed March 13, 2024).

SSA. 2024f. *SSI monthly statistics, January 2024*. https://www.ssa.gov/policy/docs/statcomps/ ssi_monthly/index.html (accessed March 13, 2024).

SSA. 2024g. *Supplemental Security Income (SSI) and eligibility for other government and state programs*. https://www.ssa.gov/ssi/text-other-ussi.htm (accessed March 13, 2024).

Straw, T. 2019. *"Direct enrollment" in marketplace coverage lacks protections for consumers, exposes them to harm*. Washington, DC: Center on Budget and Policy Priorities. https:// www.cbpp.org/research/direct-enrollment-in-marketplace-coverage-lacks-protections-for- consumers-exposes-them-to (accessed March 13, 2024).

Strong, A. 2022. *Beginning January 1, 2023–New rules for hospital patient discharge information reporting (2021 Session E2SHB 1272)*. Seattle, WA: Washington State Hospital Association. https://www.wsha.org/articles/beginning-january-1-2023-new-rules-for-hos- pital-patient-discharge-information-reporting-2021-session-e2shb-1272/ (accessed March 13, 2024).

TRICARE. 2023. *Beneficiaries eligible for TRICARE and Medicare*. Falls Church, VA: Defense Health Agency. https://www.tricare.mil/Plans/Eligibility/MedicareEligible (accessed March 13, 2024).

Truman, J., and R. Morgan. 2022. *Statistical brief: Violent victimization by sexual orientation and gender identity, 2017–2020*. Washington, DC: U.S. Department of Justice. https://bjs. ojp.gov/content/pub/pdf/vvsogi1720.pdf (accessed March 13, 2024).

VA (U.S. Department of Veterans Affairs). 2021. *TRICARE and Veterans Affairs: An overview of how TRICARE and the Department of Veterans Affairs work together to provide health benefits*. Presentation for the Department of Defense, Defense Health Agency. https://www.health.mil/Reference-Center/Presentations/2021/11/01/TRICARE-and- Veterans-Affairs-Slides (accessed March 13, 2024).

VA. 2022. *VA/DoD Health Affairs, VA & TRICARE information*. https://www.va.gov/ VADODHEALTH/TRICARE.asp (accessed March 13, 2024).

VA. 2023. *Veterans Health Administration, about VHA.* https://www.va.gov/health/aboutvha. asp (accessed March 13, 2024).

Ubri, P. S., L. Bailey, M. Gonsahn, K. Ford, and J. Murillo. 2023. *Data collection in Medicaid to advance health equity: Findings from interviews with state Medicaid agencies and managed care organizations.* Chicago, IL: NORC at the University of Chicago. https://www.norc.org/content/dam/norc-org/pdfs/HE%20Data%20Collection_Full%20Report.pdf (accessed March 13, 2024).

VHA (Veterans Health Administration). 2018. *VHA directive 1341(3): Providing health care for transgender and intersex veterans.* Washington, DC: Department of Veterans Affairs. https://www.patientcare.va.gov/LGBT/docs/directives/VHA_DIRECTIVE_1341.pdf (accessed March 13, 2024).

VHA. 2022. *Transgender and gender diverse veteran healthcare: Birth sex and gender identity.* Washington, DC: Department of Veteran Affairs. https://www.patientcare.va.gov/LGBT/docs/2022/Birth-Sex-Gender-Identity-FactSheet-for-Veterans-2022.pdf (accessed March 13, 2024).

Washington State Health Care Authority. 2022a. *Application for health care coverage.* Olympia, WA. https://www.hca.wa.gov/assets/free-or-low-cost/18-001P.pdf (accessed March 12, 2024).

Washington State Health Care Authority. 2022b. *CR-103P (December 2017) (Implements RCW 34.05.360).* Olympia, WA. https://doh.wa.gov/sites/default/files/2022-07/WSR%20 22-13-187.pdf?uid=62f6c59d3485c (accessed March 13, 2024).

Washington State Health Care Authority. 2024. *Gender identity information.* Olympia, WA. https://www.hca.wa.gov/about-hca/other-administrative-activities/gender-identity-information (accessed March 12, 2024).

Wolfe, H. L., T. L. Boyer, J. C. Shipherd, M. R. Kauth, G. K. Jasuja, and J. R. Blosnich. 2023. Barriers and facilitators to gender-affirming hormone therapy in the Veterans Health Administration. *Annals of Behavioral Medicine* 57(12):1014–1023. https://doi.org/10.1093/abm/kaad035.

Zylla, E., and E. Lukanen. 2024. *Sexual orientation and gender identity data: New and updated information on federal guidance and Medicaid data collection practices.* Minneapolis, MN: State Health Access Data Assistance Center. https://www.shvs.org/wp-content/uploads/2024/03/SHVS_Collection-of-Sexual-Orientation-and-Gender-Identity-Data_FINAL.pdf (accessed March 12, 2024).

Part II

Affirming Treatment and Care for Transgender and Gender Diverse People and People with Variations in Sex Traits

Part of understanding disability for transgender and gender diverse (TGD) people and people with variations in sex traits (VSTs) is understanding the affirming care interventions they may receive and how these interventions may impact disability determinations. In response to questions in the statement of task, the three chapters that form this part of the report focus on the broad and variable area of clinical care for TGD people and people with VSTs.

Chapter 5 provides an overview of gender-affirming care for TGD people across the lifespan, examining developmentally appropriate support for prepubescent gender diverse children; gender-affirming medical care for people who have delayed puberty and/or accessed gender-affirming hormone therapy (GAHT) during puberty; gender-affirming medical care for people who initiated GAHT and other care after puberty; gender-affirming surgery; nonmedical gender-affirming interventions; and psychosocial support and mental health care for TGD people and their families. Chapter 6 builds on this knowledge by describing various co-occurring conditions that may have a disproportionate impact on TGD populations and what this may mean for chronic disease and disability. Chapter 7 examines the numerous diagnoses that may fall under the category of VSTs and describes appropriate care for these populations, focusing on initial management of people with VSTs, hormone therapy, psychosocial and mental health supports, surgical interventions, and long-term care.

A theme running through these chapters is the wide variability in appropriate care across the life course. While existing guidelines put forward the highest standard of care, care for TGD people and people with VSTs is highly individualized and diverse. Each patient has a unique situation and personal goals for treatment, and there is no "one size fits all" approach. In addition, as described in Part I of this report, TGD people and people with VSTs encounter considerable challenges and inequalities in their ability to access competent health care services. For individual patients, these challenges and inequalities may impact appropriate medical monitoring and follow-up, resulting in considerable variability in treatment histories and outcomes. The committee notes this variability to describe for the Social Security Administration the range of care that may be documented in an applicant's medical record and the uneven or inadequate access to care that may impact health and chronic disease in ways that are often beyond the applicant's control.

5

Gender-Affirming Care for Transgender and Gender Diverse People

This chapter provides an overview of gender-affirming care for transgender and gender diverse (TGD) people across the lifespan in response to questions in the statement of task. The chapter begins with a discussion of developmentally appropriate support for prepubescent gender diverse children; in contrast with prepubescent children with variations in sex traits (VSTs) (as described in Chapter 7), prepubescent gender diverse children do not require any gender-affirming medical interventions. However, psychosocial support for gender diverse children and their families may be critical to ensure a safe environment for these children to thrive, and this chapter describes these important interventions.

Next, the chapter describes gender-affirming medical care for people who have accessed puberty-delaying medication and/or gender-affirming hormone therapy (GAHT) during puberty, including treatment with gonadotropin-releasing hormone (GnRH) analogs, exogenous testosterone, or estrogens. This is followed by an overview of gender-affirming medical care for people who initiated GAHT and other care after puberty. The committee separated these two TGD populations—those that receive GAHT during puberty and those that receive it after—as their developmental and health trajectories may differ in some known respects (e.g., with regard to physical appearance and mental health), while the long-term benefits and risks of early medical intervention are under study and not yet fully understood. However, research to date clearly indicates that gender-affirming medical interventions during puberty and adolescence lead to reduced gender

143

dysphoria and increased mental health for TGD youth (Connolly et al., 2016; de Vries and Cohen-Kettenis, 2012; de Vries et al., 2011; Van Der Miesen et al., 2020).

Following this discussion, the chapter examines gender-affirming surgery, reviewing facial, breast, chest, and genital surgeries. Next, the chapter briefly discusses nonmedical gender-affirming interventions, such as chest binding, packing, and the practice of silicone injections—the latter not uncommon and with potential disabling consequences.

In addition to the medical interventions of hormone therapy and surgery, psychosocial support and mental health care are, for many TGD people and their families, of utmost importance in coping with gender dysphoria, as well as the social stigma attached to nonconformity in gender identity and expression. The latter leads to minority stress, which has been shown to negatively affect TGD people's mental health and physical well-being (Delozier et al., 2020; Gosling et al., 2022; Pellicane and Ciesla, 2022; Pellicane et al., 2023; Valentine and Shipherd, 2018). The chapter provides an overview of TGD people's identity development across the lifespan, and how families, peers, and mental health professionals can play an important role in facilitating resilience, health, and well-being. Finally, the chapter describes the wide variability in gender-affirming care accessed by TGD people across the life course.

PREPUBESCENT GENDER DIVERSE CHILDREN: DEVELOPMENTALLY APPROPRIATE PSYCHOSOCIAL SUPPORT

Until relatively recently, little attention has been directed toward prepubescent gender diverse children, most likely because, particularly in the United States, gender-affirming health care has been limited for minors of all ages. It is only more recently that gender health centers have proliferated in the United States, typically following the model of prioritizing medical care, and therefore serving only postpubertal children and their families. Nevertheless, the distribution of these centers varies significantly by geographic location, with less access to care in southern portions of the United States. Thus, care for gender diverse prepubescent children—who do not qualify for any medical interventions to affirm their gender diversity—has been less well understood clinically and empirically than care for older youth and adults.

More recently, however, increased attention has prioritized the experiences and needs of gender diverse children prior to puberty, although characterization of this population through research remains undeveloped. For the first time, the World Professional Association for Transgender Health (WPATH) included a separate chapter on best practices and recommmendations for the care of prepubescent gender diverse children in the

Standards of Care Version 8 (SOC-8) (Coleman et al., 2022). This section of the SOC-8, based on an understanding of ethics, a review of research, and clinical expert consensus, draws on several foundational principles and frameworks extracted from clinical and developmental psychology, including ecological models and principles of developmental psychopathology. The text stipulates that gender diversity is an expected developmental variation and not a mental health disorder, and that attempts to "convert" a gender diverse child to be more gender typical of any given culture risks significant harm and should not be attempted. The chapter also emphasizes that gender expressions and identities may evolve over the course of childhood and later, and that children should be supported in gender fluidity over time.

Frameworks for Understanding the Development of Transgender and Gender Diverse Children

An ecological model of child development is rooted in the understanding that a child's well-being and safety should be prioritized in all settings in which the child functions (e.g., home, school) (Belsky, 1993; Bronfenbrenner, 1979; Lynch and Cicchetti, 1998) in order to foster positive mental health and adaptation over time. Additionally, a developmental psychopathology framework, established by a wealth of empirical research, demonstrates that childhood experiences are linked to trajectories of well-being that can continue from childhood through adolescence and into adulthood; these early life experiences may be predictive of resilience or the exacerbation of vulnerabilities and risks over time.

Early childhood is an important developmental period in many ways. Childhood is a time when a young person develops a schema or understanding of the world and of themselves, often based on their earliest relationships. As one example, much research demonstrates that secure caregiver–child relationships early in life are fundamental to positive development and continuing relationship stability over time (Hong and Park, 2012). When stress and adversity disrupt a child's well-being and relationships, the effects can be broad and can negatively impact most or all aspects of the child's mental health and function, including social, academic, emotional regulation, and somatic well-being (Nelson et al., 2020; Nurius et al., 2015). Thus, positive support and safety are important for a child's quality of life, but also for ensuring that a child has the resilience, confidence, and support to adapt during important life transitions, including that from childhood to adolescence. Thus, the prepubescent years offer an opportunity to nurture characteristics—such as confidence, optimism, and a strong sense of self—that will facilitate a child's resilience. Conversely, early-life adversities are harmful to children and are linked to a significant array of negative mental and physical health outcomes, including trauma (Anda et al., 2010; CDC, 2021; Masten and Cicchetti, 2010; Shonkoff and Garner, 2012).

TGD youth experience significantly higher rates of adversity, such as family rejection, maltreatment, and bullying, relative to their cisgender peers, with risks for continuing and accumulating mental health disabilities. Research indicates that this type of chronic stress is associated with somatic/medical morbidities as well, both from direct exposure to violence to the impacts of chronic stress on somatic well-being. In addition, TGD children often encounter persisting gender minority stressors, including lack of recognition of their gender diversity (such as deliberate misgendering), exclusion from normative peer-related activities, and ostracism within and outside of families. Although risks associated with exposure to detrimental experiences are high, research also demonstrates that family and peer acceptance can mitigate these risks to well-being for TGD children (Cardona et al., 2023; Olson et al., 2016; Pariseau et al., 2019), and children supported in their diverse identities have been shown to be well adjusted (Olson et al., 2016).

Gender Stability

At this point, researchers are unable to reliably predict the stability of a diverse gender identity expressed during childhood. Much of the research published on the stability/instability of gender identity has been criticized, particularly for not using assessment measures in childhood that clearly and validly differentiate measures of gender identity from gender expression, and some of which measure only binary (versus nonbinary) gender identities (Ehrensaft et al., 2018; Olezeski et al., 2020). The invalidity of earlier research and the limited ability to measure diversity in gender identity in childhood create obstacles to identifying rates of TGD identity in prepubescent children and to understanding the needs of these children. Research on gender stability among prepubescent TGD children is limited but suggests that children who are the most assertive about their gender diverse identity experience more identity stability compared with their less assertive peers (Olson et al., 2022; Rae et al., 2019; Steensma et al., 2013). It is likely, however, that social context and acceptance may influence a child's comfort and sense of safety in asserting a noncisgender identity, which may then complicate understanding of the occurrence and stability of gender diversity in these children. In general, as recommended in the recently published WPATH SOC-8, it is important to recognize that young TGD children may experience gender fluidity or gender evolution over time, which may be represented by inconsistencies in gender designations in medical records (Coleman et al., 2022).

Gender-Affirming Care for Prepubescent Children

The WPATH SOC-8, as well as a corresponding article (Tishelman and Rider, 2023), provides important recommendations for mental health approaches to protective care for prepubescent children. Mental health intervention is not mandatory for young TGD children. Whether to seek mental health guidance is a decision typically made by caregivers, sometimes with strong recommendations from medical providers, teachers, or others. Assessment and therapeutic supports can be critical for many purposes, including advocacy and support for safety across environments; help in reducing family conflict and increasing family acceptance and positive communication; aid in strategizing whether and how to implement a social transition process (a process by which a child manifests changes in gender expression, including pronoun preferences, name changes, and so on); assistance with caregiver support and guidance; screening for mental health adjustment and risks in the child and other family members; increasing the child's and family members' gender-related knowledge and body literacy, including preparation for changes associated with puberty; decision making about potential medical interventions at the time of puberty and after; supporting the child and family members in developing positive coping strategies; and fostering resilience.

GENDER-AFFIRMING CARE FOR PEOPLE WHO INITIATE MEDICAL INTERVENTIONS DURING PUBERTY

Gender-affirming care for TGD people is multidisciplinary and includes both medical care and psychosocial support. In this section, the committee focuses on the medical care of TGD people who have delayed puberty through the use of GnRH analogs and/or received masculinizing or feminizing hormone therapy during puberty (i.e., during childhood and adolescence). The goal of these hormonal treatments is to align the physical characteristics of TGD youth with their gender identity. These medical interventions can help reduce gender dysphoria and improve quality of life for TGD people (Coleman et al., 2022; Van Der Miesen et al., 2020). However, medical interventions are not necessary for all TGD people (Coleman et al., 2022). Some TGD youth may be comfortable with their bodies or find other ways of expressing their authentic self and gender identity. Ideally, the decision to pursue medical interventions is made in consultation with a multidisciplinary team of health care professionals with expertise in gender-affirming care. Members of the health care team typically include adolescent medicine specialists, pediatric endocrinologists, behavioral health specialists, social workers, and nursing support staff (Coyne et al., 2023).

Gender-affirming medical care for TGD people should be patient centered, such that clinicians respect patients' autonomy, preferences, values, dignity, individuality, and goals. Such standards are applicable to all health care situations. Patient-centered care is particularly important for gender-affirming care since, as discussed in Chapter 3, many TGD people experience barriers to care (e.g., difficulty locating care, disrespect, stigma in health care environments, discriminatory laws that prohibit gender-affirming care). The medical care of TGD people should be evidence based, culturally competent, and tailored to the individual needs and circumstances of each patient (Coleman et al., 2022; Salas-Humara et al., 2019).

With minors, psychologists, psychiatrists, and/or other behavioral health specialists are often asked to collaborate with patients and their families to aid in understanding their needs—which is necessary for making informed decisions about gender-affirming interventions (medical, psychosocial, or both)—and to facilitate access to these services. These clinicians also can aid in facilitating appropriate assent and consent processes[1] to ensure that youth and their parents/caregivers understand the short- and long-term implications of treatment decisions, even when assent and consent are complex because of disabilities or other factors (Shumer and Tishelman, 2015). The SOC-8 strongly emphasizes the need for a process of biopsychosocial assessment and decision making prior to the initiation of gender-affirming medical care for adolescents; typically, this process will occur with a mental health provider trained in this type of assessment. Thus, the medical care of TGD people involves much more than gender-affirming hormonal and surgical interventions; clinicians also provide accurate information, offer emotional support, help with shared decision making, and coordinate care across different settings and disciplines.

For prepubescent children, hormone therapy, surgeries, and other treatment options described in this chapter are not appropriate (Hembree et al., 2017; Salas-Humara et al., 2019). For these young children, the only

---

[1] Consent may only be given by individuals who have reached the legal age of consent (in the United States, this is typically age 18). "Assent" is an agreement by an individual who is not competent to give legally valid informed consent (e.g., a child aged 7–17 or cognitively impaired person). As part of the assent process, minors receive developmentally appropriate information about medical interventions to help them decide whether they want to take part. The American Academy of Pediatrics Committee on Bioethics (1995) describes appropriate assent as including the following: (1) Helping the patient achieve a developmentally appropriate awareness of the nature of their condition; (2) Telling the patient what he or she can expect with tests and treatment(s); and (3) Making a clinical assessment of the patient's understanding of their condition and what, if any, outside factors may be influencing the patient's response (including whether there is inappropriate pressure to accept treatment).

care choices are nonmedical and involve psychosocial interventions when needed, as described above (Coleman et al., 2022; Salas-Humara et al., 2019). For hormonal and surgical interventions, minors under age 18 provide assent and their parents or legal guardians provide consent before the intervention proceeds (Coleman et al., 2022; Salas-Humara et al., 2019). Individuals aged 18 and older can provide consent for hormonal and surgical interventions (Coleman et al., 2022; Salas-Humara et al., 2019).

Puberty-Delaying Medication

Puberty begins when increased GnRH is secreted from the hypothalamus, which causes the pituitary gland to secrete hormones known as gonadotropins (Abdel-Aziz et al., 2021). The gonadotropins cause the gonads (ovaries and testes) to produce the sex steroids estrogen and testosterone, respectively, which leads to the development of secondary sex characteristics. Puberty-delaying medications[2] (also referred to as puberty blockers or puberty suppression) are GnRH analogs that act on the pituitary gland to prevent release of the gonadotropins, thereby forestalling the hormonal and physical changes of puberty (Salas-Humara et al., 2019). These medications have been used for many years to treat some forms of precocious (early) puberty and have been found to be safe and effective (Conn and Crowley, 1991; Martinerie et al., 2020). Importantly, use of these medications to treat these specific forms of precocious puberty does not cause infertility in adulthood (Kim, 2015).

When given early in puberty, GnRH analogs can ease "gender dysphoria"—the distress TGD adolescents may experience when their body does not align with their gender identity (Achille et al., 2020; Chakraborty et al., 2023; de Vries et al., 2011; Kuper et al., 2020; Van Der Miesen et al., 2020). Gender dysphoria can negatively affect adolescents' general mental health, hamper their social development, and increase their vulnerability to self-harm and suicide (Marconi et al., 2023). By causing puberty delay, treatment with GnRH analogs may prevent these adverse outcomes, provide relief of psychological distress, and allow more time for psychosocial exploration of gender identity and expression (Achille et al., 2020; Allen et al., 2019). GnRH analogs prevent pubertal changes such as breast development and deepening of the voice, which are irreversible, thus alleviating dysphoria and reducing the need for future gender-affirming chest or voice

---

[2] It should be noted that puberty delay as described in terms of gender-affirming care is not the same thing as "delayed puberty." "Delayed puberty" is a medical condition in which puberty happens later than it is supposed to as part of a physical health condition. "Puberty-delaying medications" are used to pause puberty for adolescents who seek this intervention as part of gender-affirming care.

surgery (Patel et al., 2020; Van De Grift et al., 2020). GnRH analogs can also prevent menses, although this can also be achieved with other medications (Mauvais-Jarvis et al., 2013).[3]

Two medications are commonly used to suppress puberty: histrelin acetate (a long-acting, flexible rod inserted under the skin of the arm that typically lasts for 1–2 years) and leuprolide acetate (a long-acting injectable medication that typically lasts for 1, 3, or 4 months at a time) (Krebs et al., 2022). These medications are given only to children who have started puberty (i.e., have begun to undergo development of breast tissue or enlargement of the testes); puberty typically begins between ages 8 and 13 for children with ovaries and between ages 9 and 14 for children with testes. As with most other medical interventions for minors, puberty delay requires assent from the minor patient and consent from parents or guardians (Shumer and Tishelman, 2015).

Puberty-delaying medications are typically continued for a few months to several years, depending on an individual's age and circumstances. This treatment provides time for youth and families to consider whether to initiate masculinizing or feminizing hormone therapy (with exogenous testosterone or estrogen, respectively), and if so, when (Guss and Gordon, 2022). Use of GnRH does not mean that gender diverse adolescents will subsequently start a course of hormone therapy: one study of 434 adolescents found that GnRH use did not increase the likelihood of subsequent use of gender-affirming hormones (Nos et al., 2022). However, findings are inconsistent, and some other research has demonstrated a high likelihood of adolescents continuing on to be prescribed gender-affirming hormones (Lee, 2023; Verroken et al., 2022).

The effects of puberty-delaying medications are generally reversible; if the youth stops taking them, puberty will resume within about 6 months (Salas-Humara et al., 2019). While physical changes may be reversible, however, there may be psychological or neurocognitive changes that are not reversible, and these important issues need additional investigation (Chen et al., 2020; Jorgensen et al., 2022). In addition, youth who began puberty-delaying medications early in puberty (e.g., Tanner Stage or sexual maturity rating 2) and who then initiate and remain on exogenous testosterone or estrogen will likely experience changes in fertility (discussed below) (Cheng et al., 2019).

Research is examining the associations between puberty-delaying medications and changes in bone density and neuronal maturation; both of these

---

[3] The American College of Obstetricians and Gynecologists (ACOG) advises that hormone therapy for menstrual suppression is safe and effective in adolescent populations. According to ACOG (2022), there are many methods for achieving menstrual suppression, including "combined oral contraceptive pills, combined hormonal patches, vaginal rings, progestin-only pills, depot medroxyprogesterone acetate, the levonorgestrel-releasing intrauterine device, and the etonogestrel implant" (p. 528).

potential associations are likely further modified by treatment with exogenous testosterone or estrogen (Ciancia et al., 2022; Van Der Loos et al., 2023). Additionally, for youth with a penis, puberty-delaying medications maintain the penis at its prepubertal size, leaving less available tissue for future vaginoplasty (Cheng et al., 2019). Any potential side effects should be carefully weighed against the benefits of alleviating and preventing gender dysphoria and improving mental health outcomes. Shared decision making by the youth, the parents (if the youth is younger than 18 years), and the health care team enables comprehensive discussions regarding the benefits and risks of specific treatment options (Mazzola et al., 2023).

Gender-Affirming Masculinizing or Feminizing Hormone Therapy during Puberty

Many, but certainly not all, TGD people initiate gender-affirming masculinizing or feminizing hormone therapy (Lane et al., 2022). Exogenously administered testosterone and estrogen help TGD people achieve, respectively, a more masculine or feminine appearance.

Testosterone

Testosterone induces changes in the body similar to those expected during typical male puberty, including increased growth of facial and body hair, deepening of the voice, and increased muscle mass and strength, as well as clitoral enlargement (Irwig, 2017; Yeung et al., 2019). The timeline for changes varies among patients, but most changes begin to take place within about 3–6 months of initiating the therapy and are fully realized after 2–5 years (Irwig, 2017). Clinicians should discuss with patients and families and monitor the potential side effects of testosterone therapy, such as increased risk of acne, male-pattern baldness (Yeung et al., 2019), increased cholesterol levels, and changes in sexual function. Testosterone also stimulates erythropoiesis, the production of red blood cells, and can unmask erythrocytosis (overproduction of red blood cells).

The most commonly used formulations of testosterone in the United States are testosterone enanthate (Delatestryl) and testosterone cypionate (Depo-Testosterone), which are injected intramuscularly or intradermally (Unger, 2016). Long-acting injectable testosterone formulations, implantable testosterone, buccal patches, and oral testosterone are available but less commonly used in the United States. Testosterone patches were discontinued in the United States in spring 2023 as they can cause contact dermatitis (itchy rash) which many patients found irritating (ASHP, 2023; Fleshner and Lawrentschuk, 2009). Testosterone gels are common but are more difficult to adjust in dose compared with other modalities (Unger, 2016). Testosterone may interact with other medications or supplements an individual may be taking, but drug–drug interactions are rare (Moyer et al., 2019). Patients should be counseled that testosterone does not prevent pregnancy, even if they are not experiencing menstrual periods; thus, contraception should still be used for birth control (e.g., condoms; or long-acting reversible contraceptives such as an intrauterine device or etonogestrel implants, which can often further suppress menstruation) (Cheng et al., 2019).

Estrogen

Estrogen therapy and the suppression of testosterone induce changes similar to those expected during typical female puberty. Effects include growth of breast tissue and redistribution of fat to the buttocks and thighs (Patel et al., 2020). Lower levels of testosterone can also result in decreases in body hair, facial hair, muscle mass, acne, and balding. Decreases in spermatogenesis result in decreased testicular mass (Sinha et al., 2021). The timeline for changes varies among patients, but changes typically begin within about 3–6 months of initiating hormone therapy and continue for 2–5 years.

Estrogen therapy is associated with increased risk of blood clots (Abou-Ismail et al., 2020; Rosendaal et al., 2002). These side effects are not unique to TGD people, as cisgender people who take estrogen therapy experience these risks as well (Abou-Ismail et al., 2020; LaVasseur et al., 2022; Rozenberg et al., 2021). The most common forms of estrogen used in the United States are oral pills, injections, and transdermal patches (Safer and Tangpricha, 2019b). The choice of formulation depends on the individual's preference, medical history, and other factors. Transdermal patches are associated with lower or no risk of blood clots but may be more expensive than other formulations (Abou-Ismail et al., 2020). Exogenous estrogen therapy does not typically interact with other medications or supplements an individual may be taking, although some binding proteins are increased that result in changes to some laboratory readings (Moyer et al., 2019).

Medical Monitoring

Given the changes and potential side effects that testosterone and estrogen can induce, individuals receiving GAHT should undergo regular monitoring, including blood work (Hembree et al., 2017). Youth who begin receiving estrogen or testosterone following pubertal delay should have their height and weight checked, ideally every 3 months, during the first year of treatment (Hembree et al., 2017). Hormone levels (i.e., testosterone or estradiol) should be monitored with blood testing to ensure adequate dosing and adherence to treatment; levels should be checked more frequently when treatment is initiated or dose adjustments are made and can be checked less frequently once patients are on a stable regimen (Hembree et al., 2017). For patients on injectable formulations, interpretation of levels should be based on the timing of the most recent dose (i.e., peak, mid, or trough levels). At least yearly during adolescence, clinicians should order a complete metabolic panel, lipid panel, and hemoglobin A1C test; collectively, these assess renal function, liver function, cholesterol levels, and risk for diabetes (Hembree et al., 2017).

Dual X-ray absorptiometry scans should be performed to assess bone mineral density, especially among TGD youth using puberty-delaying medications without gender-affirming masculinizing or feminizing hormone therapy. Treatment with GnRH analogs followed by long-term gender-affirming masculinizing hormone therapy has been shown to be safe with respect to bone health in TGD people receiving testosterone (Ciancia et al., 2022); whether that is true for feminizing regimens remains to be established (Van Der Loos et al., 2023).

Fluidity of Gender Identity and Provider Response

Recent research has indicated that gender identity may evolve or be fluid for some adolescents (Katz-Wise et al., 2023a); thus, teens may experience shifts in needs and desires for medical interventions, with implications for a slower process of decision making for some (Cohen et al., 2023). Although understudied, some research also indicates that individuals may sometimes reflect upon the need or desire for continuing previously initiated GAHT, and mental health assistance may support individuals with decision making regarding care needs across time (MacKinnon et al., 2023).

Fertility Preservation

Before initiating gender-affirming hormone therapy, clinicians need to explain to youth and families that youth who receive puberty blockers followed by exogenous testosterone or estrogen may experience reduced fertility (Cheng et al., 2019; Choi and Kim, 2022). Specifically, puberty-delaying medications suppress germ cell maturation in ovaries and testes. Subsequently, sustained therapy with exogenous testosterone (in an individual with ovaries) prevents ovulation and menses, and sustained therapy with exogenous estrogen (in an individual with testes) prevents sperm development (Greenwald et al., 2021). Stimulated egg retrieval has been achieved in patients who started GnRH agonists early. In addition, in vitro fertilization (IVF) pregnancy has occurred with eggs retrieved from patients who did not stop testosterone (Greenwald et al., 2021). Thus, clinicians should present fertility preservation options to youth and their families, specifically cryopreservation of ova and sperm. Ova and sperm can be retrieved once youth are midpuberty or at any time thereafter, and ideally before initiation of puberty-delaying medications (Choi and Kim, 2022). Fertility preservation may be possible for youth with ovaries who are prepubertal or in early puberty, but clinically available fertility preservation options for youth with testes do not exist unless spermatogenesis has occurred. Later in life, ova and sperm can be used for IVF (Choi and Kim, 2022). Individuals without a functional uterus typically require that a surrogate carrier with a functional uterus carry the pregnancy (Cheng et al., 2019).

Many clinicians refer youth and their families to an interdisciplinary fertility clinic that can offer integrated medical and psychosocial care. Limited access to and the cost of high-quality fertility services may be prohibitive for some families—such services are often not covered by health insurance—thus contributing to disparities in care.

Long-Term Follow-Up

During the initiation of GAHT, patients should return at least every 3 months for monitoring of their hormonal levels and assessment of whether treatment is meeting their goals (Hembree et al., 2017). After the first year of therapy, visits can be spaced to approximately every 6 months or even longer, provided that hormone treatment doses are stable, the therapy is meeting the patient's goals, and the patient is not experiencing significant side effects or other complications. Ongoing support and care coordination from the clinician/health care team are beneficial, as gender-affirming care involves more than hormones. Thus, patients and their families should be supported in meeting with members of their health care team more frequently than every 6 months if requested. Additionally, when a multidisciplinary team is involved, and especially when care involves minors, patients may visit more frequently for psychosocial support and therapy, as well as coordination with medical intervention. More frequent visits can be particularly helpful for youth taking puberty-delaying medications who may need to decide whether and when to initiate gender-affirming masculinizing or feminizing hormone therapy, in collaboration with the team endocrinologist. Moreover, psychosocial support and therapy can benefit youth greatly in addressing social or emotional challenges that may arise. As discussed above, research indicates that it is not uncommon for adolescents' gender identities to evolve over time (Cohen et al., 2023; Katz-Wise et al., 2023b), and gender-affirming mental health professionals can help youth and families, when appropriate, to consider their evolving gender-affirming care priorities as they develop.

GENDER-AFFIRMING MEDICAL CARE FOR PEOPLE WHO INITIATE GENDER-AFFIRMING HORMONE THERAPY AND OTHER CARE AFTER PUBERTY

Many TGD people do not seek gender-affirming medical care until after puberty. For some, this may be shortly after puberty is complete (which typically occurs in late adolescence or young adulthood and may occur before or after attaining the age of majority); others may access gender-affirming care later in life, long after puberty is complete. The reasons to wait to seek gender-affirming care until after puberty are varied: for some, postpubertal initiation of gender-affirming care reflects their personal choice, but others may lack information about possible interventions until adulthood, may not have the familial support and financial resources required, and/or may lack access to appropriate providers, all of which may prohibit initiation of gender-affirming care at an earlier stage (Puckett et al., 2018). Postpuberty, TGD people may seek any one of a number of gender-affirming interventions (as described further in this chapter), including GAHT. This section describes common GAHT regimens for these groups of TGD people, modifications to GAHT regimens to meet individual patient goals, and long-term follow-up for this patient population.

Gender-Affirming Masculinizing or Feminizing Hormone Therapy Postpuberty

As in the use of GAHT during puberty, the primary therapeutic goal for GAHT postpuberty is to allow for the acquisition of secondary sex characteristics (e.g., voice, facial hair, breast size, distribution of body fat and muscle) more aligned with an individual's gender identity. For TGD people who seek gender-affirming medical care after puberty, masculinizing hormone therapy usually consists of exogenous testosterone to increase testosterone levels to the typical range of cisgender men (300–1,000 ng/dL). Feminizing hormone therapy usually consists of exogenous estrogen, along with other antiandrogens used adjunctively, to decrease testosterone to the typical range of cisgender women (<50 ng/dL). The literature describes commonly used masculinizing and femininizing hormone regimens, and these are presented briefly in the sections below (Ramsay and Safer, 2023; Safer and Tangpricha, 2019a,b). Boxes 5-1 and 5-2 display common GAHT regimens for TGD people that may be referred to in medical records.

Masculinizing Hormone Therapy

Both transgender men and other gender diverse individuals (including nonbinary and bigender people) may seek masculinizing hormone therapy

---

BOX 5-1
Common Masculinizing Hormone Therapy Regimens That May Be Referred to in Medical Records

Parenteral
- Testosterone ester (enanthate or cypionate)
- Testosterone undecanoate

Transdermal or transbuccal
- Testosterone gel
- Testosterone patch
- Testosterone buccal patch

Oral
- Testosterone undecanoate

SOURCE: Safer and Tangpricha, 2019b.

---

with the goal of developing typical male secondary sex characteristics, while minimizing sex characteristics typically associated with females. The use of GAHT in these populations is very similar to the hormone replacement therapy that cisgender men may need for hypogonadism (where the testes produce little or no hormones),[4] with some dosing modifications.

As shown in Box 5-1, testosterone can be administered orally, transdermally, or parenterally, and regimens consist of gels, patches, injectable esters, and long-acting implanted testosterone (Barbonetti et al., 2020; Ramsay and Safer, 2023). Exogenous testosterone preparations currently used in the United States are chemically equivalent to the testosterone secreted from human testes (Barbonetti et al., 2020; Shoskes et al., 2016). The most popular formulation is a testosterone ester (enanthate or cypionate) 50–200 mg weekly administered intramuscularly or subcutaneously (Safer and Tangpricha, 2019b; Spratt et al., 2017), although some patients may prefer higher doses (100–200 mg) administered less frequently. Transdermal testosterone gel (2.5–10 g/day) can achieve the same virilizing effects as injection testosterone, but poor absorption may prove frustrating, especially to larger patients (Safer and Tangpricha, 2019a). Although not widely used,

---

[4] "Hypogonadism" occurs when the body's sex glands (the testes or ovaries) produce little or no hormones. Some types of hypogonadism can be treated with hormone replacement therapy (Kumar et al., 2010).

oral testosterone undecanoate (160–240 mg/day), long-acting implanted testosterone pellets, and long-acting injectable testosterone are also available (Safer and Tangpricha, 2019b). There is no indication for adjunct antiestrogens therapy.

Over the first 3–12 months, response to testosterone treatment may include increased facial/body hair, male-pattern balding, increased acne, increased libido, increased muscle mass, clitoromegaly, deepening of the voice, and redistribution of fat (Safer and Tangpricha, 2019b). Menses cease in most individuals within 6 months of starting treatment.

Feminizing Hormone Therapy

Both transgender women and other gender diverse individuals (including nonbinary and bigender people) may seek femininizing hormone therapy with the goal of developing typical female secondary sex characteristics, while minimizing sex characteristics typically associated with males. Commonly used exogenous estradiol can suppress testosterone levels via central feedback while avoiding hypogonadism. The use of GAHT in these populations is similar to hormone replacement therapy that cisgender women use to treat menopausal symptoms, with some dosing modifications (Safer and Tangpricha 2019a; Vigneswaran and Hamoda, 2022).

Like testosterones, estrogens can be administered orally, transdermally, or parenterally, as shown in Box 5-2. The primary class of exogenous estrogen used in feminizing hormone therapy, 17-beta estradiol, is chemically identical to estradiol, a naturally occurring hormone produced by the ovaries. Oral 17-beta estradiol (2–10 mg) daily is a popular regimen because it is easy to use and readily available. Also, 17-beta estradiol can be delivered via transdermal patch. Data suggest that this approach may reduce the risk of venous thromboembolism (blood clots) associated with exogenous estradiol use,[5] and WPATH guidelines recommend transdermal estradiol in doses up to 100 mcg/daily for individuals aged 45 and older (Coleman et al., 2022). In addition, estradiol can be administered orally as conjugated estrogens (2.5–7.5 mg) or parenterally as estradiol valerate or cypionate (5–20 mg intramuscularly every 2 weeks or 2–10 mg intramuscularly every week). Each formulation may result in metabolites that can confound the measurement of hormone levels. Ethinyl estradiol should be

---

[5] There may be a slightly elevated potential for venous thromboembolism with exogenous estrogens. The risk is relatively low with estrogens in current use for TGD people. Therefore, for transgender women and nonbinary individuals seeking feminizing hormone treatment with a history of venous thromboembolism, it may be most effective to maintain the hormone treatment regimen and to follow prophylaxis protocols (Abou-Ismail et al., 2020).

BOX 5-2
Common Feminizing Hormone Therapy Regimens That May Be Referred to in Medical Records

Estrogens

Oral
- Estradiol (17-beta estradiol)
- Conjugated estrogens

Transdermal
- Estradiol patch

Parenteral
- Estradiol valerate

Androgen-lowering or inhibiting agents

Spironolactone
Cyproterone acetate
gonadotropin-releasing hormone (GnRH) agonists (e.g., leuprolide)

SOURCE: Safer and Tangpricha, 2019b.

---

avoided because of its increased risk of venous thromboembolism (Hembree et al., 2017; Safer and Tangpricha, 2019b).

Incorporating in the hormone regimen an adjunctive antiandrogen (which suppresses testosterone) is thought to allow for lower doses of estrogen, decreasing the dose-related risk of venous thromboembolism. Spironolactone—an aldosterone receptor antagonist that can also inhibit the secretion of testosterone—is the most commonly prescribed adjunct antiandrogen agent because it is the least costly (Ramsay and Safer, 2023). Spironolactone is typically administered to TGD people in doses of 100–200 mg daily. GnRH analogs, such as leuprolide (3.75 mg administered subcutaneously monthly), are another common androgen-lowering agent, working to inhibit the production of luteinizing hormone and follicle-stimulating hormone, and therefore testosterone (Ramsay and Safer, 2023). GnRH analogs are the preferred adjunct to estrogens in the United Kingdom, but they are more expensive than spironolactone and must be given by injection. Cyproterone acetate, a progestin, was historically the most popular adjunct gender-affirming hormone treatment in Continental Europe (although not available in the United States). However, side effects associated with cyproterone acetate—including elevations in prolactin levels (the hormone that enables breast milk production), worsening of lipid profiles, and rare meningioma (benign brain tumor) growth—have all served to decrease its popularity (Burinkul et al., 2021; Hage et al., 2022). Nonetheless, these adjunctive antiandrogens may still be in use by some patients and could be listed in medical records.

In the first 3–12 months of feminizing hormone therapy, patients should expect decreased rate of growth of facial/body hair, decreased libido, decreased spontaneous erections, decreased skin oiliness, decreased muscle mass, redistribution of fat, and breast development. Breast growth may continue for the first 2 years of therapy.

Lower-Dose Regimens

Some patients may request treatment with lower doses of testosterone or estrogens than would be needed to achieve typical male or female hormone levels; some patients term this "microdosing." The cautions with lower-dose regimens are twofold. First, in patients who do not have endogenous hormone production, exogenous hormone doses should not be so low that they are insufficiently protective of bone density (Safer and Tangpricha, 2019a). However, if there is sufficient sex hormone circulating (testosterone and estrogens combined), there is no medical reason to favor a hormone profile that is more typically female, versus one that is more typically male, versus one that is along the continuum in between. Second, even lower hormone therapy doses can have dramatic physical consequences for some people, and patients who seek lower-dose regimens should be aware that they may be more sensitive than anticipated and may have irreversible physical responses (e.g., more significant than expected beard growth and voice lowering from testosterone, more significant than expected breast growth from estrogen-induced testosterone lowering). Patients should be counseled accordingly, with a review of their specific needs and goals before treatment begins.

Both patients who have a binary identity (e.g., as transgender men or transgender women) and patients who identify as nonbinary or bigender may seek lower-dose hormone treatments. Also, TGD patients, regardless of terms used to describe themselves, may seek conventional binary hormone regimens. Thus, it is important to determine independently both a patient's self-identified gender identity and a patient's hormone regimen.

Additional Hormone Regimens

The WPATH *Standards of Care* (Coleman et al., 2022) and such practice guidelines as the Endocrine Society of North America's *Guidelines for Endocrine Treatment of Gender-Dysphoric/Gender-Incongruent Persons*

(Hembree et al., 2017) reflect recommended and commonly used practices, as described above. However, not all hormone regimens used by TGD patients are accounted for in these evidence-based guidelines—for example, because of a lack of efficacy data, insufficient data in TGD populations, or safety concerns. However, TGD people may access various alternative hormone regimens, as may be reflected in medical records.

Additional Approaches to Administering Masculinizing Hormone Therapy

These approaches include testosterone pellets, testosterone nasal spray, and oral testosterone undecanoate. None of these are known to be superior to the more popular injectable testosterone esters and topical testosterone gel. Concerns with the nasal spray relate to the irritation observed with other nasal spray products with other active ingredients (Acerus Pharmaceuticals Corporation, 2016). Testosterone pellets are typically reserved for people who already have an established dose because titrating pellets (especially down-titrating) can be a challenge.

Additional Approaches to Administering Feminizing Hormone Therapy

These approaches include sublingual estradiol (Doll et al., 2022; Sarvaideo et al., 2022) and estrogen pellets. Sublingual estradiol can result in higher peak levels followed by lower trough levels (Doll et al., 2022), with unknown benefits or detriments. For those patients concerned with thrombolytic events, sublingual estradiol may be useful because it avoids a first pass through the liver. Alternatively, if the major cause for increased thromboembolic risk with exogenous estrogens is associated with the total dose received, sublingual estradiol may best be avoided (Doll et al., 2020). Estrogen pellets are typically reserved for people who already have an established dose because, as noted above, titrating pellets (especially down-titrating) can be a challenge.

Additional Approaches to Androgen-Suppressing Medications

These approaches may include bicalutamide (Neyman et al., 2019; Wilde et al., 2024), dutasteride (Gao et al., 2023), and flutamide. Bicalutamide has gained interest because it is inexpensive, and it blocks the androgen receptor. However, bicalutamide has been associated with a small number of cases of fulminant hepatitis and death (O'Bryant et al., 2008; Wilde et al., 2024; Yun et al., 2016). Although rare, cases of hepatitis and death came without warning and were not dose related; currently, there are no options for monitoring these risks. Therefore, the WPATH SOC-8 guidelines note that the use of bicalutamide is not recommended (Coleman et al., 2022).

Progesterone

Available medications for administration of progesterone include medroxyprogesterone acetate and micronized progesterone (Bahr et al., 2024). There are no quality data demonstrating any benefit from progestogens used in gender-affirming hormone treatment. All data on progestogens to date show harm with agents used over many years (Coleman et al., 2022). Specifically, medroxyprogesterone is associated with increased breast cancer and increased heart disease in postmenopausal cisgender women (Chlebowski et al., 2020; Rossouw et al., 2002). A range of progestogens are associated with increased thromboembolic risk when combined with estrogens (the most common examples being birth control pills for cisgender women) (Dragoman et al., 2018). Cyproterone acetate has been associated with worse lipid profile, slight prolactin elevation, and a small increased risk of meningiomas in transfeminine people (Millward et al., 2022).

Selective Estrogen Receptor Modulators

These agents, such as tamoxifen, raloxifene, and lasofoxifene, also known as estrogen receptor agonists/antagonists, have different effects in various tissues (Xu et al., 2021). These medications have been proposed for TGD people who want some of the effects of estrogens, such as softer skin and a gynoid fat distribution, but not others, such as breast growth (Xu et al., 2021). There are no data showing the efficacy of these agents and no data to support the risks of heart disease, bone harm, or hot flash symptoms (depending on the agent chosen) outside of indicated uses (e.g., for breast cancer).

Minoxidil

Topical minoxidil has been used off-label to facilitate facial hair growth in transgender men whose response to testosterone has been limited (Pang et al., 2021). Oral minoxidil has been used off-label to treat androgenetic hair loss in TGD people exposed to higher levels of testosterone either endogenously from testicular production or exogenously as part of masculinizing hormone therapy (Motosko and Tosti, 2021).

Fertility and Gender-Affirming Hormone Therapy

GAHT may reduce fertility, but does not necessarily eliminate it (Amato, 2016). TGD people on testosterone have reduced fertility, but if a uterus and ovaries are still present, pregnancies can occur. Similarly, estrogen and antiandrogens can cause diminished spermatogenesis and testicular atrophy (Cheng et al., 2019). Because ovulation and spermatogenesis may continue in the presence of hormone therapy, all TGD people who engage in sexual activity that could result in pregnancy should be counseled on the need for contraception (Amato, 2016).

GAHT likely affects fertility only temporarily (Coleman et al., 2022), although infertility can be permanent (Amato, 2016). The extent to which fertility can return is unresearched, but some TGD people do reproduce (Keuroghlian et al., 2022; Light et al., 2014; Thornton and Mattatall, 2021). Some transgender men may wish to carry a pregnancy and stop using testosterone to facilitate doing so safely; anecdotally, fertility may return 3–6 months after cessation of GAHT (Amato, 2016). Transgender women may wish to use their sperm for pregnancy and can often do so after stopping GAHT.

However, gender-affirming surgeries that remove the gonads (ovaries or testes) result in infertility, as does hysterectomy. Guidelines recommend thorough counseling with a patient who wishes to undergo gonadectomy (Amato, 2016). Fertility preservation options for storing eggs or sperm allow for future reproductive choices (Cheng et al., 2019).

Long-Term Follow-Up

It is important to monitor hormone levels in patients receiving GAHT to ensure that levels reach the target range for specific patients. Guidelines suggest monitoring hormone levels in transgender patients with each adjustment in hormone dose (approximately every 3 months during the first year) and once or twice yearly after target levels have been achieved, or whenever the dose is changed (Hembree et al., 2017; Safer and Tangpricha, 2019b).

In addition, long-term follow-up of patients on GAHT includes monitoring other factors, as transgender men and nonbinary individuals who access GAHT may have a risk of erythrocytosis (high concentration of red blood cells), and transgender women and nonbinary individuals may have an increased risk of blood clots while on GAHT (Ramsay and Safer, 2023). Because androgens are known to stimulate erythrocytosis, hematocrit (or hemoglobin) levels in transgender men and nonbinary individuals should be monitored with dose titration, typically every 3 months, and once or twice annually thereafter (Madsen et al., 2021; Ramsay and Safer, 2023). Dose adjustment and/or other interventions, such as phlebotomy, may be required if erythrocytosis is unmasked and a reversible explanation (e.g., hypoxia, obstructive sleep apnea, polycythemia rubra vera, renal cell carcinoma) is not found. For transgender women and nonbinary individuals who receive spironolactone, routine monitoring of serum potassium is advised because of the potential risk of hyperkalemia (high potassium); serum potassium levels should be checked upon initiation of spironolactone therapy and with changes in dose (often with titration every 3 months until steady-state hormone levels have been achieved). Although some guidelines still suggest monitoring serum prolactin levels, elevated prolactin levels have been noted only in patients using adjunct cyproterone acetate, not in those using other adjunct treatments or in those using estrogens alone (Bisson et al., 2018).

In addition, testing of bone mineral density may be important for TGD patients who have had prolonged periods of hypogonadism or have other risk factors for osteoporosis. Overall, there is no evidence of major bone loss with GAHT (Verroken et al., 2022), and bone mineral density may increase for TGD people using testosterone (Radix et al., 2016; Stevenson and Tangpricha, 2019). Medicare data show lower rates of osteoporosis in TGD (8.2 percent) than in cisgender (15.7 percent) people (Dragon et al., 2017). There are no consistent guidelines for optimal frequency of bone density screening for cisgender people, and there is not enough evidence to guide recommendations on bone density testing for TGD adults (Radix et al., 2016).

Routine cancer screening is important for TGD patients in accordance with guidelines established for the general population, but screening should be performed on the tissues and organs present, not those related to gender identity or sex as recorded in the medical record. Additional considerations for cancer screening in TGD people are discussed below.

Finally, and importantly, providers should monitor patients to determine the need for mental health support. Psychosocial supports are described in further detail below.

GENDER-AFFIRMING SURGERY AND POSTOPERATIVE CARE

Gender-affirming surgery comprises a constellation of medically necessary procedures intended to align people's bodies with their identity. While some TGD people do not undergo gender-affirming surgery, such surgery is considered safe and effective and results in reduced gender dysphoria and improved quality of life (Almazan and Keuroghlian, 2021; Coleman et al., 2022; Departmental Appeals Board, 2014). The decision to pursue the surgery today is based on a thoughtful and multidisciplinary evaluation following WPATH's SOC-8 (Coleman et al., 2022). This evaluation allows for an individualized approach using shared decision making to optimize preparedness for surgical interventions.

This section examines preoperative preparation and assessment, describes surgical aftercare, and details common surgical procedures (including facial surgery, breast surgery, chest surgery, vaginoplasty, metoidioplasty, and phalloplasty). The section ends with a discussion of considerations for customizing gender-affirming surgery for individual patients.

Preoperative Preparation and Assessment

The WPATH SOC-8 guidelines offer best practices for providing evidence-based care to TGD people. The overarching goal for gender-affirming care—including surgical interventions—is to maximize overall health, psychological well-being, and self-fulfillment (Coleman et al., 2022). For this reason, surgical care for gender dysphoria is best approached with a multidisciplinary team. The diagnosis of gender dysphoria is generally made by mental health providers or primary care professionals with expertise in TGD health. These providers then refer appropriate candidates for gender-affirming surgery. Communication between the surgeon and mental health and primary care professionals helps the surgeon understand the unique needs of each individual. Discussion with other treating medical providers (endocrinologists, allied health practitioners, and other surgeons) can also provide insight into the patient's goals. Open dialogue should extend beyond the preoperative period; the surgeon should relay information regarding surgical findings and postoperative care to relevant members of the health care team (Schechter, 2009). In recent years, the multidisciplinary care team has expanded to include other disciplines, such as physical therapy for pelvic health, sex therapy, and voice therapy. This comprehensive approach helps individuals realize the optimal positive impact of the surgery.

While preoperative mental health evaluation has historically been criticized for "gate-keeping" access to gender-affirming surgery, the current role of mental health professionals has evolved. Mental health professionals can help individuals with decision making about surgical and other care options, provide counseling on reproductive and sexual goals, and collaborate with surgeons to provide counseling in preparation for surgery. In addition, mental health professionals can help prepare a patient for surgery and postoperative life by identifying and building support systems and by informing expectations regarding the impact of the surgery on other aspects of life (e.g., family, friends, intimate relationships, work) (Roblee et al., 2023). The importance of evaluating and addressing psychosocial needs is seen in other fields, such as organ transplantation, in which poor social support and other vulnerabilities are associated with less favorable outcomes (Maldonado, 2019). Additionally, preoperative assessment of psychosocial measures strengthens the informed-consent process by helping individuals understand and internalize the expected effects of surgery.

Aftercare

Development of an aftercare plan prior to surgery not only facilitates care coordination but also helps optimize surgical outcomes (Roblee et al., 2023). Social workers and/or care navigators can work with patients to assemble a detailed aftercare plan, which includes identifying physical, mental, social, and financial resources, as well as surgical follow-up. For example, social workers might verify local lodging after discharge to allow for follow-up care (especially if a patient is traveling from out of town), confirm social support during the postoperative period, and verify that travel logistics have been arranged (Coleman et al., 2022).

Surgical Procedures

Surgery for TGD people includes several options and may involve procedures to enlarge, reduce, or remove the breasts, various genital surgeries, and facial or other body-contouring procedures to create a more feminine or masculine appearance. Facial and breast surgeries may sometimes be performed prior to GAHT as a way to facilitate social transition (Altman, 2021; Davis and St. Amand, 2014; Olson-Kennedy et al., 2018; Van Boerum et al., 2019).

The principles of gender-affirming genital surgery are based on anatomy and embryology. The external genitalia are homologous structures (there is a corresponding anatomic part in each of the biological sexes), and the corresponding anatomic tissues are used to create the relevant anatomy. Figure 5-1 illustrates the embryology of the external genitalia, while Figure 5-2 shows the anatomy of common approaches to gender-affirming surgery. In vaginoplasty procedures, the glans clitoris is formed from the glans penis, the labia majora are formed from the scrotum, and the penile urethra is shortened to form the urethra and vestibule. Conversely, in a phalloplasty, the clitoro-vulvar anatomy is reconfigured, and additional tissues are used to reconstruct the penis; the perineal and penile urethra; and the scrotum, constructed from the labia majora.

The relationship between GAHT, especially estrogen, and the risk of perioperative venous thromboembolism (VTE) following gender-affirming surgery continues to evolve. Historically, surgeons discontinued GAHT in the perioperative period to decrease the risk of VTE (Hontscharuk et al., 2021). However, abrupt cessation of GAHT may negatively affect well-being (Hontscharuk et al., 2021). While additional research on mitigating the risk of VTE in gender-affirming surgical care is needed, recent research has not found significant risk of perioperative VTE in TGD people on estrogen therapy (Kozato et al., 2021), and current evidence does not support routine discontinuation of GAHT prior to surgery for all patients (Boskey et al., 2019).

The subsections below provide a brief description of facial, breast, chest, and genital gender-affirming surgical procedures.

Facial Surgery

Facial surgery can be feminizing or masculinizing. Feminizing procedures often focus on areas of the forehead, nose, malar region, mandible, and thyroid cartilage. For example, brow lift with advancement of the frontal hairline and frontal bone reduction is frequently performed. A feminizing rhinoplasty can involve dorsal hump reduction, cephalic trim, elevation of

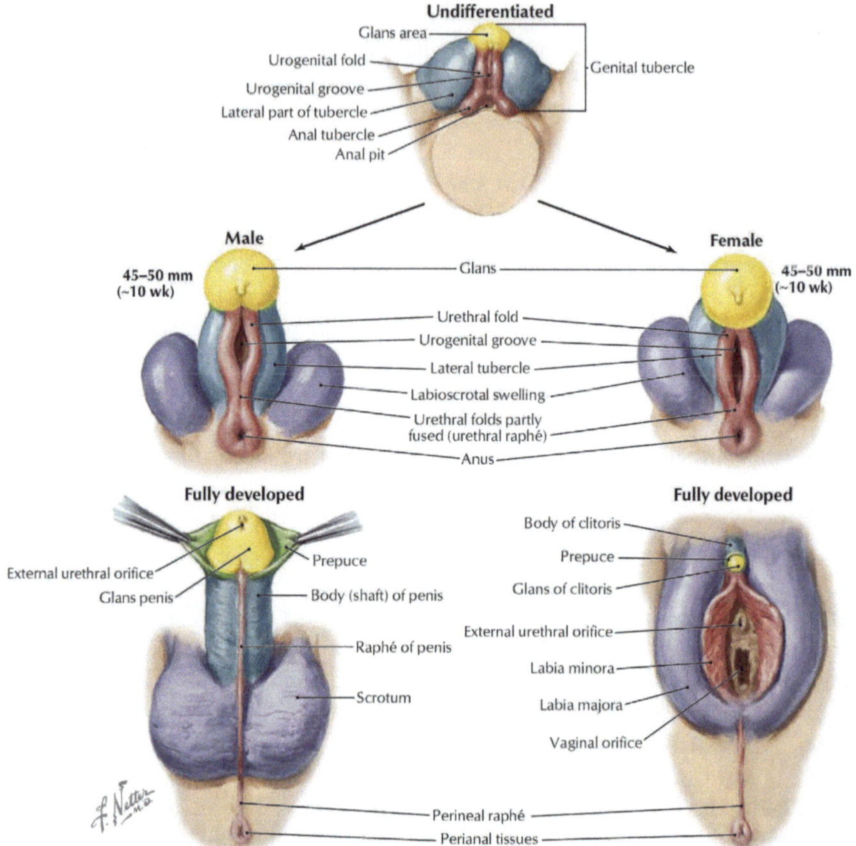

FIGURE 5-1 Embryology of the external genitalia.
NOTE: The male and female external genitalia are considered homologous structures; that is, there is a corresponding anatomic part in each of the biological sexes. In transgender females who receive gender-affirming surgery, the component parts of the typical male anatomy are reassembled to construct the relevant typical female anatomy. Conversely, in transgender males, the typical female anatomy is removed and reassembled to construct portions of the typical male anatomy.
SOURCE: Schechter, 2016. Used with permission of Elsevier; from *Surgical management of the transgender patient,* 1st Edition, Copyright © 2016: permission conveyed through Copyright Clearance Center, Inc.

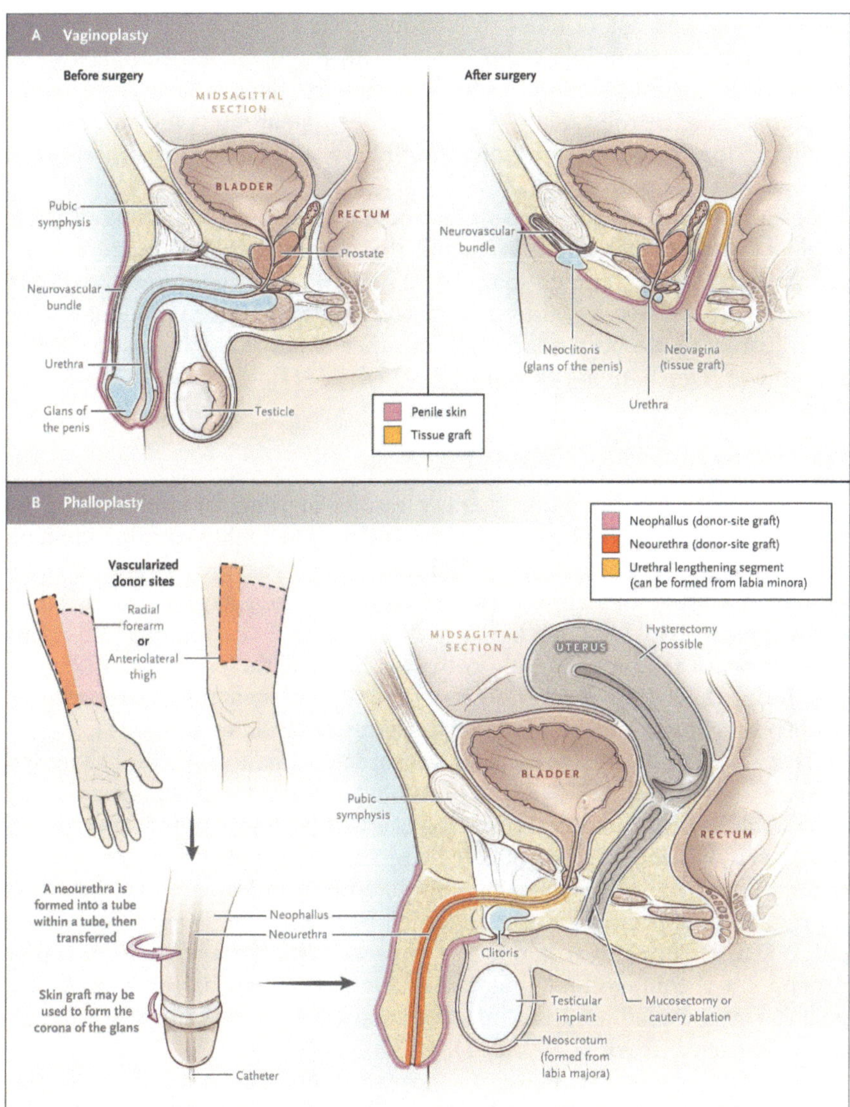

FIGURE 5-2 Anatomy of common approaches to gender-affirming surgery. NOTE: The term "mucosectomy" used in the figure in reference to ablation of the vaginal lining is not correct. The vaginal lining is epithelium (not mucus membrane). SOURCE: Safer and Tangpricha, 2019b. From New England Journal of Medicine, Care of Transgender Persons, 381(25):2451–2460 Copyright © 2018 Massachusetts Medical Society. Reprinted with permission from Massachusetts Medical Society.

the nasal tip, and osteotomies to narrow the nasal pyramid. Feminization of the chin and mandible often involves an osteoplastic genioplasty and mandibular angle reduction. Reduction thyroid chondroplasty can reduce the appearance of the "Adam's apple." Nonsurgical interventions, such as lipofilling (or "fat grafting"), injectable fillers, and hair transplantation or removal, may be performed as well.

Masculinizing facial procedures include chin and mandibular angle implants and/or augmentation of the thyroid cartilage to create a more prominent "Adam's apple" (Safa et al., 2019). This continues to be an emerging area of surgery, although the techniques for developing masculine facial features have been adapted from other types of facial plastic surgery procedures (Deschamps-Braly et al., 2017).

Breast Surgery

While estrogen hormone therapy results in some breast growth, the degree of breast growth is often limited and may be highly variable (de Blok et al., 2018; Patel et al., 2021). Additionally, the breast growth is frequently similar to a "tuberous" breast (where breasts do not have a round shape) and may consist of a constricted lower pole and "herniation" of breast tissue beneath the nipple-areola complex. Because these results can be disappointing, breast augmentation is commonly pursued among transgender women to achieve a more feminine appearance (Patel et al., 2021).

A person whose sex at birth was recorded as male and who has undergone an androgen puberty (e.g., a person who did not access pubertal delay and GAHT during puberty) typically has a wider chest than that of a person whose sex was recorded as female at birth. The nipple-areola complex is smaller, the distance between the nipple and the inframammary crease is shorter, and the pectoral muscle is larger. Because of these anatomic differences, a wider implant is commonly chosen. Location and incision choice depend on the individual, but a sublandular, subfacial, or subpectoral pocket may be used, and the inframammary crease incision is most commonly chosen (Brown et al., 2021).

Pre- and postoperative breast cancer screening guidelines depend upon age, family history, genetic risk, duration of hormone use, and physical examination (Claes et al., 2018).

Chest Surgery

Chest masculinization surgery is the most commonly requested masculinizing gender-affirming surgery. Goals of chest surgery include removing breast tissue and excess skin, reducing and repositioning the nipple-areola complex, releasing the inframammary crease, and minimizing chest scars

(Monstrey et al., 2008).[6] Choice of incision depends on breast volume, degree of breast ptosis (sagging of the breasts), nipple-areola size and position, amount of excess skin, and skin elasticity. A periareolar incision may be adequate for small breasts with good skin elasticity and without ptosis, whereas larger breasts often require the traditional "double incision" (i.e., transverse incision along the origin of the pectoral muscle) with nipple-areola grafts. Liposuction may be a useful adjunct to further contour the chest. Drains and elastic compression are used in the postoperative period (Brown et al., 2021).

Vaginoplasty

The use of pedicled penile flaps was described more than 40 years ago and serves as the foundation for feminizing genital surgery (Hage et al., 2007; Hontscharuk et al., 2021). Surgical options for vaginoplasty include penile inversion vaginoplasty, intestinal vaginoplasty, and/or peritoneal flaps. Penile inversion vaginoplasty is most commonly performed for primary surgery, while other techniques are used in revisions or in cases involving inadequate penile tissue. Penile inversion vaginoplasty uses an anterior pedicled penile skin flap combined with a scrotal skin graft. Prior to surgery, removal of hair on the scrotum and penile shaft is recommended to reduce intravaginal hair growth. The vaginoplasty procedure requires lifelong vaginal dilation to maintain vaginal depth and width. Intestinal vaginoplasty, typically using the sigmoid colon, creates a 12–15 cm vagina with moist lining due to mucus production from goblet cells. This procedure requires intra-abdominal surgery with a bowel anastomosis. While the intestinal approach may lessen the need for vaginal dilation and lubrication, significant discharge may require use of a pad in the underwear. Nongenital flaps (i.e., peritoneum) may also be employed. In these cases, the peritoneal lining is advanced to form the apex of the vaginal canal.

Additional options include vulvoplasty (construction of clitorovulvar structures) without creation of a vaginal canal. This surgery may be performed in individuals who do not anticipate receptive vaginal intercourse, are unable or do not want to dilate the vaginal canal or have medical

---

[6] While chest masculinization is very similar to mastectomy, the goals are different. Mastectomy is most often performed as part of breast cancer treatment or prevention and involves removal of the entire breast (and sometimes other nearby tissues, such as lymph nodes). The goal of chest masculinization surgery is to shape the skin and tissue of the chest to match the contour of a male chest; residual breast tissue (used to aid in masculine chest contour) may remain and, for this reason, individuals may continue to carry risk for breast cancer.

contraindications to construction of the vaginal canal (i.e., previous pelvic surgery and/or radiation).

Following vaginoplasty, in addition to dilation of the surgically created vaginal canal, vaginal rinsing (or "douching") is also recommended to cleanse the canal, as desquamated skin or mucus secretions may be retained.

Metoidioplasty and Phalloplasty

Masculinizing genital surgery requires understanding the goals of the individual, as reconstruction may or may not include urethral reconstruction, colpectomy/colpocleisis, and various flap options. Surgery may range from clitoral release (metoidioplasty) with or without urethral lengthening (to allow for voiding while standing) to phalloplasty, which allows for sexual penetration following placement of implantable penile prostheses.

Metoidioplasty, first described by Hage (1996), involves lengthening the hormonally hypertrophied clitoris by releasing the suspensory ligament, resecting the ventral chordee, and lengthening the urethra (see also Heston et al., 2019). Hysterectomy, oophorectomy, and colpectomy with colpocleisis may also be performed. Scrotoplasty and testicular implants are often performed in a secondary surgical procedure to reduce the risk of infection and wound-healing complications (Kocjancic and Iacovelli, 2018).

Phalloplasty techniques include pedicled flaps and free flaps. Pedicled flaps transfer tissue from the thigh, groin, or lower abdomen, whereas free flaps involve microsurgical transfer of tissue from a remote location, typically the forearm. The radial forearm free flap is the most common technique used for phalloplasty (Gottlieb, 2018; Schechter and Facque, 2021). This procedure transfers tissue, including blood vessels and nerves, from the forearm to reconstruct a sensate phallus and urethra, when requested. Drawbacks of the forearm procedure include the visibility of the donor site and the need for microsurgical skills. The second most common technique entails use of tissue from the thigh, known as the anterolateral thigh flap (Schechter and Facque, 2021; Xu and Watt, 2018). In some cases, however, thick subcutaneous thigh tissue may preclude this technique. In both the anterolateral thigh flap and the radial forearm free flap, the urethra is formed by a skin-lined tube; as a result, preoperative electrolysis may be required for hair removal.

Following phalloplasty, an implantable penile prosthesis may be placed to achieve rigidity and allow for penetrative intercourse. The metoidioplasty does not create a phallus of sufficient dimensions to allow placement of a prosthesis. Testicular implants may be placed in a surgically created scrotal sac following either metoidioplasty or phalloplasty.

Complications following metoidioplasty/phalloplasty are not uncommon and can include urethral problems (e.g., stricture, fistula) and wound-healing complications (Nikolavsky et al., 2018). Lifelong urological follow-up is recommended following the surgery (Coleman et al., 2022).

Individually Customized Surgery

TGD people, particularly those who self-identify as nonbinary, may have surgical goals and expectations that differ from the more binary options reviewed above. Therefore, gender-affirming surgical procedures need to be individualized (Schechter and Facque, 2021). For example, patients may opt for phallus-preserving vaginoplasty, vagina-preserving phalloplasty, penile subincision, or penile bisection (Chen et al., 2021; Salgado et al., 2021).

As with all individuals considering surgery, the patient and multidisciplinary team need to work together in a shared decision making process to ensure that the patient's goals are realistic and achievable, as well as safe and technically feasible (Coleman et al., 2022). In addition, the medical record should clearly document surgeries undertaken and organs that are still present.

Sexual Function Postsurgery

Sexual function is an important consideration for many people undergoing genital gender-affirming surgery, and preoperative sexual function tends to correlate with postoperative sexual function. Studies of sexual function following masculinizing genital surgery (metoidioplasty and phalloplasty) report high sexual function satisfaction: one study found that 87.63 percent of patients surveyed were satisfied with overall sexual function (Vukadinovic et al., 2014). Other studies have found similarly high rates of retained sexual function among transgender males (Garcia et al., 2014; Van de Grift et al., 2019). Vaginoplasty results in similar levels of high satisfaction among transgender females (Hadj-Moussa et al., 2018; Holmberg et al., 2019; Horbach et al., 2015; Zavlin et al., 2018). In a study of patients years after vaginoplasty, sexual satisfaction was related to neoclitoral sensitivity, and less to vaginal sensitivity or depth (Jerome et al., 2022).

Complications following surgery may impair sexual function. Lack of erogenous sensation and complications with prosthetics (required for the phallus to achieve rigidity) have been reported among transgender males (Elfering et al., 2021; Khorrami et al., 2022). Complications regarding prosthetics (malfunction, extrusion, infection, dislodgement) are not uncommon.

Among transgender females, a small percentage of patients (2–6 percent) report painful intercourse (dyspareunia) (Horbach et al., 2015).

NONMEDICAL MODALITIES

Gender-affirming interventions may include nonmedical modalities that can have an impact on physical health, including important implications for disability evaluations. These interventions include binding, tucking, packing, and non–medically supervised injection of soft-tissue fillers. These interventions may be used on their own or in combination with GAHT and/or surgery, depending on individual patient preference.

Binding

Transgender males and nonbinary people whose sex was recorded female at birth may choose to bind the breasts (including with commercial binders or by wearing one or more sports bras, tape, cloth, plastic wrap or elastic bandages) to create a flat and more masculine appearance (Coleman et al., 2022). Chest binding is associated with reduced chest dysphoria, improved mental health outcomes, and increased sense of safety in public, and may be undertaken prior to or in lieu of gender-affirming chest reconstruction surgery (Lee et al., 2019; Peitzmeier et al., 2017). Many individuals who bind do so daily and for extended periods of time, often exceeding 10 hours each day (Julian et al., 2021; Peitzmeier et al., 2017). Adverse effects associated with binding in a large cross-sectional survey included pain (back, chest, shoulder, and abdominal) (74 percent); skin and soft-tissue complaints, including tenderness, skin infection, scarring, and itching (76.3 percent); shortness of breath (46.6 percent); and lightheadedness or dizziness (27.8 percent). Musculoskeletal changes related to binding may include muscle wasting (5.4 percent), rib fractures (2.8 percent), or other rib/spine changes (11.6 percent) (Peitzmeier et al., 2017).

Chest binding may impact spirometry testing. In a small study of TGD people, wearing a binder reduced chest circumference and resulted in significant declines in forced vital capacity and slow vital capacity compared with not wearing a binder (Cumming et al., 2016). Chapter 8 describes respiratory health, spirometry measurement, and chest binding in greater detail.

Tucking

Tucking refers to the process of creating a flat appearance by compressing or hiding the external genitalia in transgender females and nonbinary people whose sex was recorded male at birth. One study of transgender female adults found that most (74.4 percent) practiced tucking, with the majority of those practicing tucking (84.5 percent) doing so daily (Malik et al., 2024). This process includes positioning the testicles close to or through the inguinal canal and tucking the penis back between the buttocks, usually accompanied by wearing a compressive undergarment (called a gaff), tape, or tight padded or layered underwear. Tucking may cause skin and soft-tissue conditions (itching, rash, fungal infections) (Huang et al., 2022), impaired semen quality, pain, and testicular torsion (de Nie et al., 2022; Debarbo, 2020; Williamson, 2010).

Packing

Transgender males and nonbinary people whose sex was recorded female at birth may use padding or a penile prosthesis ("packer") to create a genital bulge. Packers can be soft or firm and are held in place with a harness or tight undergarments or skin adhesive. Some packers may allow the individual to urinate while standing ("stand-to-pee" packer). Packers may be associated with skin irritation and excoriation (Huang et al., 2022; Williamson, 2010).

Silicone

Transgender females and nonbinary people whose sex was recorded male at birth may inject soft-tissue fillers, including free silicone, into the breasts, buttocks, and hips to create a more feminine appearance. This process can result in migration of silicone and pigment changes (Bertin et al., 2019; Soliman, 2023), skin and soft tissue infection (Bertin et al., 2019), granulomas (Ohnona et al., 2016; Pando et al., 2022), hypercalcemia (Pando et al., 2022), chronic ulceration (Soliman, 2023), immune reconstitution inflammatory syndrome (van der Pluijm et al., 2022), pneumonitis, and alveolar hemorrhage (Bejarano et al., 2020). It may also lead to concerns about bloodborne pathogens, such as HIV, hepatitis B, and hepatitis C, due to sharing of needles.

CANCER SCREENING CONSIDERATIONS

As noted earlier, patients should in general be screened for cancers in the tissues they have present, rather than being screened based on data on sex or gender identity recorded in medical records. TGD people who have accessed gender-affirming care interventions—including GAHT, gender-affirming surgery, and nonmedical modalities—may require modifications to routine preventive cancer screenings. This section describes considerations for screening for breast, prostate, and cervical cancer. Additional considerations for TGD people who have prostate or cervical cancer or other cancers of the reproductive system are described in Chapter 11 of this report.

Breast Cancer Screening

TGD people with breast tissue should undergo breast cancer screening based on the same clinical practice guidelines used for cisgender women, including digital breast tomosynthesis and mammography (Brown et al., 2021; Coleman et al., 2022). Individuals who have had chest surgery to remove the breasts have a lower incidence of breast cancer compared with cisgender women (standardized incidence ratio 0.2, 95% confidence interval [CI] 0.1–0.5) (de Blok et al., 2019), and screening for low-risk individuals with mammography is usually not appropriate (Brown et al., 2021). However, breast cancer screening following mastectomy depends on the mastectomy technique employed. Some surgeons resect all gross breast tissue, while others leave some breast tissue (whether in an effort to preserve nipple-areola sensation or for contouring purposes). Breast cancer has been diagnosed in transgender men who have had bilateral breast removal (Deutsch et al., 2017; Fehl et al., 2019). If the baseline level of risk for such individuals is high (e.g., based on a prior diagnosis, family history, and/ or genetic factors), providers may advise routine breast cancer screening, despite the challenges of obtaining a mammography.

TGD people who have received estrogen as part of GAHT have a higher risk of breast cancer compared with cisgender men (standardized incidence ratio [SIR] 46.7, 95% CI 27.2–75.4), but a lower risk compared with cisgender women (SIR 0.3, 95 percent CI 0.2–0.4) (de Blok et al., 2019). The current WPATH guidelines suggest that screening guidelines for cisgender women be followed in these populations (Coleman et al., 2022). The American College of Radiology states that digital breast tomosynthesis or mammography starting at age 40 is appropriate for those at average risk with duration of current or past use of hormones equal to or greater than 5 years (Brown et al., 2021). Transgender women who have injected silicone into the breasts may require contrast-enhanced magnetic resonance imaging as the preferred breast cancer screening modality when silicone and soft-tissue injection and related issues, such as granulomas, obscure breast tissue on mammography (Brown et al., 2021).

Prostate Cancer Screening

The prostate is not removed during gender-affirming vaginoplasty. Therefore, TGD people who have undergone this procedure will retain the prostate unless it has been removed for another reason (e.g., treatment of benign prostatic hyperplasia). Prostate cancer is uncommon in transgender women who have had long-term androgen suppression, either as a result of androgen blockers and estradiol or gonadectomy (removal of the gonads). However, there have been case reports of prostate cancer in this population (Deebel et al., 2017). Examination of the prostate is performed by palpating the anterior vaginal wall after vaginoplasty. Prostate-specific antigen levels are unreliable in individuals who have suppressed testosterone levels with androgen blockade or use of 5 alpha reductase inhibitors (Bertoncelli Tanaka et al., 2022). Some screening guidelines recommend screening for all people with a prostate (American Cancer Society, 2021; Wei et al., 2023), although individual TGD patients and their providers may engage in shared decision making to discuss the benefits, harms, and effectiveness of prostate cancer screening using physical examination and measuring prostate-specific antigen levels.

Cervical Cancer Screening

TGD people with a cervix should follow guidelines for cervical cancer screening for cisgender women (Coleman et al., 2022). There is no evidence that testosterone increases the risk for cervical cancer, although testosterone use has been associated with inadequate cytology using Papanicolaou (Pap) tests in one community health center (Peitzmeier et al., 2014). Transgender women who have had a vaginoplasty do not have a cervix, and cervical cancer screening is unnecessary. However, patients who opt to have a vagina-preserving phalloplasty may retain a cervix, and so require cervical screening. Squamous cell carcinoma has been reported in transgender women after penile-inversion vaginoplasty (Fierz et al., 2019), and neovaginal adenocarcinoma is a remote possibility in those who have had intestinal vaginoplasty (Yamada et al., 2018); however, there are no screening guidelines for these cancers.

PSYCHOSOCIAL SUPPORT ACROSS THE LIFESPAN

Gender-affirming care is not limited to the gender-affirming medical interventions of puberty delay, feminizing or masculinizing hormone therapy, and/or surgery; it also includes mental health care, adding to the interdisciplinary nature of gender-affirming care. Distress related to the incongruence between gender identity and sex recorded at birth (i.e., gender dysphoria) experienced by many (but not all) TGD people at some point in their lives often has both a physical and a psychosocial component. The physical component typically involves psychological distress related to sex characteristics not congruent with gender identity, including not only breasts/chest and genitalia, but also body hair, height and bone structure, distribution of body fat, and voice. The psychosocial component typically involves gender expression, gender role, and the associated societal norms and expectations. Although gender diversity has generally become more visible in U.S. society, and public accommodation of TGD people has improved, gender remains a key structuring factor in society—for example, in identity documents (driver's license, passport), sports, and public restrooms, as well as health care. On a very regular basis in everyday life, TGD people must navigate social categories of boy/man and girl/woman, which may include both efforts to conform and, inevitably, challenges to prevailing gender norms. Mental health providers play a critical role in supporting patients with TGD experience in navigating these aspects of society and coping with the cumulative impact of stigma, discrimination, and isolation (Bockting et al., 2016; McCann and Sharek, 2016; Reisner et al., 2016).

Stigma, Stress, and Gender Identity

Erikson (1994) postulated a number of psychosocial developmental tasks and related stages across the lifespan. These include trust versus mistrust, autonomy versus shame and doubt, initiative versus guilt, industry versus inferiority, identity versus identity confusion, intimacy versus isolation, generativity versus stagnation, and integrity versus despair. For TGD people, the challenges inherent in these developmental tasks are compounded by (1) the distress associated with having a gender identity that differs significantly from sex recorded at birth (see above) both physically and socially, and (2) the stigma attached to nonconformity with prevailing gender norms and gendered expectations (Bockting et al., 2013; Jackman et al., 2018).

Over the years, a number of stage models have been postulated to describe the development of gender diverse identities across the lifespan within this context (Bockting, 2014; Bockting and Ehrbar, 2006; Devor, 2004; Gagne et al., 1997; Lewins, 1995). For example, Bockting and colleagues (2016) distinguish five developmental stages (see also Bockting, 2014). During *pre-coming out*, the young person becomes aware of being different and seeks to understand privately what this means. During *coming out*, this sense of being different is acknowledged first to self and then to others; reactions of these others, including health care providers, are of paramount importance during this stage. What follows is a period of *exploration*, often characterized by immersion in online and offline community resources—including TGD peers. This exploration then extends into interpersonal relationships, where experiences of *intimacy* further shape identity. Finally, there are different levels of *integration* of a TGD identity with other identities, such as that of a family member, partner, community member, citizen, or professional. The added stress associated with these developmental stages, as well as the resilience that is fostered along the way, has been shown to explain health disparities, particularly in mental health, found among U.S. gender minority populations (Bockting et al., 2013; Caceres et al., 2022; Delozier et al., 2020; Gosling et al., 2022; Jackman et al., 2018; Nuttbrock et al., 2014a,b; Pellicane and Ciesla, 2022; Pellicane et al., 2023; Valente et al., 2020, 2022; Valentine and Shipherd, 2018).

The minority stress model postulates that social stigma attached to gender nonconformity, whether in the form of actual experiences of discrimination, bullying, and violence—which are prevalent among TGD people in the United States (e.g., Bockting et al., 2013; Hughto et al., 2015)—or internalized as shame and fear, has a negative impact on the health and well-being of TGD people (Bockting et al., 2016; Hendricks and Testa, 2012; Lefevor et al., 2019; Meyer, 2003). Indeed, numerous studies have shown the association between gender minority stress and psychological distress, substance use, nonsuicidal self-injury, and suicidal ideation and attempts (Bockting et al., 2013; Gosling et al., 2022; Jackman et al., 2018; Kaufman et al., 2023; Kidd et al., 2021; Nuttbrock et al., 2014a,b; Pellicane et al., 2023; Price et al., 2024; Puckett et al., 2023; Srivastava et al., 2021; Valente et al., 2020, 2022; Valentine and Shipherd, 2018). Additional evidence is emerging that associates gender minority stress with physical health (Flentje et al., 2022; Wilson, 2023).

Older TGD adults may be particularly vulnerable, as this population is more likely to have grown up in a historical context in which their gender identity elicited greater social stigma. Research in this population is limited, but indicates that older TGD adults are at higher risk for poor physical health, disability, depressive symptomatology, and perceived stress compared with their cisgender LGB counterparts (Fredriksen-Goldsen et al., 2014). In the U.S. Behavioral Risk Factor Surveillance System, older TGD adults were also more likely than cisgender adults to report subjective cognitive decline (Lambrou et al., 2020). Needs assessment studies reveal loneliness and isolation and substantial fears about appropriate accommodation of and respect for their identities in assisted living and long-term care facilities (Putney et al., 2018; Walker et al., 2023). Gender dysphoria, developmental challenges, and minority stress evolve during the life course, and likely have a cumulative effect on health and aging (Fredriksen-Goldsen et al., 2023). Discrimination, isolation, psychological distress, and barriers to care can be expected to take their toll, and to compound aging-related health problems and medical morbidities.

Conversely, assets such as social support, progress in identity development, and access to gender-affirming and general health care have been shown to be protective, or to moderate or buffer the negative impact of minority stress on health in TGD populations (Bockting et al., 2013; Johnson et al., 2021; Katz-Wise et al., 2021; Tebbe and Budge, 2022; Trujillo et al., 2017; Valente et al., 2020, 2022).

Role of Mental Health Professionals in Gender-Affirming Care

Given the considerable challenges faced by many TGD people in navigating society, interpersonal relationships, stigma, and discrimination, the role of mental health professionals in the lives of their TGD patients is not limited to screening candidates for hormones and surgery, but includes gender-affirming mental health care and the clinical management of coexisting mental health concerns.

The aim of gender-affirming mental health care is to facilitate the development of gender identity, with particular focus on its psychosocial aspects. Accomplishing this aim involves enhancing gender literacy (i.e., knowledge about gender identity and diversity and about the experience of TGD people throughout history and today); facilitating exploration (of gender identity, gender expression, and reproductive goals, as well as sexuality); establishing support from family, peers, and communities; providing support in gaining lived experience in navigating gender in all aspects of daily life; and facilitating shared decision making, preparation, and coordination for gender-affirming medical interventions that may or may not be medically necessary or desired along the way.

Largely as a result of the social stigma attached to gender nonconformity, but also as a result of the impact of gender dysphoria on overall psychosocial and sexual development, TGD people are at increased risk for such mental health concerns as anxiety, depression, substance use, nonsuicidal self-injury, and suicide (Bockting et al., 2013; Gosling et al., 2022; Jackman et al., 2018; Kaufman et al., 2023; Kidd et al., 2021; Nuttbrock et al., 2014a,b; Pellicane et al., 2023; Price et al., 2023; Puckett et al., 2023; Srivastava et al., 2021; Valente et al., 2020, 2022; Valentine and Shipherd, 2018). A robust literature indicates that exposures to adversity in youth are associated with high rates of both mental health and medical morbidities and earlier mortality (CDC, 2021), while a spate of literature documents the elevated rates of adversities experienced by TGD youth as compared to cisgender counterparts, including physical neglect and emotional, psychological, physical, and sexual abuse (Schnarrs et al., 2019; Thoma et al., 2021). Additionally, bullying predicts suicidality for all youth (Koyanagi et al., 2019), and bullying rates are higher for TGD youth than for cisgender youth, posing considerable risk to the well-being of this population (Smith et al., 2022). Gender-affirming medical interventions alone are unlikely to alleviate many of these concerns. After all, such medical interventions are first and foremost designed to alleviate gender dysphoria. Fortunately, an arsenal of evidence-based treatment strategies (e.g., cognitive-behavioral therapy, dialectical behavior therapy, psychotropic medications) is available to help address any coexisting mental health concerns, including trauma.

Supports

Support from family, peers, and communities, and providers who can address neurocognitive needs can help TGD people deal with the challenges described above.

Family Support

Particularly for TGD children and adolescents, but also for youth and adults of all ages, family support is critical (Fuller and Riggs, 2018; Samrock et al., 2021). Families are integrally involved in child and adolescent patients' clinical decision making, particularly with respect to gender-affirming medical interventions. Indeed, according to WPATH's *Standards of Care, Version 8 (SOC-8)*, support and consent from parents or guardians are required for adolescents to access puberty-delaying medications, masculinizing or feminizing hormone therapy, or surgery (e.g., chest surgery). Additionally, WPATH SOC-8 recommends that all youth engage in a biopsychosocial assessment prior to receiving medical interventions, which can also be thought of as a collaborative needs assessment, to help the family and young person engage in careful decision making and, if medical intervention is needed and desired, help with any family conflicts, advocate for safety and brainstorm transition-related psychosocial concerns for the child and family members. Moreover, for TGD people of any age, family of origin, chosen family, and/or immediate family (e.g., partner, children) are essential sources of support (Bariola et al., 2015; Bockting et al., 2013; Durwood et al., 2021; Puckett et al., 2019). Mental health professionals have an important role to play in assisting TGD people in including their families in the changes they may need to make in their lives to alleviate dysphoria and reach their full potential. This assistance may consist of guidance in individual psychotherapy, family therapy, group therapy, or support specifically designed for family and caregivers. In addition, mental health collaboration can help an individual at any age if they decide to retransition or otherwise consider alternative care needs that may or may not involve a continued desire for medical intervention.

Support from Peers and Communities

In addition to support from family, TGD people can benefit greatly from support from peers and their communities, both online and offline (e.g., Dowers et al., 2020). The minority stress model hypothesizes that a community of similar others can serve as an important buffer against the negative impact of gender minority stress on mental health and other stress-related health outcomes.[7] Research has shown that peer and community support can indeed moderate the impact of minority stress on mental health and well-being (Bockting et al., 2013; Kia et al., 2021; Nuttbrock et al., 2015). Mental health providers can be instrumental helping TGD people establish support from peer and community networks.

Support for Neurocognitive Needs

A robust body of literature indicates a unique overlap between autism and gender identity (Strang et al., 2023). In many situations, it may be crucial for a TGD autistic[8] individual to have access to both well-informed gender care providers and autism care specialists. When possible, these roles can be filled by the same mental health provider, or they can be filled by different providers in the same interdisciplinary clinic. This continuity can ensure that provider–patient communication is attuned to the autistic person, and that any special needs (e.g., for extra assistance with social transition) can be identified and appropriate supports provided.

VARIABILITY OF PRACTICE

Over the years, gender-affirming care has gradually evolved, as reflected in revisions of the WPATH *Standards of Care* from its first version in 1979 to its eighth, most recent version, adopted in 2022. Evolving standards mean that current gender-affirming care practices, as described above, may not have been accessible to all patients at critical junctures in their care, while other practices that are no longer included in guidelines may have formed the care experience for some patients. Moreover, it is important to acknowledge that access to care has ebbed and flowed and remains variable across the country and internationally. Not until recently has gender-affirming care

---

[7] Originally, the approach to gender-affirming care followed a binary paradigm in which TGD people were strongly encouraged to find community among cisgender women and men (and were often encouraged to "life stealth"—i.e., pass as cisgender and keep their TGD identity hidden). Over the years—and particularly since the 1990s—TGD people empowered themselves; formed strong transgender communities; and reestablished a strong coalition with their gay, lesbian, and bisexual cisgender peers. With the advent of the Internet, access to role models and peer and community support has become ubiquitous, providing a rich environment and multiple communities for TGD people to explore and express their gender identities. Support is extended to families through, for example, TGD networks affiliated with the advocacy group PFLAG.

[8] "Autistic people" (identity-first language) rather than "people with autism" (person-first language) is a conscious choice in line with autistic activists and advocates. This parallels "transgender people" (identity first) rather than "people with gender dysphoria" or "people with transness."

for adults been more widely available in the United States. With respect to care for children and particularly adolescents, the last 10 years have seen a dramatic increase in the availability of services across the country, in part in response to a sharp increase in demand (Denaro et al., 2023; Zhang et al., 2020). As discussed in Chapter 3, however, barriers to high-quality care from competent providers are substantial, and the care experience for many TGD patients may be patchy and inconsistent. All of these factors, coupled with patient choice—in pursuing one form of gender-affirming care over others or in engaging in alternative hormone regimens or non–medically supervised practices (e.g., binding, tucking)—lead to great variability in gender-affirming care. Still, the care TGD persons have received, even outside of current standards of care, may be relevant to their health today and to the Social Security Administration in making appropriate disability determinations.

Finally, health care standards and care delivery systems are largely segregated by sex recorded at birth, and TGD-specific clinical treatment guidelines are largely lacking. Chapter 6 describes common co-occurring conditions in TGD people and describes the lack of research on and guidelines for care to address these conditions appropriately. Part III of this report describes the uneven and sometimes arbitrary care decisions that providers make where research and guidelines fail to inform how to assess chronic disease for TGD patients appropriately. These factors lead to further variability in care, especially where lack of information may cause providers to recommend that patients cease gender-affirming care before they can pursue treatment for chronic conditions.

SUMMARY OF KEY POINTS

Gender-affirming care must be wide-ranging and comprehensive to address the multifaceted impact of growing up and living life with a TGD identity in a world that has far to go to rediscover the diversity in gender identity and expression that is universal and as old as time (Feinberg, 1997). As described in this chapter, gender-affirming care addresses, with both medical and mental health interventions, the visceral experience of incongruence between identity and body; the challenges of navigating a largely binary world in which gender remains a defining factor; and the social stigma—both enacted in discrimination and violence and internalized—attached to nonconformity in gender identity and expression.

Given that every patient is unique, considerable variability is observed in gender-affirming care for TGD individuals and their families across the country. The care provided may differ based on when it was provided (both in history and across the lifespan), differences in access to care, and tailoring of care to the individual needs of patients. The result is different treatment plans and varied levels of monitoring and follow-up, which in turn lead to considerable variability in outcomes.

As examined in Part III of this report, access to and timing of certain gender-affirming care services—in particular, hormone therapy—may impact functional assessment for TGD populations with chronic care needs. High-quality gender-affirming care is provided by a multidisciplinary team that communicates well and guides patients through all their care needs, including care for chronic disease. However, as described in Chapter 3, given substantial barriers to affirming health care of consistent quality faced by many TGD people, patients may not have access to chronic disease providers who know about or understand their journey with gender-affirming care; accordingly, documentation of gender-affirming care may not be present in medical records pertaining to chronic disease. Thus, having a sufficiently complete medical record of gender-affirming care is important for disability adjudication for TGD applicants, as understanding the nature of any gender-affirming care (along with its timing and duration) may be important details that improve understanding of functional measurement and eligibility for disability benefits.

REFERENCES

Abdel-Aziz, M. I., A. H. Neerincx, S. J. H. Vijverberg, S. Hashimoto, P. Brinkman, M. Gorenjak, A. A. Toncheva, S. Harner, S. Brandstetter, C. Wolff, J. Perez-Garcia, A. M. Hedman, C. Almqvist, P. Corcuera-Elosegui, J. Korta-Murua, O. Sardón-Prado, M. Pino-Yanes, U. Potočnik, M. Kabesch, A. D. Kraneveld, and A. H. Maitland-van der Zee. 2021. A system pharmacology multi-omics approach toward uncontrolled pediatric asthma. *Journal of Personalized Medicine* 11(6):484.

Abou-Ismail, M. Y., D. Citla Sridhar, and L. Nayak. 2020. Estrogen and thrombosis: A bench to bedside review. *Thrombosis Research* 192:40–51.

Acerus Pharmaceuticals Corporation. 2016. *Natesto (testosterone) nasal gel CIII.* https://www.natesto.com/pdfs/natesto-full-prescribing-information.pdf (accessed February 29, 2024).

Achille, C., T. Taggart, N. R. Eaton, J. Osipoff, K. Tafuri, A. Lane, and T. A. Wilson. 2020. Longitudinal impact of gender-affirming endocrine intervention on the mental health and well-being of transgender youths: Preliminary results. *International Journal of Pediatric Endocrinology* 2020(8).

ACOG (American College of Obstetricians and Gynecologists). 2022. *General approaches to medical management of menstrual suppression.* Committee on Clinical Consensus-Gynecology. *Obstetrics and Gynecology* 140(3):528–541. https://www.acog.org/-/media/project/acog/acogorg/clinical/files/clinical-consensus/articles/2022/09/general-approaches-to-medical-management-of-menstrual-suppression.pdf (accessed March 5, 2024).

Allen, L. R., L. B. Watson, A. M. Egan, and C. N. Moser. 2019. Well-being and suicidality among transgender youth after gender-affirming hormones. *Clinical Practice in Pediatric Psychology* 7(3):302–311.

Almazan, A. N., and A.S. Keuroghlian. 2021. Association between gender-affirming surgeries and mental health outcomes. *JAMA Surgery* 156(7):611–618.

Altman, K. 2021. Facial feminization surgery: Current state of the art. *International Journal of Oral and Maxillofacial Surgery* 41(8):885–894.

Amato, P. 2016. Fertility options for transgender persons. In *UCSF transgender care & treatment guidelines*, edited by M. B. Deutsch. San Francicso, CA: UCSF Gender Affirming Health Program, Department of Family and Community Medicine, University of California, San Francisco.

American Academy of Pediatrics, Committee on Bioethics. 1995. Informed consent, parental permission, and assent in pediatric practice. *Pediatrics* 95(2):314–317.

American Cancer Society. 2021. *Cancer care for transgender and gender nonconforming people for health care professionals.* https://www.cancer.org/content/dam/cancer-org/cancer-control/en/booklets-flyers/cancer-care-for-transgender-and-gender-nonconforming-people.pdf (accessed May, 14 2024).

Anda, R. F., A. Butchart, V. J. Felitti, and D. W. Brown. 2010. Building a framework for global surveillance of the public health implications of adverse childhood experiences. *American Journal of Preventive Medicine* 39(1):93–98.

ASHP (American Society of Health-System Pharmacists). 2023. *Testosterone transdermal system.* https://www.ashp.org/drug-shortages/current-shortages/drug-shortage-detail.aspx?id=925&loginreturnUrl=SSOCheckOnly# (accessed February 27, 2024).

Bahr, C., J. Ewald, R. Dragovich, and M. D. Gothard. 2024. Effects of progesterone on gender affirmation outcomes as part of feminizing hormone therapy. *Journal of the American Pharmacists Association* 64(1):268–272.

Barbonetti, A., S. D'Andrea, and S. Francavilla. 2020. Testosterone replacement therapy. *Andrology* 8(6):1551–1566.

Bariola, E., A. Lyons, W. Leonard, M. Pitts, P. Badcock, and M. Couch. 2015. Demographic and psychosocial factors associated with psychological distress and resilience among transgender individuals. *American Journal of Public Health* 105(10):2108–2116.

Bejarano, A., D. F. Bautista, L. F. Sua, B. Perez, J. Lores, M. Aguirre, and L. Fernandez-Trujillo. 2020. Acute pneumonitis and diffuse alveolar hemorrhage secondary to silicone embolism: A case report. *Medicine* 99(24):e20578.

Belsky, J. 1993. Etiology of child maltreatment: A developmental-ecological analysis. *Psychological Bulletin* 114(3):413–434.

Bertin, C., R. Abbas, V. Andrieu, F. Michard, C. Rioux, V. Descamps, Y. Yazdanpanah, and F. Bouscarat. 2019. Illicit massive silicone injections always induce chronic and definitive silicone blood diffusion with dermatologic complications. *Medicine* 98(4):e14143.

Bertoncelli Tanaka, M., K. Sahota, J. Burn, A. Falconer, M. Winkler, H. U. Ahmed, and T. G. Rashid. 2022. Prostate cancer in transgender women: What does a urologist need to know? *BJU International* 129(1):113–122.

Bisson, J. R., K. J. Chan, and J. D. Safer. 2018. Prolactin levels do not rise among transgender women treated with estradiol and spironolactone. *Endocrine Practice* 24(7):646–651.

Bockting, W. 2014. The impact of stigma on transgender identity development and mental health. In *Gender dysphoria and disorders of sex development: Progress in care and knowledge, Focus on Sexuality Research.* New York: Springer Science + Business Media. Pp. 319–330.

Bockting, W. O., and R. D. Ehrbar. 2006. Commentary: Gender variance, dissonance, or identity disorder? *Journal of Psychology & Human Sexuality* 17(3-4):125–134.

Bockting, W. O., M. H. Miner, R. E. Swinburne Romine, A. Hamilton, and E. Coleman. 2013. Stigma, mental health, and resilience in an online sample of the U.S. transgender population. *American Journal of Public Health* 103(5):943–951.

Bockting, W., E. Coleman, M. B. Deutsch, A. Guillamon, I. Meyer, W. Meyer, 3rd, S. Reisner, J. Sevelius, and R. Ettner. 2016. Adult development and quality of life of transgender and gender nonconforming people. *Current Opinion in Endocrinology, Diabetes & Obesity* 23(2):188–197.

Boskey, E. R., A. Tahinga, and O. Ganor. 2019. Association of surgical risk with exogenous hormone use in transgender patients: A systematic review. *JAMA Surgery* 154(2):159–169.

Bronfenbrenner, U. 1979. Contexts of child rearing: Problems and prospects. *American Psychologist* 34(10):844–850.

Brown, A., A. P. Lourenco, B. L. Niell, B. Cronin, E. H. Dibble, M. L. DiNome, M. S. Goel, J. Hansen, S. L. Heller, M. S. Jochelson, B. Karrington, K. A. Klein, T. S. Mehta, M. S. Newell, L. Schechter, A. R. Stuckey, M. E. Swain, J. Tseng, D. S. Tuscano, and L. Moy. 2021. ACR appropriateness criteria® transgender breast cancer screening. *Journal of the American College of Radiology* 18(11):S502–S515.

Burinkul, S., K. Panyakhamlerd, A. Suwan, P. Tuntiviriyapun, and S. Wainipitapong. 2021. Anti-androgenic effects comparison between cyproterone acetate and spironolactone in transgender women: A randomized controlled trial. *Journal of Sexual Medicine* 18(7):1299–1307.

Caceres, B. A., K. B. Jackman, J. Belloir, J. Dworkin, C. Dolezal, D. T. Duncan, and W. O. Bockting. 2022. Examining the associations of gender minority stressors with sleep health in gender minority individuals. *Sleep Health* 8(2):153–160.

Cardona, N., M. Nauphal, E. Pariseau, R. Clapham, L. Edwards-Leeper, and A. Tishelman. 2023. Social supports, social stressors, and psychosocial functioning in a sample of transgender youth seeking gender-affirming clinical services. *Psychology of Sexual Orientation and Gender Diversity. Advanced Online Publication.* https://doi.org/10.1037/sgd0000659.

CDC (Centers for Disease Control and Prevention). 2021. *Adverse childhood experiences (ACEs): Preventing early trauma to improve adult health.* https://www.cdc.gov/vitalsigns/aces (accessed March 11, 2024).

Chakraborty, B., J. Byemerwa, T. Krebs, F. Lim, C. Y. Chang, and D. P. McDonnell. 2023. Estrogen receptor signaling in the immune system. *Endocrine Reviews* 44(1):117–141.

Chen, D., J. F. Strang, V. D. Kolbuck, S. M. Rosenthal, K. Wallen, D. P. Waber, L. Steinberg, C. L. Sisk, J. Ross, T. Paus, S. C. Mueller, M. M. McCarthy, P. E. Micevych, C. L. Martin, B. P. C. Kreukels, L. Kenworthy, M. M. Herting, A. Herlitz, I. Haraldsen, R. Dahl, E. A. Crone, G. J. Chelune, S. M. Burke, S. A. Berenbaum, A. M. Beltz, J. Bakker, L. Eliot, E. Vilain, G. L. Wallace, E. E. Nelson, and R. Garofalo. 2020. Consensus parameter: Research methodologies to evaluate neurodevelopmental effects of pubertal suppression in transgender youth. *Transgender Health* 5(4):246–257.

Chen, W., I. Cylinder, A. Najafian, D. D. Dugi III, and J. U. Berli. 2021. An option for shaft-only gender-affirming phalloplasty: Vaginal preservation and vulvoscrotoplasty: A technical description. *Plastic and Reconstructive Surgery* 147(2):480–483.

Cheng, P. J., A. W. Pastuszak, J. B. Myers, I. A. Goodwin, and J. M. Hotaling. 2019. Fertility concerns of the transgender patient. *Translational Andrology and Urology* 8(3):209–218.

Chlebowski, R. T., G. L. Anderson, A. K. Aragaki, J. E. Manson, M. L. Stefanick, K. Pan, W. Barrington, L. H. Kuller, M. S. Simon, D. Lane, K. C. Johnson, T. E. Rohan, M. L. S. Gass, J. A. Cauley, E. D. Paskett, M. Sattari, and R. L. Prentice. 2020. Association of menopausal hormone therapy with breast cancer incidence and mortality during long-term follow-up of the women's health initiative randomized clinical trials. *JAMA* 324(4):369–380.

Choi, J. Y., and T. J. Kim. 2022. Fertility preservation and reproductive potential in transgender and gender fluid population. *Biomedicines* 10(9):2279.

Ciancia, S., V. Dubois, and M. Cools. 2022. Impact of gender-affirming treatment on bone health in transgender and gender diverse youth. *Endocrine Connections* 11(11).

Claes, K., S. D'Arpa, and S. J. Monstrey. 2018. Chest surgery for transgender and gender nonconforming individuals. *Clinics in Plastic Surgery* 45(3):369–380.

Cohen, A., V. Gomez-Lobo, L. Willing, D. Call, L. F. Damle, L. J. D'Angelo, A. Song, and J. F. Strang. 2023. Shifts in gender-related medical requests by transgender and gender-diverse adolescents. *Journal of Adolescent Health* 72(3):428–436.

Coleman, E., A. E. Radix, W. P. Bouman, G. R. Brown, A. L. C. De Vries, M. B. Deutsch, R. Ettner, L. Fraser, M. Goodman, J. Green, A. B. Hancock, T. W. Johnson, D. H. Karasic, G. A. Knudson, S. F. Leibowitz, H. F. L. Meyer-Bahlburg, S. J. Monstrey, J. Motmans, L. Nahata, T. O. Nieder, S. L. Reisner, C. Richards, L. S. Schechter, V. Tangpricha, A. C. Tishelman, M. A. A. Van Trotsenburg, S. Winter, K. Ducheny, N. J. Adams, T. M. Adrián, L. R. Allen, D. Azul, H. Bagga, K. Başar, D. S. Bathory, J. J. Belinky, D. R. Berg, J. U. Berli, R. O. Bluebond-Langner, M. B. Bouman, M. L. Bowers, P. J. Brassard, J. Byrne, L. Capitán, C. J. Cargill, J. M. Carswell, S. C. Chang, G. Chelvakumar, T. Corneil, K. B. Dalke, G. De Cuypere, E. De Vries, M. Den Heijer, A. H. Devor, C. Dhejne, A. D'Marco, E. K. Edmiston, L. Edwards-Leeper, R. Ehrbar, D. Ehrensaft, J. Eisfeld, E. Elaut, L. Erickson-Schroth, J. L. Feldman, A. D. Fisher, M. M. Garcia, L. Gijs, S. E. Green, B. P. Hall, T. L. D. Hardy, M. S. Irwig, L. A. Jacobs, A. C. Janssen, K. Johnson, D. T. Klink, B. P. C. Kreukels, L. E. Kuper, E. J. Kvach, M. A. Malouf, R. Massey, T. Mazur, C. McLachlan, S. D. Morrison, S. W. Mosser, P. M. Neira, U. Nygren, J. M. Oates, J. Obedin-Maliver, G. Pagkalos, J. Patton, N. Phanuphak, K. Rachlin, T. Reed, G. N. Rider, J. Ristori, S. Robbins-Cherry, S. A. Roberts, K. A. Rodriguez-Wallberg, S. M. Rosenthal, K. Sabir, J. D. Safer, A. I. Scheim, L. J. Seal, T. J. Sehoole, K. Spencer, C. St. Amand, T. D. Steensma, J. F. Strang, G. B. Taylor, K. Tilleman, G. G. T'Sjoen, L. N. Vala, N. M. Van Mello, J. F. Veale, J. A. Vencill, B. Vincent, L. M. Wesp, M. A. West, and J. Arcelus. 2022. Standards of care for the health of transgender and gender diverse people: Version 8. *International Journal of Transgender Health* 23(Suppl 1):S1–S259.

Conn, P. M., and W. F. Crowley, Jr. 1991. Gonadotropin-releasing hormone and its analogues. *New England Journal of Medicine* 324(2):93–103.

Connolly, M. D., M. J. Zervos, C. J. Barone, C. C. Johnson, and C. L. M. Joseph. 2016. The mental health of transgender youth: Advances in understanding. *Journal of Adolescent Health* 59(5):489–495.

Coyne, C. A., B. T. Yuodsnukis, and D. Chen. 2023. Gender dysphoria: Optimizing healthcare for transgender and gender diverse youth with a multidisciplinary approach. *Neuropsychiatric Disease and Treatment* 19:479–493.

Cumming, R., K. Sylvester, and J. Fuld. 2016. P257: Understanding the effects on lung function of chest binder use in the transgender population. *Thorax* 71:A227–A227.

Davis, S. A., and C. St. Amand. 2014. Effects of testosterone treatment and chest reconstruction surgery on mental health and sexuality in female-to-male transgender people. *International Journal of Sexual Health* 26(2):113–128.

de Blok, C. J. M., M. Klaver, C. M. Wiepjes, N. M. Nota, A. C. Heijboer, A. D. Fisher, T. Schreiner, G. T'Sjoen, and M. den Heijer. 2018. Breast development in transwomen after 1 year of cross-sex hormone therapy: Results of a prospective multicenter study. *Journal of Clinical Endocrinology & Metabolism* 103(2):532–538.

de Blok, C. J. M., C. M. Wiepjes, N. M. Nota, K. van Engelen, M. A. Adank, K. M. A. Dreijerink, E. Barbé, I. R. H. M. Konings, and M. den Heijer. 2019. Breast cancer risk in transgender people receiving hormone treatment: Nationwide cohort study in the Netherlands. *BMJ* 365:l1652.

de Nie, I., J. Asseler, A. Meissner, I. A. C. Voorn-de Warem, E. H. Kostelijk, M. den Heijer, J. Huirne, and N. M. van Mello. 2022. A cohort study on factors impairing semen quality in transgender women. *American Journal of Obstetrics and Gynecology* 226(3):390. e391–390.e310.

de Vries, A. L. C., and P. T. Cohen-Kettenis. 2012. Clinical management of gender dysphoria in children and adolescents: The Dutch approach. *Journal of Homosexuality* 59(3):301–320.

de Vries, A. L., T. D. Steensma, T. A. Doreleijers, and P. T. Cohen-Kettenis. 2011. Puberty suppression in adolescents with gender identity disorder: A prospective follow-up study. *Journal of Sexual Medicine* 8(8):2276–2283.

Debarbo, C. J. M. 2020. Rare cause of testicular torsion in a transwoman: A case report. *Urology Case Reports* 33:101422.

Deebel, N. A., J. P. Morin, R. Autorino, R. Vince, B. Grob, and L. J. Hampton. 2017. Prostate cancer in transgender women: Incidence, etiopathogenesis, and management challenges. *Urology* 110:166–171.

Delozier, A. M., R. C. Kamody, S. Rodgers, and D. Chen. 2020. Health disparities in transgender and gender expansive adolescents: A topical review from a minority stress framework. *Journal of Pediatric Psychology* 45(8):842–847.

Denaro, A., C. M. Pflugeisen, T. Colglazier, D. DeWine, and B. Thompson. 2023. Lessons from grassroots efforts to increase gender-affirming medical care for transgender and gender diverse youth in the community health care setting. *Transgender Health* 8(3):207–212.

Departmental Appeals Board. 2014. *NCD 140.3, Transsexual surgery: Docket no. A-13-87: Decision no. 2576.* May 30, 2014. Washington, DC: U.S. Department of Health and Human Services. https://www.hhs.gov/sites/default/files/static/dab/decisions/board-decisions/2014/dab2576.pdf (accessed May 21, 2024).

Deschamps-Braly, J. C., C. L. Sacher, J. Fick, and D. K. Ousterhout. 2017. First female-to-male facial confirmation surgery with description of a new procedure for masculinization of the thyroid cartilage (Adam's apple). *Plastic and Reconstructive Surgery* 139(4):883e–887e.

Deutsch, M. B., A. Radix, and L. Wesp. 2017. Breast cancer screening, management, and a review of case study literature in transgender populations. *Seminars in Reproductive Medicine* 35(5):434–441.

Devor, A. H. 2004. Witnessing and mirroring: A fourteen stage model of transsexual identity formation. *Journal of Gay & Lesbian Psychotherapy* 8(1-2):41–67.

Doll, E. E., I. Gunsolus, N. Lamberton, V. Tangpricha, and J. L. Sarvaideo. 2020. SUN-LB9 pharmacokinetics of sublingual versus oral estradiol in transgender women. *Journal of the Endocrine Society* 4(Suppl 1):SUN-LB9.

Doll, E., I. Gunsolus, A. Thorgerson, V. Tangpricha, N. Lamberton, and J. L. Sarvaideo. 2022. Pharmacokinetics of sublingual versus oral estradiol in transgender women. *Endocrine Practice* 28(3):237–242.

Dowers, E., C. White, K. Cook, and J. Kingsley. 2020. Trans, gender diverse and non-binary adult experiences of social support: A systematic quantitative literature review. *International Journal of Transgender Health* 21(3):242–257.

Dragoman, M. V., N. K. Tepper, R. Fu, K. M. Curtis, R. Chou, and M. E. Gaffield. 2018. A systematic review and meta-analysis of venous thrombosis risk among users of combined oral contraception. *International Journal of Gynecology & Obstetrics* 141(3):287–294.

Dragon, C. N., P. Guerino, E. Ewald, and A. M. Laffan. 2017. Transgender Medicare beneficiaries and chronic conditions: Exploring fee-for-service claims data. *LGBT Health* 4(6):404–411.

Durwood, L., L. Eisner, K. Fladeboe, C. G. Ji, S. Barney, K. A. McLaughlin, and K. R. Olson. 2021. Social support and internalizing psychopathology in transgender youth. *Journal of Youth and Adolescence* 50(5):841–854.

Ehrensaft, D., S. Giammattei, K. Storck, A. Tishelman, and C. St. Amand. 2018. Prepubertal social gender transitions: What we know; what we can learn—A view from a gender affirmative lens. *International Journal of Transgenderism* 19:1–18.

Elfering, L., T. C. van de Grift, M. Al-Tamimi, F. W. Timmermans, K. B. de Haseth, G. L. S. Pigot, B. I. Lissenberg-Witte, M. B. Bouman, and M. G. Mullender. 2021. How sensitive is the neophallus? Postphalloplasty experienced and objective sensitivity in transmasculine persons. *Sexual Medicine* 9(5):100413.

Erikson, E. H. 1994. *Identity and the life cycle.* New York: W.W. Norton & Company.

Fehl, A., S. Ferrari, Z. Wecht, and M. Rosenzweig. 2019. Breast cancer in the transgender population. *Journal of the Advanced Practitioner in Oncology* 10(4):387–394.

Feinberg, L. 1997. *Transgender warriors: Making history from Joan of Arc to Marsha P. Johnson and beyond.* Boston: Beacon Press.

Fierz, R., G. P. Ghisu, and D. Fink. 2019. Squamous carcinoma of the neovagina after male-to-female reconstruction surgery: A case report and review of the literature. *Case Reports in Obstetrics and Gynecology* 2019:4820396.

Flentje, A., K. D. Clark, E. Cicero, M. R. Capriotti, M. E. Lubensky, J. Sauceda, T. B. Neilands, M. R. Lunn, and J. Obedin-Maliver. 2022. Minority stress, structural stigma, and physical health among sexual and gender minority individuals: Examining the relative strength of the relationships. *Annals of Behavioral Medicine* 56(6):573–591.

Fredriksen-Goldsen, K. I., L. Cook-Daniels, H. J. Kim, E. A. Erosheva, C. A. Emlet, C. P. Hoy-Ellis, J. Goldsen, and A. Muraco. 2014. Physical and mental health of transgender older adults: An at-risk and underserved population. *Gerontologist* 54(3):488–500.

Fredriksen-Goldsen, K., A. Prasad, H. J. Kim, and H. Jung. 2023. Lifetime violence, lifetime discrimination, and microaggressions in the lives of LGBT midlife and older adults: Findings from aging with pride: National health, aging, and sexuality/gender study. *LGBT Health* 10(S1):S49–S60.

Fuller, K. A., and D. W. Riggs. 2018. Family support and discrimination and their relationship to psychological distress and resilience amongst transgender people. *International Journal of Transgenderism* 19(4):379–388.

Gagne, P., R. Tewksbury, and D. McGaughey. 1997. Coming out and crossing over: Identity formation and proclamation in a transgender community. *Gender and Society* 11(4):478–508.

Gao, J. L., C. G. Streed, Jr., J. Thompson, E. D. Dommasch, and J. K. Peebles. 2023. Androgenetic alopecia in transgender and gender diverse populations: A review of therapeutics. *Journal of the American Academy of Dermatology* 89(4):774–783.

Garcia, M. M., N. A. Christopher, F. De Luca, M. Spilotros, and D. J. Ralph. 2014. Overall satisfaction, sexual function, and the durability of neophallus dimensions following staged female to male genital gender confirming surgery: The Institute of Urology, London U.K. experience. *Translational Andrology and Urology* 3(2):156–162.

Gosling, H., D. Pratt, H. Montgomery, and J. Lea. 2022. The relationship between minority stress factors and suicidal ideation and behaviours amongst transgender and gender non-conforming adults: A systematic review. *Journal of Affective Disorders* 303:31–51.

Gottlieb, L. 2018. Radial forearm. *Clinics in Plastic Surgery* 45(3):391–398.

Greenwald P., B. Dubois, J. Lekovich, J. H. Pang, and J. Safer. 2021. Successful in vitro fertilization in a cisgender female carrier using oocytes retrieved from a transgender man maintained on testosterone. *AACE Clinical Case Reports* 16(8):19–21.

Guss, C., and C. M. Gordon. 2022. Pubertal blockade and subsequent gender-affirming therapy. *JAMA Network Open* 5(11):e2239763.

Hadj-Moussa, M., D. A. Ohl, and W. M. Kuzon, Jr. 2018. Feminizing genital gender-confirmation surgery. *Sexual Medicine Reviews* 6(3):457–468.e452.

Hage, J. 1996. Metaidoioplasty: An alternative phalloplasty technique in transsexuals. *Plastic and Reconstructive Surgery* 97(1):161–167.

Hage, J., R. Karim, and D. Laub, Sr. 2007. On the origin of pedicled skin inversion vaginoplasty: Life and work of Dr. Georges Burou of Casablanca. *Annals of Plastic Surgery* 59(6):723–729.

Hage, M., O. Plesa, I. Lemaire, and M. L. Raffin Sanson. 2022. Estrogen and progesterone therapy and meningiomas. *Endocrinology* 163(2):bqab259.

Hembree, W. C., P. T. Cohen-Kettenis, L. Gooren, S. E. Hannema, W. J. Meyer, M. H. Murad, S. M. Rosenthal, J. D. Safer, V. Tangpricha, and G. G. T'Sjoen. 2017. Endocrine treatment of gender-dysphoric/gender-incongruent persons: An endocrine society clinical practice guideline. *Journal of Clinical Endocrinology & Metabolism* 102(11):3869–3903.

Hendricks, M. L., and R. J. Testa. 2012. A conceptual framework for clinical work with transgender and gender nonconforming clients: An adaptation of the minority stress model. *Professional Psychology: Research and Practice* 43(5):460–467.

Heston, A. L., N. O. Esmonde, D. D. Dugi III, and J. U. Berli. 2019. Phalloplasty: Techniques and outcomes. *Translational Andrology and Urology* 8(3):254–265.

Holmberg, M., S. Arver, and C. Dhejne. 2019. Supporting sexuality and improving sexual function in transgender persons. *Nature Reviews Urology* 16(2):121–139.

Hong, Y. R., and J. S. Park. 2012. Impact of attachment, temperament and parenting on human development. *Korean Journal of Pediatrics* 55(12):449–454.

Hontscharuk, R., B. Alba, C. Manno, E. Pine, M. Deutsch, D. Coon, and L. Schechter. 2021. Perioperative transgender hormone management: Avoiding venous thromboembolism and other complications. *Plastic and Reconstructive Surgery* 147(4):1008–1017.

Horbach, S. E., M. B. Bouman, J. M. Smit, M. Özer, M. E. Buncamper, and M. G. Mullender. 2015. Outcome of vaginoplasty in male-to-female transgenders: A systematic review of surgical techniques. *Journal of Sexual Medicine* 12(6):1499–1512.

Huang, C., S. Gold, R. Radi, S. Amos, and H. Yeung. 2022. Managing dermatologic effects of gender-affirming therapy in transgender adolescents. *Adolescent Health, Medicine and Therapeutics* 13:93–106.

Hughto, J. M. W., S. L. Reisner, and J. E. Pachankis. 2015. Transgender stigma and health: A critical review of stigma determinants, mechanisms, and interventions. *Social Science & Medicine* 147:222–231.

Irwig, M. S. 2017. Testosterone therapy for transgender men. *The Lancet Diabetes & Endocrinology* 5(4):301–311.

Jackman, K. B., C. Dolezal, B. Levin, J. C. Honig, and W. O. Bockting. 2018. Stigma, gender dysphoria, and nonsuicidal self-injury in a community sample of transgender individuals. *Psychiatry Research* 269:602–609.

Jerome, R. R., M. K. Randhawa, J. Kowalczyk, A. Sinclair, and I. Monga. 2022. Sexual satisfaction after gender affirmation surgery in transgender individuals. *Cureus* 14(7):e27365.

Johnson, E. E. H., S. M. J. Wilder, C. V. S. Andersen, S. A. Horvath, H. M. Kolp, C. A. Gidycz, and R. C. Shorey. 2021. Trauma and alcohol use among transgender and gender diverse women: An examination of the stress-buffering hypothesis of social support. *Journal of Primary Prevention* 42(6):567–581.

Jorgensen, S. C. J., P. K. Hunter, L. Regenstreif, J. Sinai, and W. J. Malone. 2022. Puberty blockers for gender dysphoric youth: A lack of sound science. *Journal of the American College of Clinical Pharmacy* 5(9):1005–1007.

Julian, J. M., B. Salvetti, J. I. Held, P. M. Murray, L. Lara-Rojas, and J. Olson-Kennedy. 2021. The impact of chest binding in transgender and gender diverse youth and young adults. *Journal of Adolescent Health* 68(6):1129–1134.

Katz-Wise, S. L., V. Sarda, S. B. Austin, and S. K. Harris. 2021. Longitudinal effects of gender minority stressors on substance use and related risk and protective factors among gender minority adolescents. *PLoS ONE* 16(6):e0250500.

Katz-Wise, S., L. Ranker, A. Kraus, Y.-C. Wang, Z. Xuan, J. Green, and M. Holt. 2023a. Fluidity in gender identity and sexual orientation identity in transgender and nonbinary youth. *Journal of Sex Research* 1–10.

Katz-Wise, S. L., L. R. Ranker, A. R. Gordon, Z. Xuan, and K. Nelson. 2023b. Sociodemographic patterns in retrospective sexual orientation identity and attraction change in the sexual orientation fluidity in youth study. *Journal of Adolescent Health* 72(3):437–443.

Kaufman, E. A., B. Meddaoui, N. E. Seymour, and S. E. Victor. 2023. The roles of minority stress and thwarted belongingness in suicidal ideation among cisgender and transgender/nonbinary LGBTQ+individuals. *Archives of Suicide Research* 27(4):1296–1311.

Keuroghlian, A. S., J. Potter, S. L. Reisner, and I. Fenway. 2022. *Transgender and gender diverse health care: The Fenway guide.* New York: McGraw-Hill.

Khorrami, A., S. Kumar, E. Bertin, R. Wassersug, C. O'Dwyer, S. Mukherjee, L. Witherspoon, P. Mankowski, K. Genoway, and A. G. Kavanagh. 2022. The sexual goals of metoidioplasty patients and their attitudes toward using PDE5 inhibitors and intracavernosal injections as erectile aids. *Sexual Medicine* 10(3):100505.

Kia, H., K. R. MacKinnon, A. Abramovich, and S. Bonato. 2021. Peer support as a protective factor against suicide in trans populations: A scoping review. *Social Science & Medicine* 279:114026.

Kidd, J. D., T. G. Goetz, E. A. Shea, and W. O. Bockting. 2021. Prevalence and minority-stress correlates of past 12-month prescription drug misuse in a national sample of transgender and gender nonbinary adults: Results from the U.S. Transgender survey. *Drug and Alcohol Dependence Reports* 219:108474.

Kim, E. Y. 2015. Long-term effects of gonadotropin-releasing hormone analogs in girls with central precocious puberty. *Korean Journal of Pediatrics* 58(1):1–7.

Kocjancic, E., and V. Iacovelli. 2018. Penile prostheses. *Clinics in Plastic Surgery* 45(3): 407–414.

Koyanagi, A., H. Oh, A. F. Carvalho, L. Smith, J. M. Haro, D. Vancampfort, B. Stubbs, and J. E. DeVylder. 2019. Bullying victimization and suicide attempt among adolescents aged 12–15 years from 48 countries. *Journal of the American Academy of Child and Adolescent Psychiatry* 58(9):907–18.e904.

Kozato, A., G. W. C. Fox, P. C. Yong, S. J. Shin, B. K. Avanessian, J. Ting, Y. Ling, S. Karim, J. D. Safer, and J. H. Pang. 2021. No venous thromboembolism increase among transgender female patients remaining on estrogen for Gender-Affirming surgery. *Journal of Clinical Endocrinology & Metabolism* 106(4):1586–1590.

Krebs, D., R. M. Harris, A. Steinbaum, S. Pilcher, C. Guss, J. Kremen, S. A. Roberts, C. Baskaran, J. Carswell, and K. Millington. 2022. Care for transgender young people. *Hormone Research in Paediatrics* 95(5):405–414.

Kumar, P., N. Kumar, D. S. Thakur, and A. Patidar. 2010. Male hypogonadism: Symptoms and treatment. *Agricultural Policy Paper* 1(3):297.

Kuper, L. E., S. Stewart, S. Preston, M. Lau, and X. Lopez. 2020. Body dissatisfaction and mental health outcomes of youth on gender-affirming hormone therapy. *Pediatrics* 145(4):e20193006.

Lambrou, N. H., C. E. Gleason, E. Cicero, and J. D. Flatt. 2020. Prevalence of subjective cognitive decline higher among transgender and gender nonbinary adults in the U.S., 2016–2018. *Alzheimer's & Dementia* 16(S10):e044298.

Lane, M., J. F. Waljee, and D. Stroumsa. 2022. Treatment preferences and gender affirmation of nonbinary and transgender people in a national probability sample. *Obstetrics & Gynecology* 140(1):77–81.

LaVasseur, C., S. Neukam, T. Kartika, B. Samuelson Bannow, J. Shatzel, and T. G. DeLoughery. 2022. Hormonal therapies and venous thrombosis: Considerations for prevention and management. *Research and Practice in Thrombosis and Haemostasis* 23(6):e12763.

Lawrentschuk, N., and N. Fleshner. 2009. Severe irritant contact dermatitis causing skin ulceration secondary to a testosterone patch. *Scientific World Journal* 20(9):333–338.

Lee, A., P. Simpson, and B. Haire. 2019. The binding practices of transgender and gender-diverse adults in Sydney, Australia. *Culture, Health & Sex* 21(9):969–984.

Lee, J. Y. 2023. Bone health in the transgender and gender diverse youth population. *Current Osteoporosis Reports* 21(4):459–471.

Lefevor, G. T., C. C. Boyd-Rogers, B. M. Sprague, and R. A. Janis. 2019. Health disparities between genderqueer, transgender, and cisgender individuals: An extension of minority stress theory. *Journal of Counseling Psychology* 66(4):385–395.

Lewins, F. W. 1995. *Transsexualism in society: A sociology of male to female transsexuals.* Australia: Macmillan Education.

Light, A. D., J. Obedin-Maliver, J. M. Sevelius, and J. L. Kerns. 2014. Transgender men who experienced pregnancy after female-to-male gender transitioning. *Obstetrics & Gynecology* 124(6):1120–1127.

Lynch, M., and D. Cicchetti. 1998. An ecological-transactional analysis of children and contexts: The longitudinal interplay among child maltreatment, community violence, and children's symptomatology. *Development and Psychopathology* 10(2):235–257.

MacKinnon, K. R., H. Kia, W. A. Gould, L. E. Ross, A. Abramovich, G. Enxuga, and J. S. H. Lam. 2023. A typology of pathways to detransition: Considerations for care practice with transgender and gender diverse people who stop or reverse their gender transition. *Psychology of Sexual Orientation and Gender Diversity.* https://doi.org/10.1037/sgd0000678.

Madsen, M. C., D. van Dijk, C. M. Wiepjes, E. B. Conemans, A. Thijs, and M. den Heijer. 2021. Erythrocytosis in a large cohort of trans men using testosterone: A long-term follow-up study on prevalence, determinants, and exposure years. *Journal of Clinical Endocrinology & Metabolism* 106(6):1710–1717.

Maldonado, J. R. 2019. Why is it important to consider social support when assessing organ transplant candidates? *American Journal of Bioethics* 19(11):1–8.

Malik, M., E. E. Cooney, J. M. Brevelle, and T. Poteat. 2024. Tucking practices and attributed health effects in transfeminine individuals. *Transgender Health* 9(1):92–97.

Marconi, E., L. Monti, A. Marfoli, G. D. Kotzalidis, D. Janiri, C. Cianfriglia, F. Moriconi, S. Costa, C. Veredice, G. Sani, and D. P. R. Chieffo. 2023. A systematic review on gender dysphoria in adolescents and young adults: Focus on suicidal and self-harming ideation and behaviours. *Child and Adolescent Psychiatry and Mental Health* 17:110.

Martinerie, L., J. De Mouzon, J. Blumberg, L. Di Nicola, P. Maisonobe, J.-C. Carel, and the PREFER Study Group. 2020. Fertility of women treated during childhood with triptorelin (depot formulation) for central precocious puberty: The PREFER study. *Hormone Research in Paediatrics* 93(9-10):529–538.

Masten, A. S., and D. Cicchetti. 2010. Developmental cascades. *Development and Psychopathology* 22(3):491–495.

Mauvais-Jarvis, F., D. J. Clegg, and A. L. Hevener. 2013. The role of estrogens in control of energy balance and glucose homeostasis. *Endocrine Reviews* 34(3):309–338.

Mazzola, A., L. M. Vaughn, G. Chelvakumar, L. A. E. Conard, D. J. Fortenberry, R. V. Voss, and E. A. Lipstein. 2023. Decision support needs for transgender and gender-diverse youth and families: A patient-centered needs assessment. *Journal of Adolescent Health* 72(3):452–459.

McCann, E., and D. Sharek. 2016. Mental health needs of people who identify as transgender: A review of the literature. *Archives of Psychiatric Nursing* 30(2):280–285.

Meyer, I. H. 2003. Prejudice, social stress, and mental health in lesbian, gay, and bisexual populations: Conceptual issues and research evidence. *Psychological Bulletin* 129(5):674–697.

Millward, C. P., S. M. Keshwara, A. I. Islim, M. D. Jenkinson, A. F. Alalade, and C. E. Gilkes. 2022. Development and growth of intracranial meningiomas in transgender women taking cyproterone acetate as gender-affirming progestogen therapy: A systematic review. *Transgender Health* 7(6):473–483.

Monstrey, S., G. Selvaggi, P. Ceulemans, K. Van Landuyt, C. Bowman, P. Blondeel, M. Hamdi, and G. De Cuypere. 2008. Chest-wall contouring surgery in female-to-male transsexuals: A new algorithm. *Plastic and Reconstructive Surgery* 121(3):849–859.

Motosko, C. C., and A. Tosti. 2021. Dermatologic care of hair in transgender patients: A systematic review of literature. *Dermatology and Therapy* 11(5):1457–1468.

Moyer, A. M., E. T. Matey, and V. M. Miller. 2019. Individualized medicine: Sex, hormones, genetics, and adverse drug reactions. *Pharmacology Research & Perspectives* 7(6):e00541.

Nelson, C. A., R. D., Scott, Z. A., Bhutta, N. B., Harris, A. Danese, and M. Samara. 2020. Adversity in childhood is linked to mental and physical health throughout life. *British Medical Journal* 371:m3048.

Neyman, A., J. S. Fuqua, and E. A. Eugster. 2019. Bicalutamide as an androgen blocker with secondary effect of promoting feminization in male-to-female transgender adolescents. *Journal of Adolescent Health* 64(4):544–546.

Nikolavsky, D., M. Hughes, and L. C. Zhao. 2018. Urologic complications after phalloplasty or metoidioplasty. *Clinics in Plastic Surgery* 45(3):425–435.

Nos, A. L., D. A. Klein, T. A. Adirim, N. A. Schvey, E. Hisle-Gorman, A. Susi, and C. M. Roberts. 2022. Association of gonadotropin-releasing hormone analogue use with subsequent use of gender-affirming hormones among transgender adolescents. *JAMA Network Open* 1(5):e2239758.

Nurius, P. S., S. Green, P. Logan-Greene, and S. Borja. 2015. Life course pathways of adverse childhood experiences toward adult psychological well-being: A stress process analysis. *Child Abuse & Neglect* 45:143–53.

Nuttbrock, L., W. Bockting, A. Rosenblum, S. Hwahng, M. Mason, M. Macri, and J. Becker. 2014a. Gender abuse and major depression among transgender women: A prospective study of vulnerability and resilience. *American Journal of Public Health* 104(11):2191–2198.

Nuttbrock, L., W. Bockting, A. Rosenblum, S. Hwahng, M. Mason, M. Macri, and J. Becker. 2014b. Gender abuse, depressive symptoms, and substance use among transgender women: A 3-year prospective study. *American Journal of Public Health* 104(11):2199–2206.

Nuttbrock, L., W. Bockting, A. Rosenblum, S. Hwahng, M. Mason, M. Macri, and J. Becker. 2015. Transgender community involvement and the psychological impact of abuse among transgender women. *Psychology of Sexual Orientation and Gender Diversity* 2(4):386–390.

O'Bryant, C., T. Flaig, and K. Utz. 2008. Bicalutamide-associated fulminant hepatotoxicity. *Pharmacotherapy: The Journal of Human Pharmacology & Drug Therapy* 28(8):1071–1075.

Ohnona, J., P. Durand, J. L. Amegnizin, and K. Kerrou. 2016. Silicone granuloma in the buttocks incidentally detected by 18F-FDG PET/CT 30 years after free liquid silicone injections. *Clinical Nuclear Medicine* 41(6):492–493.

Olezeski, C., E. Pariseau, W. Bamatter, and A. Tishelman. 2020. Assessing gender in young children: Constructs and considerations. *Psychology of Sexual Orientation and Gender Diversity* 7(3):293–303.

Olson, K. R., L. Durwood, M. DeMeules, and K. A. McLaughlin. 2016. Mental health of transgender children who are supported in their identities. *Pediatrics* 137(3):e20153223.

Olson, K. R., L. Durwood, R. Horton, N. M. Gallagher, and A. Devor. 2022. Gender identity 5 years after social transition. *Pediatrics* 150(2):01.

Olson-Kennedy, J., J. Warus, V. Okonta, M. Belzer, and L. F. Clark. 2018. Chest reconstruction and chest dysphoria in transmasculine minors and young adults: Comparisons of nonsurgical and postsurgical cohorts. *JAMA Pediatrics* 172(5):431–436.

Pando, B. L., B. Goldsmith, A. L. Webb, K. Kinger, and B. Helmly. 2022. Free silicone-induced granulomatosis and hypercalcemia in a transgender female. *HCA Healthcare Journal of Medicine* 3(3):161–166.

Pang, K. C., T. P. Nguyen, and R. Upreti. 2021. Case report: Successful use of minoxidil to promote facial hair growth in an adolescent transgender male. *Frontiers in Endocrinology* 12:e725269.

Pariseau, E. M., L. Chevalier, K. A. Long, R. Clapham, L. Edwards-Leeper, and A. C. Tishelman. 2019. The relationship between family acceptance-rejection and transgender youth psychosocial functioning. *Clinical Practice in Pediatric Psychology* 7(3):267–277.

Patel, H., V. Arruarana, L. Yao, X. Cui, and E. Ray. 2020. Effects of hormones and hormone therapy on breast tissue in transgender patients: A concise review. *Endocrine* 68(1): 6–15.

Patel, H., Y. Samaha, G. Ives, T.-Y. Lee, X. Cui, and E. Ray. 2021. Chest feminization in male-to-female transgender patients: A review of options. *Transgender Health* 6(5): 244–255.

Peitzmeier, S. M., S. L. Reisner, P. Harigopal, and J. Potter. 2014. Female-to-male patients have high prevalence of unsatisfactory paps compared to non-transgender females: Implications for cervical cancer screening. *Journal of General Internal Medicine* 29(5):778–784.

Peitzmeier, S., I. Gardner, J. Weinand, A. Corbet, and K. Acevedo. 2017. Health impact of chest binding among transgender adults: A community-engaged, cross-sectional study. *Culture, Health, and Sexuality* 19(1):64–75.

Pellicane, M. J., and J. A. Ciesla. 2022. Associations between minority stress, depression, and suicidal ideation and attempts in transgender and gender diverse (TGD) individuals: Systematic review and meta-analysis. *Clinical Psychology Review* 91:102113.

Pellicane, M. J., M. E. Quinn, and J. A. Ciesla. 2023. Transgender and gender-diverse minority stress and substance use frequency and problems: Systematic review and meta-analysis. *Transgender Health* preprint. https://doi.org/10.1089/trgh.2023.0025.

Price, M. A., N. L. Hollinsaid, S. McKetta, E. J. Mellen, and M. Rakhilin. 2024. Structural transphobia is associated with psychological distress and suicidality in a large national sample of transgender adults. *Social Psychiatry and Psychiatric Epidemiology* 59(2):285–294.

Puckett J. A., P. Cleary, K. Rossman, M. E. Newcomb, and B. Mustanski. 2018. Barriers to gender-affirming care for transgender and gender nonconforming individuals. *Sexuality Research and Social Policy* 15(1):48–59.

Puckett, J. A., E. Matsuno, C. Dyar, B. Mustanski, and M. E. Newcomb. 2019. Mental health and resilience in transgender individuals: What type of support makes a difference? *Journal of Family Psychology* 33(8):954–964.

Puckett, J. A., C. Dyar, M. R. Maroney, B. Mustanski, and M. E. Newcomb. 2023. Daily experiences of minority stress and mental health in transgender and gender-diverse individuals. *Journal of Psychopathology and Clinical Science* 132(3):340–350.

Putney, J. M., S. Keary, N. Hebert, L. Krinsky, and R. Halmo. 2018. "Fear runs deep:" The anticipated needs of LGBT older adults in long-term care. *Journal of Gerontological Social Work* 61(8):887–907.

Radix, A., J. Sevelius, and M. B. Deutsch. 2016. Transgender women, hormonal therapy and HIV treatment: A comprehensive review of the literature and recommendations for best practices. *Journal of the International AIDS Society* 19(3 Suppl 2):e20810.

Rae, J. R., S. Gülgöz, L. Durwood, M. DeMeules, R. Lowe, G. Lindquist, and K. R. Olson. 2019. Predicting early-childhood gender transitions. *Psychological Science* 30(5): 669–681.

Ramsay, A., and J. D. Safer. 2023. Update in adult transgender medicine. *Annual Review of Medicine* 74:117–124.

Reisner, S., T. Poteat, J. Keatley, M. Cabral, T. Mothopeng, E. Dunham, C. Holland, R. Max, and S. Baral. 2016. Global health burden and needs of transgender populations: A review. *The Lancet* 388(10042):412–436.

Roblee, C., A. Hamidian Jahromi, B. Ferragamo, A. Radix, G. De Cuypere, J. Green, A. H. Dorafshar, R. Ettner, S. Monstrey, and L. Schechter. 2023. Gender-affirmative surgery: A collaborative approach between the surgeon and mental health professional. *Plastic and Reconstructive Surgery* 152(5):e953–e961.

Rosendaal, F. R., F. M. Helmerhorst, and J. P. Vandenbroucke. 2002. Female hormones and thrombosis. *Arteriosclerosis, Thrombosis, and Vascular Biology* 22(2):201–210.

Rossouw, J. E., G. L. Anderson, R. L. Prentice, A. Z. LaCroix, C. Kooperberg, M. L. Stefanick, R. D. Jackson, S. A. Beresford, B. V. Howard, K. C. Johnson, J. M. Kotchen, J. Ockene, and the Writing Group for the Women's Health Initiative Investigators. 2002. Risks and benefits of estrogen plus progestin in healthy postmenopausal women: Principal results from the Women's Health Initiative randomized controlled trial. *JAMA* 288(3):321–333.

Rozenberg, S., V. De Pietrantonio, J. Vandromme, and C. Gilles C. 2021. Menopausal hormone therapy and breast cancer risk. *Best Practice & Research Clinical Endocrinology & Metabolism* 35(6):101577.

Safa, B., W. C. Lin, A. M. Salim, J. C. Deschamps-Braly, and M. M. Poh. 2019. Current concepts in masculinizing gender surgery. *Plastic and Reconstructive Surgery* 143(4):e857–e871.

Safer, J. D., and V. Tangpricha. 2019a. Care of the transgender patient. *Annals of Internal Medicine* 171(1):ITC1–ITC16.

Safer, J. D., and V. Tangpricha. 2019b. Care of transgender persons. *New England Journal of Medicine* 381(25):2451–2460.

Salas-Humara, C., G. M. Sequeira, W. Rossi, and C. P. Dhar. 2019. Gender affirming medical care of transgender youth. *Current Problems in Pediatric & Adolescent Health Care* 49(9):e100683.

Salgado, C. J., K. Yu, and M. J. Lalama. 2021. Vaginal and reproductive organ preservation in trans men undergoing gender-affirming phalloplasty: Technical considerations. *Journal of Surgical Case Reports* 2021(12):rjab553.

Samrock, S., K. Kline, and A. K. Randall. 2021. Buffering against depressive symptoms: Associations between self-compassion, perceived family support and age for transgender and nonbinary individuals. *International Journal of Environmental Research and Public Health* 18(15):7938.

Sarvaideo, J., E. Doll, and V. Tangpricha. 2022. More studies are needed to establish the safety and efficacy of sublingual estradiol in transgender women. *Endocrine Practice* 28(3):353–354.

Schechter, L. 2009. The surgeon's relationship with the physician prescribing hormones and the mental health professional: Review for version 7 of the world professional association for transgender health's standards of care. *International Journal of Transgenderism* 11(4):222–225.

Schechter, L. 2016. *Surgical management of the transgender patient, 1st ed.* Amsterdam, Netherlands: Elsevier.

Schechter, L. S., and A. R. Facque. 2021. Surgical anatomy: Phalloplasty. In *Urological care for the transgender patient*, edited by D. Nikolavsky and S. A. Blakely. New York: Springer.

Schnarrs, P. W., A. L. Stone, R. Salcido, Jr., A. Baldwin, C. Georgiou, and C. B. Nemeroff. 2019. Differences in adverse childhood experiences (ACEs) and quality of physical and mental health between transgender and cisgender sexual minorities. *Journal of Psychiatric Research* 119:1–6.

Shonkoff, J. P., and A. S. Garner. 2012. The lifelong effects of early childhood adversity and toxic stress. *Pediatrics* 129(1):e232–246.

Shoskes, J. J., M. K. Wilson, and M. L. Spinner. 2016. Pharmacology of testosterone replacement therapy preparations. *Translational Andrology and Urology* 5(6):834–843.

Shumer, D. E., and A. C. Tishelman. 2015. The role of assent in the treatment of transgender adolescents. *International Journal of Transgender Health* 16(2):97–102.

Sinha, A., L. Mei, and C. Ferrando. 2021. The effect of estrogen therapy on spermatogenesis in transgender women. *F&S Reports* 2(3):347–351.

Smith, T. E., L. A. Bauerband, D. Aguayo, C. S. McCall, F. L. Huang, W. M. Reinke, and K. C. Herman. 2022. School bullying and gender minority youth: Victimization experiences and perceived prevalence. *School Psychology Review* 1–14.

Soliman, S. B. 2023. Liquid silicone filler migration following illicit gluteal augmentation. *Radiology Case Reports* 18(3):984–990.

Spratt, D. I., I. I. Stewart, C. Savage, W. Craig, N. P. Spack, D. W. Chandler, L. V. Spratt, T. Eimicke, and J. S. Olshan. 2017. Subcutaneous injection of testosterone is an effective and preferred alternative to intramuscular injection: Demonstration in female-to-male transgender patients. *Journal of Clinical Endocrinology & Metabolism* 102(7): 2349–2355.

Srivastava, A., J. A. Rusow, and J. T. Goldbach. 2021. Differential risks for suicidality and mental health symptoms among transgender, nonbinary, and cisgender sexual minority youth accessing crisis services. *Transgender Health* 6(1):51–56.

Steensma, T. D., J. K. McGuire, B. P. Kreukels, A. J. Beekman, and P. T. Cohen-Kettenis. 2013. Factors associated with desistence and persistence of childhood gender dysphoria: A quantitative follow-up study. *Journal of the American Academy of Child and Adolescent Psychiatry* 52(6):582–590.

Stevenson, M. O., and V. Tangpricha. 2019. Osteoporosis and bone health in transgender persons. *Endocrinology & Metabolism Clinics of North America* 48(2):421–427.

Strang, J. F., A. I. R. Van der Miesen, A. L. Fischbach, M. Wolff, M. C. Harris, and S. E. Klomp. 2023. Common intersection of autism and gender diversity in youth: Clinical perspectives and practices. *Child and Adolescent Psychiatric Clinics of North America* 32(4):747–760.

Tebbe, E. A., and S. L. Budge. 2022. Factors that drive mental health disparities and promote well-being in transgender and nonbinary people. *Nature Reviews Psychology* 1(12):694–707.

Thoma, B. C., T. L. Rezeppa, S. Choukas-Bradley, R. H. Salk, and M. P. Marshal. 2021. Disparities in childhood abuse between transgender and cisgender adolescents. *Pediatrics* 148(2):e2020016907.

Thornton, K. G. S., and F. Mattatall. 2021. Pregnancy in transgender men. *Canadian Medical Association Journal* 193(33):E1303. Assessment of gender diverse children: Incorporating the Standard of Care, 8th edition. *Child and Adolescent Psychiatric Clinics of North America* 32(4):719–730.

Tishelman, A., and G. N. Rider. 2023. Assessment of gender diverse children: Incorporating the Standard of Care, 8th edition. *Child and Adolescent Psychiatric Clinics of North America* 32(4):719–730.

Trujillo, M. A., P. B. Perrin, M. Sutter, A. Tabaac, A., and E. G. Benotsch. 2017. The buffering role of social support on the associations among discrimination, mental health, and suicidality in a transgender sample. *International Journal of Transgenderism* 18(1):39–52.

Unger, C. A. 2016. Hormone therapy for transgender patients. *Translational Andrology and Urology* 5(6):877–884.

Valente, P. K., E. W. Schrimshaw, C. Dolezal, A. J. LeBlanc, A. A. Singh, and W. O. Bockting. 2020. Stigmatization, resilience, and mental health among a diverse community sample of transgender and gender nonbinary individuals in the U.S. *Archives of Sexual Behavior* 49(7):2649–2660.

Valente, P. K., J. D. Dworkin, C. Dolezal, A. A. Singh, A. J. LeBlanc, and W. O. Bockting. 2022. Prospective relationships between stigma, mental health, and resilience in a multi-city cohort of transgender and nonbinary individuals in the United States, 2016–2019. *Social Psychiatry and Psychiatric Epidemiology* 57(7):1445–1456.

Valentine, S. E., and J. C. Shipherd. 2018. A systematic review of social stress and mental health among transgender and gender non-conforming people in the United States. *Clinical Psychology Review* 66:24–38.

Van Boerum, M. S., A. A. Salibian, R. Bluebond-Langner, and C. Agarwal. 2019. Chest and facial surgery for the transgender patient. *Translational Andrology and Urology* 8(3):219–227.

Van De Grift, T. C., G. L. S. Pigot, B. P. C. Kreukels, M.-B. Bouman, and M. G. Mullender. 2019. Transmen's experienced sexuality and genital gender-affirming surgery: Findings from a clinical follow-up study. *Journal of Sex & Marital Therapy* 45(3):201–205.

Van De Grift, T. C., Z. J. Van Gelder, M. G. Mullender, T. D. Steensma, A. L. C. De Vries, and M.-B. Bouman. 2020. Timing of puberty suppression and surgical options for transgender youth. *Pediatrics* 146(5):e20193653.

Van Der Loos, M. A. T. C., M. C. Vlot, D. T. Klink, S. E. Hannema, M. Den Heijer, and C. M. Wiepjes. 2023. Bone mineral density in transgender adolescents treated with puberty suppression and subsequent gender-affirming hormones. *JAMA Pediatrics* 177(12):1332.

Van Der Miesen, A. I. R., T. D. Steensma, A. L. C. De Vries, H. Bos, and A. Popma. 2020. Psychological functioning in transgender adolescents before and after gender-affirmative care compared with cisgender general population peers. *Journal of Adolescent Health* 66(6):699–704.

Van der Pluijm, R. W., B. W. Haak, J. Kers, T. L. S. van Heukelom, and M. van Vugt. 2022. Immune reconstitution inflammatory syndrome induced by gluteal silicones in a transgender woman living with HIV. *International Journal of STD & AIDS* 33(6):625–627.

Verroken, C., S. Collet, B. Lapauw, and G. T'Sjoen. 2022. Osteoporosis and bone health in transgender individuals. *Calcified Tissue International* 110(5):615–623.

Vigneswaran, K., and H. Hamoda. 2022. Hormone replacement therapy: Current recommendations. *Best Practice & Research Clinical Obstetrics & Gynaecology* 81:8–21.

Vukadinovic, V., B. Stojanovic, M. Majstorovic, and A. Milosevic. 2014. The role of clitoral anatomy in female to male sex reassignment surgery. *Scientific World Journal* 2014:e437378.

Walker, R. V., S. M. Powers, and T. M. Witten. 2023. Transgender and gender diverse people's fear of seeking and receiving care in later life: A multiple method analysis. *Journal of Homosexuality* 70(14):3374–3398.

Wei, J. T., D. Barocas, S. Carlsson, F. Coakley, S. Eggener, R. Etzioni, S. W. Fine, M. Han, S. K. Kim, E. Kirkby, B. R. Konety, M. Miner, K. Moses, M. G. Nissenberg, P. A. Pinto, S. S. Salami, L. Souter, I. M. Thompson, and D. W. Lin. 2023. Early detection of prostate cancer: AUA/SUO guideline part I: Prostate cancer screening. *Journal of Urology* 210(1): 46–53.

Wilde, B., J. B. Diamond, T. J. Laborda, L. Frank, M. A. O'Gorman, and I. Kocolas. 2024. Bicalutamide-induced hepatotoxicity in a transgender male-to-female adolescent. *Journal of Adolescent Health* 74(1):202–204.

Williamson, C. 2010. Providing care to transgender persons: A clinical approach to primary care, hormones, and HIV management. *Journal of the Association of Nurses in AIDS Care* 21(3):221–229.

Wilson, L. C. 2023. Physical health in transgender and nonbinary adults: The roles of minority stress and general psychological processes. *Transgender Health* preprint. https://doi.org/10.1089/trgh.2023.0079.

Xu, J. Y., M. A. O'Connell, L. Notini, A. S. Cheung, S. Zwickl, and K. C. Pang. 2021. Selective estrogen receptor modulators: A potential option for non-binary gender-affirming hormonal care? *Frontiers in Endocrinology* 12:e701364.

Xu, K. Y., and A. J. Watt. 2018. The pedicled anterolateral thigh phalloplasty. *Clinics in Plastic Surgery* 45(3):399–406.

Yamada, K., D. Shida, T. Kato, H. Yoshida, S. Yoshinaga, and Y. Kanemitsu. 2018. Adenocarcinoma arising in sigmoid colon neovagina 53 years after construction. *World Journal of Surgical Oncology* 16(1):88.

Yeung, H., B. Kahn, B. C. Ly, and V. Tangpricha. 2019. Dermatologic conditions in transgender populations. *Endocrinology and Metabolism Clinics of North America* 48(2):429–440.

Yun, G. Y., S. H. Kim, S. W. Kim, J. S. Joo, J. S. Kim, E. S. Lee, B. S. Lee, S. H. Kang, H. S. Moon, J. K. Sung, H. Y. Lee, and K. H. Kim. 2016. Atypical onset of bicalutamide-induced liver injury. *World Journal of Gastroenterology* 22(15):4062–4065.

Zavlin, D., J. Schaff, J. D. Lellé, K. T. Jubbal, P. Herschbach, G. Henrich, B. Ehrenberger, L. Kovacs, H. G. Machens, and N. A. Papadopulos. 2018. Male-to-female sex reassignment surgery using the combined vaginoplasty technique: Satisfaction of transgender patients with aesthetic, functional, and sexual outcomes. *Aesthetic Plastic Surgery* 42(1):178–187.

Zhang, Q., M. Goodman, N. Adams, T. Corneil, L. Hashemi, B. Kreukels, J. Motmans, R. Snyder, and E. Coleman. 2020. Epidemiological considerations in transgender health: A systematic review with focus on higher quality data. *International Journal of Transgender Health* 21(2):125–137.

6

Common Co-occurring Conditions and Impacts of Gender-Affirming Care on Chronic Conditions in Transgender and Gender Diverse Populations

Research demonstrates that, compared with cisgender populations, transgender and gender diverse (TGD) people suffer from more chronic health conditions, experience higher rates of health problems related to substance use and mental illness, and have higher prevalence and earlier onset of chronic disease (Cicero et al., 2020; Pinna et al., 2022; Reisner et al., 2016a; Rich et al., 2020; Scheim et al., 2022). The statement of task asks the committee to describe common co-occurring conditions among individuals seeking, undergoing, or under the effects of gender-affirming care. This chapter presents the available evidence on common chronic health conditions that may co-occur across the life course for TGD populations compared with cisgender populations and describes how gender-affirming treatment and care can impact these conditions. In addition, within each section, the chapter examines appropriate assessment of these conditions among TGD populations and describes substantial research gaps that limit understanding of appropriate management, outcomes, and disparities.

The chapter begins with an examination of co-occurring mental health conditions, followed by chronic conditions related to physical health. It concludes by examining how multilevel stigma and structural factors shape the disproportionate burden of disease in this population and describing several theories or frameworks that are useful in conceptualizing and understanding TGD health disparities, including those among multiply marginalized groups.

Several additional and important co-occurring conditions are not explored in this chapter because they are discussed elsewhere in the report. Chapter 5 describes the impact of gender-affirming care on a number of

197

important health issues, including cancer, bone health/osteoporosis, fertility, and sexual function. Part III of this report examines specific chronic conditions—including respiratory disorders (Chapter 8), chronic kidney disease (Chapter 10), and cancers of the reproductive tract (Chapter 11)—all of which could be considered co-occurring conditions for TGD people. Finally, Chapter 12 reviews certain gynecological manifestations of HIV, whereas this chapter includes a discussion of HIV as a more general concern for TGD people.

This chapter does not explore co-occurring conditions for people with variations in sex traits (VSTs). Some VSTs have notable co-occurring conditions, and where relevant, these are described in Chapter 7 and in the disease-specific chapters in Part III. Given the heterogeneity of conditions under the umbrella of VSTs, however, it is not feasible to draw broad conclusions about co-occurring conditions that span populations with VSTs. Therefore, this chapter focuses only on TGD people.

CO-OCCURRING MENTAL HEALTH CONDITIONS

Mental health is one of the most highly researched categories of health conditions in TGD populations. In a systematic review of global chronic disease burden in TGD people, Rich and colleagues (2020) found that mental health (specifically anxiety and mood disorders) and substance use disorders were the focus of most research—80 percent of studies included in the review (74 of 96 studies)—among TGD people (Rich et al., 2020). Overall, studies indicate a high prevalence of mental health conditions among TGD people compared with cisgender controls.[1]

The following sections present an overview of the data related to depression and anxiety, suicidality and nonsuicidal self-harm, posttraumatic stress disorder (PTSD), substance use disorders, and eating disorders in TGD populations. Throughout, this section describes how multilevel stigma shapes the disproportionate burden of mental health in the TGD population.

---

[1] Co-occurring mental health conditions (and physical health conditions as well) may appear to be more common in TGD populations because much of the research identifies TGD individuals using International Classification of Diseases and Related Health Problems (ICD) codes among clinical populations (i.e., populations that have sought gender-affirming care and, thus, have a related ICD code present in their medical record, as described in detail Chapter 3 of this report). The true prevalence of health conditions in the population at large may differ, as TGD populations who have *not* sought gender-affirming care (because of personal preferences or lack of access/resources) are not represented in most available studies (as this population is unlikely to have a TGD-identifying ICD code in their medical record). TGD populations that seek gender-affirming care potentially have more opportunity to receive various other diagnoses, as compared to the general TGD population, through repeated contact with clinicians and greater engagement with the health care system.

Prevalence

Depression and Anxiety

In a large cohort of TGD veterans (N = 5,135) identified in the Veterans Health Administration's (VHA's) electronic health record database for 1996–2013 (hereafter referred to as the "VHA TGD cohort"), statistically significant disparities were present between TGD veterans and cisgender veteran controls for *major depression* (adjusted odds ratio [aOR] 4.03; 95% confidence interval [CI] 3.73–4.35), *other depression* (aOR 4.55; 95% CI 4.21–4.92), and *panic disorder* (aOR 2.06; 95% CI 1.80–2.36) (Brown and Jones, 2016). Other large cohort studies have found similarly high rates of depression and anxiety in TGD people. In a large cohort of TGD Medicare beneficiaries (N = 7,454) (hereafter referred to as the "TGD Medicare cohort"), Dragon and colleagues (2017) found that TGD beneficiaries compared with their cisgender counterparts had higher observed percentages of depression (76.3 vs. 28.8 percent in cisgender beneficiaries) and anxiety (62.4 vs. 20.2 percent). Finally, in a U.S. retrospective/prospective cohort of TGD people (hereafter referred to as the "STRONG cohort"), baseline rates of depression and anxiety were much higher for both transgender females (Table 6-1) and transgender males (Table 6-2) (Quinn et al., 2017). A 2023 cross-sectional analysis using data from the National Institutes of Health All of Us Research Program (N = 372,082) (hereafter referred to as "All of Us Research Program") adds to the literature showing higher odds of anxiety and depression among TGD populations compared with cisgender and heterosexual controls (Tran et al., 2023).

TABLE 6-1 Frequency of Health Outcomes in the STRONG Transgender Female (TF) Cohort Relative to Matched Reference (Ref.) Groups

Health Outcome	TF Cohort, n (%)[a]	Ref. Males, n (%)	Ref. Females, n (%)
Anxiety	1,337 (38)	4,323 (13)	7,485 (22)
Depression	1,705 (49)	4,721 (14)	8,726 (25)
Self-inflicted injury[b]	75 (2.2)	100 (0.3)	204 (0.6)
Suicidal ideation	175 (5.0)	157 (0.5)	194 (0.6)
Substance abuse disorder	524 (15)	2,860 (8.3)	1,680 (4.9)

[a] Percentages do not add to 100% because of overlapping categories.
[b] Combined diagnoses of self-inflicted injury, self-inflicted injury/poisoning, and possible self-inflicted injury.
SOURCE: Adapted from Quinn et al., 2017.

TABLE 6-2 Frequency of Health Outcomes in the STRONG Transgender Male (TM) Cohort Relative to Matched Reference (Ref.) Groups

Health Outcome:	TM Cohort, n (%)[a]	Ref. Males, n (%)	Ref. Females, n (%)
Anxiety	1,323 (46)	3,583 (13)	6,089 (21)
Depression	1,594 (55)	3,806 (13)	6,813 (24)
Self-inflicted injury[b]	121 (4.2)	109 (0.4)	181 (0.6)
Suicidal ideation	193 (6.7)	160 (0.6)	186 (0.7)
Substance abuse disorder	418 (14)	2,391 (8.4)	1,523 (5.3)

[a] Percentages do not add to 100% because of overlapping categories.
[b] Combined diagnoses of self-inflicted injury, self-inflicted injury/poisoning, and possible self-inflicted injury.
SOURCE: Adapted from Quinn et al., 2017.

Suicidality and Nonsuicidal Self-Harm

Both suicidality (ideation, planning, attempt, and completion) and self-harm are more common among TGD people, especially TGD youth, than among cisgender people. The TransPop study, the first national probability sample of TGD adults in the United States, found high rates of recent suicidal ideation (44.4 percent; 95% CI 35.8–53.0), recent suicide attempt (6.9 percent; 95% CI 2.3–11.5), and recent nonsuicidal self-injury (21.4 percent; 95% CI 14.5–28.4) (Kidd et al., 2023). Compared with a cisgender comparison sample in TransPop, TGD participants had 5 times higher odds of recent suicidal ideation (aOR 5.1; 95% CI 2.7–9.6), almost 7 times the odds of lifetime suicidal ideation (aOR 6.7; 95% CI 3.8–11.7), more than 4 times the odds of lifetime suicide attempts (aOR 4.4; 95% CI 2.4–8.0), and 13 times the odds of nonsuicidal self-injury (aOR 13.0; 95% CI 4.8–35.1).

As shown in Tables 6-1 and 6-2, the STRONG cohort study found a higher baseline prevalence of suicidal ideation (6.7 percent) and self-harm (4.2 percent) in transgender male participants compared with transgender female participants (suicidal ideation: 5.0 percent; self-harm: 2.2 percent), and prevalence in both TGD groups was higher than in comparison groups (Quinn et al., 2017). Three systematic reviews further indicate that TGD people compared with cisgender people have consistently higher rates of suicidality and nonsuicidal self-injury, and that transgender men versus transgender women have higher rates of nonsuicidal self-injury (Marconi et al., 2023; Marshall et al., 2016; Pinna et al., 2022).

Posttraumatic Stress Disorder (PTSD)

The authors of a recent systematic review and meta-analysis of 27 studies (N = 31,903) estimate that LGBT study participants had higher odds of PTSD compared with cisgender, heterosexual controls (odds ratio [OR] 2.20; 95% CI 1.85–2.60), and that TGD study participants had even higher odds of PTSD compared with their lesbian, gay, and bisexual peers (OR 2.52; 95% CI 2.22–2.87) (Marchi et al., 2023). The VHA TGD cohort indicated that TGD veterans had nearly three times higher odds of having PTSD compared with cisgender controls (aOR 2.82; 95% CI 2.60–3.06) (Brown and Jones, 2016). In the TGD Medicare cohort, 22.7 percent of TGD Medicare beneficiaries had PTSD, compared with 1.6 percent of cisgender beneficiaries (Dragon et al., 2017). Similar results were found in a retrospective medical record review (N = 79), with PTSD affecting up to 22.8 percent of TGD adolescents who were seeking care from a large, urban multidisciplinary gender program (Nahata et al., 2017).

Substance Use Disorders

TGD populations have higher rates of substance and alcohol abuse and tobacco use relative to their cisgender counterparts. In the VHA TGD cohort, for example, TGD veterans had higher odds of alcohol abuse (aOR 1.68; 95% CI 1.55–1.82) and tobacco use (aOR 1.46; 95% CI 1.37–1.57) compared with cisgender controls (Brown and Jones, 2016), and within the TGD Medicare cohort, TGD Medicare beneficiaries had higher observed percentages of substance use disorders than were observed among cisgender beneficiaries (26.6 vs. 4.2 percent) (Dragon et al., 2017).

A review that included 41 studies found "high and excess prevalence of substance use" in TGD people compared with cisgender people, but could not pool any of the effect sizes (Connolly and Gilchrist, 2020). Such findings may be skewed by unrepresentative convenience samples, however (Scheim et al., 2022). The author of one review reported that community surveys of TGD substance use found high rates of smoking, alcohol abuse, and drug use (Scheim et al., 2022). In a scoping review examining substance use in TGD youth (aged 10–24), findings showed high to moderate use of alcohol, binge drinking, cigarettes and e-cigarettes, and marijuana (Fahey et al., 2023). In contrast to these studies, Kidd and colleagues (2023) found alcohol and drug use outcomes to be similar for TGD and cisgender adults in an analysis using TransPop study data (N = 274). While these authors report hazardous drinking among TGD people (28.2 percent; 95% CI 21.2–35.2 percent) and problematic drug use (31.2 percent; 95% CI 23.8–38.7 percent), these rates were similar to those among cisgender groups. In addition, some research has found *lower* rates of substance use among certain TGD populations:

while data from All of Us Research Program show that gender diverse people assigned male at birth (aOR 1.76; 95% CI 1.15–2.67) and transgender women (aOR 2.02; 95% CI 1.54–2.65) had significantly higher odds of having a substance use disorder compared with cisgender heterosexual women, the data revealed gender diverse people assigned female at birth (aOR 0.35; 95% CI 0.24–0.52) and transgender men (aOR 0.65; 95% CI 0.49–0.87) had *lower* odds of substance use disorder compared with cisgender heterosexual men (Tran et al., 2023). Further research is needed to understand differences in substance use among various TGD populations.

Eating Disorders

TGD populations have consistently higher prevalence of eating disorders and disordered eating compared with cisgender populations, although prevalence estimates vary (Coelho et al., 2019; Heiden-Rootes et al., 2023; Jones et al., 2016; Rasmussen et al., 2023). In the VHA TGD cohort, transgender veterans had double the odds of having an eating disorder compared with matched cisgender controls (aOR 2.01; 95% CI 1.58–2.54) (Brown and Jones, 2016). A systematic review (24 studies) and meta-analysis (14 studies) calculated an overall eating disorder prevalence of 17.7 percent in TGD people (Rasmussen et al., 2023). This figure is significantly higher when compared with the general population, as a previous meta-analysis estimated a 1.01 percent (95% CI 0.54–1.89 percent) lifetime eating disorder prevalence in the general population (Qian et al., 2013). Another review estimated that 20–50 percent of TGD people had disordered eating, more than 30 percent screened positive for eating disorders, and 2–12 percent had an eating disorder diagnosis (Keski-Rahkonen, 2023).

Eating disorders do not affect TGD populations evenly: one systematic review revealed that transgender men tend to experience a higher prevalence of eating disorders compared with transgender women (Rasmussen et al., 2023). Another study showed that transgender youth aged 8–25 were more likely than their cisgender counterparts to be diagnosed with an eating disorder, with an estimated prevalence of 2–18 percent (Coelho et al., 2019). Subpopulations not well represented in the research on eating disorders include nonbinary people, racially and ethnically minoritized groups, neurodivergent groups, and TGD people living in specific family and cultural contexts that have standards of femininity and masculinity that may impact eating behaviors (Heiden-Rootes et al., 2023; Obarzanek and Munyan, 2021).

Risk and Protective Factors

The gender minority stress model posits that gender minorities experience anticipated, internalized, and enacted stigma because of the stigma society places on minority gender identities, which leads to worse physical and mental health outcomes (Connolly and Gilchrist, 2020; Testa et al., 2015). For TGD youth especially, these repeated traumatic experiences compound over time, leading to substance use, depression, stress, shame, and loneliness (Ramos and Marr, 2023). In TGD youth, victimization experiences both related and unrelated to gender identity were found to be associated with substance use (Fahey et al., 2023). For racial minority groups and others with stigmatized identities (e.g., disability, neurodivergence), these stressors affect them synergistically, leading to even worse physical and mental health outcomes and increased barriers to care (Bowleg, 2012; Crenshaw, 1991; Mulcahy et al., 2022; Wesp et al., 2019). Specific research related to suicidality, PTSD, and eating disorders is presented below.

Suicidality and Nonsuicidal Self-Injury

Minority stress, stigma, discrimination, social rejection (Marconi et al., 2023), and thwarted belongingness are associated with increased suicidality and nonsuicidal self-injury (Phillip et al., 2022). One meta-analysis tested the associations of constructs of the minority stress model (internalized transphobia, expectations of rejection, identity concealment) with suicidality and self-harm, finding that expectations of rejection and internalized transphobia most strongly predicted suicidal ideation (Pellicane and Ciesla, 2022). TGD youth are especially vulnerable, as they may face family rejection without yet having built a strong social circle of chosen family to support them. Nonsuicidal self-injury was also found to be associated with psychopathology, interpersonal problems, and low social support (Marshall et al., 2016). Conversely, social support, parental support, having at least one personal identification document with the appropriate gender marker, and ability to obtain gender-affirming medical care are all protective against suicidal ideation (Bauer et al., 2015).

Post-Traumatic Stress Disorder (PTSD)

Higher prevalence of PTSD in TGD people is due to several factors, including both acute and chronic exposures to traumatic stressors, marginalization, and discrimination (Ramos and Marr, 2023). Factors related to gender minority stress and intersectionality, noted above, are especially pertinent here, and partially explain the higher prevalence of PTSD. Other mental health issues discussed in this section, such as eating disorders, depression, anxiety, self-harm, suicide, and substance use, are interrelated with PTSD (Ramos and Marr, 2023).

TGD youth especially have higher rates of interpersonal and community-level trauma compared with their cisgender peers.

Vulnerabilities particular to TGD youth include higher adverse childhood experience scores, higher rates of family rejection (leading to substance use, mental illness, and homelessness), more childhood abuse targeted at gender nonconformity, and more bullying and victimization (Ramos and Marr, 2023).

The gender minority stress model also emphasizes that minoritized groups form community identity, pride, and resilience (Testa et al., 2015), and TGD youth often access social support, skills-building, and affirming trauma-informed services (Ramos and Marr, 2023). Support from parents, especially at younger ages, and school, peer, and community connectedness are key protective factors against trauma for TGD youth (Ramos and Marr, 2023). Similarly, community connections and social supports are important for TGD adults, as these connections may help mitigate negative experiences of violence and other traumatic stressors (Pflum et al, 2015; Sherman et al., 2020, 2022).

Eating Disorders

There are several hypotheses as to why TGD versus cisgender populations have higher rates of eating disorders. Body dissatisfaction related to gender dysphoria and the desire to appear less gendered by becoming either thinner or heavier is a common explanation (Jones et al., 2016; Obarzanek and Munyan, 2021). A desire to be recognized as their affirmed gender may cause TGD people to adopt unhealthy behaviors in an effort to prove manliness or womanliness (McGregor et al., 2023). Disordered eating may also be an attempt to regain control, especially when there are barriers to gender-affirming care (McGregor et al., 2023). Youth may use disordered eating in an attempt to delay or prevent puberty (Coelho et al., 2019); transgender men may use it to induce amenorrhea; and transgender women may internalize societal pressure for thinness in women (Obarzanek and Munyan, 2021). One review cautions providers to be aware that body dissatisfaction is not always related to sex-specific body parts (genitals), but more to chest, curves, shoulders, body hair, and other secondary sex characteristics (Jones et al., 2016). Lastly, the high stigma, discrimination, and minority stress TGD people face, and the higher burden of mental illness as a result, likely have a large impact on eating disorders and disordered eating in these populations (Keski-Rahkonen, 2023; Obarzanek and Munyan, 2021).

Social affirmation/transition and gender-affirming hormone therapy may ameliorate body image issues and eating disorders in TGD people (Heiden-Rootes et al., 2023; Jones et al., 2016; McGregor et al., 2023; Obarzanek and Munyan, 2021; Rasmussen et al., 2023). Family, peer, school connectedness, and social support may also help, but more research is needed in this area (McGregor et al., 2023; Obarzanek and Munyan, 2021; Rasmussen et al., 2023).

Assessments

Common assessments for mental health disorders such as anxiety, depression, psychological distress, and suicidal ideation have been widely used in both cisgender and TGD populations. These assessments are not sex based, so their interpretation is the same for all populations. In the case of PTSD, however, a common assessment known as the Clinician-Administered PTSD Scale (from the *Diagnostic and Statistical Manual of Mental Disorders, Fifth Edition*) may not be appropriate for TGD people. A 2023 study tested and qualitatively explored limitations of the Clinician-Administered PTSD Scale for TGD patients; findings suggest that there may be overpathologizing or underdetection of symptoms for TGD people because discrimination-related experiences may threaten the assessment's accuracy (Valentine et al., 2023). Instead of identifying trauma, for example, the assessment may link patient symptoms to internalized transphobia or gender identity/expression (Valentine et al., 2023).

Common assessments of substance use may also have drawbacks for these populations. While the Alcohol Use Disorder Identification Test and AUDIT-Consumption appear to be reliable for TGD populations (Dermody et al., 2023; Kuhns et al., 2020; Williams et al., 2021), they include sex-specific cutoff scores. Presently, moreover, no guidance is available for health care providers on the use of sex recorded at birth or the patient's gender when using the Alcohol Use Disorder Identification Test (Flentje et al., 2020).

Likewise, common assessments for eating disorders may be inappropriate and inaccurate for TGD people, as they are centered on young, White, cisgender women. The traditional Eating Disorder Inventory, for example, includes items that could indicate either disordered eating or gender dysphoria, and so should not be used (McGregor et al., 2023). Instead, the SCOFF[2] questionnaire is genderless and can be used for TGD populations (Morgan et al., 2000), and a short seven-item version of the Eating Disorder Exam Questionnaire has been validated for gender minorities (Keski-Rahkonen, 2023).

Clinical Management and Gender-Affirming Care

The Callen-Lorde Community Health Center (2018) recommends counseling TGD patients on the potential impact of gender-affirming hormone

---

[2] The acronym "SCOFF" is taken from the five questions asked in the assessment. See Morgan et al., 2000.

therapy (GAHT) on depression and anxiety, as these conditions may be either ameliorated or exacerbated by hormones. It also recommends that patients with active psychosis or a suicidal or homicidal plan be treated and stabilized before initiating GAHT. The Callen-Lorde guidelines note further that the mental health treatment plan should be with a trans-competent provider, as delay of GAHT may worsen distress (Callen-Lorde Community Health Center, 2018). The World Professional Association of Transgender Health (WPATH) guidelines approach mental health in a general way, encouraging appropriate care, support, and empowerment (Coleman et al., 2022).

Research shows that gender-affirming medical and/or surgical treatments can help reduce suicide risk: in one study, TGD people on hormone therapy were about half as likely to have considered suicide (relative risk 0.52; 95% CI 0.37–0.75) as those who wished to use hormones as part of gender-affirming care but were unable to access this care (Bauer et al., 2015). Even among those who have had GAHT and/or gender-affirming surgery, however, suicide attempts and deaths may remain elevated compared with the cisgender population (Asscheman et al., 2011; Dhejne et al., 2011), in part because of minority stressors (including internalized transphobia, victimization, bullying, or negative family treatment), which are significantly associated with suicidal ideation and suicide attempts among TGD individuals (de Lange et al., 2022; Pellicane and Ciesla, 2022).

Best practices for mental health providers include assessing for and treating nonsuicidal self-injury and trauma (Dickey et al., 2017), and all medical providers need to screen TGD patients for childhood trauma and toxic stress symptoms (Ramos and Marr, 2023). Neither nonsuicidal self-injury nor trauma is considered a contraindication for gender-affirming care (Dickey et al., 2017). All medical care for TGD people, not just gender-affirming care, should use trauma-informed approaches (Dickey et al., 2017; Ramos and Marr, 2023), and medical providers should assume that all TGD people have experienced trauma, including in the health care setting.

While there are guidelines for treating many mental health concerns among TGD people, research on treating substance use disorders is lacking in these populations. Multiple studies, including randomized controlled trials, have tested various treatment programs for transgender populations, targeting alcohol, tobacco, meth, stimulants, and substance use generally (Chapa Montemayor and Connolly, 2023; Coffin et al., 2020; Keuroghlian et al., 2015; Kuhns et al., 2020; Lee et al., 2014; Matson et al., 2022; Zhang et al., 2018). In many cases, although substance use treatment programs can be feasibly adapted for use in TGD populations, no rigorous outcome evaluations exist, and more research is needed in this area.

In the case of eating disorders, there are no consensus guidelines for treating TGD people, although toolkits on managing eating disorders in LGBTQ+ communities exist (Joy et al., 2023; White et al., 2023). Given the high co-occurrence of these disorders in TGD people, however, researchers recommend screening TGD youth in gender dysphoria clinics for eating disorders, and vice versa (McGregor et al., 2023). TGD people do benefit from treatment for eating disorders, but providers must be attuned to transgender-competent care, understand minority stress, recognize co-occurring mental illness, and minimize dysphoria (Keski-Rahkonen, 2023; McGregor et al., 2023). Current treatment standards for marking progress (i.e., return of menses) may be distressing for transgender men and irrelevant for transgender women; treatment and markers of progress need to be sensitive to gender dysphoria and be individualized (Geilhufe et al., 2021). Qualitative findings indicate that TGD people have had highly negative experiences in eating disorder clinics, hide their identity or get misgendered, and find that providers do not have trans-competent knowledge (McGregor et al., 2023). As gender-affirming care may help with symptoms, TGD people with eating disorders may seek GAHT or other care concurrently with treatment for an eating disorder (Keski-Rahkonen, 2023).

Research Limitations and Gaps

As described above, anxiety and depression are well represented in the transgender health literature, while other mental health conditions, such as schizophrenic/psychotic disorders, bipolar disorder, personality disorders, and PTSD are less well studied. It should be noted that the cross-sectional nature of most studies reporting on suicidality and nonsuicidal self-injury limit the ability to interpret the study findings and establish temporality (e.g., when and why nonsuicidal self-injury occurs in TGD people). For example, prospective studies could elucidate whether nonsuicidal self-injury decreases with gender-affirming care and social acceptance.

Additional data are needed to better understand substance use among TGD populations. Many community-based studies of substance abuse rely on higher-risk, multiply marginalized populations, for whom substance use is likely higher than it is in the general TGD population (Connolly and Gilchrist, 2020). Trans-specific programming, education, and cessation resources are important (Turner et al., 2021), and high-quality, representative studies of substance use rates in TGD populations are lacking.

In the case of PTSD in TGD people, the research base is growing: in their review, Rich and colleagues (2020) included 24 studies that addressed PTSD (Rich et al., 2020), compared with only 3 such studies in a previous global review of transgender health (Reisner et al., 2016a). None of the major guidelines for TGD treatment and care address or provide recommendations for PTSD. Further research is warranted, especially among groups who are multiply marginalized.

To date, available data on eating disorders are based mostly on cross-sectional convenience samples with small sample sizes, and some of these data are not disaggregated by gender identity. Longitudinal studies that also include nonbinary people, racialized minority groups, neurodivergent people, and overweight and obese TGD people are needed (Obarzanek and Munyan, 2021; Rasmussen et al., 2023).

AUTISM AND OTHER NEURODEVELOPMENTAL DIAGNOSES

Several recent studies have estimated the prevalence of gender dysphoria in autistic people[3] and the prevalence of autism/autism spectrum disorder (ASD) in TGD people. All studies concur that there is an overrepresentation of autism in transgender people (Bouzy et al., 2023) and a need to raise awareness about this association.

Prevalence

A 2023 systematic review and meta-analysis of 25 studies of children, adolescents, and adults (N = 8,662) found that ASD occurs frequently in TGD people, with a prevalence of 11 percent (95% CI, 8–16 percent), compared with approximately 1 percent in the general population (Kallitsounaki and Williams, 2023). In a large U.S. cohort study conducted in eight pediatric hospitals with more than 900,000 adolescents aged 9–18, gender dysphoria was more prevalent in autistic youth (1.1 percent) than in neurotypical (nonautistic) youth (0.6 percent). There were greater odds of a gender dysphoria diagnosis among youth with an ASD diagnosis versus those without (aOR 3.00; 95% CI 2.72–3.31) (Kahn et al., 2023). In another systematic review, 7.8 percent of children and adolescents seeking care for gender dysphoria had an ASD diagnosis—four times higher than in the general population (Bouzy et al., 2023). This review reported wide ranges for estimated ASD in TGD youth (5.5–29.6 percent in transgender adults; 6.3–27.1 percent in children/adolescents with gender dysphoria) and for gender dysphoria in autistic people (0.07–31.0 percent in adults; 0.07–5.40 percent in children/ adolescents) (Bouzy et al., 2023).

Associated Factors

A variety of theories—biological, genetic, social, and psychological/ cognitive—attempt to explain the high co-occurrence of ASD and gender

---

[3] "Autistic people" (identity-first language) rather than "people with autism" (person-first language) is a conscious choice in line with autistic activists and advocates. This parallels "transgender people" (identity first) rather than "people with gender dysphoria" or "people with transness."

dysphoria. While certain subpopulations are overrepresented in autism diagnoses (i.e., White, middle class, assigned male sex at birth), this does not indicate the absence of autism in all other populations. A cohort study by Kahn and colleagues (2023) showed that while White youth were significantly more likely than Black or Asian youth to have co-occurring ASD and gender dysphoria, White youth in the cohort also had greater access to gender clinics and to private insurance, both of which increased the likelihood of a gender dysphoria diagnosis. The authors posit that the lack of documentation of ASD and gender dysphoria co-occurrence among Black and Asian youth could be due to disparities in health services or other demographic differences (Hadland et al., 2023; Kahn et al., 2023). Additional research is needed to determine disparities and outcomes faced by youth of color with ASD.

This same study also revealed co-occurring ASD and gender dysphoria diagnoses to be more prevalent in youth with female sex recorded at birth versus male sex recorded at birth (aOR 1.77, 95% CI 1.45–2.16) (Kahn et al., 2023). This finding stands in contrast to a body of literature showing that, overall, ASD diagnoses are higher among cisgender men compared with cisgender women; male-skewed ASD diagnoses have been attributed to possible bias in ASD diagnostic criteria toward male-typical behaviors (Haney, 2016). Kahn and colleagues (2023), therefore, posit that youth with female sex recorded at birth who exhibit male-typical behavior and/or identify as male may be more likely to be diagnosed with ASD compared with other youth with female sex recorded at birth, given current diagnostic criteria. Further research is needed to understand these possible differences by sex and what they may mean for ASD diagnosis among TGD youth.

Assessments

Strang and colleagues (2018) offer initial clinical guidelines for combined assessment of gender dysphoria and autism. Investigators encourage gender clinics to screen for autism, and for autism clinics to screen for gender dysphoria (Bouzy et al., 2023; Kallitsounaki and Williams, 2023; Strang et al., 2018). WPATH addresses autism only in the context of diagnosis of gender dysphoria in children and adolescents and the need for taking extra care to support autistic youth in fully understanding their dysphoria and transition options and consequences (Coleman et al., 2022). Others agree that TGD autistic people may need extra support with respect to tolerance of change, flexibility, planning, and social skills during the changes involved in transition, and offer ideas for ensuring that gender clinics are autism friendly (Bouzy et al., 2023). Researchers also note that LGBTQ+ autistic people (including adults) are often discredited and infantilized and told that they cannot know their LGBTQ+ identities. ASD diagnosis does not invalidate someone's TGD identity, and it is not appropriate to use an ASD diagnosis to prevent care; GAHT can improve difficulties associated with autism and does not exacerbate autistic traits (Bouzy et al., 2023; Hadland et al., 2023; Nobili et al., 2018).

Clinical Management and Gender-Affirming Care

As noted above, co-occurrence of ASD and gender dysphoria is not a contraindication for gender-affirming care (Bouzy et al., 2023). Rather, additional cultural sensitivity and specialized care to meet the needs associated with both autism and gender dysphoria is necessary, as both being transgender and being autistic are stigmatized, compounding minority stress and the risk of discrimination (Hadland et al., 2023) and increasing the risk of anxiety and depression (Bouzy et al., 2023). The first preliminary clinical guidelines for co-occurring autism and TGD identity in adolescents were developed using the Delphi method in 2018 (Strang et al., 2018). These guidelines provide recommendations for assessment and treatment and address some primary clinical and psychosocial challenges that may be faced by autistic TGD adolescents (Strang et al., 2018). The National LGBTQIA+ Health Education Center (2024) offers a webinar for providers on neurodiversity and the gender diverse experience.

Research Limitations and Gaps

Most attention around autism is aimed at children and adolescents, ignoring adults' experiences and needs. Tailored services and interventions for autistic TGD people of all ages are needed, in addition to those for children and adolescents. Screening autistic people for gender dysphoria and TGD people for autism would help them access appropriate care earlier (Kallitsounaki and Williams, 2023). The disparities in access and care among racialized minorities need to be addressed as well.

There are also large gaps in research on the co-occurrence of other neurotypes and conditions, such as attention-deficit/hyperactivity disorder. Two systematic reviews on this topic found only a handful of studies (Goetz and Adams, 2022; Thrower et al., 2020).

CO-OCCURRING PHYSICAL HEALTH CONDITIONS

While the majority of the data on the health of TGD populations comes from studies focused on mental health concerns, there are some data related to chronic physical health conditions. The following sections present research data on human immunodeficiency virus/acquired immuno-deficiency syndrome (HIV/AIDS), cardiovascular conditions, metabolic and endocrine disorders, and chronic liver disease. As mentioned above, other important chronic health conditions—including cancer, respiratory disorders, and chronic kidney disease—are addressed elsewhere in this report.

HIV/AIDS

Transgender individuals continue to be disproportionately burdened by HIV, with both transgender women and transgender men showing elevated rates of HIV infection worldwide. The unique HIV prevention and care needs among TGD people are an important consideration for the health of this population.

Prevalence

Transgender women have the highest prevalence of HIV of any TGD group. Serious racial disparities exist among transgender women. According to Centers for Disease Control and Prevention (2021) estimates, 17 percent of White, 62 percent of Black, and 35 percent of Latina transgender women in the United States are living with HIV. In a systematic review of studies reporting HIV prevalence among TGD people published between January 2000 and January 2019, Stutterheim and colleagues (2021) found that transgender women were 66 times more likely to have HIV (95% CI 51.4–84.8) compared with the general population over age 15. Transgender men were almost 7 times more likely to have HIV (95% CI 3.6–13.1), compared with the general population over age 15. HIV prevalence among nonbinary and other gender diverse people is unknown.

Risk and Protective Factors

Although the majority of research on HIV among TGD people centers on transgender women, all TGD people can be at risk for acquiring or transmitting HIV, depending on type of sexual exposure (anal, vaginal, oral), presence of sexually transmitted infection and/or inflammation, and genital surgery type (e.g., neovagina risk is not well known) (Poteat et al., 2016, 2017). Research shows that transgender women are likely to engage in sexually risky behaviors (e.g., condomless sex, high number of sexual partners, sex work) that elevate HIV risk (Guadamuz et al., 2011; Naz-McLean et al., 2022; Salazar et al., 2017; Silva-Santisteban et al., 2012). Although research on transgender men is less available, it indicates sexually risky behaviors in this population as well (Bauer et al., 2012; McFarland et al., 2017, 2018; Reisner and Murchison, 2016).

In addition, changes in transgender men brought by testosterone therapy, such as vaginal dryness, may increase susceptibility to HIV infection (Reisner et al., 2016b).

The social contexts of racism, sexism, and transphobia contribute to HIV vulnerability among TGD people (Baral et al., 2013; Sevelius, 2013). Stigma and discrimination reduce access to employment opportunities, and for some, these circumstances may reach the point where sex work becomes the only option available for income (Poteat et al., 2015). The circumstances of social oppression and psychological distress may increase engagement in high-risk behavior (e.g., exchange sex, sex with a person of known HIV status, illicit injection of hormones or silicone) (Habarta et al., 2015; Poteat et al., 2017). Social gender affirmation (living full-time in one's identified gender, with or without gender-affirming care) may also play an important role in sexual risk behavior for transgender men who have sex with cisgender men; here, transgender men may face the same social stigma and stressors that put cisgender men who have sex with men at increased risk of HIV infection (Reisner et al., 2016b).

Inadequate and uneven access to HIV testing and treatment is another important disparity to consider for TGD people living with HIV. TGD people are reported to have lower lifetime rates of HIV testing compared with cisgender gay and bisexual men (Pitasi et al., 2017). In one study examining data from the 2015 U.S. Transgender Survey (N = 26,927), 45 percent of respondents had never been tested for HIV (Olakunde et al., 2022). In another U.S. study of transgender and nonbinary people (N = 539), 26.2 percent of survey respondents had never been tested for HIV (Lacombe-Duncan et al., 2022). While rates of HIV screening in the general population are also low—in 2022, only 36.3 percent of U.S. adults over age 18 reported having ever been tested for HIV (KFF, 2022)—given the higher HIV risk profile of TGD people, HIV testing in this population is suboptimal. However, HIV testing varies between subgroups: corroborating other research (Sevelius et al., 2020), a survey conducted by Lacombe-Duncan and colleagues (2022) found that Black survey participants had a greater likelihood of having had a previous HIV test compared with White participants (aOR 0.28; 95% CI 0.09–0.86). The survey also found that participants who had experienced sexual violence were more likely to have had an HIV test (aOR 0.38; 95% CI 0.21–0.67); participants who had access to an inclusive, trans-affirming primary care provider also had increased likelihood of HIV testing (aOR 0.29; 95% CI 0.17–0.49).

These findings point to the need for trans-inclusive HIV testing practices, particularly at the point of sexual violence intervention, and the importance of educating primary care providers to be more trans affirming. Other studies show that TGD people are more likely to access HIV testing in community-based, non–health care settings, highlighting difficulties in access to HIV prevention within the health care system and the need for expanding targeted HIV testing for TGD people outside of traditional settings (Habarta et al., 2015).

In addition, research points to the need to expand use of pre-exposure prophylaxis (PrEP) as an important part of HIV prevention among TGD people. PrEP is a safe and effective way to prevent HIV (Grant et al., 2010; Molina et al., 2015), but among TGD people eligible for PrEP, only 3 percent take it up (3.2 percent of eligible transgender women and 2.3 percent of eligible transgender men) (Sevelius et al., 2020). Furthermore, rates of PrEP discontinuation among TGD people are high: one study found 35–40 percent annual discontinuation of PrEP among sexual and gender minority people, citing housing instability and prior history of PrEP discontinuation as predictors of discontinuation (Guo et al., 2024).

Beyond testing and sustained PrEP use, TGD people may lack access to HIV treatment upon diagnosis. While limited outcomes data exist, research indicates that TGD people living with HIV are less likely to receive and adhere to antiretroviral treatment and have poorer viral suppression compared with cisgender people living with HIV (Kalichman et al., 2017; Klein et al., 2020; Melendez et al., 2006; Mizuno et al., 2015, 2017; Xia et al., 2019). In addition, some TGD people may fear that HIV medications could interfere with their GAHT, causing some to forgo HIV medication in favor of hormone therapy (Braun et al., 2017; Sevelius et al., 2016).

Taken together, all of these impediments may lead to delayed diagnosis and poorer outcomes for TGD people with HIV.

Assessments

When assessing vulnerability to HIV, University of California, San Francisco (UCSF) guidelines encourage providers and other practitioners not to assume gender or body parts or history of surgeries in TGD people or their partners (Poteat, 2016; UCSF, 2016). Gender identity and sexual orientation are two separate concepts, and TGD people can have any sexual orientation. Furthermore, TGD people can have partners of any gender identity—men, women, nonbinary, etc.—and any gender modality—transgender, cisgender, etc. (Rioux et al., 2022). Anatomy-specific questions should be asked with sensitivity (Poteat, 2016).

Clinical Management and Gender-Affirming Care

There are no clinically significant contraindications for current medications for prevention or treatment of HIV in patients receiving GAHT (Cespedes et al., 2022; Poteat, 2016). Chapter 12 examines the impact of GAHT and other gender-affirming care on HIV in greater depth.

Limitations and Gaps

Although HIV/AIDS is one of the most researched topics in transgender health, gaps in knowledge remain. The biomedical tools for filling these gaps are available, but structural barriers limit access; attention to dismantling these structural barriers is key (Poteat et al., 2017). Cisgender male partners of transgender women and men are understudied, but likely have high HIV risk—especially those who conceal their relationships and behaviors because of stigma (Poteat et al., 2021). Research on transgender men is nascent, and research on nonbinary people and HIV is nonexistent.

Cardiovascular Conditions

Prevalence

Data on cardiovascular mortality and morbidity risk in TGD populations are inconsistent and incomplete. While some studies have found a higher prevalence of myocardial infarction and cerebrovascular disease rates among transgender females relative to the general population, others have found no increased risk of myocardial infarction, stroke, or venous thromboembolism in transgender females (Asscheman et al., 2011; Dhejne et al., 2011; Getahun et al., 2018; Tran et al., 2023; Wierckx et al., 2013). For transgender men and gender nonconforming people, the risk of myocardial infarction may be the same as for the general population (Nokoff et al., 2018).

In the STRONG cohort, baseline prevalence for five cardiovascular outcomes—venous thromboembolism, stroke, myocardial infarction, peripheral artery disease, and unstable angina—was reported separately for transgender females and males (see Tables 6-3 and 6-4, respectively).

TABLE 6-3 Frequency of Cardiovascular Disease Health Outcomes in the STRONG Transgender Female (TF) Cohort Relative to Matched Reference (Ref.) Groups

Health Outcome	TF Cohort, n (%)[a]	Ref. Males, n (%)	Ref. Females, n (%)
Venous thromboembolism	86 (2.5)	670 (1.9)	677 (2.0)
Stroke	88 (2.5)	943 (2.7)	674 (2.0)
Myocardial infarction	61 (1.8)	664 (1.9)	319 (0.9)
Peripheral artery disease	106 (3.1)	879 (2.6)	645 (1.9)
Unstable angina	64 (1.8)	656 (1.9)	336 (1.0)

[a] Percentages do not add to 100% because of overlapping categories.
SOURCE: Adapted from Quinn et al., 2017.

TABLE 6-4 Frequency of Cardiovascular Disease Health Outcomes in the STRONG Transgender Male (TM) Cohort Relative to Matched Reference (Ref.) Groups

Health Outcome	TM Cohort, n (%)[a]	Ref. Males, n (%)	Ref. Females, n (%)
Venous thromboembolism	45 (1.6)	266 (0.9)	356 (1.2)
Stroke	42 (1.5)	360 (1.3)	250 (0.9)
Myocardial infarction	17 (0.6)	210 (0.7)	88 (0.3)
Peripheral artery disease	38 (1.3)	309 (1.1)	242 (0.8)
Unstable angina	20 (0.7)	215 (0.8)	123 (0.4)

[a] Percentages do not add to 100% because of overlapping categories.
SOURCE: Adapted from Quinn et al., 2017.

In both populations prevalence in all categories was similar to that in the general population (Quinn et al., 2017).

On the other hand, the TGD Medicare cohort study showed *lower* rates of five cardiovascular conditions in TGD compared with cisgender beneficiaries, as shown in Table 6-5 (Dragon et al., 2017).

Still other analyses have shown higher cardiovascular disease risk in TGD people. Analyses of the Behavioral Risk Factor Surveillance System have revealed that transgender men have a greater than 2-fold higher rate of myocardial infarction compared with cisgender men (aOR 2.53; 95% CI 1.14–5.63) and a 4-fold higher rate compared with cisgender women (aOR 4.90; 95% CI 2.21–10.90) (Alzahrani et al., 2019). For transgender women, Alzahrani and colleagues (2019) found a higher rate of myocardial infarction compared with cisgender women (aOR 2.56; 95% CI 1.78–3.68), but no significant difference compared with cisgender men. In addition, the VHA TGD cohort showed higher odds for several cardiovascular conditions compared with non-TGD counterparts, as shown in Table 6-6 (Brown and Jones, 2016).

TABLE 6-5 Percentage of Medicare Beneficiaries with Cardiovascular Conditions

Condition	Transgender and Gender Diverse Beneficiaries (%)	Cisgender Beneficiaries (%)
Cardiac arrhythmia	6.3	11.4
Congestive heart failure	16.0	19.7
Coronary artery disease	30.4	35.7
Stroke	9.0	11.2
Hyperlipidemia	61.1	61.6

SOURCE: Dragon et al., 2017.

TABLE 6-6 Adjusted Odds Ratio (aOR) of Cardiovascular Diseases for Transgender Veterans Seeking Veterans Health Administration Care, 1996–2013

Condition	aOR	95% Confidence Interval (CI)
Acute myocardial infarction	1.36	1.10–1.69
Cardiac arrest	1.72	1.20–2.47
Cerebral vascular disease	1.41	1.24–1.60
Congestive heart failure	1.35	1.19–1.54
Hypercholesterolemia	1.58	1.47–1.70
Hypertension	1.51	1.40–1.61
Ischemic heart disease	1.49	1.36–1.63

SOURCE: Brown and Jones, 2016.

Risk and Protective Factors

A review by the American Heart Association examined the literature related to TGD people with respect to common cardiovascular risk factors (including tobacco use, physical activity, body mass index [BMI], lipid profile, and diabetes). The review found a lack of data across all factors, which limited the ability to determine disparities in cardiovascular health among TGD populations (Streed et al., 2021).

HIV is associated with increased risk for cardiovascular disease, given the high prevalence of cardiovascular risk behaviors among people living with HIV and the physiological effects of HIV disease itself (Feinstein et al., 2019). Given significantly higher rates of HIV among TGD people (as described above), it might be expected that cardiovascular disease risk would be higher in this population. While data are limited, existing research suggests that TGD people with HIV may be at higher risk for cardiovascular-related disease compared with cisgender people with HIV (Gosiker et al., 2020).

Assessments

Assessment of risk for atherosclerotic cardiovascular disease (ASCVD) is commonly used in clinical practice to aid in decision making surrounding primary prevention therapies. Assessment tools for ASCVD use either male or female reference sex when calculating risk, leaving health care providers who care for TGD people to make these decisions without clinical guidance on how best to assess these populations (Poteat et al., 2023). Likewise, other common assessments of risk for cardiovascular disease, including the

Framingham Risk Score and the Reynolds Risk Score, use sex-specific risk factor algorithms (National Cholesterol Education Program Expert Panel, 2001; Ridker et al., 2007). As a result, TGD populations are subject to miscalculation of risk for cardiovascular disease (Poteat et al., 2023).

Clinical Management and Gender-Affirming Care

WPATH recommends taking detailed histories to assess for traditional cardiovascular and cerebrovascular risk factors, along with past and present hormone use and presence or absence of gonads, to tailor management of cardiovascular health (Coleman et al., 2022). Given that masculinizing GAHT (testosterone) may exacerbate hypertension, sleep apnea, and polycythemia (an excess of red blood cells that reduces blood flow), monitoring of blood pressure and lipid profiles is important; changes may require medications and/ or alterations in diet to reduce risk (Coleman et al., 2022). As with cisgender people who use hormone therapy, GAHT may alter the lipid profile of TGD people, particularly transgender men, with important implications for cholesterol and cardiovascular health; changes in lipid profile among transgender women are less well understood (Nokoff et al., 2020; Streed et al., 2021).

Feminizing hormone therapy (estrogen) carries an increased risk of thromboembolism (Khan et al., 2019), as described further in Chapter 5 of this report, but changes can be made to counteract this risk. Modifiable risk factors include smoking, obesity, and sedentariness. If there are nonmodifiable risk factors, a transdermal formulation of estrogen is available; use of anticoagulants is also recommended based on limited data (Coleman et al., 2022; Defreyne et al., 2019).

Research Limitations and Gaps

The impact of GAHT on heart disease risk is unknown (Safer, 2021). There are no prospective cohorts of TGD people (other than STRONG) for whom cardiovascular conditions are tracked. One systematic review found only retrospective studies, and those were all conducted in Europe (Defreyne et al., 2019). For better understanding of cardiovascular conditions in TGD populations, as for other chronic conditions, prospective cohorts with sufficient sample sizes of TGD people need to be studied.

Metabolic and Endocrine Disorders

In a systematic review by Rich and colleagues (2020), metabolic and endocrine disorders accounted for 22 percent of the included studies and 6 percent of the data points; studies reported mainly on obesity, diabetes, polycystic ovarian syndrome, and metabolic syndrome.

Prevalence

Rich and colleagues (2020) report that the prevalence of diabetes was as low as <1 percent to as high as 6 percent in studies relying on self-report (vs. 30.2 percent in cisgender patients). The TGD Medicare cohort study found diabetes in 27–31 percent of Medicare clinical diagnoses among TGD beneficiaries (Dragon et al., 2017). The VHA TGD cohort study also found higher odds of type 2 diabetes among that cohort compared with cisgender veterans (aOR 1.34; 95% CI 1.23–1.45) (Brown and Jones, 2016). In contrast, the California Health Interview Survey (2015–2016) found no statistically significant difference in diabetes prevalence between TGD and cisgender people (Herman et al., 2017), and a recent analysis of data from the All of Us Research Program found slightly lower prevelance of diabetes among TGD populations (Tran et al., 2023). Another systematic review showed no increased odds of diabetes in one included study and higher prevalence in another, but the diagnoses were made before the initiation of GAHT; the authors of the review hypothesize that diabetes prevalence may be higher in the latter study partly because TGD people are more likely to be screened in the process of receiving gender-affirming care, and this finding may not represent a true disparity (Defreyne et al., 2019; Wesp, 2016).

Questions about diabetes prevalence can best be answered in prospective cohort studies: in the STRONG cohort study, at baseline, 5.3 percent of transgender male and 9.0 percent of transgender female participants had type 2 diabetes (Quinn et al., 2017). After 9 years of follow-up of 2,869 transgender female and 2,133 transgender male patients, review of medical records revealed that the transgender female cohort had higher prevalence (OR 1.3; 95% CI 1.1–1.5) and incidence of type 2 diabetes (OR 1.4 95% CI 1.1–1.8). There was no significant difference between transgender and cisgender male patients (Islam et al., 2022).

Studies have shown an increased prevalence of type 1 diabetes in TGD children and adults (Defreyne et al., 2017; Logel et al., 2020). One study indicates that TGD youth have increased risk of developing type 1 diabetes, and its authors hypothesize that this is due to minority stress. In that study, 9.9/1,000 U.S. TGD youth had diabetes versus 1.93/1,000 cisgender youth (Maru et al., 2021).

Like the diabetes research, data on obesity are mixed. In the TGD Medicare cohort, TGD patients had a higher prevalence of obesity diagnosis compared with cisgender patients—31.3 percent versus 17.2 percent, respectively (Dragon et al., 2017). Likewise, in the VHA TGD cohort, TGD veterans had higher odds of obesity relative to cisgender controls (aOR 1.58; 95% CI 1.48–1.70) (Brown and Jones, 2016). On the other hand, a systematic review found that TGD people on GAHT were not more likely to be obese compared with age-matched cisgender controls (Defreyne et al., 2019).

Risk and Protective Factors

Risk factors for overweight TGD people include socioeconomic barriers to health care access; disparities in healthy behaviors (e.g., less exercise, perhaps due to lack of safe access to gyms and locker rooms); comorbid physical and mental health conditions; and gender minority stress (Taormina and Iwamoto, 2023). Polycystic ovarian syndrome (PCOS) is a risk factor for developing type 2 diabetes, but the prevalence of PCOS among transgender men is not well known. Two studies included in a review by Rich and colleagues (2020) found an estimated prevalence in transgender men of 32–26 percent, but neither study was based on U.S. populations (Baba et al., 2011; Becerra-Fernandez et al., 2014).

Assessments

Testing for (pre)diabetes includes measuring hemoglobin A1C, which does not differ by sex, and no concerns have been reported about the appropriateness of the test for TGD populations. However, BMI is often used to assess overweight and obesity, and it is unclear which sex standard, if any, should be applied to TGD people (AMA, 2023). Some surgeons place restrictions on BMI before gender-affirming surgery, but this practice is not evidence based (Taormina and Iwamoto, 2023).

Clinical Management and Gender-Affirming Care

The UCSF guidelines state that providers should monitor fasting glucose and hemoglobin A1C when initiating or adjusting hormone therapy (Wesp, 2016). WPATH and the Endocrine Society recommend that preexisting conditions, including diabetes, be "reasonably well controlled" before GAHT is initiated (Coleman et al., 2022; Hembree et al., 2017). UCSF notes that starting GAHT may help patients better control their diabetes. The UCSF guidelines advise that diabetes management be the same for TGD as for cisgender people, regardless of GAHT use (Wesp, 2016). Similarly, USCF prefers that patients with diabetes seeking gender-affirming surgery have normal glucose, but abnormal glucose is not a contraindication for surgery (Wesp, 2016).

Research Limitations and Gaps

The effects of GAHT on diabetes risk is unknown, including in youth using gonadotropin-releasing hormone (GnRH) agonists (medications to delay puberty, as discussed in Chapter 5); little evidence is available on this subject, and what is available is mixed (Islam et al., 2022). The management of diabetes in TGD people has not yet been studied, and UCSF's guidelines are the only ones to address this overlap (Moverley et al., 2021; Wesp, 2016). PCOS is a known risk factor for insulin resistance and type 2 diabetes in cisgender women, but impacts in transgender men are unknown (Moverley et al., 2021; Wesp, 2016). Additionally, evidence is lacking on trans-oriented weight loss programs, medications, and bariatric surgeries (Taormina and Iwamoto, 2023).

Chronic Liver Disease

Prevalence

Very little data on chronic liver disease are available. The systematic review by Rich and colleagues (2020) reports that liver outcomes constituted the lowest proportion of available studies examining health among TGD people. However, some research does exist. In the TGD Medicare cohort, TGD beneficiaries fared worse than cisgender beneficiaries with regard to measures of liver disease: 8.6 percent of TGD beneficiaries had a diagnosis of hepatitis, compared with 1.7 percent of cisgender beneficiaries (Dragon et al., 2017). In the same study, the prevalence of nonhepatitis liver conditions was also high in TGD beneficiaries—12 percent compared with 7.3 percent in cisgender beneficiaries (Dragon et al., 2017). On the other hand, the VHA TGD cohort study found that cirrhosis of the liver was less common in TGD than in cisgender veterans (aOR 0.77; 95% CI 0.61–0.96) (Brown and Jones, 2016). Other systematic reviews on transgender health do not report on liver disparities and outcomes (Scheim et al., 2022), and more research is needed in this area.

Risk and Protective Factors

For TGD populations, how GAHT may impact the liver is unknown. Increased substance use (as described above) and lower levels of physical activity among TGD people may contribute to poor liver function; however, there is no empirical evidence to support or refute this hypothesis (Streed at al., 2021). Barriers to adopting liver-healthy behaviors may be challenging to overcome for TGD people. Exercise, for example, may be more challenging because of discomfort with the body; socioeconomic status; mental health issues, such as depression; and lack of safe access to sports teams, sport facilities, and locker rooms.

Assessments

The Model for End-Stage Liver Disease calculation was recently updated to version 3, which added "female sex" as a variable (Newman et al., 2023).

Previously, sex had not been factored into the calculation. The implications of this change for TGD people with chronic liver disease have not yet been studied (Newman et al., 2023). As for other sex-specific measures described in this report, which sex marker to use for TGD people, including those receiving hormone therapy, is unclear. As with other sex-based guidelines, it is possible that a combination of sex and gender identity will lead to a more accurate interpretation; but again, this possibility is untested and unknown.

Clinical Management and Gender-Affirming Care

There are sex-based differences in nonalcoholic fatty liver disease, and estrogen affects metabolic states and hepatic adenomas. Whether GAHT affects liver outcomes is unknown, however (Newman et al., 2023). Among the major transgender standards of care, only the Callen-Lorde Community Health Center (2018) guidelines address management of liver disease. These guidelines direct that liver function be tested regularly if the patient has a self-limited hepatic infection, such as acute hepatitis A and B, and advise waiting to initiate hormone therapy until the patient has recovered and transaminase levels are normalized. Hepatitis C should be treated the same for TGD and cisgender people. For chronic liver disease, Callen-Lorde (2018) recommends that the primary care provider ensure that all relevant vaccinations are up to date and encourage behavioral interventions to minimize further risk.

Research Limitations and Gaps

Virtually nothing is known about chronic liver disease in TGD populations except that it may be more prevalent than in cisgender populations. Data on GAHT management in the context of liver transplantation are needed; there is risk of thromboembolism in the postoperative period, but stopping GAHT has to be weighed against risks of gender dysphoria and mental health sequalae (Newman et al., 2023). Newman and colleagues (2023) recommend prospective research with biobank specimens before and after GAHT initiation to generate data on impacts on the liver.

CO-OCCURING CONDITIONS AND MULTIMORBIDITY

As alluded to throughout this chapter, TGD people are at higher risk than cisgender people of experiencing multimorbidities of both mental and physical health outcomes via syndemics. The term "syndemic" denotes the overlapping, mutually reinforcing combination of two or more diseases or other conditions in a population, especially when caused and reinforced by social inequities and power imbalance (Poteat et al., 2016). The term has been used to describe the synergistic co-occurrence of substance abuse, mental health conditions, HIV, sexually transmitted infections, violence, racism, poverty, and daily trauma experienced by many TGD people (Poteat et al., 2016).

Analysis of data from the Behavioral Risk Factor Surveillance System indicates that participants in all transgender subgroups experienced worse mental and physical health compared with cisgender participants, while gender nonbinary participants had higher odds of multiple chronic conditions, and poor quality of life compared with both binary transgender and all cisgender participants (Downing and Przedworski, 2018). Another analysis of the same data set found that 36.7 percent of transgender women, 33.8 percent of transgender men, and 40.9 percent of nonbinary participants had two or more chronic health conditions; these participants were also highly likely to be unemployed: aOR 2.39; 95% CI 1.73–3.31). Many participants also had three or more health problems or impairments (transgender women 15 percent, transgender men 17 percent, and nonbinary people 21 percent), and they had much higher odds of not working (aOR 5.18; 95% CI 2.92–9.19) (Cicero et al., 2020). These results are corroborated by Abramovich and colleagues (2020), who found comorbid chronic health conditions were higher among the TGD population studied compared with cisgender controls (702 [33.7%] vs. 2,941 [28.2%]; p < .001.

In another study, older nonbinary adults and transgender women were found to be less likely to have a personal doctor or to have had a checkup in the past 2 years. Older nonbinary adults were also more likely than cisgender controls to have poor mental and physical health, depression, and asthma (Pharr, 2021).

The Amsterdam Cohort of Gender Dysphoria Study reported on all-cause mortality over 5 decades of follow-up. The statistics and causes of death are telling: transgender women were 80 percent and transgender men 280 percent more likely to die compared with cisgender men and cisgender women, respectively (standardized mortality ratio [SMR] 1.8; 95% CI 1.6–2.0, and 2.8; 95% CI 2.5–3.1, respectively). Their top causes of death were cardiovascular disease, lung cancer, HIV, and suicide. Transgender men were 80 percent more likely to die compared with cisgender women (SMR 1.8; 95% CI 1.3–2.4); their top causes of death were nonnatural causes (e.g., suicide). Over the 5 decades of follow-up, mortality risk did not decrease for TGD people (de Blok et al., 2021).

From disparities in the burden of chronic physical conditions and risk (e.g., cardiovascular disease, HIV) to disparities in the burden of mental health conditions (e.g., depression, anxiety), multiple studies demonstrate how multilevel stigma and structural factors (e.g., antitransgender policies, practices, and laws)—which could be addressed by interventions—contribute to the disproportionate burden of disease for TGD people (Bockting et al.,

2013; Brown and Jones, 2016; Caceres et al., 2020; Feldman et al., 2021; Poteat et al., 2016; Streed et al., 2021; Stutterheim et al., 2021; Tebbe and Budge, 2022; White Hughto et al., 2015), and may cause or contribute to chronic disease morbidity over the life course.

Along with growing recognition of the magnitude and breadth of health inequities facing TGD people, an emerging health literature addresses resilience at the TGD individual and community levels (Edwards et al., 2020; McCann and Brown, 2017; Tankersley et al., 2021). Resilience, which includes coping skills, strategies, and social support systems that help mitigate adversity, is a key consideration for TGD health and well-being (Bockting et al., 2020; Puckett et al., 2024; Reisner et al., 2016a). Importantly, resilience as an individual-level solution to structural drivers of inequity has been critiqued as inappropriate and inadequate (Suslovic and Lett, 2023). Instead, addressing structural barriers to TGD health through systems-level changes more closely matches the solution to the problem and better promotes health equity.

When considering the disproportionate burden of chronic disease experienced by TGD people, it is essential to identify the fundamental causes of these disparities (Link and Phelan, 1995, 2001; Williams et al., 2019). As noted, a growing body of evidence indicates that stigma and discrimination, including harmful laws and practices, drive health inequities in TGD populations (Caceres et al., 2020; Dragon et al., 2017; Meyer et al., 2017; Reisner et al., 2016b; Streed et al., 2021; White Hughto et al., 2015). Several key concepts, models, and frameworks have been used to advance an understanding of how stigma and discrimination, at multiple levels and across multiple minoritized identities, lead to health inequities across the life course (Crenshaw, 1991; Homan et al., 2021; Smith et al., 2022; Wesp et al., 2019). Table 6-7 provides brief definitions of salient concepts for TGD populations.

SUMMARY OF KEY POINTS

This chapter has examined a range of co-occurring conditions that may be common among TGD people, presenting data on the high co-occurrence of several conditions, including various mental health conditions, ASD, and HIV. Other important co-occurring conditions are described throughout this report, including cancers, osteoporosis, fertility, respiratory disorders, and chronic kidney disease. Taken together, this evidence shows that TGD people have a disproportionate level of co-occurring chronic diseases and mental health conditions. These significant health concerns do not occur in a vacuum: multilevel stigma and structural factors shape the disproportionate burden of disease in TGD people, potentially putting them at greater risk of disease with reduced ability to seek the services they need for

TABLE 6-7 Conceptual Frameworks and Explanatory Models Salient for Health for Transgender and Gender Diverse People

Concept	Definition/Description
Stigma	This social process of labeling, stereotyping, and rejecting human differences has been described as a fundamental cause of poorer health among TGD people because of its indirect effects on health-promoting factors, including power and wealth, as well as its direct impact on stress. Structural stigma includes societal norms, conditions, laws, and practices that disproportionately disadvantage TGD people. Examples include lack of health insurance due to employment discrimination and restrictions on access to medically necessary gender-affirming care. Interpersonal stigma includes explicit and implicit biases against TGD individuals due to perceptions of nonconformity (Bockting et al., 2013; Link and Phelan, 2001; Valdiserri et al., 2019).
Minority Stress	The gender minority stress framework describes how experiences such as gender nonaffirmation, enacted stigma, rejection, and/or gender-based victimization and violence cause greater stress for TGD people relative to cisgender people. This additional stress then leads to poorer behavioral, mental, and physical health outcomes.
Ecosocial Theory, Social Determinants of Health	These terms describe a conceptual framework for understanding how social factors—such as discrimination, economic disadvantage—become embodied and manifest as health inequality (Krieger, 1994, 2016; OASH, n.d.; Smart et al., 2022).
Intersectionality	The concept of intersectionality posits that multiple social categories—such as race, ethnicity, gender, sexual orientation—intersect at the level of individual experience to reflect multiple interlocking systems of power at the structural level, such as racism, sexism, cissexism, and heterosexism (Bowleg, 2021; Smith et al., 2022). These systems lead to unequal distribution of the social determinants of health that drive poorer health outcomes, especially among people in multiple disadvantaged social categories, such as TGD people of color (Bowleg, 2012, 2019; Homan et al., 2021; Lett et al., 2023; Richman and Zucker, 2019; Wesp et al., 2019).
Syndemics Model	This theory examines why certain diseases cluster among specific groups, and the ways in which conditions of social inequality and injustice contribute to disease clustering and interaction, as well as to vulnerability.
Weathering Hypothesis, Allostatic Load	This theory postulates that minoritized individuals' poorer health outcomes are due in part to the accumulation of stress response to structural inequalities that accrue uniquely to minoritized individuals (Geronimus et al., 2006). The similar concept of allostatic load describes the cumulative wear and tear on the body's systems owing to repeated adaptation to social stressors (McEwen, 2000). Several studies of TGD people provide evidence for the effects of minority stress on physiologic regulation of body systems (Dubois, 2012; DuBois and Juster, 2022).

TABLE 6-7 (Continued)

Concept	Definition/Description
Medical Distrust	This has been a well-described impediment to research participation, health service utilization, and health care satisfaction among racial and ethnic minority and other minoritized individuals (Boulware et al., 2003; Corbie-Smith et al., 2002; Jaiswal and Halkitis, 2019; LaVeist et al., 2009; Mohottige and Boulware, 2020). Operating as a similar product of current and historical experiences of discrimination, mistrust exacerbates the underrepresentation of TGD individuals in research, leaving a gap in knowledge of intervention efficacy in this population and creating barriers to engagement in health care (D'Avanzo et al., 2019; Perez-Brumer et al., 2021).

SOURCES: Bockting et al., 2013; Boulware et al., 2003; Bowleg, 2012, 2019, 2021; Corbie-Smith et al., 2002; D'Avanzo et al., 2019; Dubois, 2012; DuBois and Juster, 2022; Geronimus et al., 2006; Homan et al., 2021; Jaiswal and Halkitis, 2019; Krieger, 1994, 2016; LaVeist et al., 2009; Lett et al., 2023; Link and Phelan, 2001; McEwen, 2000; Mohottige and Boulware, 2020; OASH, n.d.; Perez-Brumer et al., 2021; Richman and Zucker, 2019; Smart et al., 2022; Smith et al., 2022; Valdiserri et al., 2019; Wesp et al., 2019.

optimal care and management. These realities may lead to delayed diagnosis and poorer outcomes for TGD people with chronic disease.

While the co-occurring conditions described in this chapter were not among the specific conditions reviewed by the committee (i.e., respiratory disease, growth failure, chronic kidney disease, reproductive cancers, and HIV), the committee notes parallels between the conditions described in this chapter and those described in Part III of this report, including notable disparities and important considerations for appropriate assessment and clinical management of TGD people with chronic disease.

Given that many of the conditions described here are categories within the Social Security Administration's (SSA's) Listings, the committee presents these data to inform SSA on how TGD people may experience various chronic health conditions that are important for disability evaluation, particularly when TGD applicants present with more than one such condition. Importantly, as discussed in Chapter 1, under SSA's disability determination process, SSA considers the combined effects of all physical and mental conditions ("impairments") when determining eligibility for benefits (SSA, 2017).[4] Two-thirds of all SSA disability beneficiaries report physical or mental health impairments in more than one impairment category, and beneficiaries with multiple impairments tend to have poorer health and more activity limitations than beneficiaries with one impairment (Walker and Roessel, 2019). Although available SSA data do not allow for analysis of impairments among TGD beneficiaries, given the body of evidence presented in this chapter that TGD people often experience physical and mental health

---

[4] 20 C.F.R. § 404.1523 (2017).

conditions at a higher rate than the cisgender population, TGD people may be particularly likely to present to SSA with multiple impairments.

Finally, as presented in this chapter, there is a great need for TGD health research outside of mental and sexual health. Data are lacking on nearly every chronic condition and across the lifespan. Age-related chronic conditions among aging TGD people need to be understood. Likewise, long-term impacts will unfold as more TGD people transition at younger ages and more TGD youth will have had a history of GnRH agonist use. Rigorous, prospective cohort studies that collect biospecimens and survey data before GnRH agonist and GAHT use and at regular intervals thereafter are key to establishing temporality and causation for a variety of conditions. Representative, probability-based samples are also important; to this end, more large and national studies need to include appropriate, sensitive, and standardized measures that capture both gender identity and sex recorded at birth. The field of transgender health needs more studies based on patient-centered outcomes and on research questions the community deems important.

REFERENCES

Abramovich A., C. de Oliveira, T. Kiran, T. Iwajomo, L. E. Ross, P. Kurdyak. 2020. Assessment of health conditions and health service use among transgender patients in Canada. *Journal of the American Medical Association Network Open* 3(8):e2015036.

Alzahrani, T., T. Nguyen, A. Ryan, A. Dwairy, J. McCaffrey, R. Yunus, J. Forgione, J. Krepp, C. Nagy, R. Mazhari, and J. Reiner. 2019. Cardiovascular disease risk factors and myocardial infarction in the transgender population. *Circulation: Cardiovascular Quality and Outcomes* 12(4):e005597.

AMA (American Medical Association). 2023. *AMA adopts new policy clarifying role of BMI as a measure in medicine.* Chicago, IL: American Medical Association.

Asscheman, H., E. J. Giltay, J. A. Megens, W. P. de Ronde, M. A. van Trotsenburg, and L. J. Gooren. 2011. A long-term follow-up study of mortality in transsexuals receiving treatment with cross-sex hormones. *European Journal of Endocrinology* 164(4):635–642.

Baba, T., T. Endo, K. Ikeda, A. Shimizu, H. Honnma, H. Ikeda, N. Masumori, T. Ohmura, T. Kiya, T. Fujimoto, M. Koizumi, and T. Saito. 2011. Distinctive features of female-to-male transsexualism and prevalence of gender identity disorder in Japan. *Journal of Sexual Medicine* 8(6):1686–1693.

Baral, S., C. H. Logie, A. Grosso, A. L. Wirtz, and C. Beyrer. 2013. Modified social ecological model: A tool to guide the assessment of the risks and risk contexts of HIV epidemics. *BMC Public Health* 13(1):482.

Bauer, G. R., R. Travers, K. Scanlon, and T. A. Coleman. 2012. High heterogeneity of HIV-related sexual risk among transgender people in Ontario, Canada: A province-wide respondent-driven sampling survey. *BMC Public Health* 12(1):292.

Bauer, G. R., A. I. Scheim, J. Pyne, R. Travers, and R. Hammond. 2015. Intervenable factors associated with suicide risk in transgender persons: A respondent driven sampling study in Ontario, Canada. *BMC Public Health* 15:525.

Becerra-Fernandez, A., G. Perez-Lopez, M. M. Roman, J. F. Martin-Lazaro, M. J. Lucio Perez, N. Asenjo Araque, J. M. Rodriguez-Molina, M. C. Berrocal Sertucha, and M. V. Aguilar Vilas. 2014. Prevalence of hyperandrogenism and polycystic ovary syndrome in female to male transsexuals. *Endocrinología y Nutrición* 61(7):351–358.

Bockting, W. O., M. H. Miner, R. E. Swinburne Romine, A. Hamilton, and E. Coleman. 2013. Stigma, mental health, and resilience in an online sample of the us transgender population. *American Journal of Public Health* 103(5):943–951.

Bockting, W., R. Barucco, A. LeBlanc, A. Singh, W. Mellman, C. Dolezal, and A. Ehrhardt. 2020. Sociopolitical change and transgender people's perceptions of vulnerability and resilience. *Sexuality Research & Social Policy* 17(1):162–174.

Boulware, L. E., L. A. Cooper, L. E. Ratner, T. A. LaVeist, and N. R. Powe. 2003. Race and trust in the health care system. *Public Health Reports* 118(4):358–365.

Bouzy, J., J. Brunelle, D. Cohen, and A. Condat. 2023. Transidentities and autism spectrum disorder: A systematic review. *Psychiatry Research* 323:115176.

Bowleg, L. 2012. The problem with the phrase women and minorities: Intersectionality—An important theoretical framework for public health. *American Journal of Public Health* 102(7):1267–1273.

Bowleg, L. 2019. Perspectives from the social sciences: Critically engage public health. *American Journal of Public Health* 109(1):15–16.

Bowleg, L. 2021. Evolving intersectionality within public health: From analysis to action. *American Journal of Public Health* 111(1):88–90.

Braun, H. M., J. Candelario, C. L. Hanlon, E. R. Segura, J. L. Clark, J. S. Currier, and J. E. Lake. 2017. Transgender women living with HIV frequently take antiretroviral therapy and/ or feminizing hormone therapy differently than prescribed due to drug-drug interaction concerns. *LGBT Health* 4(5):371–375.

Brown, G. R., and K. T. Jones. 2016. Mental health and medical health disparities in 5135 transgender veterans receiving healthcare in the Veterans Health Administration: A case-control study. *LGBT Health* 3(2):122–131.

Caceres, B. A., K. B. Jackman, D. Edmondson, and W. O. Bockting. 2020. Assessing gender identity differences in cardiovascular disease in U.S. adults: An analysis of data from the 2014–2017 BRFSS. *Journal of Behavioral Medicine* 43(2):329–338.

Callen-Lorde Community Health Center. 2018. *Callen-Lorde protocols for the provision of hormone therapy.* https://static1.squarespace.com/static/5ac6a3e825bf0250fa23d6cb/t/ 5beceba240ec9a141594abe7/1542253481054/Callen-Lorde-TGNC-Hormone-Therapy-Protocols-2018.pdf (accessed January 4, 2024).

Centers for Disease Control and Prevention. 2021. *HIV infection, risk, prevention, and testing behaviors among transgender women–national HIV behavioral surveillance–7 U.S. Cities, 2019–2020.* Atlanta, GA.

Cespedes, M. S., M. Das, J. Yager, M. Prins, I. Krznaric, J. de Jong, D. Xiao, Y. Shao, P. Wong, A. Kintu, C. Carter, E. Hoornenborg, P. Ruane, J. Phoenix, I. Younis, and J. Halperin. 2022. Gender affirming hormones do not affect the exposure and efficacy of F/TDF or F/TAF for HIV preexposure prophylaxis: A subgroup analysis from the discover trial. *Transgender Health* 9(1).

Chapa Montemayor, A. S., and D. J. Connolly. 2023. Alcohol reduction interventions for transgender and non-binary people: A prisma-SCR-adherent scoping review. *Addictive Behaviors* 145:107779.

Cicero, E. C., S. L. Reisner, E. I. Merwin, J. C. Humphreys, and S. G. Silva. 2020. The health status of transgender and gender nonbinary adults in the United States. *PLoS ONE* 15(2):e0228765.

Coelho, J. S., J. Suen, B. A. Clark, S. K. Marshall, J. Geller, and P. Y. Lam. 2019. Eating disorder diagnoses and symptom presentation in transgender youth: A scoping review. *Current Psychiatry Reports* 21(11):107.

Coffin, P. O., G. M. Santos, J. Hern, E. Vittinghoff, J. E. Walker, T. Matheson, D. Santos, G. Colfax, and S. L. Batki. 2020. Effects of mirtazapine for methamphetamine use disorder among cisgender men and transgender women who have sex with men: A placebo-controlled randomized clinical trial. *JAMA Psychiatry* 77(3):246–255.

Coleman, E., A. E. Radix, W. P. Bouman, G. R. Brown, A. L. C. de Vries, M. B. Deutsch, R. Ettner, L. Fraser, M. Goodman, J. Green, A. B. Hancock, T. W. Johnson, D. H. Karasic, G. A. Knudson, S. F. Leibowitz, H. F. L. Meyer-Bahlburg, S. J. Monstrey, J. Motmans, L. Nahata, T. O. Nieder, S. L. Reisner, C. Richards, L. S. Schechter, V. Tangpricha, A. C. Tishelman, M. A. A. Van Trotsenburg, S. Winter, K. Ducheny, N. J. Adams, T. M. Adrián, L. R. Allen, D. Azul, H. Bagga, K. Başar, D. S. Bathory, J. J. Belinky, D. R. Berg, J. U. Berli, R. O. Bluebond-Langner, M. B. Bouman, M. L. Bowers, P. J. Brassard, J. Byrne, L. Capitán, C. J. Cargill, J. M. Carswell, S. C. Chang, G. Chelvakumar, T. Corneil, K. B. Dalke, G. De Cuypere, E. de Vries, M. Den Heijer, A. H. Devor, C. Dhejne, A. D'Marco, E. K. Edmiston, L. Edwards-Leeper, R. Ehrbar, D. Ehrensaft, J. Eisfeld, E. Elaut, L. Erickson-Schroth, J. L. Feldman, A. D. Fisher, M. M. Garcia, L. Gijs, S. E. Green, B. P. Hall, T. L. D. Hardy, M. S. Irwig, L. A. Jacobs, A. C. Janssen, K. Johnson, D. T. Klink, B. P. C. Kreukels, L. E. Kuper, E. J. Kvach, M. A. Malouf, R. Massey, T. Mazur, C. McLachlan, S. D. Morrison, S. W. Mosser, P. M. Neira, U. Nygren, J. M. Oates, J. Obedin-Maliver, G. Pagkalos, J. Patton, N. Phanuphak, K. Rachlin, T. Reed, G. N. Rider, J. Ristori, S. Robbins-Cherry, S. A. Roberts, K. A. Rodriguez-Wallberg, S. M. Rosenthal, K. Sabir, J. D. Safer, A. I. Scheim, L. J. Seal, T. J. Sehoole, K. Spencer, C. St. Amand, T. D. Steensma, J. F. Strang, G. B. Taylor, K. Tilleman, G. G. T'Sjoen, L. N. Vala, N. M. Van Mello, J. F. Veale, J. A. Vencill, B. Vincent, L. M. Wesp, M. A. West, and J. Arcelus. 2022. Standards of care for the health of transgender and gender diverse people, version 8. *International Journal of Transgender Health* 23(Suppl 1):S1–S259.

Connolly, D., and G. Gilchrist. 2020. Prevalence and correlates of substance use among transgender adults: A systematic review. *Addictive Behaviors* 111:106544.

Corbie-Smith, G., S. B. Thomas, and D. M. St George. 2002. Distrust, race, and research. *Archives of Internal Medicine* 162(21):2458–2463.

Crenshaw, K. 1991. Mapping the margins: Intersectionality, identity politics, and violence against women of color. *Stanford Law Review* 43(6):1241–1299.

D'Avanzo, P. A., S. B. Bass, J. Brajuha, L. Gutierrez-Mock, N. Ventriglia, C. Wellington, and J. Sevelius. 2019. Medical mistrust and prep perceptions among transgender women: A cluster analysis. *Behavioral Medicine* 45(2):143–152.

de Blok, C. J., C. M. Wiepjes, D. M. van Velzen, A. S. Staphorsius, N. M. Nota, L. J. Gooren, B. P. Kreukels, and M. den Heijer. 2021. Mortality trends over five decades in adult transgender people receiving hormone treatment: A report from the Amsterdam cohort of gender dysphoria. *The Lancet Diabetes & Endocrinology* 9(10):663–670.

de Lange, J., L. Baams, D. D. van Bergen, H. M. W. Bos, and R. J. Bosker. 2022. Minority stress and suicidal ideation and suicide attempts among LGBT adolescents and young adults: A meta-analysis. *LGBT Health* 9(4):222–237.

Defreyne, J., D. De Bacquer, S. Shadid, B. Lapauw, and G. T'Sjoen. 2017. Is type 1 diabetes mellitus more prevalent than expected in transgender persons? A local observation. *Sexual Medicine* 5(3):e215–e218.

Defreyne, J., L. D. L. Van de Bruaene, E. Rietzschel, J. Van Schuylenbergh, and G. G. R. T'Sjoen. 2019. Effects of gender-affirming hormones on lipid, metabolic, and cardiac surrogate blood markers in transgender persons. *Clinical Chemistry* 65(1):119–134.

Dermody, S. S., A. Uhrig, A. Moore, T. Raessi, and A. Walker. 2023. A narrative systematic review of the gender inclusivity of measures of harmful drinking and their psychometric properties among transgender adults. *Addiction* 118(9):1649–1660.

Dhejne, C., P. Lichtenstein, M. Boman, A. L. Johansson, N. Langstrom, and M. Landen. 2011. Long-term follow-up of transsexual persons undergoing sex reassignment surgery: Cohort study in Sweden. *PLoS ONE* 6(2):e16885.

Dickey, L. M., A. A. Singh, and D. Walinsky. 2017. Treatment of trauma and nonsuicidal self-injury in transgender adults. *Psychiatry Clinics of North America* 40(1):41–50.

Downing, J. M., and J. M. Przedworski. 2018. Health of transgender adults in the U.S., 2014–2016. *American Journal of Preventive Medicine* 55(3):336–344.

Dragon, C. N., P. Guerino, E. Ewald, and A. M. Laffan. 2017. Transgender Medicare beneficiaries and chronic conditions: Exploring fee-for-service claims data. *LGBT Health* 4(6):404–411.

Dubois, L. Z. 2012. Associations between transition-specific stress experience, nocturnal decline in ambulatory blood pressure, and c-reactive protein levels among transgender men. *American Journal of Human Biology* 24(1):52–61.

Dubois, L. Z., and R. P. Juster. 2022. Lived experience and allostatic load among transmasculine people living in the United States. *Psychoneuroendocrinology* 143:105849.

Edwards, L. L., A. Torres Bernal, S. M. Hanley, and S. Martin. 2020. Resilience factors and suicide risk for a sample of transgender clients. *Family Process* 59(3):1209–1224.

Fahey, K. M. L., K. Kovacek, A. Abramovich, and S. S. Dermody. 2023. Substance use prevalence, patterns, and correlates in transgender and gender diverse youth: A scoping review. *Drug and Alcohol Dependence* 250:110880.

Feinstein, M. J., P. Y. Hsue, L. A. Benjamin, G. S. Bloomfield, J. S. Currier, M. S. Freiberg, S. K. Grinspoon, J. Levin, C. T. Longenecker, and W. S. Post. 2019. Characteristics, prevention, and management of cardiovascular disease in people living with HIV: A scientific statement from the American Heart Association. *Circulation* 140(2):e98–e124.

Feldman, J. L., W. E. Luhur, J. L. Herman, T. Poteat, and I. H. Meyer. 2021. Health and health care access in the US transgender population health (transpop) survey. *Andrology* 9(6):1707–1718.

Flentje, A., B. T. Barger, M. R. Capriotti, M. E. Lubensky, M. Tierney, J. Obedin-Maliver, and M. R. Lunn. 2020. Screening gender minority people for harmful alcohol use. *PLoS ONE* 15(4):e0231022.

Geilhufe, B., O. Tripp, S. Silverstein, L. Birchfield, and M. Raimondo. 2021. Gender-affirmative eating disorder care: Clinical considerations for transgender and gender expansive children and youth. *Pediatric Annals* 50(9):e371–e378.

Geronimus, A. T., M. Hicken, D. Keene, and J. Bound. 2006. "Weathering" and age patterns of allostatic load scores among blacks and whites in the United States. *American Journal of Public Health* 96(5):826–833.

Getahun, D., R. Nash, W. D. Flanders, T. C. Baird, T. A. Becerra-Culqui, L. Cromwell, E. Hunkeler, T. L. Lash, A. Millman, V. P. Quinn, B. Robinson, D. Roblin, M. J. Silverberg, J. Safer, J. Slovis, V. Tangpricha, and M. Goodman. 2018. Cross-sex hormones and acute cardiovascular events in transgender persons: A cohort study. *Annals of Internal Medicine* 169(4):205–213.

Goetz, T. G., and N. Adams. 2022. The transgender and gender diverse and attention deficit hyperactivity disorder nexus: A systematic review. *Journal of Gay & Lesbian Mental Health* 28(1):2–19.

Gosiker, B. J., C. R. Lesko, A. J. Rich, H. M. Crane, M. M. Kitahata, S. L. Reisner, K. H. Mayer, R. J. Fredericksen, G. Chander, W. C. Mathews, and T. C. Poteat. 2020. Cardiovascular disease risk among transgender women living with HIV in the United States. *PLoS ONE* 15(7):e0236177.

Grant, R. M., J. R. Lama, P. L. Anderson, V. McMahan, A. Y. Liu, L. Vargas, P. Goicochea, M. Casapía, J. V. Guanira-Carranza, M. E. Ramirez-Cardich, O. Montoya-Herrera, T. Fernández, V. G. Veloso, S. P. Buchbinder, S. Chariyalertsak, M. Schechter, L. G.Bekker, K. H. Mayer, E. G. Kallás, K. R. Amico, K. Mulligan, L. R. Bushman, R. J. Hance, C. Ganoza, P. Defechereux, B. Postle, F. Wang, J. J. McConnell, J. H. Zheng, J. Lee, J. F. Rooney, H. S. Jaffe, A. I. Martinez, D. N. Burns, D. V. Glidden, and the iPrEx Study Team. 2010. Preexposure chemoprophylaxis for HIV prevention in men who have sex with men. *New England Journal of Medicine* 363(27):2587–99.

Guadamuz, T. E., W. Wimonsate, A. Varangrat, P. Phanuphak, R. Jommaroeng, J. M. McNicholl, P. A. Mock, J. W. Tappero, and F. van Griensven. 2011. HIV prevalence, risk behavior, hormone use and surgical history among transgender persons in Thailand. *AIDS & Behavior* 15(3):650–658.

Guo, Y., D. A. Westmoreland, A. D'Angelo, C. Mirzayi, M. Dearolf, P. B. Carneiro, M. Ray, D. W. Pantalone, A. W. Carrico, V. V. Patel, S. A. Golub, S. Hirshfield, D. Hoover, D. Nash, and C. Grov. 2024. PrEP discontinuation in a U.S. national cohort of sexual and gender minority populations, 2017–22. *Health Affairs* 43(3):443–451.

Habarta, N., G. Wang, M. S. Mulatu, and N. Larish. 2015. HIV testing by transgender status at Centers for Disease Control and Prevention-funded sites in the United States, Puerto Rico, and U.S. Virgin Islands, 2009–2011. *American Journal of Public Health* 105(9):1917–1925.

Hadland, S. E., E. D. Solomon, and C. E. Guss. 2023. Affirming care for autism and gender diversity. *Pediatrics* 152(2).

Haney, J. L. 2016. Autism, females, and the DSM-5: Gender bias in autism diagnosis. *Social Work in Mental Health* 14(4):396–407.

Heiden-Rootes, K., W. Linsenmeyer, S. Levine, M. Oliveras, and M. Joseph. 2023. A scoping review of research literature on eating and body image for transgender and nonbinary youth. *Journal of Eating Disorders* 11(1):168.

Hembree, W. C., P. T. Cohen-Kettenis, L. Gooren, S. E. Hannema, W. J. Meyer, M. H. Murad, S. M. Rosenthal, J. D. Safer, V. Tangpricha, and G. G. T'Sjoen. 2017. Endocrine treatment of gender-dysphoric/gender-incongruent persons: An Endocrine Society* clinical practice guideline. *Journal of Clinical Endocrinology & Metabolism* 102(11):3869–3903.

Herman, J. L., B. D. Wilson, and T. Becker. 2017. Demographic and health characteristics of transgender adults in California: Findings from the 2015–2016 California Health Interview Survey. *Policy Brief UCLA Center for Health Policy Research* (8):1–10.

Homan, P., T. H. Brown, and B. King. 2021. Structural intersectionality as a new direction for health disparities research. *Journal of Health and Social Behavior* 62(3):350–370.

Islam, N., R. Nash, Q. Zhang, L. Panagiotakopoulos, T. Daley, S. Bhasin, D. Getahun, J. Sonya Haw, C. McCracken, M. J. Silverberg, V. Tangpricha, S. Vupputuri, and M. Goodman. 2022. Is there a link between hormone use and diabetes incidence in transgender people? Data from the strong cohort. *Journal of Clinical Endocrinology & Metabolism* 107(4):e1549–e1557.

Jaiswal, J., and P. N. Halkitis. 2019. Towards a more inclusive and dynamic understanding of medical mistrust informed by science. *Behavioral Medicine* 45(2):79–85.

Jones, B. A., E. Haycraft, S. Murjan, and J. Arcelus. 2016. Body dissatisfaction and disordered eating in trans people: A systematic review of the literature. *International Review of Psychiatry* 28(1):81–94.

Joy, P., O. Ferlatte, M. Aston, H. Minzloff, and J. Hillis. 2023. Wicked bodies: A health and well-being toolkit addressing eating disorders within LGBTQIA2S+ communities. *Health Promotion Practice* 24(2):258–260.

Kahn, N. F., G. M. Sequeira, M. M. Garrison, F. Orlich, D. A. Christakis, T. Aye, L. A. E. Conard, N. Dowshen, A. E. Kazak, L. Nahata, N. J. Nokoff, R. V. Voss, and L. P. Richardson. 2023. Co-occurring autism spectrum disorder and gender dysphoria in adolescents. *Pediatrics* 152(2).

Kalichman, S. C., D. Hernandez, S. Finneran, D. Price, and R. Driver. 2017. Transgender women and HIV-related health disparities: Falling off the HIV treatment cascade. *Sexual Health* 14(5):469–476.

Kallitsounaki, A., and D. M. Williams. 2023. Autism spectrum disorder and gender dysphoria/incongruence. A systematic literature review and meta-analysis. *Journal of Autism and Developmental Disorders* 53(8):3103–3117.

Keski-Rahkonen, A. 2023. Eating disorders in transgender and gender diverse people: Characteristics, assessment, and management. *Current Opinions in Psychiatry* 36(6):412–418.

Keuroghlian, A. S., S. L. Reisner, J. M. White, and R. D. Weiss. 2015. Substance use and treatment of substance use disorders in a community sample of transgender adults. *Drug and Alcohol Dependence* 152:139–146.

KFF. 2022. *Adults who report ever receiving an HIV test by race/ethnicity; KFF analysis of the Centers for Disease Control and Prevention (CDC)'s 2013–2022 Behavioral Risk Factor Surveillance System (BRFSS).* https://www.kff.org/other/state-indicator/adults-who-report-ever-receiving-an-hiv-test-by-race-ethnicity/?currentTimeframe=0&sortModel=%7B%22c olId%22:%22Location%22,%22sort%22:%22asc%22%7DK (accessed April 29, 2024).

Khan, J., R. L. Schmidt, M. J. Spittal, Z. Goldstein, K. J. Smock, and D. N. Greene. 2019. Venous thrombotic risk in transgender women undergoing estrogen therapy: A systematic review and metaanalysis. *Clinical Chemistry* 65(1):57–66.

Kidd, J. D., N. A. Tettamanti, R. Kaczmarkiewicz, T. E. Corbeil, J. D. Dworkin, K. B. Jackman, T. L. Hughes, W. O. Bockting, and I. H. Meyer. 2023. Prevalence of substance use and mental health problems among transgender and cisgender U.S. Adults: Results from a national probability sample. *Psychiatry Research* 326:115339.

Klein, P. W., P. Demetrios, J. Xavier, and S. Cohen. 2020. HIV-related outcome disparities between transgender women living with HIV and cisgender people living with HIV served by the Health Resources and Services Administration's Ryan White HIV/aids program: A retrospective study. *PLoS Medicine* 17(5):e1003125.

Krieger, N. 1994. Epidemiology and the web of causation: Has anyone seen the spider? *Social Science & Medicine* 39(7):887–903.

Krieger, N. 2016. Living and dying at the crossroads: Racism, embodiment, and why theory is essential for a public health of consequence. *American Journal of Public Health* 106(5):832–833.

Kuhns, L. M., N. Karnik, A. Hotton, A. Muldoon, G. Donenberg, K. Keglovitz, M. McNulty, J. Schneider, F. Summersett-Williams, and R. Garofalo. 2020. A randomized controlled efficacy trial of an electronic screening and brief intervention for alcohol misuse in adolescents and young adults vulnerable to HIV infection: Step up, test up study protocol. *BMC Public Health* 20(1):30.

Lacombe-Duncan, A., L. Kattari, S. K. Kattari, A. I. Scheim, F. Alexander, S. Yonce, and B. A. Misiolek. 2022. HIV testing among transgender and nonbinary persons in Michigan, United States: Results of a community-based survey. *Journal of the International AIDS Society* (Suppl 5):e25972.

LaVeist, T. A., L. A. Isaac, and K. P. Williams. 2009. Mistrust of health care organizations is associated with underutilization of health services. *Health Services Research* 44(6):2093–2105.

Lee, J. G., A. K. Matthews, C. A. McCullen, and C. L. Melvin. 2014. Promotion of tobacco use cessation for lesbian, gay, bisexual, and transgender people: A systematic review. *American Journal of Preventive Medicine* 47(6):823–831.

Lett, E., C. H. Logie, and D. Mohottige. 2023. Intersectionality as a lens for achieving kidney health justice. *Nature Reviews Nephrology* 19(6):353–354.

Link, B. G., and J. C. Phelan. 1995. Social conditions as fundamental causes of disease. *Journal of Health and Social Behavior* Spec No:80–94.

Link, B. G., and J. C. Phelan. 2001. Conceptualizing stigma. *Annual Review of Sociology* 27(27):363–385.

Logel, S. N., M. T. Bekx, and J. L. Rehm. 2020. Potential association between type 1 diabetes mellitus and gender dysphoria. *Pediatric Diabetes* 21(2):266–270.

Marchi, M., A. Travascio, D. Uberti, E. De Micheli, P. Grenzi, E. Arcolin, L. Pingani, S. Ferrari, and G. M. Galeazzi. 2023. Post-traumatic stress disorder among LGBTQ people: A systematic review and meta-analysis. *Epidemiology and Psychiatric Sciences* 32:e44.

Marconi, E., L. Monti, A. Marfoli, G. D. Kotzalidis, D. Janiri, C. Cianfriglia, F. Moriconi, S. Costa, C. Veredice, G. Sani, and D. P. R. Chieffo. 2023. A systematic review on gender dysphoria in adolescents and young adults: Focus on suicidal and self-harming ideation and behaviours. *Child and Adolescent Psychiatry and Mental Health* 17(1):110.

Marshall, E., L. Claes, W. P. Bouman, G. L. Witcomb, and J. Arcelus. 2016. Non-suicidal self-injury and suicidality in trans people: A systematic review of the literature. *International Review of Psychiatry* 28(1):58–69.

Maru, J., K. Millington, and J. Carswell. 2021. Greater than expected prevalence of type 1 diabetes mellitus found in an urban gender program. *Transgender Health* 6(1):57–60.

Matson, T. E., A. H. S. Harris, J. A. Chen, A. T. Edmonds, M. C. Frost, A. D. Rubinsky, J. R. Blosnich, and E. C. Williams. 2022. Influence of a national transgender health care directive on receipt of alcohol-related care among transgender Veteran Health Administration patients with unhealthy alcohol use. *Journal of Substance Use and Addiction Treatment* 143:108808.

McCann, E., and M. Brown. 2017. Discrimination and resilience and the needs of people who identify as transgender: A narrative review of quantitative research studies. *Journal of Clinical Nursing* 26(23-24):4080–4093.

McEwen, B. S. 2000. Allostasis and allostatic load: Implications for neuropsychopharmacology. *Neuropsychopharmacology* 22(2):108–124.

McFarland, W., E. C. Wilson, and H. F. Raymond. 2017. HIV prevalence, sexual partners, sexual behavior and HIV acquisition risk among trans men, San Francisco, 2014. *AIDS & Behavior* 21(12):3346–3352.

McFarland, W., E. C. Wilson, and H. Fisher Raymond. 2018. How many transgender men are there in San Francisco? *Journal of Urban Health* 95(1):129–133.

McGregor, K., J. L. McKenna, E. P. Barrera, C. R. Williams, S. M. Hartman-Munick, and C. E. Guss. 2023. Disordered eating and considerations for the transgender community: A review of the literature and clinical guidance for assessment and treatment. *Journal of Eating Disorders* 11(1):75.

Melendez, R. M., T. A. Exner, A. A. Ehrhardt, B. Dodge, R. H. Remien, M. J. Rotheram-Borus, M. Lightfoot, and D. Hong. 2006. Health and health care among male-to-female transgender persons who are HIV positive. *American Journal of Public Health* 96(6):1034–1037.

Meyer, I. H., T. N. Brown, J. L. Herman, S. L. Reisner, and W. O. Bockting. 2017. Demographic characteristics and health status of transgender adults in select us regions: Behavioral risk factor surveillance system, 2014. *American Journal of Public Health* 107(4):582–589.

Mizuno, Y., E. L. Frazier, P. Huang, and J. Skarbinski. 2015. Characteristics of transgender women living with HIV receiving medical care in the United States. *LGBT Health* 2(3):228–234.

Mizuno, Y., L. Beer, P. Huang, and E. L. Frazier. 2017. Factors associated with antiretroviral therapy adherence among transgender women receiving HIV medical care in the United States. *LGBT Health* 4(3):181–187.

Mohottige, D., and L. E. Boulware. 2020. Trust in American medicine: A call to action for health care professionals. *Hastings Center Report* 50(1):27–29.

Molina J. M., C. Capitant, B. Spire, G. Pialoux, L. Cotte, I. Charreau, C. Tremblay, J. M. Le Gall, E. Cua, A. Pasquet, F. Raffi, C. Pintado, C. Chidiac, J. Chas, P. Charbonneau, C. Delaugerre, M. Suzan-Monti, B. Loze, J. Fonsart, G. Peytavin, A. Cheret, J. Timsit, G. Girard, N. Lorente, M. Préau, J.F. Rooney, M. A. Wainberg, D. Thompson, W. Rozenbaum, V. Doré, L. Marchand, M. C. Simon, N. Etien, J. P. Aboulker, L. Meyer, and J. F. Delfraissy. 2015. ANRS IPERGAY study group. On-demand preexposure prophylaxis in men at high risk for HIV-1 infection. *New England Journal of Medicine* 373(23):2237–2246.

Morgan, J. F., F. Reid, and J. H. Lacey. 2000. The SCOFF questionnaire: A new screening tool for eating disorders. *Western Journal of Medicine* 172(3):164–165.

Moverley, J., S. Loebner, B. Carmona, and D. Vuu. 2021. Considerations for transgender people with diabetes. *Clinical Diabetes* 39(4):389–396.

Mulcahy, A., C. G. G. Streed, A. M. Wallisch, K. Batza, N. Kurth, J. P. P. Hall, and D. J. McMaughan. 2022. Gender identity, disability, and unmet healthcare needs among disabled people living in the community in the United States. *International Journal of Environmental Research and Public Health* 19(5):2588.

Nahata, L., G. P. Quinn, N. M. Caltabellotta, and A. C. Tishelman. 2017. Mental health concerns and insurance denials among transgender adolescents. *LGBT Health* 4(3):188–193.

National Cholesterol Education Program Expert Panel. 2001. Expert panel on detection, evaluation, and treatment of high blood cholesterol in adults. Executive summary of the third report of the National Cholesterol Education Program (NCEP) expert panel on detection, evaluation, and treatment of high blood cholesterol in adults (adult treatment panel III). *Journal of the American Medical Association* 285(19):2486–2497.

National LGBTQIA+ Health Education Center. 2024. *Neurodiversity and the gender-diverse experience.* Recorded Webinar. Boston, MA: The Fenway Institute. https://www.lgbtqia-healtheducation.org/courses/neurodiversity-and-the-gender-diverse-experience/ (accessed Jan 18, 2024).

Naz-McLean, S., J. L. Clark, S. L. Reisner, J. C. Prenner, B. Weintraub, L. Huerta, X. Salazar, J. R. Lama, K. H. Mayer, and A. Perez-Brumer. 2022. Decision-making at the intersection of risk and pleasure: A qualitative inquiry with trans women engaged in sex work in Lima, Peru. *AIDS & Behavior* 26(3):843–852.

Newman, K. L., C. Vélez, S. Paul, A. E. Radix, C. G. Streed, and L. E. Targownik. 2023. Research considerations in digestive and liver disease in transgender and gender-diverse populations. *Clinical Gastroenterology and Hepatology* 21(10):2443–2449.e2442.

Nobili, A., C. Glazebrook, W. P. Bouman, D. Glidden, S. Baron-Cohen, C. Allison, P. Smith, and J. Arcelus. 2018. Autistic traits in treatment-seeking transgender adults. *Journal of Autism and Developmental Disorders* 48(12):3984–3994.

Nokoff, N. J., S. Scarbro, E. Juarez-Colunga, K. L. Moreau, and A. Kempe. 2018. Health and cardiometabolic disease in transgender adults in the United States: Behavioral Risk Factor Surveillance System (BRFSS) 2015. *Journal of the Endocrine Society* 2(4):349–360.

Nokoff, N. J., S. L. Scarbro, K. L. Moreau, P. Zeitler, K. J. Nadeau, E. Juarez-Colunga, and M. M. Kelsey. 2020. Body composition and markers of cardiometabolic health in transgender youth compared with cisgender youth. *Journal of Clinical Endocrinology & Metabolism* 105(3):e704–714.

OASH (Office of the Assistant Secretary for Health). n.d. *Healthy People 2030.* https://health.gov/healthypeople/objectives-and-data/browse-objectives/lgbt (accessed February 21, 2024).

Obarzanek, L., and K. Munyan. 2021. Eating disorder behaviors among transgender individuals: Exploring the literature. *Journal of the American Psychiatric Nurses Association* 27(3):203–212.

Olakunde, B. O., J. R. Pharr, D. A. Adeyinka, and D. F. Conserve. 2022. Non-uptake of HIV testing among transgender populations in the United States: Results from the 2015 U.S. Transgender Survey. *Transgender Health* 7(5):430–439.

Pellicane, M. J., and J. A. Ciesla. 2022. Associations between minority stress, depression, and suicidal ideation and attempts in transgender and gender diverse (TGD) individuals: Systematic review and meta-analysis. *Clinical Psychology Reviews* 91:102113.

Perez-Brumer, A., S. Naz-McLean, L. Huerta, X. Salazar, J. R. Lama, J. Sanchez, A. Silva-Santisteban, S. L. Reisner, K. H. Mayer, and J. L. Clark. 2021. The wisdom of mistrust: Qualitative insights from transgender women who participated in prep research in Lima, Peru. *Journal of the International AIDS Society* 24(9):e25769.

Pflum, S. R., R. J. Testa, K. F. Balsam, P. B. Goldblum, and B. Bongar. 2015. Social support, trans community connectedness, and mental health symptoms among transgender and gender nonconforming adults. *Psychology of Sexual Orientation and Gender Diversity* 2(3):281–286.

Pharr, J. R. 2021. Health disparities among lesbian, gay, bisexual, transgender, and nonbinary adults 50 years old and older in the United States. *LGBT Health* 8(7):473–485.

Phillip, A., A. Pellechi, R. DeSilva, K. Semler, and R. Makani. 2022. A plausible explanation of increased suicidal behaviors among transgender youth based on the interpersonal theory of suicide (IPTS): Case series and literature review. *Journal of Psychiatric Practice* 28(1):3–13.

Pinna, F., P. Paribello, G. Somaini, A. Corona, A. Ventriglio, C. Corrias, I. Frau, R. Murgia, S. El Kacemi, G. M. Galeazzi, M. Mirandola, F. Amaddeo, A. Crapanzano, M. Converti, P. Piras, F. Suprani, M. Manchia, A. Fiorillo, and B. Carpiniello. 2022. Mental health in transgender individuals: A systematic review. *International Review of Psychiatry* 34(3-4):292–359.

Pitasi, M. A., E. Oraka, H. Clark, M. Town, and E. A. DiNenno. 2017. HIV testing among transgender women and men—27 states and Guam, 2014–2015. *Morbidity & Mortality Weekly Report* 66(33):883–887.

Poteat, T. 2016. Transgender health and HIV. In *UCSF transgender care and treatment guidelines*, edited by M. B. Deutsch. San Francicso, CA: UCSF Gender Affriming Health Program, Department of Family and Community Medicine, University of California San Francisco.

Poteat, T., A. L. Wirtz, A. Radix, A. Borquez, A. Silva-Santisteban, M. B. Deutsch, S. I. Khan, S. Winter, and D. Operario. 2015. HIV risk and preventive interventions in transgender women sex workers. *The Lancet* 385(9964):274–286.

Poteat, T., A. Scheim, J. Xavier, S. L. Reisner, and S. Baral. 2016. Global epidemiology of HIV infection and related syndemics affecting transgender people. *Journal of Acquired Immune Deficiency Syndromes* 72:S210–S219.

Poteat, T., M. Malik, A. Scheim, and A. Elliott. 2017. HIV prevention among transgender populations: Knowledge gaps and evidence for action. *Current HIV/AIDS Reports* 14(4):141–152.

Poteat, T., E. Cooney, M. Malik, A. Restar, D. T. Dangerfield, and J. White. 2021. HIV prevention among cisgender men who have sex with transgender women. *AIDS and Behavior* 25(8):2325–2335.

Poteat, T., E. Lett, A. Rich, H. Jiang, A. Wirtz, A. Radix, S. Reisner, A. Harris, J. Malone, W. La Cava, C. Lesko, K. Mayer, and C. Streed. 2023. Effects of race and gender classifications on atherosclerotic cardiovascular disease risk estimates for clinical decision-making in a cohort of black transgender women. *Health Equity* 7(1):803–808.

Puckett, J. A., S. Domínguez, and E. Matsuno. 2024. Measures of resilience: Do they reflect the experiences of transgender individuals? *Transgender Health* 9(1):1–13.

Qian, J., Q. Hu, Y. Wan, T. Li, M. Wu, Z. Ren, and D. Yu. 2013. Prevalence of eating disorders in the general population: A systematic review. *Shanghai Archives of Psychiatry.* 25(4):212–223.

Quinn, V. P., R. Nash, E. Hunkeler, R. Contreras, L. Cromwell, T. A. Becerra-Culqui, D. Getahun, S. Giammattei, T. L. Lash, A. Millman, B. Robinson, D. Roblin, M. J. Silverberg, J. Slovis, V. Tangpricha, D. Tolsma, C. Valentine, K. Ward, S. Winter, and M. Goodman. 2017. Cohort profile: Study of Transition, Outcomes and Gender (STRONG) to assess health status of transgender people. *BMJ Open* 7(12):e018121.

Ramos, N., and M. C. Marr. 2023. Traumatic stress and resilience among transgender and gender diverse youth. *Child and Adolescent Psychiatry Clinics of North America* 32(4):667–682.

Rasmussen, S. M., M. K. Dalgaard, M. Roloff, M. Pinholt, C. Skrubbeltrang, L. Clausen, and G. Kjaersdam Telleus. 2023. Eating disorder symptomatology among transgender individuals: A systematic review and meta-analysis. *Journal of Eating Disorders* 11(1):84.

Reisner, S. L., and G. R. Murchison. 2016. A global research synthesis of HIV and STI biobehavioural risks in female-to-male transgender adults. *Global Public Health* 11(7-8):866–887.

Reisner, S., T. Poteat, J. Keatley, M. Cabral, T. Mothopeng, E. Dunham, C. Holland, R. Max, and S. Baral. 2016a. Global health burden and needs of transgender populations: A review. *The Lancet* 388(10042):412–436.

Reisner, S. L., J. M. White Hughto, D. Pardee, and J. Sevelius. 2016b. Syndemics and gender affirmation: HIV sexual risk in female-to-male trans masculine adults reporting sexual contact with cisgender males. *International Journal of STD and AIDS* 27(11):955–966.

Rich, A. J., A. I. Scheim, M. Koehoorn, and T. Poteat. 2020. Non-HIV chronic disease burden among transgender populations globally: A systematic review and narrative synthesis. *Preventive Medicine Reports* 20:101259.

Richman, L. S., and A. N. Zucker. 2019. Quantifying intersectionality: An important advancement for health inequality research. *Social Science & Medicine* 226:246–248.

Ridker, P. M., J. E. Buring, N. Rifai, and N. R. Cook. 2007. Development and validation of improved algorithms for the assessment of global cardiovascular risk in women: The Reynolds Risk Score. *Journal of the American Medical Association* 297(6):611–619.

Rioux, C., A. Pare, K. London-Nadeau, R. P. Juster, S. Weedon, S. Levasseur-Puhach, M. Freeman, L. E. Roos, and L. M. Tomfohr-Madsen. 2022. Sex and gender terminology: A glossary for gender-inclusive epidemiology. *Journal of Epidemiology and Community Health* 76(8):764–768.

Safer, J. D. 2021. Research gaps in medical treatment of transgender/nonbinary people. *Journal of Clinical Investigation* 131(4):e142029.

Salazar, L. F., R. A. Crosby, J. Jones, K. Kota, B. Hill, and K. E. Masyn. 2017. Contextual, experiential, and behavioral risk factors associated with HIV status: A descriptive analysis of transgender women residing in Atlanta, Georgia. *International Journal of STD and AIDS* 28(11):1059–1066.

Scheim, A. I., K. E. Baker, A. J. Restar, and R. L. Sell. 2022. Health and health care among transgender adults in the United States. *Annual Reviews of Public Health* 43:503–523.

Sevelius, J. M. 2013. Gender affirmation: A framework for conceptualizing risk behavior among transgender women of color. *Sex Roles* 68(11-12):675–689.

Sevelius, J. M., T. Poteat, W. E. Luhur, S. Reisner, and I. H. Meyer. 2020. HIV testing and PrEP use in a national probability sample of sexually active transgender people in the United States. *Journal of Acquired Immune Deficiency Syndromes* 84(5):437–442.

Sherman, A. D. F., K. D. Clark, K. Robinson, T. Noorani, and T. Poteat. 2020. Trans community connection, health, and wellbeing: A systematic review. *LGBT Health* 7(1):1–14.

Sherman, A. D. F., S. Allgood, K. A. Alexander, M. Klepper, M. S. Balthazar, M. Hill, C. M. Cannon, D. Dunn, T. Poteat, and J. Campbell. 2022. Transgender and gender diverse community connection, help-seeking, and mental health among black transgender women who have survived violence: A mixed-methods analysis. *Violence Against Women* 28(3-4):890–921.

Silva-Santisteban, A., H. F. Raymond, X. Salazar, J. Villayzan, S. Leon, W. McFarland, and C. F. Caceres. 2012. Understanding the HIV/AIDS epidemic in transgender women of Lima, Peru: Results from a sero-epidemiologic study using respondent driven sampling. *AIDS & Behavior* 16(4):872–881.

Smart, B. D., L. Mann-Jackson, J. Alonzo, A. E. Tanner, M. Garcia, L. Refugio Aviles, and S. D. Rhodes. 2022. Transgender women of color in the U.S. South: A qualitative study of social determinants of health and healthcare perspectives. *International Journal of Transgender Health* 23(1-2):164–177.

Smith, L. R., V. V. Patel, A. C. Tsai, M. L. Mittal, K. Quinn, V. A. Earnshaw, and T. Poteat. 2022. Integrating intersectional and syndemic frameworks for ending the U.S. HIV epidemic. *American Journal of Public Health* 112(S4):S340–S343.

SSA (Social Security Administration). 2017. Revisions to rules regarding the evaluation of medical evidence. *Federal Register* 82(5869).

Strang, J. F., H. Meagher, L. Kenworthy, A. L. C. de Vries, E. Menvielle, S. Leibowitz, A. Janssen, P. Cohen-Kettenis, D. E. Shumer, L. Edwards-Leeper, R. R. Pleak, N. Spack, D. H. Karasic, H. Schreier, A. Balleur, A. Tishelman, D. Ehrensaft, L. Rodnan, E. S. Kuschner, F. Mandel, A. Caretto, H. C. Lewis, and L. G. Anthony. 2018. Initial clinical guidelines for co-occurring autism spectrum disorder and gender dysphoria or incongruence in adolescents. *Journal of Clinical Child and Adolescent Psychology* 47(1):105–115.

Streed, C. G., Jr., L. B. Beach, B. A. Caceres, N. L. Dowshen, K. L. Moreau, M. Mukherjee, T. Poteat, A. Radix, S. L. Reisner, and V. Singh, on behalf of the American Heart Association Council on Peripheral Vascular Disease; Council on Arteriosclerosis, Thrombosis and Vascular Biology; Council on Cardiovascular and Stroke Nursing; Council on Cardiosvascular Radiology and Intervention; Council on Hypertension; and Stroke Council. 2021. Assessing and addressing cardiovascular health in people who are transgender and gender diverse: A scientific statement from the American Heart Association. *Circulation* 144(6):e136–e148.

Stutterheim, S. E., M. van Dijk, H. Wang, and K. J. Jonas. 2021. The worldwide burden of HIV in transgender individuals: An updated systematic review and meta-analysis. *PLoS ONE* 16(12):e0260063.

Suslovic, B., and E. Lett. 2024. Resilience is an adverse event: A critical discussion of resilience theory in health services research and public health. *Community Health Equity Research and Policy* 44(3):339–343.

Tankersley, A. P., E. L. Grafsky, J. Dike, and R. T. Jones. 2021. Risk and resilience factors for mental health among transgender and gender nonconforming (TGNC) youth: A systematic review. *Clinical Child and Family Psychology Review* 24(2):183–206.

Taormina, J. M., and S. J. Iwamoto. 2023. Filling a gap in care: Addressing obesity in transgender and gender diverse patients. *International Journal of Obesity (London)* 47(9):761–763.

Tebbe, E. A., and S. L. Budge. 2022. Factors that drive mental health disparities and promote well-being in transgender and nonbinary people. *Nature Reviews Psychology* 1(12):694–707.

Testa, R. J., J. Habarth, J. Peta, K. Balsam, and W. Bockting. 2015. Development of the gender minority stress and resilience measure. *Psychology of Sexual Orientation and Gender Diversity* 2(1):65–77.

Thrower, E., I. Bretherton, K. C. Pang, J. D. Zajac, and A. S. Cheung. 2020. Prevalence of autism spectrum disorder and attention-deficit hyperactivity disorder amongst individuals with gender dysphoria: A systematic review. *Journal of Autism and Developmental Disorders* 50(3):695–706.

Tran, N. K., M. R. Lunn, C. E. Schulkey, S. Tesfaye, S. Nambiar, S. Chatterjee, D. Kozlowski, P.Lozano, F. T. Randal, Y. Mo, S. Qi, E. Hundertmark, C. Eastburn, A. T. Pho, Z. Dastur, M. E. Lubensky, A. Flentje, and J. Obedin-Maliver. 2023. Prevalence of 12 common health conditions in sexual and gender minority participants in the all of U.S. research program. *JAMA Network Open* 6(7):e2324969.

Turner, G. A., N. J. Amoura, and H. M. Strah. 2021. Care of the transgender patient with a pulmonary complaint. *Annals of the American Thoracic Society* 18(6):931–937.

UCSF (University of California, San Francisco). 2016. *UCSF transgender care & treatment guidelines*. 2nd ed. San Francisco, CA: UCSF Gender Affriming Health Program, Department of Family and Community Medicine.

Valdiserri, R. O., D. R. Holtgrave, T. C. Poteat, and C. Beyrer. 2019. Unraveling health disparities among sexual and gender minorities: A commentary on the persistent impact of stigma. *Journal of Homosexuality* 66(5):571–589.

Valentine, S. E., A. M. Smith, K. Miller, L. Hadden, and J. C. Shipherd. 2023. Considerations and complexities of accurate PTSD assessment among transgender and gender diverse adults. *Psychological Assessment* 35(5):383–395.

Walker, E., and E. Roessel. 2019. Social Security Disability Insurance and Supplemental Security Income beneficiaries with multiple impairments. *Social Security Bulletin* 79(3). https://www.ssa.gov/policy/docs/ssb/v79n3/v79n3p21.html#:~:text=Two%2Dthirds%20of%20all%20beneficiaries,more%20than%20two%20impairment%20categories (accessed May 1, 2024).

Wesp, L. M. 2016. Diabetes mellitus. In *UCSF transgender care & treatment guidelines*, edited by M. B. Deutsch. San Francisco, CA: UCSF Gender Affirming Health Program, Department of Family and Community Medicine, University of California, San Francisco. https://transcare.ucsf.edu/guidelines/diabetes (accessed May 1, 2024).

Wesp, L. M., L. H. Malcoe, A. Elliott, and T. Poteat. 2019. Intersectionality research for transgender health justice: A theory-driven conceptual framework for structural analysis of transgender health inequities. *Transgender Health* 4(1):287–296.

White, M., S. Jones, and P. Joy. 2023. Safe, seen, and supported: Navigating eating disorders recovery in the 2SLGBTQ+ communities. *Canadian Journal of Dietetic Practice and Research* 84(2):84–92.

White Hughto, J. M., S. Reisner, and J. Pachankis. 2015. Transgender stigma and health: A critical review of stigma determinants, mechanisms, and interventions. *Social Science & Medicine* 147:222–231.

Wierckx, K., E. Elaut, E. Declercq, G. Heylens, G. De Cuypere, Y. Taes, J. M. Kaufman, and G. T'Sjoen. 2013. Prevalence of cardiovascular disease and cancer during cross-sex hormone therapy in a large cohort of trans persons: A case-control study. *European Journal of Endocrinology* 169(4):471–478.

Williams, D. R., J. A. Lawrence, B. A. Davis, and C. Vu. 2019. Understanding how discrimination can affect health. *Health Services Research* 54(Suppl 2):1374–1388.

Williams, E. C., M. C. Frost, A. D. Rubinsky, J. E. Glass, C. L. Wheat, A. T. Edmonds, J. A. Chen, T. E. Matson, O. V. Fletcher, K. Lehavot, and J. R. Blosnich. 2021. Patterns of alcohol use among transgender patients receiving care at the Veterans Health Administration: Overall and relative to nontransgender patients. *Journal of Studies on Alcohol and Drugs* 82(1):132–141.

Xia, Q., S. Seyoum, E. W. Wiewel, L. V. Torian, and S. L. Braunstein. 2019. Reduction in gaps in high CD4 count and viral suppression between transgender and cisgender persons living with HIV in New York City, 2007–2016. *American Journal of Public Health* 109(1):126–131.

Zhang, S. X., S. Shoptaw, C. J. Reback, K. Yadav, and A. M. Nyamathi. 2018. Cost-effective way to reduce stimulant-abuse among gay/bisexual men and transgender women: A randomized clinical trial with a cost comparison. *Public Health* 154:151–160.

7

Care for Individuals with Variations in Sex Traits

Society and biology generally view sex as a "binary." Typically, a baby's sex as "girl" or "boy" is identified in the delivery room immediately after birth based on the appearance of the baby's external genitalia. Increasingly, the baby's sex is being ascertained through prenatal ultrasound imaging and/or noninvasive prenatal screening studies. Sometimes, however, the appearance of the external genitalia does not inform determination of the infant's biological sex because of unconventional or atypical appearance of the external genital anatomy.[1] In these cases, ascertaining or labeling a child's sex may be challenging. Diverse and heterogeneous etiologies can affect development of the reproductive tract, resulting in atypical genital development.

Atypical genitalia are estimated to occur in approximately 1 in 4,500 live births. Several terms are used interchangeably to describe this condition (Hughes, 2007). These terms include "ambiguous genitalia," "variations of sex development," "variants of sex traits" (VSTs), "variations in sex characteristics," "intersex," and "differences of sex development" (DSD). For the purposes of this report, the committee uses the term "variations in sex

---

[1] Infants with atypical external genitalia may have a "phallus," the term used to describe both a clitoris and a penis. In the usual situation, 46,XY fetuses secrete testosterone from their testes, causing the phallus to develop into a penis, whereas in 46,XX fetuses, the absence of testosterone causes the phallus to develop into a clitoris. Where the genitalia are ambiguous, the phallus may not have fully developed. Infants with variations in sex traits may also have the urethral meatus on the perineum and nonpalpable gonads. Other infants may have an asymmetric appearance of the external genitalia, with an ostensibly rugated scrotum and palpable gonad on one side and an apparent labia majora and nonpalpable gonad on the other side.

239

traits," or "VSTs," when describing people with atypical genital development and other clinical presentations as described in this chapter.[2]

In some instances, the clinical presentation of a VST condition occurs beyond infancy, during childhood, adolescence, or adulthood. In total, estimates of the percentage of the population born with VSTs vary from 0.05 to 1.7 percent, depending on the definition used for VST (e.g., restricting the definition to include only those with atypical genitalia or taking a broader approach to include other differences in characteristics or reproductive anatomy) and the type of study conducted (medical or general population study) (Blackless et al., 2000). Overall, the statistics for the occurrence of VST are possibly inaccurate, given the difficulty patients with VSTs face in accessing knowledgeable medical providers and the variability in medical documentation.

Much variability exists in clinical presentations and precise etiologies. Sex determination and sex development involve complex sequential biologic networks with carefully orchestrated time-based interactions between specific molecular signals and hormones, and cross-talk between these signaling pathways. Hence, clinical features, age at presentation, diagnostic evaluations, appropriate health care interventions, clinical course, and specific etiologies are quite variable. Given the global perception of biological sex as perpetually binary, affected individuals, clinicians, parents or other caregivers, and family members often struggle when confronted with these conditions. While appropriate care may include hormonal treatment (or, in some cases, surgical treatment), behavioral/mental/psychosocial support, guidance, and counseling are essential for children, adolescents, emerging adults, and adults with VSTs and their caregivers and family members.

This chapter provides an overview of many of the conditions included under the VST rubric, describes common care management for people with VSTs, reviews potential hormonal and surgical interventions, and examines psychosocial/mental health/behavioral health care for this population.

---

[2] The committee chose to use the term "variations in sex traits" (VSTs) for this report to describe individuals with variations in development of the reproductive system (sex determination and sex development). The term "differences of sex development" (DSD) is commonly used in medical records and in the medical literature. However, some patients and clinicians consider the term "DSD" to be inaccurate and distasteful. "Intersex" is another commonly used term, but some individuals take issue with the notion that their reproductive anatomy falls between the binary and question this terminology. "Variations in sex traits," therefore, is intended to encompass all variations in reproductive tract development while being attentive to patient lived experience. However, the committee acknowledges that stakeholders have different and varied opinions on appropriate terminology, and, as is true for other terminology in this report, this terminology is likely to evolve over time. Table 2-3 in Chapter 2 displays a range of terms that may be present in medical records to describe VSTs, including some terms that have fallen out of popular use and may be considered offensive (including "pseudohermaphroditism" and "hermaphroditism"); however, these terms may still be found in older medical records.

Long-term health concerns and considerations are reviewed. While this chapter refers to guidelines and common care practices, it is not within the charge of this committee to recommend preferred practices; rather the committee's charge in response to the statement of task is to present the range of care practices that may exist and therefore may be seen in medical records submitted to the Social Security Administration (SSA) as part of a disability application.

CLASSIFICATIONS OF VARIATIONS IN SEX TRAITS

In 2005, recognizing inconsistences in terminology and health care among people with VSTs, an expert consensus meeting was held in Chicago to examine the vocabulary and health care for individuals with VSTs from a broad perspective (Hughes et al., 2006). The participating experts reviewed available patient outcomes, medical treatments, psychosocial management, potential surgical considerations, and gender concerns. Discussions focused on improving diagnostic approaches, expanding patient and family participation in medical decision making, involving multidisciplinary health care teams, and advancing medical management strategies. This conference represented a milestone in improving health care for individuals with VSTs, especially the introduction of a multidisciplinary team approach.

The consensus meeting concluded that rigid algorithms and guidelines were inappropriate because of the need for individualized treatment, and that additional outcome data were essential to developing future clinical guidelines (Lee et al., 2016). The "Consensus Statement on Management of Intersex Disorders" surfaced from this meeting, which proposed a classification system with three major categories to assist with the VST diagnostic process. Outlined in Box 7-1, these categories are sex chromosome DSD; 46,XX DSD; and 46,XY DSD (Hughes et al., 2006). Importantly, for some VST conditions, the manifestations are limited to the reproductive system, whereas other conditions may have additional features, such as renal agenesis, hearing loss, and developmental delay (Cox et al., 2014). Box 7-1 defines the three major DSD categories, with subcategories underneath.

Critiques of the 2006 Consensus Statement[3] prodded stakeholders to continue to modify the terminology and classification of VSTs to better categorize the underlying genetic etiologies (Aaronson and Aaronson, 2010;

---

[3] Criticisms of the DSD classification system presented in Box 7-1 are that it does not achieve its goals of bringing clarity and precision to VST diagnosis or care, and that terms used (particularly "disorder" or other pathologizing terms) may medicalize nonpathological variations. In addition, VST scholars and organizations have criticized the 2006 consensus statement process for failing to adequately involve persons with lived experience, who, research demonstrates, have different and varied opinions on appropriate terminology and categorization (Lundberg et al., 2018).

BOX 7-1
Consensus Statement on Management
of Intersex Disorders, 2006

Sex Chromosome DSD: A category of VSTs that includes any condition in which there is an atypical number/arrangement of the sex chromosomes.

   (A)   45,X (Turner syndrome and variants)
   (B)   47,XXY (Klinefelter syndrome and variants)
   (C)   45,X/46,XY (mixed gonadal dysgenesis, ovotesticular DSD)
   (D)   46,XX/46,XY (chimeric, ovotesticular DSD)

46,XY DSD: Children born with XY chromosomes (46,XY) usually develop male physical sex characteristics. However, some have underdeveloped gonads or cannot produce or respond to sex hormones to develop the typical male physical characteristics.

   (A)   Disorders of gonadal (testicular) development
   (B)   Disorders in androgen synthesis or action
   (C)   Other

46,XX DSD: Children born with two X chromosomes (46,XX) usually develop female physical sex characteristics. However, some were exposed before birth to excess male sex hormones that led to genitals that appear atypical.

   (A)   Disorders of gonadal (ovarian) development
   (B)   Androgen excess
   (C)   Other

SOURCE: Adapted from Hughes et al. (2006).

Acién and Acién, 2020; Davies et al., 2011; Lee et al., 2016). This committee does not offer commentary on the appropriate categorization of VSTs; however, medical records since 2006 often use the classification system displayed in Box 7-1 when describing patients with VSTs because this classification provides a system for organizing the many different VST conditions (Pasterski et al., 2010). Terminology used prior to 2006 was often inconsistent and mainly descriptive; therefore, older medical records may not use the 2006 terminology.

The following sections examine the VSTs within each of the three major categories displayed in Box 7-1. This presentation does not represent an exhaustive listing of every possible VST, but a description of many common conditions. In the discussion in Chapter 3 of the codes of the International Classification of Diseases and Related Health Problems (ICD), the report presents numerous ICD codes that may be used in medical records to indicate a VST.

Sex Chromosome DSD

Sex chromosome DSD is characterized by sex chromosome aneuploidy (or atypical number/arrangement of the sex chromosomes). Subcategories include Turner syndrome, Klinefelter syndrome, and 47,XYY, as described in the subsections below (Tallaksen et al., 2023). The sex chromosome DSD category also includes individuals with mosaic karyotypes (e.g., 45,X/46,XY; 45,X/46,XY/47,XXX), which are associated with multiple distinct peripheral blood cell lines. This condition is known as mosaicism; people with "mosaic" chromosomes have different chromosome patterns in some cells of the body as a result of random differences in how cells divide while an embryo is growing (McCoy, 2017). Importantly, sex chromosome aneuploidy may not be detected in all cells because of the variable presence of these multiple cell lines.

Turner Syndrome

Turner syndrome is characterized by the absence or structural abnormalities of an X chromosome. The incidence of Turner syndrome is approximately 1 in 2,500 live female births (Gravholt et al., 2023a; Yoon et al., 2023). Common clinical features include short stature, congenital heart disease, horseshoe kidney, webbed neck, and premature ovarian insufficiency. Premature ovarian insufficiency usually presents as complete absence of pubertal development in a pubertal-aged girl and leads to infertility. Girls and women with Turner syndrome have an increased risk for autoimmune disorders, hypertension, type 2 diabetes, lymphedema, chronic ear infections, neurosensory hearing loss, numerous nevi, and osteoporosis (Augoulea et al., 2019; De Sanctis and Khater, 2019; Mitsch et al., 2023; Sandahl et al., 2020). Most girls and women with Turner syndrome have intelligence levels that mirror the spectrum seen in the general population. However, many struggle with educational challenges, developmental delay, and features of autism spectrum disorder (ASD) (Hutaff-Lee et al., 2019). Anxiety, low self-esteem, neurocognitive dysfunction, and poor social skills often occur. External genital development is typical female; median age of diagnosis is 15 years. Girls with Turner syndrome typically present for health care because of short stature, delayed puberty, or infertility (Gravholt et al., 2023a).

Klinefelter Syndrome

Klinefelter syndrome is characterized by the presence of additional X chromosomes in an individual carrying a Y chromosome. The most common karyotype is 47,XXY. Reported prevalence is approximately 1.5 in 1,000 live births (Morris et al., 2008). Median age at diagnosis is 27 years; the presenting complaint is often infertility due to impaired testicular function. Some boys are diagnosed during evaluation for behavioral abnormalities, such as attention-deficit/hyperactivity disorder (ADHD), dyslexia, ASD, or poor school performance. Boys may present with delayed onset of or failure to complete puberty.[4] In addition to hypogonadism and infertility, health concerns include neurocognitive dysfunction, anxiety, depression, flat feet (pes planus), gynecomastia, hypotonia, extragonadal germ cell neoplasia, osteopenia, and autoimmune disorders (Foland-Ross et al., 2023; Jordan et al., 2023). Men with Klinefelter syndrome have increased risk for diabetes, thromboembolic events, and cardiovascular disease (Gravholt et al., 2023b).

47,XYY Karyotypes

The phenotypes of patients with 47,XYY karyotypes are poorly characterized, largely because of underdiagnosis. Reported clinical features include tall stature; scoliosis; learning difficulties, including ADHD; and autism. The reported incidence is approximately 1 in 1,000 men (Davis et al., 2020; El-Dahtory and Elsheikha, 2009). Median age at diagnosis is 15 years. In contrast with Klinefelter syndrome, pubertal development tends to be normal. Subfertility is common. Men with 47,XYY karyotypes have increased risk for diabetes, dyslipidemia, asthma, and obstructive lung disease (Riddler et al., 2023). In a longitudinal Danish study, men with 47,XYY had better fertility, increased mortality, and lower socioeconomic status compared with men with Klinefelter syndrome (47,XXY) (Berglund et al., 2020; Ridder et al., 2023).

Among the Million Veteran Program cohort,[5] approximately 1 in 370 men were found to have sex chromosome aneuploidy, with an additional X or Y chromosome being present in 145 and 125 per 100,000 males,

---

[4] It should be noted that "delayed puberty" as described here is not the same thing as puberty delay induced by medications, as described in Chapter 5. Delayed puberty is a medical condition, where puberty happens later than expected or never starts as part of atypical development. Puberty-delaying medications are used to delay puberty in adolescents who seek this intervention as part of gender-affirming care. These medications may also be used for cisgender children to treat precocious puberty (marked by breast development before age 8 or testes growth before age 9).

[5] The Veteran's Health Administration Million Veteran Program is a voluntary population-based study of genetic determinants of various illnesses and health outcomes for individuals who have served in the U.S. military.

respectively (Davis et al., 2023). This prevalence is comparable to population estimates. Thus, men with sex chromosomal aneuploidy, either 47,XXY or 47,XYY, are often underdiagnosed and unrecognized.

45,X/46,XY, Mixed Gonadal Dysgenesis

Individuals with 45,X/46,XY mixed gonadal dysgenesis have a mosaic karyotype consisting of at least two distinct cell lines: 45,X and 46,XY. Development of the internal and external genital structures can vary (Lindhardt Johansen et al., 2012). The external genitalia may range from appearing like those of girls to those of relatively typical-appearing phenotypic boys. Specific clinical features (phenotype) vary. Individuals with this karyotype may have short stature and, like girls with Turner syndrome (discussed later in this chapter), may benefit from growth hormone treatment (Lindhardt Johansen et al., 2012). Based on an older study evaluating neonatal chromosome analyses, many individuals with this karyotype appear as phenotypic males (Hsu, 1989).

Gonadal development is usually aberrant in individuals with mosaic karyotypes, resulting in "streak" (underdeveloped) gonads and/or abnormal testicular development (Acién and Acién, 2020). Typically, one gonad is a streak gonad and the other a dysgenetic testes. In some instances, a gonad is considered to be an "ovotestis" because of the presence of both ovarian and testicular elements, as indicated by the presence of both oogonia and seminiferous tubules. Individuals with 45,X/46,XY karyotypes often present for medical evaluation because of asymmetric external genitalia. Importantly, the risk for gonadal germ cell neoplasia is high in these individuals, necessitating early gonadectomy (Berklite et al., 2019).

Chimeric 46,XX/46,XY

Chimeric 46,XX/46,XY individuals are extremely rare. Phenotypes range from typical girl to typical male appearance. Gonadal histology is also variable and may show ovotestis in which a gonad has both ovarian follicles and seminiferous tubules.

46,XY DSD

The category of 46,XY DSD encompasses anomalous testicular development, defective testosterone synthesis, abnormal cellular response to testosterone (androgen insensitivity disorders), and abnormal synthesis of or response to anti-Müllerian hormone. These disorders occur in both complete and partial forms. The complete forms are more often referred for medical evaluations because of the severity of their symptoms. The appearance of the external genitalia may be atypical in individuals with aberrant testicular development, defective testosterone synthesis, and androgen insensitivity. The appearance of the external genitalia can range from female to underdeveloped male.

Studies in the 1950s suggested that an infant's sex could be assigned if the external genitalia and upbringing corresponded to that sex (Money, 1952). Based on this hypothesis, males born with underdevelopment of their external genital structures, such as aphallia, were assigned to female sex for rearing and underwent gonadectomy (Wisniewski et al., 2019; Witchel et al., 2022). Parents were instructed never to share information about the "sex reversal" with anyone, especially the affected individual. Thus, medical records for older individuals may indicate sex reassignment (boy to girl), gonadectomy, and reconstructive surgery of the external genital structures. Indeed, because of past practices regarding secrecy, some affected individuals may be unaware of the full extent of surgical interventions performed during their early childhood.

Clinical observations led to questioning and eventual discarding of this hypothesis. A 2004 study involving the follow-up of genetic males with cloacal exstrophy treated with sex reversal and gonadectomy exposed the importance of prenatal androgen exposure to gender identity; 8 of 14 individuals assigned female sex at birth subsequently transitioned to male (Reiner and Gearhart, 2004). Hence, with the exception of individuals with complete androgen insensitivity syndrome, most 46,XY individuals with underdeveloped male external genitalia are currently raised as male and provided with testosterone replacement therapy as needed (Wisniewski, 2012; Witchel et al., 2022).

Aberrant Testicular Development

Testicular testosterone production results from a series of enzymatic steps occurring within the testes. Genetic variants in these enzymes can interfere with in utero testosterone production, resulting in fetal testosterone deficiency and underdevelopment of the external genitalia. The phenotype of the external genitalia in these 46,XY infants ranges from essentially female to small penis and hypospadias (Domenice et al., 2022). Genetic variants in two specific enzymes—17-beta hydroxysteroid dehydrogenase type 3 (*HSD17B3*) and 5-alpha reductase type 2 (*SRD5A2*)—warrant additional discussion because affected infants have atypical genitalia at birth and virilize with the onset of puberty (Bergougnoux et al., 2023). In some areas of the world, infants with *HSD17B3* or *SRD5A2* variants are raised as girls and transition to a male role during puberty (Imperato-McGinley et al., 1991). However, male assignment at birth often occurs with early identification and diagnosis.

Disorders of Androgen Synthesis or Action

Individuals with androgen insensitivity syndrome (AIS) are born with typical testes that secrete testosterone (Tyutyusheva et al., 2021). However, the cells of these individuals do not respond typically to the testosterone they produce. AIS appears on a spectrum, whereby some individuals have complete AIS (their bodies cannot react to testosterone), and others have partial AIS (their bodies have a reduced response to testosterone). In individuals with complete AIS, the external genitalia appear consistent with typical female genitalia, apart from palpable gonads within the labia. These individuals have a vaginal pouch and lack a uterus. People with partial AIS may be born with undescended or partially descended testes and with various genital differences (e.g., a shallow vaginal opening, a phallus that may be perceived as a large clitoris or a small penis). The prevalence of complete AIS has been estimated to be 1 in 20,000–64,000 XY (karyotypically male) births; the prevalence for partial AIS is unknown (Mendoza and Motos, 2013).

Complete AIS is due most commonly to genetic variants located in the androgen receptor gene (Gottlieb et al., 2012). Typically, individuals with complete AIS are raised as girls. In the past, gonadectomies were performed at young ages. Today, with observations that the risk for gonadal tumor is low and that pubertal testicular testosterone secretion is converted to estrogens (enabling spontaneous pubertal breast development), gonadectomy is often postponed or avoided (Barros et al., 2021; Chaudhry et al., 2017). Some women with complete AIS choose to retain and internally relocate the gonads to improve tumor surveillance imaging (Tack et al., 2018). If gonadectomy is performed, estrogen therapy is essential to preserve bone health (Ko et al., 2017). If gonadectomy was performed in childhood, estrogen treatment will also be needed for breast development (Sultan et al., 2014). Women with complete AIS often perform self-vaginal dilatation to elongate their vaginal pouches to enable sexual intercourse. A uterine transplant, although rare, may enable a person to carry a pregnancy. Individualized health care is essential for patients with AIS, especially those with partial AIS, to accord with individual preferences and phenotypic heterogeneity (Chen et al., 2023).

Disorders of Anti-Müllerian Hormone Synthesis or Action

During fetal male development, the testes secrete anti-Müllerian hormone (AMH) in addition to testosterone. This hormone promotes degradation of the fetal Müllerian ducts. The phenotype of a 46,XY individual with genetic variants in either the AMH gene or the AMH receptor (*AMHR2*) gene shows typical male phallus; typical placement of the urethra meatus;

and, usually, inguinal (groin) hernia and undescended testes. Internally, uterine tissue is present. This rare autosomal recessive entity is called persistent Müllerian duct syndrome and has been reported in only a few hundred cases in the literature (Brunello and Rey, 2022; Da Aw et al., 2016). Infertility is common because the vas deferens travels through the uterine tissue. However, fatherhood may be achieved by testicular aspiration followed by intracytoplasmic sperm injection (Fang et al., 2021). Rarely, uterine tissue is identified during abdominal surgery in an otherwise typically developed man. Women carrying variants on both alleles have no obvious clinical features.

46,XX DSD

46,XX DSD in Females

In females, the category 46,XX DSD encompasses anomalous ovarian development, disorders of androgen excess, and vaginal or uterine atresia.

Anomalous ovarian development

The list of genetic variants associated with impaired ovarian development and/or function continues to expand. Individuals with these variants have typical female external genitalia at birth; they typically present for evaluation during the adolescent years with delayed or failed onset of female pubertal development (Yatsenko and Rajkovic, 2019). These women have premature ovarian insufficiency (previously referred to as premature ovarian failure). They require hormone replacement therapy with estrogens and usually progestogens to promote pubertal development, support menstrual cycles, and maintain bone health. Typically, these women possess a uterus and can carry a pregnancy using modern reproductive technology, such as in vitro fertilization.

Disorders of androgen excess

The most frequent cause of 46,XX DSD is congenital adrenal hyperplasia, a group of autosomal recessive genetic disorders that affect the adrenal glands (leading to impaired adrenal cortisol biosynthesis and excessive adrenal androgen [C19 steroid] production). A spectrum of phenotypes occurs, reflecting the consequences of the genetic variant for enzyme function, resulting in much clinical heterogeneity. The most common "classic" form of congenital adrenal hyperplasia is 21-hydroxylase deficiency due to deleterious variants in the 21-hydroxylase (*CYP21A2*) gene. The incidence of the classic (and more severe) form of 21-hydroxylase deficiency (salt-losing and simple virilizing) is approximately 1 in 14,000 to 1 in 18,000 live births worldwide (Claahsen-van der Grinten et al., 2022). The incidence of the milder (or nonclassic) form is approximately 1 in 200 White American individuals (Hannah-Shmouni et al., 2017). While deficiencies related to 21-hydroxylase account for 90–95 percent of congenital adrenal hyperplasias (Momodu et al., 2023), other enzyme deficiencies that may cause this condition include 11β-hydroxylase deficiency due to *CYP11B1* variants, 3β-hydroxysteroid dehydrogenase type 2 deficiency due to *HSD3B2* variants, and P450-oxidoreductase deficiency due to *POR* genetic variants (Miller and Auchus, 2011). Genetic variants in the 17α-hydroxylase/17-20, lyase (*CYP17A1*) in 46,XX (and 46,XY) individuals are associated with typical female external genital appearance at birth. Because of their inability to produce cortisol, androgens, and estrogens, these individuals may present with hypertension and delayed puberty (Auchus, 2022).

The 21-hydroxylase form of congenital adrenal hyperplasia is typically associated with mineralocorticoid deficiency, which if unrecognized is associated with neonatal deaths and morbidities due to acute adrenal insufficiency (Speiser et al., 2018). Affected 46,XX infants have atypical genitalia at birth. The excessive circulating prenatal androgen concentrations cause virilization of the external genital structures of affected 46,XX fetuses. A small number of 46,XX individuals with 21-hydroxylase deficiency and extensive male external genital development have been assigned male sex at birth (Mazur et al., 2023).

As 21-hydroxylase deficiency is an autosomal recessive disorder, affected 46,XY fetuses have typical male external genitalia at birth (Speiser et al., 2018). Individuals (both 46,XX and 46,XY) with extremely deleterious *CYP21A2* genetic variants typically develop acute adrenal insufficiency within the first 2 weeks of life. If these infants are not promptly recognized and treated with appropriate hormone replacement therapy, significant morbidity or mortality may occur. Newborn screening programs exist in all 50 states and many other countries to detect infants with the classic forms of 21-hydroxylase deficiency (Therrell, 2001). Given the possibility of false negative tests in the immediate newborn period, some states have instituted a second screen during the first month of life. However, newborn screening protocols vary widely (Conlon et al., 2023).

Milder (nonclassic) forms of 21-hydroxylase deficiency present in childhood with premature development of pubic hair, phallic (clitoris or penis) enlargement, increased linear growth velocity, and accelerated skeletal maturation. As a result of the nature of the hyperandrogenic symptoms, the mildest form presents predominantly in adolescent and adult women (Claahsen-van der Griten et al., 2022).

Vaginal or uterine atresia

Individuals with uterine/vaginal anomalies may experience pubertal onset with breast development and present for evaluation of primary amenorrhea and/or hydrometrocolpos (Grant et al., 2023; Porsius et al., 2022). This group of anomalies is labeled as the Mayer-Rokitansky-Küster-Hauser (MRKH) syndrome or Müllerian agenesis, which occurs in approximately 1 in 5,000 46,XX women (Herlin et al., 2020). This syndrome is characterized by incomplete development of the female reproductive tract and may involve the uterus, cervix, and upper vagina. MRKH is subclassified as isolated uterine/vaginal anomalies (Type I) or syndromic (Type II) (Herlin et al., 2020). The syndromic form is associated with other anomalies, such as renal, skeletal, and facial anomalies; the "MURCS" association is a severe form of MRKH characterized by Müllerian duct, renal, and cervicothoracic spine abnormalities. Like people with complete androgen insensitivity syndrome, people with MRKH may seek a uterine transplant to give them the opportunity to bear a biological child (Brännström et al., 2015). Uterine and vaginal agenesis are included in this category. At birth, 46,XX infants with aberrant ovarian development and/or uterine/vaginal anomalies have typical female external genitalia appearance.

46,XX DSD in Males

46,XX males have a male phenotype despite a 46,XX karyotype. There are two different forms of 46,XX DSD in males: *SRY* (sex-determining region on Y chromosome)–positive or *SRY*-negative (Wu et al., 2014). Approximately 90 percent of XX males are *SRY*-positive and have a translocation of the *SRY* gene to another chromosome, typically the X chromosome. These patients present with micropenis, atypical external genital development, delayed/failed puberty, and/or infertility. The *SRY*-negative group reflects the consequence of aberrant testicular differentiation. One example of XX sex reversal involves variants in the R-Spondin1 (*RSPO1*) gene, which is associated with palmoplantar keratoderma, congenital bilateral corneal opacities, nail dystrophy, and hearing impairment (Tomaselli et al., 2008). Other genes associated with *SRY*-negative XX males include *SOX9*, *SOX3*, and *FOXL2* (Grinspon and Rey, 2019). One in every 20,000 male births is thought to be 46,XX, and this condition accounts for approximately 2 percent of male infertility cases (Adrião et al., 2020).

Nonhormonal Variations in Sex Traits

In addition to the conditions discussed above and listed in Box 7-1, it is important to recognize disorders associated with atypical genital development that are not caused by hormones or gonadal function. These are primarily anatomic malformation disorders of the genitourinary tract that include caudal regression syndrome, mild epispadias, cloacal exstrophy, omphalocele-exstrophy-imperforate anus-spinal defects complex, and aphallia. These disorders are usually associated with typical gonadal function congruent with the sex chromosomes. Although these conditions are rare, affected individuals require substantial medical, behavioral health, and surgical treatments to address the structural and functional impairments of the genitourinary, gastrointestinal, and neurologic systems. These conditions typically require lifelong care such that affected individuals may need assistance with activities of daily living either transiently or permanently. These individuals often suffer from urinary and bowel incontinence (Maruf et al., 2020). Urinary incontinence may be treated with a catherizable stoma. Many patients require bowel diversion surgery to achieve bowel continence. Renal anomalies may also coexist. In some instances, the renal anomalies are associated with deteriorating renal function (Bolduc et al., 2002). Skeletal anomalies include scoliosis, hip dysplasia, and clubfeet; affected individuals may require osteotomies. Aberrant development of the uterus and vagina is commonly associated with these malformations. For males, the penis and scrotum are bifid typically with testes palpable within the hemiscrotum. Individuals with these disorders experience numerous challenges, including multiple surgeries, bladder/bowel diversions complicated by foul odor and infections, sexual dysfunction, and embarrassment (Van den Eede et al., 2023). In a group of 63 patients, anxiety and/or depression were noted in 52.4 percent (Haney et al., 2024).

INITIAL MANAGEMENT OF VARIATIONS IN SEX TRAITS

Individuals suspected of having VSTs are often referred to expert and experienced health care professionals. A multidisciplinary team offers the optimal management for such individuals and their families. Members of this team may include pediatric endocrinologists, pediatric urologists/surgeons, geneticists, neonatologists, radiologists, behavioral health specialists, social workers, and pediatric nurse educators (Ahmed et al., 2011; Coleman et al., 2022). The multidisciplinary team provides individualized care in the context of enabling the affected individual to enjoy "the best life possible" (Wilkins et al., 1955; Witchel et al., 2022). Some pediatric hospitals have ongoing family support committees to help with the shared decision making and management of children with VSTs. Figure 7-1 depicts the many types of clinical experts and community supports that may be involved in care for people with VSTs.

Prenatal Diagnosis

VSTs may be suspected prenatally based on fetal ultrasound findings. More recently, noninvasive prenatal screening (NIPS) has increasingly been

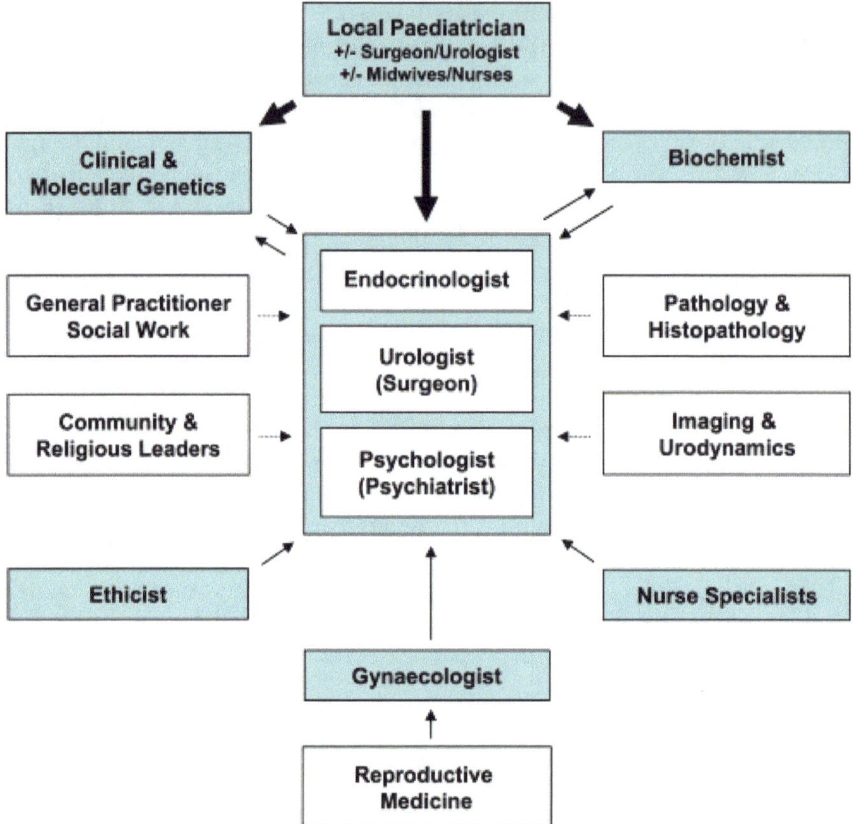

FIGURE 7-1 Overview of the multidisciplinary team that may be involved in the initial and ongoing care of people with variations in sex traits.
NOTE: Specialists in adolescent medicine are often an important part of the multidisciplinary team. These specialists are included within the local pediatrician box in the schematic.
SOURCE: Brain et al., 2010. CC BY 3.0.

used to determine some VSTs (and other conditions) prenatally (Gregg et al., 2016; Saulnier et al., 2021). This test, which involves a single blood sample obtained from the pregnant person, is used to examine the fetal (placental) cell-free DNA in circulation. NIPS results may differ from those inferred from the ultrasound appearance of the fetal genitalia. When genital ambiguity is evident on the fetal ultrasound exam or discordant results from NIPS/genetic testing are obtained, prenatal consultation with a multidisciplinary team needs to be arranged immediately.

Initial Evaluation by the Multidisciplinary Team

As described above, some people with VSTs are diagnosed prenatally, others at birth, and others later in life (during puberty or adulthood). Regardless of chronologic age at presentation, initial evaluation of VSTs by a multidisciplinary team often includes a comprehensive medical history comprising prenatal, family, and psychosocial histories and information about potential environmental exposures (Brain et al., 2010; Coleman et al., 2022; Cools et al., 2024; Moran and Karkazis, 2012). A thorough physical examination with detailed observation of the external genitalia is performed. Box 7-2 offers examples of common inquiries providers may have during the physical exam.

Next, laboratory and imaging studies, and increasingly genetic studies, are performed. The specific studies performed depend on the patient history and physical examination.

Laboratory Studies

Blood samples are collected to measure hormone concentrations, determine functioning of the adrenal and pituitary glands (adrenocorticotropic hormone stimulation), and/or measure the amount of sex hormones being produced in the body naturally (human chorionic gonadotropin [hCG] stimulation) (Mayo Clinic, 2018). Blood and, occasionally, urine samples are used to determine the karyotype and assess for chromosomal abnormalities. Over time, the methodology for measuring blood and urine hormone concentrations

---

BOX 7-2
Common Inquiries During Physical Examination
to Determine Variations in Sex Traits

- Are the labioscrotal folds fused or not?
- Are gonads palpable?
- Are the external genital structures symmetric?
- What is the appearance of the phallus (clitorophallus)?
- Where is the urethral meatus?
- How many orifices are present on the perineum?
- Are other anomalies present?
- In adolescents and young adults, what clinical features of puberty are present or absent?

SOURCE: Adapted from Ahmed et al., 2011; Lee et al., 2006.

has changed as a result of improved technology. In the past, radioimmunoassays were used to measure hormone concentrations. Given the potential for variable results, these methods are used less commonly today (Braunstein, 2022; Ghazal et al., 2022; Tomlinson et al., 2004). More recently, liquid chromatography–tandem mass spectroscopy is increasingly being used; this method is more accurate and can measure multiple analytes simultaneously (Andrieu et al., 2022; Wudy et al., 2018). However, some hospitals may not have access to liquid chromatography–tandem mass spectroscopy methods. It is important to acknowledge that biotin (a compound commonly used in skin/hair products and vitamins) can interfere with some assays (Samarasinghe et al., 2017).

Imaging Studies

Imaging studies can include ultrasound, magnetic resonance imaging, and computed tomography imaging. The goal of imaging studies is to determine the status of the internal genital structures (e.g., presence or absence of uterus) and to assess for additional anomalies such as renal agenesis (absence of one or both kidneys) (Grinspon et al., 2023). Due to the technical limitations of current imaging modalities, laparoscopic surgery may be necessary to visualize the internal genital structures and, when needed, obtain gonadal biopsies to assess gonadal histology and risk for malignancy (Ahmed et al., 2011; Farrugia et al., 2013).

Genetic Studies

Increasingly, genetic studies are performed as the first-line study, especially in individuals with atypical genitalia and 46,XY karyotypes (Ahmed et al., 2022). Yet despite the increased knowledge and understanding of genetic variants in VSTs, the specific genetic diagnosis remains unknown in many patients (Persani et al., 2022). In addition, not all genetic variants are deleterious or disease-causing. Some genetic variants are characterized as "variants of unknown significance," which means that available data are insufficient to ascertain the functional significance of a variant (i.e., whether it has any functional consequences for health). Establishing the functional consequences of such variants is often challenging. For this reason, specific standards and guidelines are followed to ascertain the likelihood that a genetic variant is deleterious (Richards et al., 2015).

Sex Assignment at Birth

One of the most difficult aspects of managing patients with VSTs is the sex assignment at birth, also referred to as sex of rearing (i.e., the child's gender-specific upbringing), which becomes the sex recorded on birth certificates and medical records. This aspect, and its associated decisions, reflects society's dogmatic insistence on classifying people by their sex. Through a shared decision-making process between the multidisciplinary care team and the child's parents or other caregivers, the goal is to select a sex that has the greatest likelihood of matching gender identity in adulthood (Sandberg et al., 2012). However, sex assignment for infants with VSTs is not straightforward, as it is often based on numerous factors, including results of laboratory, imaging, and genetic studies; specific VST diagnosis; phallus length; psychological orientation; the possibility of fertility and sexual functionality; expectation or wishes of the family; and consensus opinion among experienced specialist providers (Campo-Engelstein et al., 2017; Gürbüz et al., 2020; Sandberg et al., 2012). In addition, as discussed previously in this report, an individual's personal gender identity develops over time.

During initial evaluation of a newborn infant with atypical genitalia, health care providers avoid any language suggesting a "sex assignment" (referring to the baby as "your baby," rather than "your daughter"/"your son"), and medical documents do not indicate "sex" at this stage. In addition, health care providers explain VSTs to parents or other caregivers with sensitivity to the family's cultural background (especially related to rituals used to celebrate births), use language at the 5th- to 8th-grade level, and repeat their explanations multiple times (Jackson et al., 2008; Lipstein et al., 2014; Sandberg et al., 2019; Weidler and Peterson, 2019). Early involvement of behavioral/mental health professionals is essential to support the family in dealing with the initial uncertainties regarding sex assignment; the diagnostic procedures; the decision-making process; final diagnosis; and discussions with extended family members, friends, and colleagues. Following these discussions and diagnostic procedures, shared decision-making conversations involving the parents or other caregivers and health care providers take place, ultimately leading to a decision about a sex assignment for the infant. Although some families elect to defer decisions regarding sex of rearing, most families are more comfortable with a binary determination.

Gender Identity

Typically, gender identity follows sex assignment for individuals with VSTs (Bakula et al., 2017; Callens et al., 2016). As defined in Chapter 2, "gender identity" refers to the term used by individuals to label themselves and their internal sense of self. People with VSTs, like anyone else, can have a gender identity that differs from their sex recorded at birth. The proportion of gender identity concerns among people with VSTs is greater than the proportion of TGD people in the general population (Dessens et al., 2005; Furtado et al., 2012; Herman et al., 2022; Hines, 2020; Meyer-Bahlburg et al., 1996; Zucker et al., 1996).

A 2021 systematic review and meta-analysis analyzed the prevalence of transgender or gender diverse (TGD) identity in adolescents and adults with VSTs, finding an overall prevalence of 15 percent (95% CI 13–17 percent), but variability in prevalence of TGD identity among different VST categories (Babu and Shah, 2021). For example, Babu and Shah found that the prevalence of gender dysphoria was 53 percent among populations with 5-alpha reductase deficiency (*SRD5A2*) who were reared as female, but only 1.7 percent among individuals with complete androgen insensitivity syndrome (all individuals identified in the review with complete androgen insensitivity syndrome were raised as female). This finding mirrors other studies that show TGD identity is rare among individuals with complete androgen insensitivity syndrome (T'Sjoen et al., 2011). However, Babu and Shah found TGD identity to be much higher in populations with partial androgen insensitivity syndrome, with gender dysphoria more common among male-raised individuals compared to female-raised individuals (25 vs. 12 percent). Sex assignment at birth is also an important factor in TGD identity for individuals with congenital adrenal hyperplasia; Babu and Shah found 4 percent gender dysphoria among individuals with congenital adrenal hyperplasia who were reared female, but 15 percent gender dysphoria among those reared male. de Jesus et al. (2019) confirm gender dysphoria is more common in male-raised individuals with congenital adrenal hyperplasia, compared to those raised female.

However, the committee notes that methodological flaws in these studies may obscure what researchers know about gender preferences in VST populations, including the use of invalid and binary measures of gender identity and collection of data when it was much rarer to assert a gender diverse or transgender identity (Pasterski et al., 2015).

As in people without VSTs, the development of the secondary sex characteristics typical of puberty may prompt discussion of gender identity in people with VSTs. Certain VSTs may cause pubertal changes that impact gender identity. For example, some 46,XY infants with aberrant testicular development are undervirilized, and they may be assigned female sex at birth (Thigpen et al., 1992). At puberty, these individuals experience phallic and testicular enlargement and may subsequently self-reassign from female to male (Costa et al., 2012; Maimoun et al., 2011). This specific autosomal recessive disorder, associated with *SRD5A2* genetic variants, is more prevalent in specific populations, such as that of the Dominican Republic, where these individuals have been labeled as "guevedoces" (which translates to "penis at 12") (Marks, 2004).

Upon VST diagnoses, reflection on gender identity may be included in conversations with patients and their care team as these patients may be more likely to question their gender because of their atypical external

---

Panelist Perspective

"And we make these kind of generalizations based on specific conditions that people have or specific variations that those people have. We also tend to make some broad brushstrokes based on someone's chromosomes or the presence of certain hormones or you know, specific hormonal levels. But we're often proven wrong. So, actually, in a clinic setting, although somebody like me who has complete androgen insensitivity syndrome we may typically identify as female most of the time. But then we'll have a patient, [or] will have a kiddo who comes in, [who] over time starts to identify as nonbinary or start to identify as male. And that would be contrary to what the medical data or a lot of the past research data would tend to tell us or tend to indicate. So, I would just want to caution everyone not to make assumptions about somebody's gender identity or the way they choose to express themselves, based on their specific traits or based on specific test result[s]."

—Statement from patient–provider panel,
presented to the committee on November 30, 2023.

---

genitalia, discordant karyotype, fertility status, romantic attractions, or medical interventions (e.g., hormone treatment and/or surgery) (Granero-Molina et al., 2023; Kreukels et al., 2018). Gender identity may be broached during discussions about initiating exogenous sex hormone treatment to induce puberty. In addition, some individuals may seek a gender assessment from a mental health provider, often initiated as a referral from an endocrinologist or medical provider.

The gender-related needs of people with VSTs may be complicated even if a self-initiated gender transition is not desired. For instance, girls with Turner syndrome may feel that they are not true females because of their body differences, need for exogenous estrogen, and likely infertility (Granero-Molina et al., 2023). Others may be concerned about having body parts that they perceive as inconsistent with their affirmed gender. These feelings may lead to poor self-esteem, shame, and confusion. Such concerns are important when considering patients' psychosocial or mental health needs (Kreukels et al., 2018).

Ongoing Shared Decision Making and Access to Providers and Services

In addition to initial evaluation and decisions about sex assignment, an important function of multidisciplinary care teams is assisting patients and parents or other caregivers with difficult choices about immediate and future care and treatment (including hormone treatment, surgery, and mental health care, as described in detail below). Health care management recommendations and choices vary even for individuals with similar conditions. Recognizing that health care for VSTs is highly variable and patient specific, coordination of care with patients and their parents or other caregivers is essential among the multidisciplinary providers (Sandberg et al., 2019).

Multidisciplinary care for people with VSTs is clearly beneficial for patients and their parents or other caregivers. Yet access to multidisciplinary care can be challenging because such expertise is limited primarily to large urban areas in the United States. Families may need to travel for many hours to meet with specialists and the multidisciplinary team. Expertise related to specific aspects of VST care may be unavailable in smaller urban and rural areas. In addition, health care providers in rural locations may lack the knowledge and expertise to offer initial VST management because of the rarity of these conditions.

Older persons with VSTs may not have had access to a multidisciplinary care arrangement in their youth and may have lacked the options in care and treatment that exist today. As discussed below, in the past, genital reconstructive surgery was performed during infancy and childhood, reflecting the prevailing hypothesis that genital anatomy needed to be consistent with sex assignment. Due to past recommendations for nondisclosure, some individuals may lack information regarding prior medical or surgical management. For these individuals, ongoing care involves decision making around future medical care and treatment, with particular focus on psychosocial well-being and follow-up care based on earlier surgeries (Berry and Monro, 2022).

HORMONE TREATMENT FOR PEOPLE WITH VARIATIONS IN SEX TRAITS

Hormone treatments may be helpful for some people with VSTs in the context of their gender identity, age, and unique medical circumstances. This section describes appropriate hormone treatment for a number of VST conditions. In addition to the hormone therapies described here, people with VSTs may also access hormone therapy as part of gender-affirming care (described in Chapter 5).

Congenital Adrenal Hyperplasia

Upon confirmation of diagnosis, individuals with congenital adrenal hyperplasia are treated with glucocorticoid replacement therapy. Typically, hydrocortisone, administered three to four times daily, is used—although other regimens may be appropriate for individual patients (Allolio, 2015; Dineen et al., 2019; Ng et al., 2020). Individuals with the "classic" salt-losing form of congenital adrenal hyperplasia are also treated with fludrocortisone, a synthetic mineralocorticoid. All individuals prescribed daily hydrocortisone treatment must be treated with extra exogenous glucocorticoid for stressful situations such as fever, acute gastroenteritis, and severe physical trauma, as well as during surgery. Initially, parents or other caregivers are responsible for providing this treatment, with eventual training for adolescents and adults. Stress doses can be administered orally if tolerated. If oral medication is not tolerated, parenteral hydrocortisone needs to be administered promptly. Parents or other caregivers and older affected individuals need to have parenteral hydrocortisone readily available and know how and when to administer this medication for acute situations. Individuals requiring hydrocortisone stress dosing need to wear medical alert ID badges (Ahmet et al., 2023; Puar et al., 2016).

Hormone Therapy for Small Penis

During infancy, some boys with a small penis are treated with small doses of testosterone for 3–6 months to promote elongation of the penis (Stancampiano et al., 2022). In some instances, hCG, which is very similar to luteinizing hormone, is administered for an hCG stimulation test to assess testicular testosterone production. Specific practices regarding the number of injections and dosing vary among physicians.

Growth Hormone Therapy

During childhood, sex steroid hormone replacement therapy is unnecessary because sex steroid levels are normally low. For individuals with short stature associated with Turner syndrome, 45,X/46,XY mosaicism, or severe intrauterine growth retardation, growth hormone therapy is beneficial to increase linear growth velocity and final adult height (Bertelloni et al., 2015; Hwang, 2014; Ranke, 1995; Ross et al., 1986; Urban et al., 1979).

Delayed/Absent Puberty

For individuals unable to experience endogenous pubertal development because of hormone deficiencies, sex steroid treatment is used to initiate secondary sex characteristics and promote bone health (De Luca et al., 2001; Klein et al., 2017; Saggese et al., 1997; Villanueva and Argente, 2014). Causes of delayed or absent puberty include hypogonadotropic hypogonadism, hypothalamic and pituitary tumors, premature ovarian insufficiency, and testicular failure (Howard and Dunkel, 2018; Klein et al., 2017; Sullivan et al., 2016). Some chronic disorders, such as celiac disease, cystic fibrosis, and sickle cell anemia, are commonly associated with delayed puberty (Johannesson et al., 1997; Rhodes et al., 2009; Saari et al., 2015).

Where appropriate, feminizing hormone treatment (small doses of estrogen) is initiated around age 10–14; the estrogen dose is increased gradually (Palmert and Dunkel, 2012). Estrogen is preferably administered using a transdermal estradiol patch; oral and parenteral estrogen are available as alternatives. Approximately 1–2 years following initiation of estrogen treatment, cyclic progestin therapy is initiated when a uterus is present to experience cyclic withdrawal bleeding. Combined estrogen/progestin therapy is important to decrease the risk for endometrial cancer later in life. In addition, experiencing regular menses is important to some patients. Estrogen also promotes uterine growth, which is essential for future pregnancies (when possible).

Where appropriate, masculinizing hormone treatment (small doses of testosterone) is initiated around age 12–15; the testosterone dose is increased gradually (Palmert and Dunkel, 2012). Testosterone is typically administered by intramuscular or subcutaneous injection. Dose titration to initiate puberty is nearly impossible for testosterone gels; in addition, other family members may be accidentally exposed to the testosterone gel. Once an adult testosterone replacement dose has been achieved, testosterone can be administered by intramuscular or subcutaneous injection or transdermal gel. In the future, oral testosterone undecanoate may prove to be beneficial in people with ongoing testosterone deficiency.

Reproduction/Fertility

Gonadotropin deficiencies in patients with congenital or acquired hypogonadotropic hypogonadism result in delayed pubertal development and inadequate stimulation of the gonads to secrete sex steroids and mature gametes (Alexander et al., 2024). Similarly, individuals with disorders affecting steroidogenesis may have hormone imbalances that affect pubertal development and ovulation/spermatogenesis (Sengupta et al., 2021). Depending on the specific diagnosis and endogenous hormone secretion, sex steroid hormone replacement therapy may be needed to promote the development of secondary sex features and maintain bone health.

Gonadal differentiation and pubertal development are abnormal in most individuals with chromosomal anomalies such as 45,X monosomy;

45,X/46,XY; 47,XXY; and other variants. Secondary sex development is delayed/absent because of the deficient secretion of gonadal sex steroid. The aberrant gonadal environment impairs maturation of oogonia and spermatogonia, resulting in subfertility/infertility. Individuals with nonpalpable gonads and Y chromosomal material have an increased risk for gonadal neoplasia. Such individuals typically undergo gonadectomy (Lucas-Herald et al., 2021).

Some individuals, such as those with congenital adrenal hyperplasia, are generally fertile; both women and men may require intensive glucocorticoid hormone replacement therapy to enable normal hypothalamic-pituitary-gonadal axis function and gametogenesis. For some, such as those with Turner syndrome and Klinefelter syndrome, infertility is typical. Depending on the specific disorder, fertility preservation may be possible (Rodriguez-Wallberg et al., 2023).

SURGICAL INTERVENTIONS

Currently, decisions regarding surgical interventions for people with VSTs are complex and involve shared decision making among the patient, parents or other caregivers, and the interdisciplinary health care team. Over the past few decades, philosophies regarding surgical interventions have been discussed and modified. It has been increasingly recognized that even minor operations may have undesirable outcomes. Most importantly, the inability to obtain informed consent from a minor child for a surgical intervention has been acknowledged. Indications for surgery generally focus on functional outcomes rather than aesthetic (Lee et al., 2006). In some instances, for example, early surgical intervention is performed because of an increased risk for urinary tract infections (Ding et al., 2023). Typically, surgery is appropriate for 46,XY individuals with hypospadias to enable standing to urinate and eventually having children (Halaseh et al., 2022). In addition, as described in further detail below, surgery is important for VSTs that cause genitourinary malformation.

While it has been believed that surgery performed for cosmetic reasons in infancy relieves parental stress and improves attachment between the child and parents, this approach lacks consistent evidence (Crawford et al., 2009; Dayner et al., 2004; Lee et al., 2006). Accordingly, many centers have moved away from surgery in early childhood when function is not impaired, and medical organizations oppose medically unnecessary genital surgeries (AAFP, 2024; Children's Hospital of Chicago, 2021). Historically, however, practices were very different, and older medical records may refer to surgeries performed that were based on best practices at the time, which, with modern understanding, may no longer be considered appropriate.[6]

In 2016, the Global DSD Update Consortium released a consensus statement on the approach to and care of individuals with VSTs (Lee et al., 2016). These guidelines reconfirm an obligation for individualized care given that evidence-based data regarding indications, timing, and need for surgery remain uncertain. The authors describe four VST procedures: (1) surgery of the genital tubercle (clitoroplasty or reconstruction), (2) surgery of the Müllerian structures, (3) surgery of the gonads (orchiopexy, removal, biopsy, or preservation), and (4) perineoplasty. When considering each procedure, patient goals, possible complications, and long-term outcomes need to be considered. Despite support for these guidelines by the experts, the levels of evidence for the recommendations were low, and the experts did not reach consensus regarding indication, timing, procedure, and evaluation of outcomes. However, consensus was achieved regarding the following points: (1) health care should be provided by centers of expertise with multidisciplinary care; (2) providers should take a conservative approach to gonadal surgery in patients with complete androgen insensitivity; (3) providers should avoid vaginal dilatation in childhood; (4) asymptomatic Müllerian remnants can remain intact during childhood and removed later if needed; (5) it is appropriate to remove biopsy-confirmed streak gonads among individuals with Y chromosomal material; and (6) in discussions of sex assignment, patients with 46,XY cloacal exstrophy should be raised as males despite anomalous anatomy.

Genitourinary Malformation Syndromes

As noted above, genitourinary malformation syndromes are often included with the differential diagnosis of atypical external genitalia. This category encompasses cloacal exstrophy, bladder exstrophy, and persistent cloaca (also known as urorectal septum malformation sequence). Cloacal

---

[6] In the 1950s, the American pediatric endocrinology community promoted the belief that a child's lived experiences as a boy or a girl, established the child's gender role and erotic orientation and that, at least in the United States, the birth of a child with atypical external genitalia was a social emergency. Parents were advised to share their child's situation only with family members. These beliefs led to the practice of assigning female sex of rearing to 46,XY infants with an undersized phallus, aphallia, or female-appearing external genital structures. In other words, nurture took precedence over nature in establishing gender identity. The sole exception was girls with congenital adrenal hyperplasia, who are known to have normal female internal genitalia; these virilized girls underwent surgical procedures to make the external genitalia appear more female. Over time, based on lived experiences, challenges arose regarding these hypotheses and the need for early surgical management. Nevertheless, older medical records may need to be reviewed to ascertain any details regarding prior surgeries. Given the past practices of concealment with respect to atypical external genital development and previous genital surgery, individual patients may not be fully aware of past surgical procedures performed during their early childhood.

exstrophy—where a portion of the large intestine lies outside the body—may be part of a more extensive malformation syndrome that includes omphalocele, spinal defects, and imperforate anus (Neel and Tarabay, 2018). It is also commonly associated with other defects of the genitourinary system, such as hydronephrosis/hydroureter, renal agenesis, cystic dysplasia of the kidneys, horseshoe kidney, and duplicated urinary collecting system (Keppler-Noreuil et al., 2017). Bladder exstrophy refers to a defect such that the bladder forms outside the body. Bladder exstrophy typically involves the digestive and reproductive systems as well as the urinary tract; it is often considered to be a milder form of cloacal exstrophy. Both appear to represent different manifestations of a primary developmental field defect in the fetus (Martínez-Frías et al., 2001). Although these are serious conditions and may require a series of operations, the long-term outcome is good for many children with appropriate surgical repair and follow-up care.

Sexual Function

For individuals with atypical external genitalia, sexual intimacy may be challenging as a result of the specific details of an individual's genital anatomy. In addition, individuals may differ in their definitions and practices for sexual intimacy.

Women with complete androgen insensitivity syndrome, some women with congenital adrenal hyperplasia, women with vaginal atresia, and women with MRKH syndrome may have vaginas inadequate for penile-vaginal intercourse. Vaginal dilatation may be helpful for individuals who desire penile–vaginal intercourse as it may help maintain the dimensions of the vaginal canal (ACOG, 2018; Callens et al., 2014). For some, surgery to construct or lengthen the vaginal canal may be the appropriate intervention. Women with altered anatomy may experience uncomfortable and awkward sexual experiences, and self-esteem and quality of life may be poor (Beisert et al., 2022; Weijenborg et al., 2019). Pelvic floor physical therapy may be beneficial to help alleviate pain and/or assist with psychosocial considerations.

Men with hypospadias, "micropenis," and other genital malformations may experience difficulty with erection, ejaculation, and orgasm (van der Zwan et al., 2013). Reconstructive surgery may be required to facilitate urinary and/or sexual function.

Sexual discomfort and dysfunction are commonly reported in people with VSTs (Kerckhof et al., 2019; Kohler et al., 2012). While some suggest that complications of surgery are the main factor contributing to dysfunction, this remains uncertain (Crouch et al., 2008; Van de Grift et al., 2022). In a large study of masculinizing surgery, sexual problems and satisfaction with sex life were similarly prevalent in individuals who did and did not undergo surgery (Van de Grift et al., 2022).

Surgical Complications

Complications following surgery for VSTs can be divided into the categories of early and late. Early complications are often related to wound healing and infection, whereas stenosis, stricture, or fistula, as well as recurrent urinary infections, can be seen long term. The need for a second and/or revision surgery is not uncommon. A lack of consistent terminology and the wide range of procedures performed for VSTs make the risk of early complications difficult to quantify.

Also challenging to measure are the long-term outcomes following surgical intervention for VSTs. Outcomes can be classified as both functional and aesthetic (Creighton et al., 2001; Crouch et al., 2008). Functional outcomes, such as voiding and/or sexual dysfunction, are likely related to underlying anatomy, as well as the complexity of the procedures. Aesthetic outcomes can be measured with patient self-reported satisfaction questionnaires. These evaluations are limited by poor response rates, however, and may be biased toward favorable or unfavorable responses (Van de Grift, 2022). Interestingly, in the case of hypospadias repair (surgery to address a problem in the opening of the penis that is present at birth), one study found that adolescents who did not recall the surgery (i.e., had the surgery before 18 months of age) were more satisfied with their overall body appearance compared with those who remembered the surgery (van der Horst and Wall, 2017). Data are inconsistent as to whether hypospadias repair later in life is associated with more complications (van der Horst and Wall, 2017). The multidisciplinary care team needs to engage patients and their families in discussions about possible outcomes, long-term complications of surgery, and quality of life.

MENTAL HEALTH INTERVENTIONS

People with VSTs may experience wide-ranging impacts on their mental and behavioral health and on their social lives. This section discusses important mental health–related considerations for patients with VSTs, relevant risk factors for these patients, mental health considerations for their parents and caregivers, and the role of mental health providers in care for people with VSTs.

Mental Health–Related Considerations for Patients

People with VSTs may have limited access to thoughtful, trained, and knowledgeable health care providers who can support their physical and mental health care needs. This can result in undesirable clinical and psychosocial outcomes. Some patients with VSTs describe stressful or even traumatic medical practices, including (1) overly frequent and uncomfortable medical/genital exams; (2) lack of privacy due to the presence of multiple providers and trainees in the room; (3) patient marginalization in medical and surgical decision making (often associated with early surgeries, but occurring for adolescents as well); (4) lack of psychosocial support; and (5) stigmatizing communications with health care providers and staff (Haghighat et al., 2023; Thyen et al., 2014). One study found that while satisfaction with health care services was lower for all people with VSTs compared with other patients with serious chronic care needs, satisfaction was lowest among those with the rarest VST conditions because of the scarcity of knowledgeable specialists (Thyen et al., 2014).

Panelist Perspective

"[Patients] encounter providers using insensitive terminology, and also with providers asking invasive questions with a lack of compassion. We are certainly finding out that for many intersex people it is uncomfortable seeking care. Many of the times as intersex adults we don't know where to seek care in terms of specialty care."

—Statement from patient–provider panel,
presented to the committee on November 30, 2023.

Navigating social relationships can also be stressful. From the time of diagnosis, many affected individuals and their parents or other caregivers are aware of their physical and medical differences compared with other children. For example, children with VSTs may need to justify to their peers and teachers their repeated absences from school to attend medical appointments. Children with congenital adrenal hyperplasia must wear medical alert ID badges indicating their special needs and must carry emergency medical supplies with them. These factors can lead to absence from important school-related functions, stigmatization, and exclusion (Claahsen-van der Grinten et al., 2022; Traino et al., 2022). Individuals requiring hormone replacement therapy for pubertal development also experience being different from their peers (Dwyer at al., 2019). In addition, some people with VSTs (e.g., patients with genitourinary malformation) need repeated surgeries to address health concerns. The recovery periods associated with such surgeries disrupt both academic and nonacademic activities, and individuals may experience pain and medically related discomforts (e.g., following bladder or bowel diversion procedures). Other VST conditions—particularly cloacal exstrophy and/or adrenal insufficiency (congenital adrenal hyperplasia)—cause frequent medical crises creating stress in patients and parents (Fleming et al., 2017).

For almost all individuals with VSTs (and their families, as described below), consideration of how and whether to share information about a VST diagnosis with others can provoke anxiety and fear of stigmatization. Children may find it difficult to explain their condition to classmates or teachers, which may hinder social development (Cools et al., 2018). Feelings of shame and fear of negative reactions can lead to social withdrawal, isolation, and poor quality of life (Mackenzie et al., 2009; Schweizer et al., 2009; van Lisdonk, 2014).

Panelist Perspective

"Mental health problems are enormous among adults with intersex variations. And I think a lot of us have come to think of this as partly an artifact of societal stigma and minority stress, but it can for a lot of people also be an artifact of the way they were treated as children navigating medical trauma, navigating complications from the treatments and surgeries that they had as children."

—Statement from patient–provider panel,
presented to the committee on November 30, 2023.

The pubertal transition from childhood to adulthood leads to particular challenges for adolescents with VSTs, especially for those who are not diagnosed with a VST until puberty fails to progress as expected (Howard and Quinton, 2024). These young people may be confronted with having to reassess their personal identity, sex, gender, medical needs, future goals, and potential for fertility.

In addition to ongoing concerns regarding sexual and urological function, older adolescents and adults often confront fear and apprehension regarding intimacy (Frank, 2018). For example, people with uterine/vaginal agenesis typically must self-dilate to elongate their vaginal "dimple" to engage in sexual intercourse. People with atypical genital development due to congenital adrenal hyperplasia and those with complete androgen insensitivity syndrome may also need to perform self-dilatation. Many feel embarrassed and challenged by this daily task and feel stressed in determining how to reveal their situation to romantic partners before being physically intimate (Batista et al., 2023; Sutton et al., 2005). In many instances, VST diagnoses are accompanied by infertility (as described above), which can be devastating for the individual and extended family (Diamond and Watson, 2004; Jones, 2020; Sutton et al., 2005). Some people with VSTs experience considerable barriers to accessing knowledgeable medical and mental health care. For some, past negative encounters with the health care system result in avoidance of needed medical care and support (Haghighat et al., 2023; Thyen et al., 2014).

For some people with VSTs, the details of their diagnosis were not shared with them until many years after diagnosis; some did not learn of the diagnosis until adulthood. These practices can contribute to feelings of betrayal, accompanied by reassessment of identity, future prospects, hopes, and dreams (Berry and Monro, 2022; Moreno-Begines et al., 2022). The practice of delayed diagnosis and "keeping secrets" has largely been abandoned by the pediatric endocrine community.

Panelist Perspective

"I think that if you're going through multiple surgeries at different medical facilities, it is traumatizing. Also, it promotes the challenges of obtaining medical records as adults because you don't know where to begin, and oftentimes we are not told about having these surgeries [as children] until we are adults, or even much older, when we see a specialist. And we're not told that this surgical procedure has happened on me."

—Statement from patient–provider panel,
presented to the committee on November 30, 2023.

Mental Health–Related Risks

As noted above, some people with VSTs experience mental and behavioral health challenges. In one survey of U.S. adults with VSTs ($N = 198$), more than half of respondents (53.6 percent) described their mental health as fair/poor, 61.1 percent reported depression, 62.6 percent an anxiety disorder, and 40.9 percent posttraumatic stress disorder (PTSD) (Rosenwohl-Mack et al., 2020). Almost a third (31.8 percent) of respondents reported a previous suicide attempt. These results are consistent with those of other studies that have documented high rates of depression, anxiety, and suicide attempts in people with VSTs (Bohet et al., 2019; D'Alberton et al., 2015; de Vries et al., 2019; Engberg et al., 2017; Falhammar et al., 2018; Rosenwohl-Mack et al., 2020; van Rijn et al., 2014). Other commonly reported clinical diagnoses and symptoms among people with VSTs are isolation, stress, low self-esteem, low sexual quality of life (e.g., low sexual

satisfaction, difficulties searching for partners), and feeling they lack identification with a community group (D'Alberton et al., 2015; Schönbucher
et al., 2012; Schweizer et al., 2009). However, these findings are only for
those individuals willing to participate in such research. Importantly, some
people with VSTs choose not to participate in research and published studies may reflect an ascertainment bias. Additional limitations include small
sample sizes and heterogeneous disorders. Further research involving more
comprehensive patient populations would help clarify the risk factors and
identify prevention strategies.

Neuropsychological disabilities and behavioral dysregulation may be
associated with specific VST diagnoses and may be noted even before
diagnosis of the VST. Individuals with Turner syndrome have an increased
prevalence of difficulties with visual-spatial reasoning, visual-spatial memory, executive functioning, and motor and math skills, as well as ADHD;
some also have ASD features (Hutaff-Lee et al., 2019). Figure 7-2 depicts
the many neuropsychological risks that may impact people with Turner
syndrome.

Individuals with Klinefelter syndrome have high rates of bipolar disorder, ASD, ADHD, and psychotic disorders compared with the general
population (Bojesen et al., 2006; Bruining et al., 2009; Cederlof et al., 2014;
van Rijn et al., 2014). Upon diagnosis of Turner or Klinefelter syndrome,
children can be evaluated, monitored, and engaged in early intervention
programs to bolster their skills and attempt to prevent risks related to
learning or other neuropsychological disabilities (Chadwick et al., 2014;

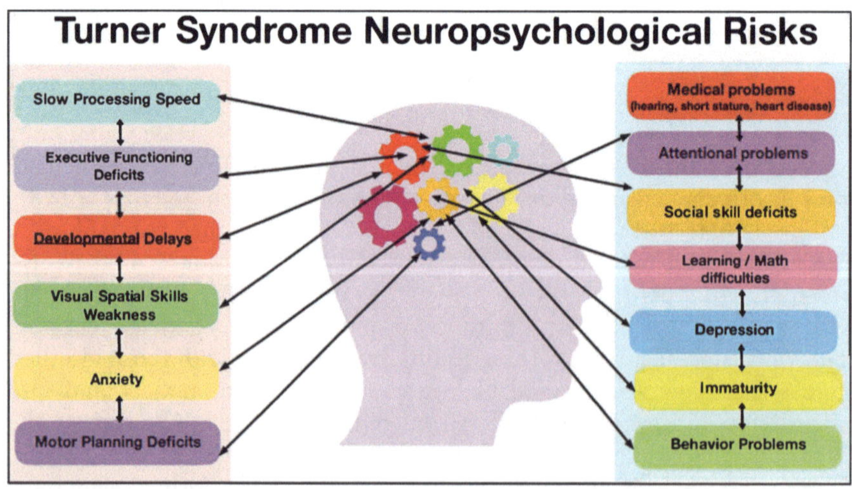

FIGURE 7-2 Neuropsychological risks associated with Turner syndrome.
SOURCE: Hutaff-Lee et al., 2019.

Hutaff-Lee et al., 2019). However, in the past and even at present, few children have been or are regularly monitored or referred for appropriate neuropsychological treatment.

Mental Health–Related Considerations for Family and Caregivers

Specific health care details for people with VSTs depend on multiple factors, such as age at diagnosis; specific VST diagnosis; cultural considerations; and the understanding, beliefs, and attitudes of parents or other caregivers about gender and sex. Upon diagnosis of a VST, parents or other caregivers may feel weighed down by the seemingly overwhelming demands for medical and surgical decision making on behalf of a child. In addition to their beliefs, the availability of counseling and provider biases may influence these complex decisions. Parents or other caregivers may be counseled about their newborn's VST when simultaneously being exhausted by trying to bond with their baby and meet the baby's care needs; indeed, they may meet the definition of having PTSD (Duguid et al., 2007; Pasterski et al., 2014).

Panelist Perspective

"The parents of children with variations of sex traits experience really significant and at times disabling mental health distress. There's some evidence that you compare populations of parents of children with VST relative to parents of children with cancer. Those populations look very similar from a psychological profile and levels of psychological distress."
—Statement from patient–provider panel, presented to the committee on November 30, 2023.

Some diagnoses are associated with a range of medical and/or neurodevelopmental disabilities that require monitoring and family support. Parents or other caregivers may be frustrated by the specialized nature of VSTs, the limited number of knowledgeable providers, and worries about their child's future. In some instances, families must travel to distant health care centers for accurate diagnosis and longitudinal follow-up. Sorting out how medical or surgical decisions may impact choices regarding the child's name, sex assignment, urinary function, potential fertility, and later sexual function is arduous. Parents or other caregivers may have different opinions and feelings about priorities related to medical and surgical decision making, which can generate family conflict and distrust.

Parents or other caregivers benefit from ongoing education and psychosocial support. However, resources for such support are often inadequate or unavailable for many families, especially in rural settings (Crissman et al., 2011; Fleming et al., 2017). Barriers include limited number of skilled health care providers and lack of financial resources to cover the costs of support (Ernst et al., 2018; Lampalzer et al., 2021). In addition, some health care providers and parents or other caregivers fail to appreciate the benefits of education and psychosocial support.

Roles of Mental Health Providers in Care for People with Variations in Sex Traits

The psychological care needs of people with VSTs and their parents or other caregivers may be wide ranging; specific needs vary among individuals. Ideally, mental health clinicians work as part of the multidisciplinary care team and can ascertain family strengths and vulnerabilities to provide guidance on a child's developmental needs (Coyne et al., 2023). Mental health providers can help parents or other caregivers understand their beliefs, priorities, and concerns for their children, as well as potential short- and long-term outcomes, in collaboration with medical and surgical clinicians, and can help families resolve conflicts or differences related to health care decisions. In addition, mental health providers can help families decide whether and how to share information about the child's diagnosis and how to impart developmentally appropriate information to the child. Concerns about what information to share and with whom may vary among family members, and mental health providers can provide support and guidance to help in assessing and resolving differences. Other important areas of discussion may include screening for mental health and emotional needs of parents or other caregivers so they can best support their child. Finally, mental health providers can support families in problem solving and managing other co-occurring life stressors, such as financial, marital, and work–life balance issues.

Older children, adolescents, and adults benefit from similar support from mental health clinicians in monitoring their psychosocial needs and well-being, family and peer supports, and academic progress. Depending on the individual and specific situations, mental health providers can help with VST-related questions that may emerge about gender and identity, fertility and family building, long- and short-term implications of their VST, and past medical and/or surgical interventions. They can help patients process their feelings about their VSTs, normalize differences, and support patients in verbalizing and coping with VST-related stressors and potential stigmatization. They can ensure that VST patients are screened for mental health risks and suicidality, provide interventions as needed, or recommend other clinicians for long-term therapeutic care. The goal of mental/behavioral health care is to build patient resilience through the development of coping strategies, to empower patients to participate in age-appropriate activities of daily living, to enable patients to educate other providers about their needs, and to teach patients how to self-advocate. Mental health clinicians can provide support for coping with urological and/or sexual dysfunction and the development of peer and intimate relations in the context of having a VST. For people with VSTs who are struggling with age-appropriate activities of daily living, psychological and/or neuropsychological assessment and intervention may be beneficial.

LONG-TERM HEALTH CONCERNS

Patients with VSTs need support in addressing their health concerns long term. Support is especially needed—and sometimes challenging to acquire—when transitioning from pediatric to adult care and when managing co-occurring conditions.

Transition of Care

Ideally, transition of care from pediatric and adolescent health care providers to adult providers needs to be an actively planned process organized by the multidisciplinary care team, addressing medical, psychosocial, educational, and vocational needs of emerging adults (Lee et al., 2006). During childhood and adolescence, parents or other caregivers typically play an active role in the medical management of their children. During the transition period, the individual's health care paradigm shifts from active supervision to self-directed management, often concomitant with varying education and work settings. Holistic patient-centered comprehensive care throughout the lifespan and especially during the transition from pediatric to adult care maximizes quality of life and promotes the individual's independence (Balagamage et al., 2023). During the transition process, relevant topics include fertility; sexuality; pathophysiology; knowledge of daily and emergency medications; medical alert ID; and potential chronic consequences, such as obesity, osteopenia, dysglycemia, cardiovascular disease, and testicular adrenal rest tissue in boys and men (Balagamage et al., 2023; Claahsen-van der Griten et al., 2022; Pofi et al., 2023).

Despite the importance of maintaining care regimens—particularly for people who require hormone therapy for management of VSTs—the escalating propensity for risk-taking behaviors in adolescence may lead to poor adherence to medications, office visits, and other aspects of care. Consequences of poor adherence include virilization among girls identified with classic forms of congenital adrenal hyperplasia, short stature, Cushingoid features,[7] and decreased bone mineral density. Individuals who fail to appropriately adhere to glucocorticoid treatment may experience dehydration, hyponatremia, hyperkalemia, hypotension, hypovolemic cardiovascular compromise, or death (Chrisp et al., 2020; Falhammar et al., 2014).

Patients are often lost to follow-up during the transition process (Zahra et al., 2023). For example, previous studies have shown that many young women with Turner syndrome are "lost in transition," suggesting that successful passage from pediatric to adult care requires a special focus in patients with Turner syndrome (Culen et al., 2017; Davies, 2010).

Additional research is needed to examine pediatric-to-adult health care transitions for people with VSTs to optimize physical and psychosocial outcomes. In addition, appropriate care—particularly mental health services needed by young adults—may not be accessible outside of larger urban areas in the United States and is typically available only in large academic pediatric centers through multidisciplinary teams (Sandberg et al., 2017). This means that for people with VSTs, access to these services becomes scarcer just as they reach maturity.

Panelist Perspective

"[It's] pretty like darn near impossible, actually, for adults in most parts of the country to be able to access adult providers who know anything about variations in sex characteristics. You create the situation in which people are experiencing health disparities and are not able to access the care they're getting and what we see in the community is those health problems become increasingly disabling over time for people."

*—Statement from patient–provider panel,
presented to the committee on November 30, 2023.*

Management of Co-Occurring Conditions

Cardiovascular Disease

Individuals with 45,X monosomy or other mosaic karyotypes—typically girls diagnosed with Turner syndrome—may have congenital heart disease.

---

[7] Cushing syndrome occurs when the body has too much of the hormone cortisol for a long time. This condition can result in people with VSTs who take glucocorticoids, which affect the body the same way as cortisol. Symptoms include a fatty hump between the shoulders, a rounded face, and pink or purple stretch marks on the skin.

Common disorders in these individuals include coarctation of the aorta, bicuspid aortic valve, and partial anomalous pulmonary venous return (Meccanici et al., 2023). Older individuals with Turner syndrome have a high propensity to develop dilatated aortic valves and aortic dissection, the latter being a catastrophic event with a high mortality rate (Thunström et al., 2023). Although congenital heart disease and cardiac surgery are more common in individuals with 45,X monosomy compared with those with other karyotypes, the risk of developing aortic dilatation is similar, necessitating regular cardiovascular surveillance (Birjiniuk et al., 2023). Cardiovascular surveillance necessitates cardiac echograms in infants and young children; adolescents and adults need cardiac magnetic resonance angiography studies.

Individuals with congenital adrenal hyperplasia have an increased risk for cardiometabolic disease. This risk is attributed to excessive glucocorticoid dosing, obesity, insulin resistance, hypertension, and dyslipidemia (Torky et al., 2021).

Hypertension is frequently identified in girls, adolescents, and adults with Turner syndrome. The etiology of hypertension in Turner syndrome is likely multifactorial; contributing factors include congenital heart disease, renal anomalies, impaired vagal tone, and high body mass index (McCarrison et al., 2023). Individuals with 21-hydroxylase deficiency congenital adrenal hyperplasia have a higher risk of developing hypertension compared with the general population. Contributing factors include excessive fludrocortisone dosage and obesity (Espinosa Reyes et al., 2023; Falhammar et al., 2011).

Bone Health

Osteopenia and osteoporosis can occur among people with VSTs. For congenital adrenal hyperplasia and other disorders requiring chronic glucocorticoid replacement therapy, monitoring of bone mass density by dual-energy X-ray absorptiometry is warranted, and treatment with calcium, vitamin D, and bisphosphonate drugs may be indicated. Individuals with congenital adrenal hyperplasia diagnosed prior to the introduction of routine newborn screening have an increased prevalence of both any fractures and fractures associated with osteoporosis (Falhammar et al., 2022).

Individuals with sex steroid hormone deficiencies, such as those associated with Turner syndrome and other VSTs, have an increased risk of osteopenia and osteoporosis. Fracture and osteoporosis pose major health challenges for women with Turner syndrome. Although estrogen hormone replacement therapy improves bone mineral density, this appropriate hormone treatment does not fully mitigate against bone loss (Ikegawa and Hasegawa, 2022).

Neoplasia

Aberrant testicular development, also known as testicular dysgenesis, and aberrant gonadal development in the presence of a Y chromosome is associated with an increased risk for gonadal germ cell tumors. For this reason, gonadectomy is performed. Gonadoblastoma have been described in infants at 3 and 5 months of age (Berklite et al., 2019). Individuals with nonpalpable gonads and Y chromosomal material have an increased risk for gonadal neoplasia. Such individuals typically undergo gonadectomy and consequently are infertile (Lucas-Herald et al., 2021; Mittal et al., 2023).

Neuropsychological and Learning-Related Needs

Girls with Turner syndrome typically have normal intelligence, apart from specific areas such as geometry and spatial relations. Some have developmental delay and autism (Björlin Avdic et al., 2021; Kremen et al., 2023). Phenotype–genotype correlation regarding intellectual abilities is poor. Boys with 47,XXY or 47,XYY karyotypes tend to have learning difficulties, psychosocial issues, and increased risk for autism (Jordan et al., 2023; Tartaglia et al., 2017). Children with congenital adrenal hyperplasia who have experienced multiple episodes of acute adrenal insufficiency with electrolyte abnormalities may have learning difficulties (Berenbaum, 2001).

Autoimmune Disorders

Women with Turner syndrome are at increased risk for autoimmune disorders, especially Hashimoto's hypothyroidism (Bakalov et al., 2012; Naessén et al., 2024). Men with Klinefelter syndrome (47,XXY) also have an increased risk of autoimmune disorders (Kanakis and Nieschlag, 2018; Seminog et al., 2015).

Metabolic Syndromes

The reported prevalence of obesity among individuals with congenital adrenal hyperplasia varies among populations. Abnormal glucose tolerance, dyslipidemia, increased thromboembolic risk, and increased carotid intima thickness have been described in these patients (Righi et al., 2023).

Other Conditions Included in This Report

Chapters 8 through 12 of this report describe a number of specific conditions investigated by this committee, including respiratory disease (asthma, chronic obstructive pulmonary disease, cystic fibrosis, and others), childhood growth failure, chronic kidney disease, cancers of the reproductive system, and certain gynecological manifestations of HIV. Overall, few studies have examined these conditions among people with VSTs. However, these chapters present a few findings. Chapter 8 describes some findings about the prevalence of respiratory disease among VST populations—for example, a study found that androgen insensitivity syndrome is strongly associated with increased asthma risk (Gaston et al., 2021). Studies have also found that men with Klinefelter syndrome are more likely to be diagnosed with pulmonary diseases than age-matched male controls (Bojesen et al., 2006), and cystic fibrosis has been linked with male hypogonadism (Yoon et al., 2019). Chapter 9 examines certain VSTs known to interfere with childhood growth, including Turner syndrome. Chapter 10 describes how some people with VSTs, such as people with testosterone deficiency (hypogonadism), may be at elevated risk of chronic kidney disease (Romejko et al., 2022); testosterone deficiency is common in patients receiving dialysis (Carrero and Stenvinkel, 2012; Edey, 2017). In addition, some women with Turner syndrome may develop impaired kidney function over time (Izumita et al., 2020; Ogawa et al., 2021). As described in Chapter 11, the literature evaluating the incidence and experience of cancers of the reproductive organs among people with VSTs is exceptionally limited and insufficient for drawing conclusions. Finally, as described in Chapter 12, the epidemiology of HIV among people with VSTs is unknown.

SUMMARY OF KEY POINTS

People with VSTs are a heterogenous group that includes individuals with genetic variations and malformation syndromes affecting the anatomy of the genitourinary and reproductive systems. The diverse VST diagnoses differ in extent and impact on health and chronic disease. Some people with VSTs experience lifelong and ongoing care needs, whereas others experience sporadic severe health crises (for example, cycling in and out of health crises or experiencing a sudden need for lengthy hospitalization, followed by periods of stability). Some individuals experience mental health conditions and neurodiversity associated with VST-related stressors. Details of health care and treatments are highly variable and patient specific, and currently, multiple gaps exist in the research surrounding health care for the VST patient population, producing an imperfect standardized approach to care. Further research is necessary to gain a deeper understanding of the impacts and implications of VSTs across a range of chronic conditions.

As examined in Part III of this report, access to and timing of services related to care for VSTs—in particular, hormone therapy that may be provided during puberty or later in life—may impact functional assessment for people with VSTs who have chronic care needs. Ideally, care for people with VSTs involves a multidisciplinary team of providers that communicates well and guides patients through all their care needs, including care for chronic disease. However, many individuals, especially in the past, have encountered substantial barriers to consistent multidisciplinary health care and lacked access to knowledgeable providers. Hence, thorough documentation of care related to past or ongoing VST treatment may not be present in medical records. In addition, medical records that merely list a VST diagnosis may fail to provide sufficient historical information for evaluating health and functional status.

Having sufficiently complete medical records that document care related to management of VSTs is important for disability adjudication for applicants with VSTs. Given that a VST diagnosis is often made during early childhood and adolescence, records from many years ago may be relevant to disability adjudication for these individuals. In addition, although available SSA data do not allow for analysis of physical and mental health conditions ("impairments") among beneficiaries with VSTs, given the body of evidence presented in this chapter that people with VSTs often experience a high burden of physical and mental health conditions, people with VSTs may be particularly likely to present to SSA with multiple impairments. Because SSA considers the combined effects of all impairments when determining eligibility for benefits (SSA, 2017),[8] records related to other mental and physical chronic health conditions experienced by applicants with VSTs are important.

Given that patients with VSTs and their parents or other caregivers often lack access to supportive health care services, SSA may better serve applicants with VSTs by explaining to them that medical records related to VST care and related chronic health conditions may be relevant to their disability application. However, the committee acknowledges that older records related to care for VSTs may be very difficult to obtain, and an undue burden would result by requiring applicants to locate such records.

REFERENCES

AAFP (American Academy of Family Physicians). 2024. *Genital surgeries in intersex children.* https://www.aafp.org/about/policies/all/genital-surgeries.html (accessed March 12, 2024).

Aaronson, I. A., and A. J. Aaronson. 2010. How should we classify intersex disorders? *Journal of Pediatric Urology* 6(5):443–446.

Acién, P., and M. Acién. 2020. Disorders of sex development: Classification, review, and impact on fertility. *Journal of Clinical Medicine* 9(11):3555.

ACOG (American College of Obstetricians and Gynecologists). 2018. *Müllerian agenesis: Diagnosis, management, and treatment.* https://www.acog.org/clinical/clinical-guidance/committee-opinion/articles/2018/01/mullerian-agenesis-diagnosis-management-and-treatment (accessed March 12, 2024).

Adrião, M., S. Ferreira, R. S. Silva, M. Garcia, S. Dória, C. Costa, C. Castro-Correia, and M. Fontoura. 2020. 46,XX male disorder of sexual development. *Clinical Pediatric Endocrinology* 29(1):43–45.

---

[8] 20 C.F.R. § 404.1523 (2017).

Ahmed, S. F., J. C. Achermann, W. Arlt, A. H. Balen, G. Conway, Z. L. Edwards, S. Elford, I. A. Hughes, L. Izatt, N. Krone, H. L. Miles, S. O'Toole, L. Perry, C. Sanders, M. Simmonds, A. M. Wallace, A. Watt, and D. Willis. 2011. UK guidance on the initial evaluation of an infant or an adolescent with a suspected disorder of sex development. *Clinical Endocrinology* 75(1):12–26.

Ahmed, S. F., M. Alimusina, R. L. Batista, S. Domenice, N. Lisboa Gomes, R. McGowan, S. Patjamontri, and B. B. Mendonca. 2022. The use of genetics for reaching a diagnosis in XY DSD. *Sexual Development* 16(2-3):207–224.

Ahmet, A., A. Gupta, J. Malcolm, and C. Constantacos. 2023. Approach to the patient: Preventing adrenal crisis through patient and clinician education. *Journal of Clinical Endocrinology & Metabolism* 108(7):1797–1805.

Alexander, E. C., D. Faruqi, R. Farquhar, A. Unadkat, K. Ng Yin, R. Hoskyns, R. Varughese, and S. R. Howard. 2024. Gonadotropins for pubertal induction in males with hypogonadotropic hypogonadism: Systematic review and meta-analysis. *European Journal of Endocrinology* 190(1):S1–S11.

Allolio, B. 2015. Extensive expertise in endocrinology: Adrenal crisis. *European Journal of Endocrinology* 172(3):R115–R124.

Andrieu, T., T. du Toit, B. Vogt, M. D. Mueller, and M. Groessl. 2022. Parallel targeted and non-targeted quantitative analysis of steroids in human serum and peritoneal fluid by liquid chromatography high-resolution mass spectrometry. *Analytical and Bioanalytical Chemistry* 414(25):7461–7472.

Auchus, R. J. 2022. The uncommon forms of congenital adrenal hyperplasia. *Current Opinion in Endocrinology, Diabetes and Obesity* 29(3):263–270.

Augoulea, A., G. Zachou, and I. Lambrinoudaki. 2019. Turner syndrome and osteoporosis. *Maturitas* 130:41–49.

Babu, R., and U. Shaw. 2021. Gender identity disorder (GID) in adolescents and adults with differences of sex development (DSD): A systematic review and meta-analysis. *Journal of Pediatric Urology* 17(1):39–47.

Bakalov, V. K., L. Gutin, C. M. Cheng, J. Zhou, P. Sheth, K. Shah, S. Arepalli, V. Vanderhoof, L. M. Nelson, and C. A. Bondy. 2012. Autoimmune disorders in women with Turner syndrome and women with karyotypically normal primary ovarian insufficiency. *Journal of Autoimmunity* 38(4):315–321.

Bakula, D. M., A. J. Mullins, C. M. Sharkey, C. Wolfe-Christensen, L. L. Mullins, and A. B. Wisniewski. 2017. Gender identity outcomes in children with disorders/differences of sex development: Predictive factors. *Seminars in Perinatology* 41(4):214–217.

Balagamage, C., A. Arshad, Y. S. Elhassan, W. Ben Said, R. E. Krone, H. Gleeson, and J. Idkowiak. 2023. Management aspects of congenital adrenal hyperplasia during adolescence and transition to adult care. *Clinical Endocrinology*. Advanced online publication. https://doi.org/10.1111/cen.14992.

Barros, B. A., L. R. Oliveira, C. R. C. Surur, A. A. Barros-Filho, A. T. Maciel-Guerra, and G. Guerra-Junior. 2021. Complete androgen insensitivity syndrome and risk of gonadal malignancy: Systematic review. *Annals of Pediatric Endocrinology & Metabolism* 26(1):19–23.

Batista, R. L., M. Inácio, V. N. Brito, M. H. P. Sircili, M. J. Bag, N. L. Gomes, E. M. F. Costa, S. Domenice, and B. B. Mendonca. 2023. Sexuality and fertility desire in a large cohort of individuals with 46,XY differences in sex development. *Clinics (Sao Paulo, Brazil)* 78:100185.

Beisert, M. J., A. M. Chodecka, K. Walczyk-Matyja, M. E. Szymańska-Pytlińska, W. Kędzia, and K. Kapczuk. 2022. Psychological correlates of sexual self-esteem in young women with Mayer-Rokitansky-Küster-Hauser syndrome. *Current Issues in Personality Psychology* 10(4):333–342.

Berenbaum, S. A. 2001. Cognitive function in congenital adrenal hyperplasia. *Endocrinology & Metabolism Clinics of North America* 30(1):173–192.

Berglund, A., K. Stochholm, and C. H. Gravholt. 2020. The epidemiology of sex chromosome abnormalities. *American Journal of Medical Genetics Part C: Seminars in Medical Genetics* 184(2):202–215.

Bergougnoux, A., L. Gaspari, M. Soleirol, N. Servant, S. Soskin, S. Rossignol, K. Wagner-Mahler, J. Bertherat, C. Sultan, N. Kalfa, and F. Paris. 2023. Virilization at puberty in adolescent girls may reveal a 46,XY disorder of sexual development. *Endocrine Connections* 12(12):e230267.

Berklite, L., S. F. Witchel, S. A. Yatsenko, F. X. Schneck, and M. Reyes-Mugica. 2019. Early bilateral gonadoblastoma associated with 45,X/46,XY mosaicism: The spectrum of undifferentiated gonadal tissue and gonadoblastoma in the first months of life. *Pediatric and Developmental Pathology* 22(4):380–385.

Berry, A. W., and S. Monro. 2022. Ageing in obscurity: A critical literature review regarding older intersex people. *Sexual and Reproductive Health Matters* 30(1):e2136027.

Bertelloni, S., G. I. Baroncelli, F. Massart, and B. Toschi. 2015. Growth in boys with 45,X/46,XY mosaicism: Effect of growth hormone treatment on statural growth. *Sexual Development* 9(4):183–189.

Birjiniuk, A., A. G. Weisman, C. Laternser, J. Camarda, W. J. Brickman, R. Habiby, and S. R. Patel. 2023. Cardiovascular manifestations of Turner syndrome: Phenotypic differences between karyotype subtypes. *Pediatric Cardiology* 45(7):1407–1414.

Björlin Avdic, H., A. Butwicka, A. Nordenström, C. Almqvist, A. Nordenskjöld, H. Engberg, and L. Frisén. 2021. Neurodevelopmental and psychiatric disorders in females with Turner syndrome: A population-based study. *Journal of Neurodevelopmental Disorders* 13(1):51.

Blackless, M., A. Charuvastra, A. Derryck, A. Fausto-Sterling, K. Lauzanne, and E. Lee. 2000. How sexually dimorphic are we?: Review and synthesis. *American Journal of Human Biology* 12(2):151–166.

Bohet, M., R. Besson, R. Jardri, S. Manouvrier, S. Catteau-Jonard, M. Cartigny, E. Aubry, C. Leroy, C. Frochisse, and F. Medjkane. 2019. Mental health status of individuals with sexual development disorders: A review. *Journal of Pediatric Urology* 15(4):356–366.

Bojesen, A., S. Juul, N. H. Birkebaek, and C. H. Gravholt. 2006. Morbidity in Klinefelter syndrome: A Danish register study based on hospital discharge diagnoses. *Journal of Clinical Endocrinology & Metabolism* 91(4):1254–1260.

Bolduc, S., G. Capolicchio, J. Upadhyay, D. J. Bagli, A. E. Khoury, and G. A. McLorie. 2002. The fate of the upper urinary tract in exstrophy. *Journal of Urology* 168(6):2579–2582.

Brain, C. E., S. M. Creighton, I. Mushtaq, P. A. Carmichael, A. Barnicoat, J. W. Honour, V. Larcher, and J. C. Achermann. 2010. Holistic management of DSD. *Best Practice & Research Clinical Endocrinology & Metabolism* 24(2):335–354.

Brännström, M., L. Johannesson, H. Bokstrom, N. Kvarnstrom, J. Molne, P. Dahm-Kahler, A. Enskog, M. Milenkovic, J. Ekberg, C. Diaz-Garcia, M. Gabel, A. Hanafy, H. Hagberg, M. Olausson, and L. Nilsson. 2015. Livebirth after uterus transplantation. *The Lancet* 385(9968):607–616.

Braunstein, G. D. 2022. Spurious serum hormone immunoassay results: Causes, recognition, management. *touchREVIEWS in Endocrinology* 18(2):141–147.

Bruining, H., H. Swaab, M. Kas, and H. van Engeland. 2009. Psychiatric characteristics in a self-selected sample of boys with Klinefelter syndrome. *Pediatrics* 123(5):e865–e870.

Brunello, F. G., and R. A. Rey. 2022. AMH and AMHR2 involvement in congenital disorders of sex development. *Sexual Development* 16(2-3):138–146.

Callens, N., G. De Cuypere, P. De Sutter, S. Monstrey, S. Weyers, P. Hoebeke, and M. Cools. 2014. An update on surgical and non-surgical treatments for vaginal hypoplasia. *Human Reproduction Update* 20(5):775–801.

Callens, N., M. Van Kuyk, J. H. van Kuppenveld, S. L. S. Drop, P. T. Cohen-Kettenis, A. B. Dessens, and the Dutch Study Group on DSD. 2016. Recalled and current gender role behavior, gender identity and sexual orientation in adults with disorders/differences of sex development. *Hormones and Behavior* 86:8–20.

Campo-Engelstein, L., D. Chen, A. B. Baratz, E. K. Johnson, and C. Finlayson. 2017. The ethics of fertility preservation for pediatric patients with differences (disorders) of sex development. *Journal of the Endocrine Society* 1(6):638–645.

Carrero, J. J., and P. Stenvinkel. 2012. The vulnerable man: Impact of testosterone deficiency on the uraemic phenotype. *Nephrology Dialysis Transplantation* 27(11):4030–4041.

Cederlof, M., A. Ohlsson Gotby, H. Larsson, E. Serlachius, M. Boman, N. Langstrom, M. Landen, and P. Lichtenstein. 2014. Klinefelter syndrome and risk of psychosis, autism and ADHD. *Journal of Psychiatric Research* 48(1):128–130.

Chadwick, P. M., A. Smyth, and L. M. Liao. 2014. Improving self-esteem in women diagnosed with Turner syndrome: Results of a pilot intervention. *Journal of Pediatric & Adolescent Gynecology* 27(3):129–132.

Chaudhry, S., R. Tadokoro-Cuccaro, S. E. Hannema, C. L. Acerini, and I. A. Hughes. 2017. Frequency of gonadal tumours in complete androgen insensitivity syndrome (CAIS): A retrospective case-series analysis. *Journal of Pediatric Urology* 13(5):e491–e498.

Chen, Z., P. Li, Y. Lyu, Y. Wang, K. Gao, J. Wang, F. Lan, and F. Chen. 2023. Molecular genetics and general management of androgen insensitivity syndrome. *Intractable & Rare Diseases Research* 12(2):71–77.

Children's Hospital of Chicago. 2021. *Update on intersex care at Lurie Children's and our sex development clinic.* https://www.luriechildrens.org/en/blog/update-on-intersex-care-at-lurie-childrens-and-our-sex-development-clinic (accessed March 12, 2024).

Chrisp, G. L., D. J. Torpy, A. M. Maguire, M. Quartararo, H. Falhammar, B. R. King, C. F. Munns, S. Hameed, and R. L. Rushworth. 2020. The effect of patient-managed stress dosing on electrolytes and blood pressure in acute illness in children with adrenal insufficiency. *Clinical Endocrinology* 93(2):97–103.

Claahsen-van der Grinten, H. L., P. W. Speiser, S. F. Ahmed, W. Arlt, R. J. Auchus, H. Falhammar, C. E. Fluck, L. Guasti, A. Huebner, B. B. M. Kortmann, N. Krone, D. P. Merke, W. L. Miller, A. Nordenstrom, N. Reisch, D. E. Sandberg, N. Stikkelbroeck, P. Touraine, A. Utari, S. A. Wudy, and P. C. White. 2022. Congenital adrenal hyperplasia-current insights in pathophysiology, diagnostics, and management. *Endocrine Reviews* 43(1):91–159.

Coleman, E., A. E. Radix, W. P. Bouman, G. R. Brown, A. L. C. de Vries, M. B. Deutsch, R. Ettner, L. Fraser, M. Goodman, J. Green, A. B. Hancock, T. W. Johnson, D. H. Karasic, G. A. Knudson, S. F. Leibowitz, H. F. L. Meyer-Bahlburg, S. J. Monstrey, J. Motmans, L. Nahata, T. O. Nieder, S. L. Reisner, C. Richards, L. S. Schechter, V. Tangpricha, A. C. Tishelman, M. A. A. Van Trotsenburg, S. Winter, K. Ducheny, N. J. Adams, T. M. Adrián, L. R. Allen, D. Azul, H. Bagga, K. Başar, D. S. Bathory, J. J. Belinky, D. R. Berg, J. U. Berli, R. O. Bluebond-Langner, M. B. Bouman, M. L. Bowers, P. J. Brassard, J. Byrne, L. Capitán, C. J. Cargill, J. M. Carswell, S. C. Chang, G. Chelvakumar, T. Corneil, K. B. Dalke, G. De Cuypere, E. de Vries, M. Den Heijer, A. H. Devor, C. Dhejne, A. D'Marco, E. K. Edmiston, L. Edwards-Leeper, R. Ehrbar, D. Ehrensaft, J. Eisfeld, E. Elaut, L. Erickson-Schroth, J. L. Feldman, A. D. Fisher, M. M. Garcia, L. Gijs, S. E. Green, B. P. Hall, T. L. D. Hardy, M. S. Irwig, L. A. Jacobs, A. C. Janssen, K. Johnson, D. T. Klink, B. P. C. Kreukels, L. E. Kuper, E. J. Kvach, M. A. Malouf, R. Massey, T. Mazur, C. McLachlan, S. D. Morrison, S. W. Mosser, P. M. Neira, U. Nygren, J. M. Oates, J. Obedin-Maliver, G. Pagkalos, J. Patton, N. Phanuphak, K. Rachlin, T. Reed, G. N. Rider, J. Ristori, S. Robbins-Cherry, S. A. Roberts, K. A. Rodriguez-Wallberg, S. M. Rosenthal, K. Sabir, J. D. Safer, A. I. Scheim, L. J. Seal, T. J. Sehoole, K. Spencer, C. St. Amand, T. D. Steensma, J. F. Strang, G. B. Taylor, K. Tilleman, G. G. T'Sjoen, L. N. Vala, N. M. Van Mello, J. F. Veale, J. A. Vencill, B. Vincent, L. M. Wesp, M. A. West, and J. Arcelus. 2022. Standards of care for the health of transgender and gender diverse people, version 8. *International Journal of Transgender Health* 23(Suppl 1):S1–S259.

Conlon, T. A., C. P. Hawkes, J. Brady, J. G. Loeber, and N. Murphy. 2023. International newborn screening practices for the early detection of congenital adrenal hyperplasia. *Hormone Research in Paediatrics* 97(2):113–125.

Cools, M., A. Nordenström, R. Robeva, J. Hall, P. Westerveld, C. Flück, B. Köhler, M. Berra, A. Springer, K. Schweizer, V. Pasterski, and COST Action BM 1303 Working Group 1. 2018. Caring for individuals with a difference of sex development (DSD): A consensus statement. *Nature Reviews Endocrinology* 14(7):415–429.

Cools, M., E. Y. Cheng, J. Hall, J. Alderson, A. M. Amies Oelschlager, A. H. Balen, Y. M. Chan, M. E. Geffner, C. H. Gravholt, T. Guran, P. Hoebeke, P. Lee, E. Magritte, D. Matos, K. McElreavey, H. F. L. Meyer-Bahlburg, R. C. Rink, A. Springer, K. M. Szymanski, E. Vilain, J. Williams, K. P. Wolffenbuttel, D. E. Sandberg, and R. Subramaniam. 2024. Multi-stakeholder opinion statement on the care of individuals born with differences of sex development: Common ground and opportunities for improvement. *Hormone Research in Paediatrics* 1–17.

Costa, E. M., S. Domenice, M. H. Sircili, M. Inacio, and B. B. Mendonca. 2012. DSD due to 5alpha-reductase 2 deficiency: From diagnosis to long term outcome. *Seminars in Reproductive Medicine* 30(5):427–431.

Cox, K., J. Bryce, J. Jiang, M. Rodie, R. Sinnott, M. Alkhawari, W. Arlt, L. Audi, A. Balsamo, S. Bertelloni, M. Cools, F. Darendeliler, S. Drop, M. Ellaithi, T. Guran, O. Hiort, P. M. Holterhus, I. Hughes, N. Krone, L. Lisa, Y. Morel, O. Soder, P. Wieacker, and S. F. Ahmed. 2014. Novel associations in disorders of sex development: Findings from the I-DSD registry. *Journal of Clinical Endocrinology & Metabolism* 99(2):E348–E355.

Coyne C. A., B. T. Yuodsnukis, and D. Chen. 2023. Gender dysphoria: Optimizing healthcare for transgender and gender diverse youth with a multidisciplinary approach. *Neuropsychiatric Disease and Treatment* 19:479–493.

Crawford, J. M., G. Warne, S. Grover, B. R. Southwell, and J. M. Hutson. 2009. Results from a pediatric surgical centre justify early intervention in disorders of sex development. *Journal of Pediatric Surgery* 44(2):413–416.

Creighton, S. M., C. L. Minto, and S. J. Steele. 2001. Objective cosmetic and anatomical outcomes at adolescence of feminising surgery for ambiguous genitalia done in childhood. *The Lancet* 358(9276):124–125.

Crissman, H. P., L. Warner, M. Gardner, M. Carr, A. Schast, A. L. Quittner, B. Kogan, and D. E. Sandberg. 2011. Children with disorders of sex development: A qualitative study of early parental experience. *International Journal of Pediatric Endocrinology* 2011(1):10.

Crouch, N. S., L. M. Liao, C. R. Woodhouse, G. S. Conway, and S. M. Creighton. 2008. Sexual function and genital sensitivity following feminizing genitoplasty for congenital adrenal hyperplasia. *Journal of Urology* 179(2):634–638.

Culen, C., D. A. Ertl, K. Schubert, L. Bartha-Doering, and G. Haeusler. 2017. Care of girls and women with Turner syndrome: Beyond growth and hormones. *Endocrine Connections* 6(4):R39–R51.

Da Aw, L., M. M. Zain, S. C. Esteves, and P. Humaidan. 2016. Persistent Mullerian duct syndrome: A rare entity with a rare presentation in need of multidisciplinary management. *International Brazilian Journal of Urology* 42(6):1237–1243.

D'Alberton, F., M. T. Assante, M. Foresti, A. Balsamo, S. Bertelloni, E. Dati, L. Nardi, M. L. Bacchi, and L. Mazzanti. 2015. Quality of life and psychological adjustment of women living with 46,XY differences of sex development. *Journal of Sexual Medicine* 12(6):1440–1449.

Davies, J. H., E. J. Knight, A. Savage, J. Brown, and P. S. Malone. 2011. Evaluation of terminology used to describe disorders of sex development. *Journal of Pediatric Urology* 7(4):412–415.

Davies, M. C. 2010. Lost in transition: The needs of adolescents with Turner syndrome. *British Journal of Obstetrics and Gynaecology* 117(2):134–136.

Davis, S. M., L. Bloy, T. P. L., Roberts, K. Kowal, A. Alston, A. Tahsin, A. Truxon, and J. L., Ross. 2020. Testicular function in boys with 47,XYY and relationship to phenotype. *American Journal of Medical Genetics: Part C, Seminars in Medical Genetics* 184(2):371–385.

Davis, S. M., C. Teerlink, J. A. Lynch, B. R. Gorman, M. Pagadala, A. Liu, M. S. Panizzon, V. C. Merritt, G. Genovese, S. Pyarajan, J. L. Ross, and R. L. Hauger. 2023. Prevalence, morbidity, and mortality of 1,609 men with sex chromosome aneuploidy: Results from the diverse Million Veteran Program cohort. *medRxiv (Cold Spring Harbor Laboratory)*. Advanced online publication. https://doi.org/10.1101/2023.07.15.23292710.

Dayner, J. E., P. A. Lee, and C. P. Houk. 2004. Medical treatment of intersex: Parental perspectives. *Journal of Urology* 172(4 Pt 2):1762–1765.

de Jesus, L. E., E. C. Costa, and S. Dekermacher. 2019. Gender dysphoria and XX congenital adrenal hyperplasia: How frequent is it? Is male-sex rearing a good idea? *Journal of Pediatric Surgery* 54(11):2421–2427.

De Luca, F., J. Argente, L. Cavallo, E. Crowne, H. A. Delemarre-Van de Waal, C. De Sanctis, S. Di Maio, E. Norjavaara, W. Oostdijk, F. Severi, G. Tonini, G. Trifiro, P. G. Voorhoeve, F. Wu, and the International Workshop on Management of Puberty for Optimum Auxological Results. 2001. Management of puberty in constitutional delay of growth and puberty. *Journal of Pediatric Endocrinology & Metabolism* 2(Suppl 14):953–957.

De Sanctis, V., and D. Khater. 2019. Autoimmune diseases in Turner syndrome: An overview. *Acta Biomedica* 90(3):341–344.

de Vries, A. L. C., R. Roehle, L. Marshall, L. Frisén, T. C. van de Grift, B. P. C. Kreukels, C. Bouvattier, B. Kohler, U. Thyen, A. Nordenström, M. Rapp, and P. T. Cohen-Kettenis. 2019. Mental health of a large group of adults with disorders of sex development in six eastern European countries. *Psychosomatic Medicine* 81(7):629–640.

Dessens, A. B., F. M. Slijper, and S. L. Drop. 2005. Gender dysphoria and gender change in chromosomal females with congenital adrenal hyperplasia. *Archives of Sexual Behavior* 34(4):389–397.

Diamond, M., and L. A. Watson. 2004. Androgen insensitivity syndrome and Klinefelter's syndrome: Sex and gender considerations. *Child and Adolescent Psychiatric Clinics of North America* 13(3):623–640, viii.

Dineen, R., P. M. Stewart, and M. Sherlock. 2019. Factors impacting on the action of glucocorticoids in patients receiving glucocorticoid therapy. *Clinical Endocrinology* 90(1):3–14.

Ding, Y., Y. Wang, Y. Lyu, H. Xie, Y. Huang, M. Wu, F. Chen, and Z. Chen. 2023. Urogenital sinus malformation: From development to management. *Intractable & Rare Diseases Research* 12(2):78–87.

Domenice, S., R. L. Batista, I. J. P. Arnhold, M. H. Sircili, E. M. F. Costa, and B. B. Mendonca. 2022. 46,XY differences of sexual development. In *Endotext [Internet]* edited by K. R. Feingold, B. Anawalt, M. R. Blackman, A. Boyce, G. Chrousos, E. Corpas, W. W. de Herder, K. Dhatariya, K. Dungan, J. Hofland, S. Kalra, G. Kaltsas, N. Kapoor, C. Koch, P. Kopp, M. Korbonits, C. S. Kovacs, W. Kuohung, B. Laferrère, M. Levy, E. A. McGee, R. McLachlan, M. New, J. Purnell, R. Sahay, A. S. Shah, F. Singer, M. A. Sperling, C. A. Stratakis, D. L. Trence, and D. P. Wilson. South Dartmouth, MA.

Duguid, A., S. Morrison, A. Robertson, J. Chalmers, G. Youngson, S. F. Ahmed, and the Scottish Genital Anomaly Network. 2007. The psychological impact of genital anomalies on the parents of affected children. *Acta Paediatrica* 96(3):348–352.

Dwyer, A. A., N. Smith, and R. Quinton. 2019. Psychological aspects of congenital hypogonadotropic hypogonadism. *Frontiers in Endocrinology* 10:353.

Edey, M. M. 2017. Male sexual dysfunction and chronic kidney disease. *Frontiers in Medicine (Lausanne)* 4:32.

El-Dahtory, F., and H. M. Elsheikha. 2009. Male infertility related to an aberrant karyotype, 47,XYY: Four case reports. *Cases Journal* 2(1):28.

Engberg, H., A. Strandqvist, A. Nordenstrom, A. Butwicka, A. Nordenskjold, A. L. Hirschberg, and L. Frisen. 2017. Increased psychiatric morbidity in women with complete androgen insensitivity syndrome or complete gonadal dysgenesis. *Journal of Psychosomatic Research* 101:122–127.

Ernst, M. M., L. M. Liao, A. B. Baratz, and D. E. Sandberg. 2018. Disorders of sex development/intersex: Gaps in psychosocial care for children. *Pediatrics* 142(2):e20174045.

Espinosa Reyes, T. M., A. K. Pesantez Velepucha, J. O. Cabrera Rego, W. Valdes Gomez, E. Dominguez Alonso, and H. Falhammar. 2023. Cardiovascular risk in Cuban adolescents and young adults with congenital adrenal hyperplasia. *BMC Endocrine Disorders* 23(1):241.

Falhammar, H., H. Filipsson Nyström, A. Wedell, and M. Thorén. 2011. Cardiovascular risk, metabolic profile, and body composition in adult males with congenital adrenal hyperplasia due to 21-hydroxylase deficiency. *European Journal of Endocrinology* 164(2):285–293.

Falhammar, H., L. Frisen, C. Norrby, A. L. Hirschberg, C. Almqvist, A. Nordenskjold, and A. Nordenstrom. 2014. Increased mortality in patients with congenital adrenal hyperplasia due to 21-hydroxylase deficiency. *Journal of Clinical Endocrinology & Metabolism* 99(12):e2715–2721.

Falhammar, H., H. Claahsen-van der Grinten, N. Reisch, J. Slowikowska-Hilczer, A. Nordenstrom, R. Roehle, C. Bouvattier, B. P. C. Kreukels, B. Kohler, and on behalf of the DSD-LIFE Group. 2018. Health status in 1040 adults with disorders of sex development (DSD): A European multicenter study. *Endocrine Connections* 7(3):466–478.

Falhammar, H., L. Frisen, A. L. Hirschberg, A. Nordenskjold, C. Almqvist, and A. Nordenstrom. 2022. Increased prevalence of fractures in congenital adrenal hyperplasia: A Swedish population-based national cohort study. *Journal of Clinical Endocrinology & Metabolism* 107(2):e475–e486.

Fang, J., G. Gao, J. Liu, L. Cai, Y. Cui, and X. Yang. 2021. A novel mutation of AMHR2 in two brothers with persistent Mullerian duct syndrome and their intracytoplasmic sperm injection outcome. *Molecular Genetics & Genomic Medicine* 9(10):e1801.

Farrugia, M. K., N. J. Sebire, J. C. Achermann, A. Eisawi, P. G. Duffy, and I. Mushtaq. 2013. Clinical and gonadal features and early surgical management of 45,X/46,XY and 45,X/47,XYY chromosomal mosaicism presenting with genital anomalies. *Journal of Pediatric Urology* 9(2):139–144.

Fleming, L., K. Knafl, G. Knafl, and M. Van Riper. 2017. Parental management of adrenal crisis in children with congenital adrenal hyperplasia. *Journal for Specialists in Pediatric Nursing* 22(4):e12190.

Foland-Ross, L. C., E. Ghasemi, V. Lozano Wun, T. Aye, K. Kowal, J. Ross, and A. L. Reiss. 2023. Executive dysfunction in Klinefelter syndrome: Associations with brain activation and testicular failure. *Journal of Clinical Endocrinology & Metabolism* 109(1):e88–e95.

Frank, S. E. 2018. Intersex and intimacy: Presenting concerns about dating and intimate relationships. *Sexuality & Culture* 22(1):127–147.

Furtado, P. S., F. Moraes, R. Lago, L. O. Barros, M. B. Toralles, and U. Barroso, Jr. 2012. Gender dysphoria associated with disorders of sex development. *Nature Reviews Urology* 9(11):620–627.

Gaston, B., N. Marozkina, D. C. Newcomb, N. Sharifi, and J. Zein. 2021. Asthma risk among individuals with androgen receptor deficiency. *JAMA Pediatrics* 175(7):743–745.

Ghazal, K., S. Brabant, D. Price, and M. L. Piketty. 2022. Hormone immunoassay interference: A 2021 update. *Annals of Laboratory Medicine* 42(1):3–23.

Gottlieb, B., L. K. Beitel, A. Nadarajah, M. Paliouras, and M. Trifiro. 2012. The androgen receptor gene mutations database: 2012 update. *Human Mutation* 33(5):887–894.

Granero-Molina, J., R. A. Roman, M. Del Mar Jimenez-Lasserrotte, M. D. Ruiz-Fernandez, M. I. Ventura-Miranda, G. Granero-Heredia, and I. M. Fernandez-Medina. 2023. "I'm still a woman": A qualitative study on sexuality in heterosexual women with Turner syndrome. *Journal of Clinical Nursing* 32(17-18):6634–6647.

Grant, A., C. P. Carpenter, B. Li, and S. J. Kim. 2023. Hydrometrocolpos: A contemporary review of the last 5 years. *Current Urology Reports* 24(12):601–610.

Gravholt, C. H., A. Ferlin, J. Gromoll, A. Juul, A. Raznahan, S. van Rijn, A. D. Rogol, A. Skakkebaek, N. Tartaglia, and H. Swaab. 2023a. New developments and future trajectories in supernumerary sex chromosome abnormalities: A summary of the 2022 3rd International Workshop on Klinefelter Syndrome, Trisomy X, and XYY. *Endocrine Connections* 12(3):e220500.

Gravholt, C. H., M. Viuff, J. Just, K. Sandahl, S. Brun, J. van der Velden, N. H. Andersen, and A. Skakkebaek. 2023b. The changing face of Turner syndrome. *Endocrine Reviews* 44(1):33–69.

Gregg, A. R., B. G. Skotko, J. L. Benkendorf, K. G. Monaghan, K. Bajaj, R. G. Best, S. Klugman, and M. S. Watson. 2016. Noninvasive prenatal screening for fetal aneuploidy, 2016 update: A position statement of the American College of Medical Genetics and Genomics. *Genetics in Medicine* 18(10):1056–1065.

Grinspon, R. P., and R. A. Rey. 2019. Molecular characterization of XX maleness. *International Journal of Molecular Sciences* 20(23):6089.

Grinspon, R. P., S. Castro, and R. A. Rey. 2023. Up-to-date clinical and biochemical workup of the child and the adolescent with a suspected disorder of sex development. *Hormone Research in Paediatrics* 96(2):116–127.

Gürbüz, F., M. Alkan, G. Çelik, A. Bişgin, N. Çekin, I. Ünal, A. K. Topaloğlu, Ü. Zorludemir, A. Avcı, and B. Yüksel. 2020. Gender identity and assignment recommendations in disorders of sex development patients: 20 years' experience and challenges. *Journal of Clinical Research in Pediatric Endocrinology* 12(4):347–357.

Haghighat, D., T. Berro, L. Torrey Sosa, K. Horowitz, B. Brown-King, and K. Zayhowski. 2023. Intersex people's perspectives on affirming healthcare practices: A qualitative study. *Social Science & Medicine* 329:e116047.

Halaseh, S. A., S. Halaseh, and M. Ashour. 2022. Hypospadias: A comprehensive review including its embryology, etiology and surgical techniques. *Cureus* 14(7):e27544.

Haney, N. M., C. C. Morrill, A. Haffar, C. Crigger, A. T. Gabrielson, L. Galansky, and J. P. Gearhart. 2024. Long-term management of problems in cloacal exstrophy: A single-institution review. *Journal of Pediatric Surgery* 59(1):26–30.

Hannah-Shmouni, F., R. Morissette, N. Sinaii, M. Elman, T. R. Prezant, W. Chen, A. Pulver, and D. P. Merke. 2017. Revisiting the prevalence of nonclassic congenital adrenal hyperplasia in U.S. Ashkenazi Jews and Caucasians. *Genetics in Medicine* 19(11):1276–1279.

Herlin, M. K., M. B. Petersen, and M. Brannstrom. 2020. Mayer-Rokitansky-Kuster-Hauser (MRKH) syndrome: A comprehensive update. *Orphanet Journal of Rare Diseases* 15(1):214.

Herman, J. L., A. R. Flores, and K. K. O'Neill. 2022. *How many adults and youth identify as transgender in the United States?* Los Angeles, CA: The Williams Institute, UCLA School of Law.

Hines, M. 2020. Human gender development. *Neuroscience Biobehavioral Reviews* 118:89–96.

Howard, S. R., and L. Dunkel. 2018. Management of hypogonadism from birth to adolescence. *Best Practice & Research Clinical Endocrinology & Metabolism* 32(4):355–372.

Howard, S. R., and R. Quinton. 2024. Outcomes and experiences of adults with congenital hypogonadism can inform improvements in the management of delayed puberty. *Journal of Pediatric Endocrinology & Metabolism* 37(1):1–7.

Hsu, L. Y. 1989. Prenatal diagnosis of 45X/46,XY mosaicism: A review and update. *Prenatal Diagnosis* 9(1):31–48.

Hughes, I. A. 2007. Early management and gender assignment in disorders of sexual differentiation. *Endocrine Development* 11:47–57.

Hughes, I. A., C. Houk, S. F. Ahmed, P. A. Lee, L. C. Group, and the LWPES/ESPE Consensus Group. 2006. Consensus statement on management of intersex disorders. *Archives of Disease in Childhood* 91(7):554–563.

Hutaff-Lee, C., E. Bennett, S. Howell, and N. Tartaglia. 2019. Clinical developmental, neuro-psychological, and social-emotional features of Turner syndrome. *American Journal of Medical Genetics Part C: Seminars in Medical Genetics* 181(1):126–134.

Hwang, I. T. 2014. Efficacy and safety of growth hormone treatment for children born small for gestational age. *Korean Journal of Pediatrics* 57(9):379–383.

Ikegawa, K., and Y. Hasegawa. 2022. Fracture risk, underlying pathophysiology, and bone quality assessment in patients with Turner syndrome. *Frontiers in Endocrinology* 13:e967857.

Imperato-McGinley, J., M. Miller, J. D. Wilson, R. E. Peterson, C. Shackleton, and D. C. Gajdusek. 1991. A cluster of male pseudohermaphrodites with 5 alpha-reductase deficiency in Papua New Guinea. *Clinical Endocrinology* 34(4):293–298.

Izumita, Y., S. Nishigaki, M. Satoh, N. Takubo, C. Numakura, I. Takahashi, S. Soneda, Y. Abe, H. Kamasaki, Y. Ohtsu, J. Igaki, Y. Hasegawa, and K. Nagasaki. 2020. Retrospective study of the renal function using estimated glomerular filtration rate and congenital anomalies of the kidney-urinary tract in pediatric Turner syndrome. *Congenital Anomalies* 60(6):175–179.

Jackson, C., F. M. Cheater, and I. Reid. 2008. A systematic review of decision support needs of parents making child health decisions. *Health Expectations* 11(3):232–251.

Johannesson, M., C. Gottlieb, and L. Hjelte. 1997. Delayed puberty in girls with cystic fibrosis despite good clinical status. *Pediatrics* 99(1):29–34.

Jones, C. 2020. Intersex, infertility and the future: Early diagnoses and the imagined life course. *Sociology of Health & Illness* 42(1):143–156.

Jordan, T. L., L. C. Foland-Ross, V. L. Wun, J. L. Ross, and A. L. Reiss. 2023. Cognition, academic achievement, adaptive behavior, and quality of life in child and adolescent boys with Klinefelter syndrome. *Journal of Developmental & Behavioral Pediatrics* 44(7):e476–e485.

Kanakis, G. A., and E. Nieschlag. 2018. Klinefelter syndrome: More than hypogonadism. *Metabolism* 86:135–144.

Keppler-Noreuil, K. M., K. M. Conway, D. Shen, A. J. Rhoads, J. C. Carey, P. A. Romitti, and National Birth Defects Prevention Study. 2017. Clinical and risk factor analysis of cloacal defects in the national birth defects prevention study. *American Journal of Medical Genetics Part A* 173(11):2873–2885.

Kerckhof, M. E., B. P. C. Kreukels, T. O. Nieder, I. Becker-Hebly, T. C. van de Grift, A. S. Staphorsius, A. Kohler, G. Heylens, and E. Elaut. 2019. Prevalence of sexual dysfunctions in transgender persons: Results from the ENIGI follow-up study. *Journal of Sexual Medicine* 16(12):2018–2029.

Klein, D. A., J. E. Emerick, J. E. Sylvester, and K. S. Vogt. 2017. Disorders of puberty: An approach to diagnosis and management. *American Family Physician* 96(9):590–599.

Ko, J. K. Y., T. F. J. King, L. Williams, S. M. Creighton, and G. S. Conway. 2017. Hormone replacement treatment choices in complete androgen insensitivity syndrome: An audit of an adult clinic. *Endocrine Connections* 6(6):375–379.

Kohler, B., E. Kleinemeier, A. Lux, O. Hiort, A. Gruters, U. Thyen, and the DSD Network Working Group. 2012. Satisfaction with genital surgery and sexual life of adults with XY disorders of sex development: Results from the German clinical evaluation study. *Journal of Clinical Endocrinology & Metabolism* 97(2):577–588.

Kremen, J., S. M. Davis, L. Nahata, H. M. Kapa, T. M. Dattilo, E. Liu, C. Hutaff-Lee, A. C. Tishelman, and C. E. Crerand. 2023. Neuropsychological and mental health concerns in a multicenter clinical sample of youth with Turner syndrome. *American Journal of Medical Genetics Part A* 191(4):962–976.

Kreukels, B. P. C., B. Kohler, A. Nordenstrom, R. Roehle, U. Thyen, C. Bouvattier, A. L. C. de Vries, P. T. Cohen-Kettenis. 2018. Gender dysphoria and gender change in disorders of sex development/intersex conditions: Results from the DSD-life study. *Journal of Sexual Medicine* 15(5):777–785.

Lampalzer, U., P. Briken, and K. Schweizer. 2021. Psychosocial care and support in the field of intersex/diverse sex development (DSD): Counselling experiences, localisation and needed improvements. *International Journal of Impotence Research* 33(2):228–242.

Lee, P. A., C. P. Houk, S. Faisal Ahmed, I. A. Hughes, and the International Consensus Conference on Intersex organized by the Lawson Wilkins Pediatric Endocrine Society and the European Society for Paediatric Endocrinology. 2006. Consensus statement on management of intersex disorders: International consensus conference on intersex. *Pediatrics* 118(2):e488–e500.

Lee, P. A., A. Nordenstrom, C. P. Houk, S. F. Ahmed, R. Auchus, A. Baratz, K. Baratz Dalke, L. M. Liao, K. Lin-Su, L. H. Looijenga, 3rd, T. Mazur, H. F. Meyer-Bahlburg, P. Mouriquand, C. A. Quigley, D. E. Sandberg, E. Vilain, S. Witchel, and the Global DSD Update Consortium. 2016. Global disorders of sex development update since 2006: Perceptions, approach and care. *Hormone Research in Paediatrics* 85(3):158–180.

Lindhardt Johansen, M., C. P. Hagen, E. Rajpert-De Meyts, S. Kjaergaard, B. L. Petersen, N. E. Skakkebaek, K. M. Main, and A. Juul. 2012. 45,X/46,XY mosaicism: Phenotypic characteristics, growth, and reproductive function: A retrospective longitudinal study. *Journal of Clinical Endocrinology & Metabolism* 97(8):e1540–e1549.

Lipstein, E. A., C. M. Dodds, and M. T. Britto. 2014. Real life clinic visits do not match the ideals of shared decision making. *Journal of Pediatrics* 165(1):178–183.E1.

Lucas-Herald, A. K., J. Bryce, A. Kyriakou, M. L. Ljubicic, W. Arlt, L. Audi, A. Balsamo, F. Baronio, S. Bertelloni, M. Bettendorf, A. Brooke, H. L. Claahsen van der Grinten, J. H. Davies, G. Hermann, L. de Vries, I. A. Hughes, R. Tadokoro-Cuccaro, F. Darendeliler, S. Poyrazoglu, M. Ellaithi, O. Evliyaoglu, S. Fica, L. Nedelea, A. Gawlik, E. Globa, N. Zelinska, T. Guran, A. Guven, S. E. Hannema, O. Hiort, P. M. Holterhus, V. Iotova, V. Mladenov, V. Jain, R. Sharma, F. Jennane, C. Johnston, G. Guerra Junior, D. Konrad, O. Gaisl, N. Krone, R. Krone, K. Lachlan, D. Li, C. Lichiardopol, L. Lisa, R. Markosyan, I. Mazen, K. Mohnike, M. Niedziela, A. Nordenstrom, R. Rey, M. Skaeil, L. J. W. Tack, J. Tomlinson, N. Weintrob, M. Cools, and S. F. Ahmed. 2021. Gonadectomy in conditions affecting sex development: A registry-based cohort study. *European Journal of Endocrinology* 184(6):791–801.

Lundberg, T., P. Hegarty, and K. Roen. 2018. Making sense of 'intersex' and 'DSD': How laypeople understand and use terminology. *Psychology & Sexuality* 9(2):161–173.

MacKenzie, D., A. Huntington, and J. A. Gilmour. 2009. The experiences of people with an intersex condition: A journey from silence to voice. *Journal of Clinical Nursing* 18(12):1775–1783.

Maimoun, L., P. Philibert, B. Cammas, F. Audran, P. Bouchard, P. Fenichel, M. Cartigny, C. Pienkowski, M. Polak, N. Skordis, I. Mazen, G. Ocal, M. Berberoglu, R. Reynaud, C. Baumann, S. Cabrol, D. Simon, K. Kayemba-Kay's, M. De Kerdanet, F. Kurtz, B. Leheup, C. Heinrichs, S. Tenoutasse, G. Van Vliet, A. Grüters, M. Eunice, A. C. Ammini, M. Hafez, Z. Hochberg, S. Einaudi, H. Al Mawlawi, C. J. Nuñez, N. Servant, A. Lumbroso, F. Paris, and C. Sultan. 2011. Phenotypical, biological, and molecular heterogeneity of 5α-reductase deficiency: An extensive international experience of 55 patients. *Journal of Clinical Endocrinology & Metabolism* 96(2):296–307.

Marks, L. S. 2004. 5alpha-reductase: History and clinical importance. *Reviews in Urology* 6(Suppl 9):S11–S21.

Martínez-Frías, M. L., E. Bermejo, E. Rodriguez-Pinilla, and J. L. Frias. 2001. Exstrophy of the cloaca and exstrophy of the bladder: Two different expressions of a primary developmental field defect. *American Journal of Medical Genetics* 99(4):261–269.

Maruf, M., R. Manyevitch, J. Michaud, J. Jayman, M. Kasprenski, M. H. Zaman, K. Benz, M. Eldridge, B. Trock, K. T. Harris, W. J. Wu, H. N. Di Carlo, and J. P. Gearhart. 2020. Urinary continence outcomes in classic bladder exstrophy: A long-term perspective. *Journal of Urology* 203(1):200–205.

Mayo Clinic. 2018. *Ambiguous genitalia.* https://www.mayoclinic.org/diseases-conditions/ambiguous-genitalia/diagnosis-treatment/drc-20369278 (accessed March 13, 2024).

Mazur, T., J. O'Donnell, and P. A. Lee. 2023. Extensive literature review of 46,XX newborns with congenital adrenal hyperplasia (CAH) and severe genital masculinization: Should they be assigned and reared male? *Journal of Research in Pediatric Endocrinology* 16(2):123–136.

McCarrison, S., A. Carr, S. C. Wong, and A. Mason. 2023. The prevalence of hypertension in paediatric Turner syndrome: A systematic review and meta-analysis. *Journal of Human Hypertension* 37(8):675–688.

McCoy, R. C. 2017. Mosaicism in preimplantation human embryos: When chromosomal abnormalities are the norm. *Trends in Genetics* 33(7):448–463.

Meccanici, F., J. W. C. de Bruijn, J. S. Dommisse, J. J. M. Takkenberg, A. E. van den Bosch, and J. W. Roos-Hesselink. 2023. Prevalence and development of aortic dilation and dissection in women with Turner syndrome: A systematic review and meta-analysis. *Expert Review of Cardiovascular Therapy* 21(2):133–144.

Mendoza, N., and M. A. Motos. 2013. Androgen insensitivity syndrome. *Gynecological Endocrinology* 29(1):1–5.

Meyer-Bahlburg, H. F., R. S. Gruen, M. I. New, J. J. Bell, A. Morishima, M. Shimshi, Y. Bueno, I. Vargas, and S. W. Baker. 1996. Gender change from female to male in classical congenital adrenal hyperplasia. *Hormones and Behavior* 30(4):319–332.

Miller, W. L., and R. J. Auchus. 2011. The molecular biology, biochemistry, and physiology of human steroidogenesis and its disorders. *Endocrine Reviews* 32(1):81–151.

Mitsch, C., E. Alexandrou, A. W. Norris, and C. T. Pinnaro. 2023. Hyperglycemia in Turner syndrome: Impact, mechanisms, and areas for future research. *Frontiers in Endocrinology* 14:e1116889.

Mittal, S., J. Weaver, A. Aghababian, R. Edwins, K. Godlewski, K. Fischer, S. Siu, D. Gruccio, J. Van Batavia, A. Srinivasan, C. Long, V. Bamba, V. Batra, T. Bhatti, and T. Kolon. 2023. Deferring gonadectomy in patients with Turner syndrome with a genetic Y component is not a safe practice. *Journal of Pediatric Urology* 19(3):e291–e294.

Momodu, I. I., B. Lee, and G. Singh. 2023. *Congenital adrenal hyperplasia.* [Updated 2023 July 17], Statpearls. Treasure Island, FL: StatPearls Publishing.

Money, J. 1952. *Hermaphroditism: An inquiry into the nature of a human paradox.* Doctoral Thesis, Harvard University.

Moran, M. E., and K. Karkazis. 2012. Developing a multidisciplinary team for disorders of sex development: Planning, implementation, and operation tools for care providers. *Advances in Urology* 2012:e604135.

Moreno-Begines, M. L. N., A. Arroyo-Rodriguez, A. Borrallo-Riego, and M. D. Guerra-Martin. 2022. Intersexuality/differences of sex development through the discourse of intersex people, their relatives, and health experts: A descriptive qualitative study. *Healthcare (Basel, Switzerland)* 10(4):671.

Morris, J. K., E. Alberman, C. Scott, and P. Jacobs. 2008. Is the prevalence of Klinefelter syndrome increasing? *European Journal of Human Genetics* 16(2):163–170.

Naessén, S., M. Eliasson, K. Berntorp, M. Kitlinski, P. Trimpou, E. Amundson, S. Thunstrom, B. Ekman, J. Wahlberg, A. Karlsson, M. Isaksson, I. Bergstrom, C. Levelind, I. Bryman, and K. Landin-Wilhelmsen. 2024. Autoimmune disease in Turner syndrome in Sweden: An up to 25 years' controlled follow-up study. *Journal of Clinical Endocrinology & Metabolism* 109(2):e602–e612.

Neel, N., and M. S. Tarabay. 2018. Omphalocele, exstrophy of cloaca, imperforate anus, and spinal defect complex, multiple major reconstructive surgeries needed. *Urology Annals* 10(1):118–121.

Ng, S. M., K. M. Stepien, and A. Krishan. 2020. Glucocorticoid replacement regimens for treating congenital adrenal hyperplasia. *Cochrane Database of Systematic Reviews* 3(3):CD012517.

Ogawa, T., F. Takizawa, Y. Mukoyama, A. Ogawa, and J. Ito. 2021. Renal morphology and function from childhood to adulthood in Turner syndrome. *Clinical and Experimental Nephrology* 25(6):633–640.

Palmert, M. R., and L. Dunkel. 2012. Clinical practice: Delayed puberty. *New England Journal of Medicine* 366(5):443–453.

Pasterski, V., P. Prentice, and I. A. Hughes. 2010. Impact of the consensus statement and the new DSD classification system. *Best Practice & Research Clinical Endocrinology & Metabolism* 24(2):187–195.

Pasterski, V., K. Mastroyannopoulou, D. Wright, K. J. Zucker, and I. A. Hughes. 2014. Predictors of posttraumatic stress in parents of children diagnosed with a disorder of sex development. *Archives of Sexual Behavior* 43(2):369–375.

Pasterski, V., K. J. Zucker, P. C. Hindmarsh, I. A. Hughes, C. Acerini, D. Spencer, S. Neufeld, and M. Hines. 2015. Increased cross-gender identification independent of gender role behavior in girls with congenital adrenal hyperplasia: Results from a standardized assessment of 4- to 11-year-old children. *Archives of Sexual Behavior* 44(5):1363–1375.

Persani, L., M. Cools, S. Ioakim, S. Faisal Ahmed, S. Andonova, M. Avbelj-Stefanija, F. Baronio, J. Bouligand, H. T. Bruggenwirth, J. H. Davies, E. De Baere, I. Dzivite-Krisane, P. Fernandez-Alvarez, A. Gheldof, C. Giavoli, C. H. Gravholt, O. Hiort, P. M. Holterhus, A. Juul, C. Krausz, K. Lagerstedt-Robinson, R. McGowan, U. Neumann, A. Novelli, X. Peyrassol, L. A. Phylactou, J. Rohayem, P. Touraine, D. Westra, V. Vezzoli, and R. Rossetti. 2022. The genetic diagnosis of rare endocrine disorders of sex development and maturation: A survey among endo-ERN centres. *Endocrine Connections* 11(12):e220367.

Pofi, R., X. Ji, N. P. Krone, and J. W. Tomlinson. 2023. Long-term health consequences of congenital adrenal hyperplasia. *Clinical Endocrinology*. Advanced online publication. https://doi.org/10.1111/cen.14967.

Porsius, E., M. Spath, K. Kluivers, W. Klein, and H. Claahsen-van der Grinten. 2022. Primary amenorrhea with apparently absent uterus: A report of three cases. *Journal of Clinical Medicine* 11(15):4305.

Puar, T. H., N. M. Stikkelbroeck, L. C. Smans, P. M. Zelissen, and A. R. Hermus. 2016. Adrenal crisis: Still a deadly event in the 21st century. *American Journal of Medicine* 129(3):e331–e339.

Ranke, M. B. 1995. Growth hormone therapy in Turner syndrome: Analysis of long-term results. *Hormone Research* 44(Suppl 3):35–41.

Reiner, W. G., and J. P. Gearhart. 2004. Discordant sexual identity in some genetic males with cloacal exstrophy assigned to female sex at birth. *New England Journal of Medicine* 350(4):333–341.

Rhodes, M., S. A. Akohoue, S. M. Shankar, I.Fleming, A. Q. An, C. Yu, S. Acra, and M. S. Buchowski. 2009. Growth patterns in children with sickle cell anemia during puberty. *Pediatric Blood & Cancer*, 53(4):635–641.

Richards, S., N. Aziz, S. Bale, D. Bick, S. Das, J. Gastier-Foster, W. W. Grody, M. Hegde, E. Lyon, E. Spector, K. Voelkerding, H. L. Rehm, and the ACMG Laboratory Quality Assurance Committee. 2015. Standards and guidelines for the interpretation of sequence variants: A joint consensus recommendation of the American College of Medical Genetics and Genomics and the Association for Molecular Pathology. *Genetics in Medicine* 17(5):405–424.

Ridder, L. O., A. Berglund, K. Stochholm, S. Chang, and C. H. Gravholt. 2023. Morbidity, mortality, and socioeconomics in Klinefelter syndrome and 47,XYY syndrome: A comparative review. *Endocrine Connections* 12(5):e230024.

Righi, B., S. R. Ali, J. Bryce, J. W. Tomlinson, W. Bonfig, F. Baronio, E. C. Costa, G. Guaragna-Filho, G. T'Sjoen, M. Cools, R. Markosyan, T. Bachega, M. C. Miranda, V. Iotova, H. Falhammar, F. Ceccato, M. R. Stancampiano, G. Russo, E. Daniel, R. J. Auchus, R. J. Ross, and S. F. Ahmed. 2023. Long-term cardiometabolic morbidity in young adults with classic 21-hydroxylase deficiency congenital adrenal hyperplasia. *Endocrine* 80(3):630–638.

Rodriguez-Wallberg, K. A., F. Sergouniotis, H. P. Nilsson, and F. E. Lundberg. 2023. Trends and outcomes of fertility preservation for girls, adolescents and young adults with Turner syndrome: A prospective cohort study. *Frontiers in Endocrinology* 14:e1135249.

Romejko, K., A. Rymarz, H. Sadownik, and S. Niemczyk. 2022. Testosterone deficiency as one of the major endocrine disorders in chronic kidney disease. *Nutrients* 14(16):3438.

Rosenwohl-Mack, A., S. Tamar-Mattis, A. B. Baratz, K. B. Dalke, A. Ittelson, K. Zieselman, and J. D. Flatt. 2020. A national study on the physical and mental health of intersex adults in the U.S. *PLoS ONE [Electronic Resource]* 15(10):e0240088.

Ross, J. L., L. M. Long, M. Skerda, F. Cassorla, D. Kurtz, D. L. Loriaux, and G. B. Cutler, Jr. 1986. Effect of low doses of estradiol on 6-month growth rates and predicted height in patients with Turner syndrome. *Journal of Pediatrics* 109(6):950–953.

Saari, A., S. Harju, O. Makitie, M. T. Saha, L. Dunkel, and U. Sankilampi. 2015. Systematic growth monitoring for the early detection of celiac disease in children. *JAMA Pediatrics* 169(3):e1525.

Saggese, G., S. Bertelloni, and G. I. Baroncelli. 1997. Sex steroids and the acquisition of bone mass. *Hormone Research* 48(Suppl 5):65–71.

Samarasinghe, S., F. Meah, V. Singh, A. Basit, N. Emanuele, M. A. Emanuele, A. Mazhari, and E. W. Holmes. 2017. Biotin interference with routine clinical immunoassays: Understand the causes and mitigate the risks. *Endocrine Practice* 23(8):989–998.

Sandahl, K., J. Wen, M. Erlandsen, N. H. Andersen, and C. H. Gravholt. 2020. Natural history of hypertension in Turner syndrome during a 12-year pragmatic interventional study. *Hypertension* 76(5):1608–1615.

Sandberg, D. E., M. Gardner, and P. T. Cohen-Kettenis. 2012. Psychological aspects of the treatment of patients with disorders of sex development. *Seminars in Reproductive Medicine* 30(5):443–452.

Sandberg, D. E., M. Gardner, N. Callens, T. Mazur, the DSD-TRN Psychosocial Workgroup, the DSD-TRN Advocacy Advisory Network, and the Accord Alliance. 2017. Interdisciplinary care in disorders/differences of sex development (DSD): The psychosocial component of the DSD-translational research network. *American Journal of Medical Genetics Seminars in Medical Genetics Part C* 175(2):279–292.

Sandberg, D. E., M. Gardner, K. Kopec, M. Urbanski, N. Callens, C. E. Keegan, B. M. Yashar, P. Y. Fechner, M. Shnorhavorian, E. Vilain, S. Timmermans, and L. A. Siminoff. 2019. Development of a decision support tool in pediatric differences/disorders of sex development. *Seminars in Pediatric Surgery* 28(5):150838.

Saulnier, K. M., H. Gallois, and Y. Joly. 2021. Prenatal genetic testing for intersex conditions in Canada. *Journal of Obstetrics and Gynaecology Canada* 43(3):369–371.

Schönbucher, V., K. Schweizer, L. Rustige, K. Schutzmann, F. Brunner, and H. Richter-Appelt. 2012. Sexual quality of life of individuals with 46,XY disorders of sex development. *Journal of Sexual Medicine* 9(12):3154–3170.

Schweizer, K., F. Brunner, K. Schützmann, V. Schönbucher, and H. Richter-Appelt. 2009. Gender identity and coping in female 46,XY adults with androgen biosynthesis deficiency (intersexuality/DSD). *Journal of Counseling Psychology* 56(1):189–201.

Seminog, O. O., A. B. Seminog, D. Yeates, and M. J. Goldacre. 2015. Associations between Klinefelter's syndrome and autoimmune diseases: English national record linkage studies. *Autoimmunity* 48(2):125–128.

Sengupta, P., S. Dutta, I. R. Karkada, and S. V. Chinni. 2021. Endocrinopathies and male infertility. *Life* 12(1):10.

Speiser, P. W., W. Arlt, R. J. Auchus, L. S. Baskin, G. S. Conway, D. P. Merke, H. F. L. Meyer-Bahlburg, W. L. Miller, M. H. Murad, S. E. Oberfield, and P. C. White. 2018. Congenital adrenal hyperplasia due to steroid 21-hydroxylase deficiency: An endocrine society clinical practice guideline. *Journal of Clinical Endocrinology & Metabolism* 103(11):4043–4088.

SSA (Social Security Administration). 2017. Revisions to rules regarding the evaluation of medical evidence. *Federal Register* 82(5869).

Stancampiano, M. R., K. Suzuki, S. O'Toole, G. Russo, G. Yamada, and S. Faisal Ahmed. 2022. Congenital micropenis: Etiology and management. *Journal of the Endocrine Society* 6(2):bvab172.

Sullivan, S. D., P. M. Sarrel, and L. M. Nelson. 2016. Hormone replacement therapy in young women with primary ovarian insufficiency and early menopause. *Fertility and Sterility* 106(7):1588–1599.

Sultan, C., P. Philibert, L. Gaspari, F. Audran, L. Maimoun, N. Kalfa, and F. Paris. 2014. Chapter 5 - androgen insensitivity syndrome. In *Genetic steroid disorders*, edited by M. I. New, O. Lekarev, A. Parsa, T. T. Yuen, B. W. O'Malley and G. D. Hammer. San Diego: Academic Press. Pp. 225–237.

Sutton, E. J., A. McInerney-Leo, C. A. Bondy, S. E. Gollust, D. King, and B. Biesecker. 2005. Turner syndrome: Four challenges across the lifespan. *American Journal of Medical Genetics Part A* 139A(2):57–66.

Tack, L. J. W., E. Maris, L. H. J. Looijenga, S. E. Hannema, L. Audi, B. Kohler, P. M. Holterhus, S. Riedl, A. Wisniewski, C. E. Fluck, J. H. Davies, G. T'Sjoen, A. K. Lucas-Herald, O. Evliyaoglu, N. Krone, V. Iotova, O. Marginean, A. Balsamo, G. Verkauskas, N. Weintrob, M. Ellaithi, A. Nordenstrom, A. Verrijn Stuart, K. B. Kluivers, K. P. Wolffenbuttel, S. F. Ahmed, and M. Cools. 2018. Management of gonads in adults with androgen insensitivity: An international survey. *Hormone Research in Paediatrics* 90(4):236–246.

Tallaksen, H. B. L., E. B. Johannsen, J. Just, M. H. Viuff, C. H. Gravholt, and A. Skakkebaek. 2023. The multi-omic landscape of sex chromosome abnormalities: Current status and future directions. *Endocrine Connections* 12(9):e230011.

Tartaglia, N. R., R. Wilson, J. S. Miller, J. Rafalko, L. Cordeiro, S. Davis, D. Hessl, and J. Ross. 2017. Autism spectrum disorder in males with sex chromosome aneuploidy: XXY/Klinefelter syndrome, XYY, and XXYY. *Journal of Developmental & Behavioral Pediatrics* 38(3):197–207.

Therrell, B. L. 2001. Newborn screening for congenital adrenal hyperplasia. *Endocrinology & Metabolism Clinics of North America* 30(1):15–30.

Thigpen, A. E., D. L. Davis, A. Milatovich, B. B. Mendonca, J. Imperato-McGinley, J. E. Griffin, U. Francke, J. D. Wilson, and D. W. Russell. 1992. Molecular genetics of steroid 5 alpha-reductase 2 deficiency. *Journal of Clinical Investigation* 90(3):799–809.

Thunström S., E. Thunström, S. Naessén, K. Berntorp, M. Laczna Kitlinski, B. Ekman, J. Wahlberg, I. Bergström, O. Bech-Hanssen, E. Krantz, C. M. Laine, I. Bryman, and K. Landin-Wilhelmsen. 2023. Aortic size predicts aortic dissection in Turner syndrome: A 25-year prospective cohort study. *International Journal of Cardiology* 373: 47–54.

Thyen, U., A. Lux, M. Jurgensen, O. Hiort, and B. Kohler. 2014. Utilization of health care services and satisfaction with care in adults affected by disorders of sex development (DSD). *Journal of General Internal Medicine* 29(Suppl 3):S752–S759.

Tomaselli, S., F. Megiorni, C. De Bernardo, A. Felici, G. Marrocco, G. Maggiulli, B. Grammatico, D. Remotti, P. Saccucci, F. Valentini, M. C. Mazzilli, S. Majore, and P. Grammatico. 2008. Syndromic true hermaphroditism due to an R-spondin1 (RSPO1) homozygous mutation. *Human Mutation* 29(2):220–226.

Tomlinson, C., H. Macintyre, C. A. Dorrian, S. F. Ahmed, and A. M. Wallace. 2004. Testosterone measurements in early infancy. *Archives of Disease in Childhood: Fetal and Neonatal Edition* 89(6):F558–F559.

Torky, A., N. Sinaii, S. Jha, J. Desai, D. El-Maouche, A. Mallappa, and D. P. Merke. 2021. Cardiovascular disease risk factors and metabolic morbidity in a longitudinal study of congenital adrenal hyperplasia. *Journal of Clinical Endocrinology & Metabolism* 106(12):e5247–e5257.

Traino, K. A., C. M. Roberts, R. S. Fisher, A. M. Delozier, P. F. Austin, L. S. Baskin, Y. M. Chan, E. Y. Cheng, D. A. Diamond, A. J. Fried, B. Kropp, Y. Lakshmanan, S. Z. Meyer, T. Meyer, C. Buchanan, B. W. Palmer, A. Paradis, K. J. Reyes, A. Tishelman, P. Williot, C. Wolfe-Christensen, E. B. Yerkes, L. L. Mullins, and A. B. Wisniewski. 2022. Stigma, intrusiveness, and distress in parents of children with a disorder/difference of sex development. *Journal of Developmental & Behavioral Pediatrics* 43(7):e473–e482.

T'Sjoen, G., G. De Cuypere, S. Monstrey, P. Hoebeke, F. K. Freedman, M. Appari, P. M. Holterhus, J. Van Borsel, and M. Cools. 2011. Male gender identity in complete androgen insensitivity syndrome. *Archives of Sexual Behavior* 40(3):635–638.

Tyutyusheva, N., I. Mancini, G. I. Baroncelli, S. D'Elios, D. Peroni, M. C. Meriggiola, and S. Bertelloni. 2021. Complete androgen insensitivity syndrome: From bench to bed. *International Journal of Molecular Sciences* 22(3):1264.

Urban, M. D., P. A. Lee, J. P. Dorst, L. P. Plotnick, and C. J. Migeon. 1979. Oxandrolone therapy in patients with Turner syndrome. *Journal of Pediatrics* 94(5):823–827.

van de Grift, T. C., M. Rapp, G. Holmdahl, L. Duranteau, A. Nordenskjold, and the DSD-LIFE Group. 2022. Masculinizing surgery in disorders/differences of sex development: Clinician- and participant-evaluated appearance and function. *BJU International* 129(3):394–405.

Van den Eede, E., M. Sterckx, K. Vangelabbeek, C. Dunford, A. Noah, D. Wood, and G. De Win. 2023. An observational study on the sexual, genital and fertility outcomes in bladder exstrophy and epispadias patients. *Journal of Pediatric Urology* 19(1):e31–e37.

van der Horst, H. J., and L. L. de Wall. 2017. Hypospadias: All there is to know. *European Journal of Pediatrics* 176(4):435–441.

van der Zwan, Y. G., N. Callens, J. van Kuppenveld, K. Kwak, S. L. Drop, B. Kortmann, A. B. Dessens, K. P. Wolffenbuttel, and the Dutch Study Group on DSD. 2013. Long-term outcomes in males with disorders of sex development. *Journal of Urology* 190(3):1038–1042.

van Lisdonk, J. 2014. *Living with intersex/DSD: An exploratory study of the social situation of persons with intersex/DSD.* The Hague, Netherlands: The Netherlands Institute for Social Research.

van Rijn, S., L. Stockmann, M. Borghgraef, H. Bruining, C. van Ravenswaaij-Arts, L. Govaerts, K. Hansson, and H. Swaab. 2014. The social behavioral phenotype in boys and girls with an extra X chromosome (Klinefelter syndrome and trisomy X): A comparison with autism spectrum disorder. *Journal of Autism and Developmental Disorders* 44(2):310–320.

Villanueva, C., and J. Argente. 2014. Pathology or normal variant: What constitutes a delay in puberty? *Hormone Research in Paediatrics* 82(4):213–221.

Weidler, E. M., and K. E. Peterson. 2019. The impact of culture on disclosure in differences of sex development. *Seminars in Pediatric Surgery* 28(5):e150840.

Weijenborg, P. T. M., K. B. Kluivers, A. B. Dessens, M. J. Kate-Booij, and S. Both. 2019. Sexual functioning, sexual esteem, genital self-image and psychological and relational functioning in women with Mayer-Rokitansky-Kuster-Hauser syndrome: A case-control study. *Human Reproduction* 34(9):1661–1673.

Wilkins, L., M. M. Grumbach, J. J. Van Wyk, T. H. Shepard, and C. Papadatos. 1955. Hermaphroditism: Classification, diagnosis, selection of sex and treatment. *Pediatrics* 16(3):287–302.

Wisniewski, A. B. 2012. Gender development in 46,XY DSD: Influences of chromosomes, hormones, and interactions with parents and healthcare professionals. *Scientifica* 2012:834967.

Wisniewski, A. B., R. L. Batista, E. M. F. Costa, C. Finlayson, M. H. P. Sircili, F. T. Denes, S. Domenice, and B. B. Mendonca. 2019. Management of 46,XY differences/disorders of sex development (DSD) throughout life. *Endocrine Reviews* 40(6):1547–1572.

Witchel, S. F., T. Mazur, C. P. Houk, and P. A. Lee. 2022. The long path to our current understanding regarding care of children with differences/disorders of sexual development. *Hormone Research in Paediatrics* 95(6):608–618.

Wu, Q. Y., N. Li, W. W. Li, T. F. Li, C. Zhang, Y. X. Cui, X. Y. Xia, and J. S. Zhai. 2014. Clinical, molecular and cytogenetic analysis of 46,XX testicular disorder of sex development with SRY-positive. *BMC Urology* 14:70.

Wudy, S. A., G. Schuler, A. Sanchez-Guijo, and M. F. Hartmann. 2018. The art of measuring steroids: Principles and practice of current hormonal steroid analysis. *Journal of Steroid Biochemistry & Molecular Biology* 179:88–103.

Yatsenko, S. A., and A. Rajkovic. 2019. Genetics of human female infertility. *Biology of Reproduction* 101(3):549–566.

Yoon, J. C., J. L. Casella, M. Litvin, and A. S. Dobs. 2019. Male reproductive health in cystic fibrosis. *Journal of Cystic Fibrosis* 18:S105–S110.

Yoon, S. H., G. Y. Kim, G. T. Choi, and J. T. Do. 2023. Organ abnormalities caused by Turner syndrome. *Cells* 12(10):1365.

Zahra, B., A. Sastry, M. Freel, M. Donaldson, and A. Mason. 2023. Turner syndrome transition clinic in the west of Scotland: A perspective. *Frontiers in Endocrinology* 14:e1233723.

Zucker, K. J., S. J. Bradley, G. Oliver, J. Blake, S. Fleming, and J. Hood. 1996. Psychosexual development of women with congenital adrenal hyperplasia. *Hormones and Behavior* 30(4):300–318.

Part III

Sex, Gender, and Disability Determinations Introduction

With an understanding of the collection of sex and gender data in clinical practice (Part I) and a foundation of care and treatment for transgender and gender diverse (TGD) people and people with variations in sex traits (VSTs) (Part II), the final portion of this report examines the specific disability Listings within the statement of task and responds to the Social Security Administration's (SSA's) questions about whether changes in disability criteria may be warranted to assess these conditions accurately for TGD applicants and applicants with VSTs, considering current guidelines and standards of care.

Chapter 8 reviews Listings for adult and childhood respiratory disorders, including asthma, chronic obstructive pulmonary disease, and cystic fibrosis. Here, the committee examines the sex-specific pulmonary function tests contained in disability criteria—including spirometry and diffusing capacity of the lungs tests—assessing whether these tests are appropriate for measuring pulmonary function among TGD people and people with VSTs, or whether alternative measures may be more appropriate.

Chapter 9 examines the pediatric weight-for-length and body mass index–for-age tables. Both are gendered and may have implications for appropriate measurement for childhood disability applicants who are TGD or who have VSTs.

Chapter 10 reviews adult and childhood kidney disease and the use of estimated glomerular filtration rate (eGFR)—a common test of kidney function that has sex-specific criteria. Here the committee assesses whether eGFR is appropriate for measuring kidney function among TGD and VST populations, or whether alternative measurements may be more appropriate.

Chapter 11 focuses on reproductive cancers, including "cancers of the female genital tract" (which includes cancers of the uterus, uterine cervix, vulva, vagina, fallopian tubes, and ovaries) and cancers of the prostate gland, testicles, and penis. Here, the committee reviews current guidelines that recommend screening based on organs rather than gender identity or sex recorded at birth, and evaluates whether the language SSA uses to describe reproductive cancers could be updated to be more inclusive of TGD people and people with VSTs.

Chapter 12 reviews the gender-specific language under the disability Listing "HIV infection manifestations specific to women," and, similar to the analysis of reproductive cancers in Chapter 11, reviews whether language under this Listing could be worded differently to capture data on TGD people and people with VSTs more accurately.

Finally, in Chapter 13, the committee gives an overview of the various types of experts who inform SSA disability determinations at different stages in the process. The committee draws a few conclusions about where, within its current policies and processes, SSA might consider opportunities to ensure that these experts have the information and tools they need to make appropriate disability determinations for TGD applicants and applicants with VSTs.

8

Chronic Respiratory Disorders

Chronic respiratory diseases affect the airways and other structures of the lungs. While there are many chronic respiratory diseases, this chapter reviews only those that appear in the disability criteria established by the Social Security Administration (SSA) under 3.00 Respiratory Disorders—Adult and 103.00 Respiratory Disorders—Childhood. SSA further specified that this committee examine only those respiratory disorders that use sex-specific diagnostic criteria. Under SSA's disability criteria, there are two primary pulmonary function tests that, under current medical guidelines, use sex-specific diagnostic criteria: (1) spirometry and (2) diffusing capacity of the lungs for carbon monoxide (DLCO). Box 8-1 outlines the SSA disability Listings examined in this chapter, all of which contain spirometry and/or DLCO test measurements in disability criteria.

While asthma is a major focus of this chapter, it should be noted that the childhood Listing for asthma is absent from Box 8-1 and from this committee's charge. As explained in the notes to Box 8-1, SSA's childhood Listings include asthma as a category (under 103.03). However, to meet criteria for having a disability due to asthma under 103.03, a child applicant is required to demonstrate asthma exacerbations or complications that require hospitalization, but not to provide the results of any pulmonary function test (such as spirometry or DLCO).[1] For this reason,

---

[1] Under 103.03, SSA criteria state that child applicants must show asthma with "exacerbations or complications requiring three hospitalizations within a 12-month period and at least 30 days apart (the 12-month period must occur within the period we are considering in connection with your application or continuing disability review). Each hospitalization must last at least 48 hours, including hours in a hospital emergency department immediately before the hospitalization" (SSA, n.d.-b).

BOX 8-1
Disability Listings for Respiratory Disorders
with Sex-Specific Diagnostic Criteria

3.00 Respiratory Disorders—Adult:
   3.02: Chronic respiratory disorders due to any cause except CF[a]
   3.03: Asthma
   3.04: Cystic fibrosis
103.00 Respiratory Disorders—Childhood:
   103.02: Chronic respiratory disorders due to any cause except CF[b]
   103.04: Cystic fibrosis

NOTES: CF = cystic fibrosis.

[a] The adult Listing "Chronic respiratory disorders due to any cause except CF" (3.02) includes chronic obstructive pulmonary disease (COPD) (chronic bronchitis and emphysema), pulmonary fibrosis, pneumoconiosis, and bronchiectasis. This category also includes asthma, which covers cases of overlap between asthma and COPD (known as asthma–COPD overlap syndrome or ACOS).

[b] The childhood Listing "Chronic respiratory disorders due to any cause except CF" (103.02), includes COPD, pulmonary fibrosis, and asthma. The childhood Listings also include chronic lung disease of infancy (also known as bronchopulmonary dysplasia) under 103.02, but measurement of this condition does not include spirometry. For this reason, this report does not address this respiratory condition.

SOURCES: Social Security Administration (SSA), n.d.-a, b.

SSA did not include this specific Listing within the committee's statement of task.[2]

This chapter describes the multiple respiratory disorders listed in Box 8-1, describes available research on the prevalence of these disorders in transgender and gender diverse (TGD) people and people with variations in sex traits (VSTs), and examines whether and how gender-affirming hormone therapy impacts these disorders and overall lung function. This chapter also reviews the current research on pulmonary function tests,

---

[2] Other respiratory disorders—including chronic pulmonary hypertension (under 3.09), lung transplant (under 3.11 and 103.11), and respiratory failure (under 3.14 and 103.14)—are not included in this committee's charge as they do not include spirometry or DLCO measurements as part of the evaluation of disability for these conditions. In addition, this chapter does not include a discussion of lung cancer; while the committee acknowledges there are sex differences in the presentation of lung cancer and disparities for the transgender and gender diverse population, SSA's Listing for lung cancer (13.14) does not include sex- or gender-specific criteria and, therefore, this condition was not included within the statement of task. SSA childhood Listing 103.06, "Growth failure due to any chronic respiratory disorder," is within the committee's purview but included in the discussions of growth failure in Chapter 9.

appropriate evaluation criteria for TGD people or people with VSTs, and what this information means for SSA disability evaluation.

CHRONIC RESPIRATORY DISEASE: PREVALENCE AMONG TRANSGENDER AND GENDER DIVERSE PEOPLE AND PEOPLE WITH VARIATIONS IN SEX TRAITS

Respiratory diseases are common. An estimated 7.7 percent of American adults and children (24.96 million) have asthma (National Center for Environmental Health, 2023), and an estimated 6.5 percent of American adults (14.2 million) have chronic obstructive pulmonary disease (COPD) (Liu et al., 2023). While other respiratory diseases are less common, the substantial symptoms experienced by people who have these conditions can cause significant impairment and disability. Some data suggest that TGD people may experience a greater burden of respiratory disease relative to the general population, but respiratory disease is not well researched in TGD people, and few studies have examined these conditions among people with VSTs.

This section reviews the prevalence of asthma, COPD, pulmonary fibrosis, pneumoconiosis, bronchiectasis, and cystic fibrosis and, where possible, describes the known research on these conditions in TGD people and people with VSTs.

Asthma (Adult Listing 3.03)

Asthma is the most common chronic respiratory disease, affecting an estimated 262 million people worldwide (Global Asthma Network, 2022), including approximately 4.7 million children and 20.3 million adults in the United States (National Center for Environmental Health, 2023). Asthma attacks cause inflamed and narrowed airways, making it more difficult for air to flow out of the lungs during exhalation.

Asthma affects people of all ages and often starts during childhood. Of importance to this study, there are well-established sex differences in the prevalence of asthma throughout the lifespan: before adolescence, the prevalence of asthma is higher in populations assigned male sex at birth, but this trend is reversed after adolescence. In addition, after puberty, asthma severity worsens in people who go through typical female puberty compared with those who go through typical male puberty. According to asthma surveillance data from the Centers for Disease Control and Prevention (CDC, 2023a), males younger than 18 are more likely than their female counterparts to have asthma, asthma-related emergency department visits and hospitalizations, and mortality due to asthma. After puberty, CDC data show a sex shift in asthma prevalence, whereby asthma becomes more common among females compared with males, asthma severity (characterized by the rate of hospitalization and emergency department visits) becomes greater for female patients, and asthma-related mortality is higher in females (CDC, 2023a; National Center for Environmental Health, 2023). Gender differences in asthma incidence, prevalence, and severity, along with the postpuberty gender switch in asthma prevalence and severity, have been reported worldwide and indicate the importance of puberty for lung development and function (Almqvist et al., 2008; de Marco et al., 2000; Fu et al., 2014; Schatz and Camargo, 2003; Siroux et al., 2004; Yung et al., 2018; Zein and Erzurum, 2015).

Asthma in Transgender and Gender Diverse Populations

A few studies have attempted to estimate asthma in TGD populations. Using data from the U.S. Transgender Population Health Survey fielded from 2016 to 2018, researchers at the Williams Institute estimate that 208,500 transgender adults in the United States have asthma (Herman and O'Neill, 2020). Overall, research finds that transgender status is associated with a significantly greater risk of lifetime asthma. A 2018 cross-sectional study with a large clinical data set assessed the prevalence of lifetime asthma among transgender people, finding that asthma prevalence was high for transgender men (odds ratio [OR] 2.62; 95% confidence interval [CI] 2.40–2.85, p < .001 and highest among transgender women (OR 3.49; 95%CI 3.18–3.84, p < .001) compared with cisgender individuals of the same birth sex (Morales-Estrella et al., 2018).

Other studies have yielded similar results. A 2023 analysis of 2020 Behavioral Risk Factor Surveillance System survey data showed significantly higher odds of lifetime asthma among transgender men compared with cisgender individuals (Job et al., 2023), and a 2017 study of chronic conditions among Medicare beneficiaries observed higher percentages of asthma among transgender beneficiaries compared with cisgender beneficiaries (29.6 vs. 13.6 percent) (Dragon et al., 2017). Finally, the Minnesota Student Survey, an anonymous statewide school-based survey on the health and well-being of student populations in Minnesota, found that transgender students reported the highest prevalence of asthma across all grades (Minnesota Department of Health, 2019).

Finding accurate data on asthma prevalence is a challenge, as CDC's most recent data on asthma prevalence are based on the 2021 National Health Interview Survey (NHIS), which did not ask survey respondents about their gender identity or sex recorded at birth. However, the 2023 NHIS includes questions about gender identity or sex recorded at birth (CDC, 2023b), so future data may provide better estimates of asthma prevalence and severity among TGD populations in the United States.

Asthma in Populations with Variations in Sex Traits

A few studies have examined asthma risk among populations with VSTs. A 2021 study found that androgen insensitivity syndrome (AIS) is strongly associated with increased asthma risk (18.4 vs. 6.8 percent; p <. 001) (Gaston et al., 2021). The study found that the risk of asthma is higher in individuals with complete AIS than in those with partial AIS, and that both pediatric and adult populations with loss of androgen receptor function are at comparable asthma risk. Men with Klinefelter syndrome (characterized by lower concentration of testosterone) are more likely to be diagnosed with pulmonary diseases compared with men without Klinefelter syndrome (Bojesen et al., 2006), and asthma is also reported in this population (Ladias and Katsenos, 2018; Nan et al., 2013). It is unclear whether the 2023 NHIS will provide any data on asthma and populations with VSTs, as the 2023 questionnaire does not ask about VSTs, and while it asks about sex recorded at birth and gender identity, it does not allow for any free-text responses to these questions where a person might disclose or explain a variation in sex trait (CDC, 2023b).

Chronic Respiratory Disorders Due to Any Cause Except CF (SSA Adult Listing 3.02 and Childhood Listing 103.02)

The SSA Listing "Chronic respiratory disorders due to any cause except CF" [cystic fibrosis] is a category of respiratory disorders that includes COPD, pulmonary fibrosis, pneumoconiosis, asthma,[3] and bronchiectasis.[4,5]

---

[3] Asthma also has its own adult Listing, 3.03, and its own childhood Listing, 103.03. Asthma is also included under the Listing "Chronic respiratory disorders due to any cause except CF" (3.02 and 103.02) in recognition of the overlap between asthma and COPD. Asthma–COPD overlap syndrome (ACOS) is diagnosed for people who have symptoms of both asthma and COPD. It may be difficult for clinicians to distinguish between the two conditions, as asthma and COPD have overlapping symptoms and features. Therefore, for the purposes of disability evaluation, listing criteria under the broader category of 3.02 or 103.02 may be appropriate (ALA, 2023c; de Marco et al., 2013).

[4] Bronchiectasis has its own adult Listing, 3.07, but it is also included under "Chronic respiratory disorders due to any cause except CF" (3.02) in recognition of the fact that while some people experience bronchiectasis on its own, many will have a dual diagnosis of COPD and bronchiectasis. For disability applicants with both COPD and bronchiectasis, listing criteria under the broader category of 3.02 may be appropriate (Martinez-Garcia and Miravitlles, 2017).

[5] The adult Listing "Chronic respiratory disorders due to any cause except CF" (3.02) includes COPD (chronic bronchitis and emphysema), pulmonary fibrosis, pneumoconiosis, asthma, and bronchiectasis. The childhood Listing "Chronic respiratory disorders due to any cause except CF" (103.02) includes COPD, pulmonary fibrosis, and asthma. The childhood Listing "Chronic lung disease of infancy" (also known as bronchopulmonary dysplasia) is also included, but measurement of this condition does not include spirometry. For this reason, this report does not address this respiratory condition (SSA, n.d.-a,b).

Chronic Obstructive Pulmonary Disease (COPD)

Of the diseases within this disability Listing, COPD is by far the most common. COPD refers to a group of diseases—including emphysema and chronic bronchitis—that cause airflow blockage and persistent breathing-related problems. In 2021, an estimated 6.5 percent of adults in the United States (14.2 million) had COPD (Liu et al., 2023). Chronic lower respiratory diseases (of which COPD is the main component) were the sixth leading cause of death in the United States in 2021 (Liu et al., 2023).

Sex-specific differences have been reported for COPD. Historically, COPD was considered a disease that impacted mainly elderly men, but in many developed countries, it is now more prevalent among women (Boers at al., 2023; Mannino and Buist, 2007). While increases in rates of smoking among females have contributed to increases in COPD among women, research shows that females compared with males may be more susceptible to developing COPD, may have more severe disease, and may experience a more rapid decline in lung function (Barnes, 2016; Rea et al., 2024; Tam et al., 2011). Given these sex differences, COPD may impact TGD people or people with VSTs differently, but there is very limited research on COPD in these populations:

- *COPD and TGD Populations.* One study of chronic conditions among Medicare beneficiaries observed higher percentages of COPD among TGD compared with cisgender beneficiaries (27.3 vs. 20.8 percent) (Dragon et al., 2017). In an analysis of electronic health record data from the Veterans Health Administration, researchers found that, among known TGD veterans who had died between October 1999 and December 2019 (N = 1,415), 15.1 percent had died of COPD, and COPD was the third leading cause of death overall (Henderson et al., 2023). As with asthma, future data may provide better estimates of COPD prevalence among TGD people since the 2023 version of the NHIS, has, for the first time, included questions about sex recorded at birth and gender identity (CDC, 2023b), which could be used to track COPD in these populations.

- *COPD and Populations with VSTs.* The committee found only one study that examined COPD among populations with VSTs. Bojesen and colleagues (2006) found that men with Klinefelter syndrome are more likely than men without Klinefelter syndrome to be diagnosed with pulmonary diseases, such as COPD. Again as with asthma, despite including questions on sex recorded at birth and gender identity, the 2023 NHIS may not shed light on COPD prevalence among populations with VSTs because the questionnaire does not ask about VSTs or allow for free-text responses, which may prevent people with VSTs from reporting about COPD.

Pulmonary Fibrosis

Pulmonary fibrosis (PF) is a rare disease that causes scarring (fibrosis) of the lungs, which can make it difficult to breathe (ALA, 2023a). Some cases of PF can be caused by other diseases, medication, and/or genetics, or by inhalation of hazardous chemicals. Most often, however, the cause of PF is unknown, and the condition can be referred to as idiopathic pulmonary fibrosis (IPF). Although IPF is the most common type of PF, IPF is considered a rare disease, with prevalence rates in North America of 2.40 to 2.98 per 10,000 persons (Maher et al., 2021). However, IPF prevalence has been increasing in recent years, possibly occurring secondary to COVID-19 (Pergolizzi et al., 2023).

IPF is found predominantly in males: in international cohorts, males had a higher prevalence, with 67.7 percent found among males in an Australian registry and 78 percent of males in a study of low-income adults in France (Jo et al., 2017; Sesé et al., 2021). Males also have higher IPF-related mortality (Sauleda et al., 2018). Given its rarity in the population overall, PF has not been studied for TGD populations or populations with VSTs.

Pneumoconiosis

Pneumoconiosis comprises a spectrum of respiratory diseases caused by the inhalation of mineral dust in the lungs, usually as the result of certain occupations. For example, coal worker's pneumoconiosis, also known as "black lung disease," occurs when exposure to airborne coal and silica dust causes lung scarring (fibrosis), impairing the ability to breathe. While coal worker's pneumoconiosis declined over time in the United States with increased workplace safety procedures for coal miners, the disease has been on the rise since 2000, an increase that may be linked to changes in coal mining technology that appear to impact lung health negatively (Shriver and Bodenhamer, 2018). Researchers estimate the prevalence of coal worker's pneumoconiosis to be more than 10 percent among miners who have worked for 25 years or more (Potera, 2019). Men have higher occupational exposures associated with the development of pneumoconiosis (Shi et al., 2020), and therefore, the condition is found predominantly in men. Pneumoconiosis has not been studied for TGD populations or populations with VSTs.

Bronchiectasis

In this chronic lung condition, the walls of the bronchi or airways become irreversibly thickened and damaged, a phenomenon associated with persistent airway inflammation, chronic cough mucus buildup, and risk of infection (Chalmers et al., 2018). While it is often linked to CF, bronchiectasis can result from other conditions, including COPD and asthma, and it can also be caused by infections such as pneumonia, pertussis (whooping cough), and tuberculosis (ALA, 2024). Non-CF bronchiectasis was once considered an orphan disease, but its prevalence is increasing worldwide as a result of improved and increased use of imaging techniques such as computed tomography (CT) scans (Imam and Duarte, 2020). In one study of data from Medicare prescription drug plans, the average annual prevalence of bronchiectasis from 2012 to 2014 was 701 per 100,000 persons (Henkle et al., 2018), and the American Lung Association (2024) estimates that bronchiectasis affects an estimated 350,000 to 500,000 adults in the United States. The risk of developing bronchiectasis increases with age, and the condition is more common in women than in men (Henkle et al., 2018; Seitz et al., 2012). However, no studies have been published on the prevalence of bronchiectasis among TGD populations and populations with VSTs.

Cystic Fibrosis

Cystic fibrosis (CF) is an autosomal recessive inherited life-limiting disease that affects more than 40,000 adults and children in the United States, according to the Cystic Fibrosis Foundation (CFF) Patient Registry (CFF, n.d.-a.), and upward of 160,000 people worldwide (Guo et al., 2022). CF is a multisystem disorder, but people with CF most commonly die of complications of progressive respiratory failure (Mall and Elborn, 2014).

Multiple epidemiologic studies show that CF is a disease of equal incidence in females and males (given its autosomal recessive nature), but that females exhibit a decreased life expectancy, largely because of more severe lung disease (Harness-Brumley et al., 2014; Rosenfeld et al., 1997). Reports using the U.S. CFF Patient Registry show worse outcomes in females relative to males, even after adjusting for confounding morphometric, nutritional, and comorbid factors. In addition, *Pseudomonas aeruginosa*, one of the most common and pathogenic bacteria in CF, is acquired earlier and associated with a more rapid decline in lung function and higher mortality in females versus males with CF (Harness-Brumley et al., 2014; Rosenfeld et al., 1997). Etiologies for this differential are likely multifactorial, but sex hormones have been implicated. Several pathophysiology studies suggest that estrogen can convert *Pseudomonas aeruginosa* to a more pathogenic mucoid form, increases mucus synthesis in airway epithelium, is associated with more pulmonary inflammation, and inhibits calcium-mediated chloride channels on the airway epithelial cell surface—all of these factors may contribute to the sex disparity in CF (Abid et al., 2017; Chotirmall et al., 2012; Coakley et al., 2008; Demko et al., 1995; Holtrop et al., 2021; Tam et al., 2014).

Cystic Fibrosis and TGD Populations

No published data exist on the prevalence of CF among TGD populations (Shaffer et al., 2021). However, researchers have estimated that 200–300 people with CF may identify as TGD (Shaffer et al., 2022).

Cystic Fibrosis and Populations with VSTs

CF is known to have a major impact on male reproductive health, and has been linked with male hypogonadism, a condition whereby the body does not produce enough testosterone during puberty (Khan et al., 2022; Yoon et al., 2019). CF is also genetically linked to congenital bilateral absence of the vas deferens, a rare obstructive anomaly that contributes to male factor infertility; nearly 95 percent of men with CF have this condition (de Souza et al., 2018; Hannema and Hughes, 2007). Cases of people with Turner syndrome and CF have been reported, but CF has not been studied in this population (Wu et al., 2022).

IMPACT OF GENDER-AFFIRMING HORMONE THERAPIES ON LUNG FUNCTION

The pathophysiology of respiratory diseases is complex, and many factors may contribute to sex differences in chronic respiratory disorders. These include the influence of sex differences on environmental factors, such as differing immune responses to viral infection (Malinczak et al., 2019), rhinitis prevalence (Pinart et al., 2017), and different exposures to asthma-causing triggers, as well as the contribution of specific genetic risk factors, which differs between males and females (Hunninghake et al., 2010; Ranjbar et al., 2020). However, since females experience greater prevalence, morbidity, and mortality for many respiratory diseases, some research has examined the role of circulating female hormones (estradiol and progesterone) and male hormones (androgen or testosterone) in these conditions. This section examines sex hormones, their impact on respiratory disease, and the potential impact of gender-affirming hormone therapy (GAHT) on lung function.

Asthma

Circulating sex hormones from endogenous and exogenous sources may influence sex differences in asthma-related outcomes in adults (McCleary et al., 2018; Zein et al., 2021). The trends observed in asthma prevalence and severity suggest that hormonal changes occurring during puberty may contribute to the increased incidence of asthma in adult females (McCleary et al.,

2018; Naeem and Silveyra, 2019; Sathish et al., 2015). In general, research shows that estrogen and progesterone aggravate asthma and other allergic diseases, whereas androgen and testosterone suppress such diseases. Studies show that androgens may have a beneficial effect on lung function and may protect against asthma in adults through systemic and airway-specific anti-inflammatory effects (Becerra-Diaz et al., 2020; Han et al., 2020; McManus et al., 2022; Mohan et al., 2015), while estrogen and progesterone may have a detrimental effect on adult lung function, increasing allergic airway inflammation (DeBoer et al., 2018; Fuseini and Newcomb, 2017; Han et al., 2020; McCleary et al., 2018).

It is important to take into account the impact of hormones on the lungs when considering lung function for TGD people who have asthma and who may have accessed GAHT in puberty or adulthood. As described in detail in Chapter 5, some TGD adolescents may elect to delay puberty (using puberty blockers) and later access GAHT to go through the puberty of their affirmed gender. Other TGD people may complete the puberty of their birth sex and later access GAHT in adulthood. These treatment decisions impact what hormones were present during puberty, which in turn may impact the eventual size and function of the lungs, along with risks for asthma or other lung conditions (Fechter-Legget, 2023).

Researchers hypothesize that because of the important role of hormones in lung development during puberty, populations who access GAHT prior to or during puberty could be expected to have lung size more aligned with their affirmed gender rather than with their sex recorded at birth (Turner et al., 2021). However, more research is needed to understand fully whether and how GAHT during puberty affects lung function and, consequently, acute and/or long-term asthma risk.

For TGD populations that access GAHT in adulthood (after first going through natal puberty), the impact of these exogenous hormones on asthma prevalence and severity is inconclusive and has not been well studied. One cross-sectional study with a large clinical data set assessed the prevalence of lifetime asthma among TGD individuals. The researchers hypothesized that transgender women (who take exogenous feminizing hormone therapy) would have a higher risk of asthma compared with transgender men (who take exogenous masculinizing hormone therapy); however, the study did not show a causative effect of gender-affirming masculinizing or feminizing hormone therapy (Morales-Estrella et al., 2018).

Studies of cisgender populations have found similar conflicting and unclear results when examining the impact of exogenous hormone therapy on asthma incidence and severity. Several studies of pre- and postmenopausal women using hormone replacement therapy show increased risk of asthma onset (Bønnelykke et al., 2015; Gómez Real et al., 2006; Shah and Newcomb, 2018; Troisi et al., 1995; Zemp et al., 2012). However, the findings of studies on this topic are inconsistent, and evidence on the role of exogenous female hormones in asthma severity in women is conflicting (Carlson et al., 2001; Naeem and Silveyra, 2019; Shah et al., 2021), with some studies showing that the use of these hormones may in fact decrease asthma risk in women (Zhang et al., 2023).

Chronic Respiratory Disorders Due to Any Cause Except CF

Studies have examined the factors that may contribute to COPD among females. As smoking and exposure to cigarette smoke are major contributors to COPD risk, studies have examined the role of sex hormones in metabolism of cigarette smoke. In studies using mice models, airways of female mice demonstrated greater injury when exposed to cigarette smoke than airways of male mice (Chichester et al., 1994; Van Winkle et al., 2002). Testosterone, on the other hand, may be protective. In a 2023 study of two separate large COPD cohorts (with baseline measurement of testosterone and longitudinal data pertaining to health outcomes in both men and women), researchers demonstrated that circulating testosterone levels are not associated with COPD exacerbations or all-cause mortality (Pavey et al., 2023).

Compared with research on asthma, research on COPD and GAHT is much more limited, with only one published case report examining COPD for a transgender female (Cortes-Puentes et al., 2023). In a 2023 scoping review of existing research on health inequities surrounding the treatment and prevention of COPD, the authors uncovered only one study examining LGBTQ+ populations with COPD and no studies researching GAHT's impact on lung function in TGD patients with COPD (Rea et al., 2024).

The impact of endogenous hormones or GAHT on pulmonary fibrosis, pneumoconiosis, and bronchiectasis has not been examined in detail.

Cystic Fibrosis

Little is known about the effect of GAHT on a person with CF. Two case reports of transgender women with CF who were treated with estrogen gender-affirming therapy show a potential decline in health. One case showed a decline in lung function as estrogen levels rose, and the other showed acquisition of *Pseudomonas aeruginosa* for the first time after initiation of the hormone therapy (Lam et al., 2020; Shaffer et al., 2021). Whether either of these findings is directly related to the hormone treatment is unknown.

Importantly, people with CF have higher rates of anxiety and depression relative to the general population, as do individuals who identify as LQBTQ+ (Guta et al., 2021; Latchford and Duff, 2013; Riekert et al., 2007). Given the impacts of mental health on health outcomes in CF, it is critical to factor in mental health when making decisions about GAHT for people with CF.

IMPACT OF CHEST BINDING ON LUNG FUNCTION

"Chest binding" is any activity that involves compressing breast tissue to create a flatter chest appearance.[6] Some TGD people assigned female sex at birth may use chest binding to reduce the appearance of their breasts as a way of achieving a more masculine gender expression (Dutton et al., 2008; Maycock and Kennedy, 2014). Some people with VSTs may also use chest binders (Jarrett et al., 2018). Chest binding is a common practice, used by 87 percent of TGD respondents in one study (Jones et al., 2015). For transgender men, chest binding is not merely an elective activity to enhance appearance, but is an essential daily practice for reducing chest dysphoria (discomfort and distress from unwanted breast development), improving mental health outcomes, and increasing the sense of safety in public (Julian et al., 2021; Lee et al., 2019; Peitzmeier et al., 2022). Chapter 5 describes chest binding in further detail.

Minimal research exists on the use of chest binders, but some studies indicate their impact on pulmonary function. One study of transgender men who had either current or previous experience with chest binding (N = 1,273, all of whom had been assigned female sex at birth or had VSTs), found that more than half (51.7 percent) had a respiratory complaint (Jarrett et al., 2018). Another study found that transgender men who wore chest binders experienced several negative physical effects that implicate lung health, such as shortness of breath (46.6 percent of survey respondents), chest pain (48.8 percent), scarring (7.7 percent), or rib fractures (2.8 percent) (Peitzmeier et al., 2017). The authors of this study caution that their chest binding survey did not measure the severity of symptoms among respondents, did not assess whether these symptoms were transient or persistent, and may not be representative of all people who bind (Peitzmeier et al., 2022). There are no published data on the impact of chest binders on specific respiratory diseases such as asthma, COPD, or CF.

RESPIRATORY DISEASE AND SSA DISABILITY DETERMINATION

In addition to being common, respiratory conditions can lead to significant impairment and disability. Many people with respiratory diseases live active lives, but some experience severe symptoms and complications that may impact their ability to work or complete certain daily activities.

Severe Asthma

The symptoms of an asthma attack—shortness of breath, chest tightness, wheezing, or coughing—can often be managed by medication and by

---

[6] Examples of chest binding include wearing one or multiple sports bras, wrapping the chest with elastic bandages, and wearing specially designed commercial binders.

avoiding the triggers that can cause an attack. When asthma is not well controlled, however, some people may require more intensive or prolonged treatment, with frequent emergency room visits or hospitalizations. Asthma accounted for 94,560 discharges from hospital inpatient care and nearly 1 million emergency department visits in 2020, and for 6.5 percent of all physician office visits in 2019 (Santo and Kang, 2023). People with severe asthma may have to limit activity because of the frequency and severity of asthma attacks.

Advanced COPD

Common COPD symptoms are shortness of breath, coughing, and difficulty breathing deeply; with advanced COPD, these symptoms can progress to the point where an individual is too breathless to leave the home (Miravitlles and Ribera, 2017). People with advanced COPD may require frequent emergency care and hospitalization: COPD accounted for 791,000 emergency department visits in 2020, and research indicates that up to 19 percent of people with COPD who experience an exacerbation will require hospital admission (Cairns and Kang, 2021), and up to 24 percent will be readmitted within 30 days of discharge (Miravitlles et al., 2023). People with COPD can have additional extrapulmonary symptoms, including muscle wasting, cardiovascular disease, depression, osteopenia, and chronic infections (Barnes, 2010). When COPD is severe, symptoms of the condition can affect a person's ability to complete certain daily activities, such as walking or performing manual tasks.

Advanced CF

The severity of CF symptoms can vary widely from person to person. Symptoms can be managed through airway clearance, inhaled medications, and regular physical activity (CFF, n.d.-a.). Those with advanced CF may have significant difficulty breathing, leading to severe discomfort and the need for daily oxygen therapy, pulmonary rehabilitation, and symptom and pain management from palliative care specialists (CFF, n.d.-b.). In addition, CF may cause recurrent infections of the lungs and sinuses and impact other organs and systems, causing pancreatic insufficiency, gastrointestinal dysmotility, CF-related diabetes, arthropathy, and bone disease (Basile et al., 2023). These symptoms and complications may cause lengthy hospitalizations: studies from the United States and United Kingdom have found that CF patients have mean lengths of hospital stays of 9 days (Bradley et al., 2013; Vadagam and Kamal, 1995). For patients at this stage of disease, it may be difficult to continue working because of time-consuming treatments and the inability to engage in physical activity because of breathing difficulties.

The significant symptoms that occur with advanced respiratory disease can cause severe impairment and disability. These factors lead people with asthma, COPD, CF, and other respiratory diseases to seek disability benefits from SSA. As a whole, respiratory diseases accounted for 2.4 percent of all Social Security Disability Income (SSDI) recipients (217,378 people) and 1.75 percent of Supplemental Security Income recipients (91,328 people) according to 2022 data published by SSA (2022, 2023).

Pulmonary Function Tests and SSA Disability Criteria

A person (child or adult) with respiratory disease must show medical evidence to SSA documenting the severity of their condition. While medical evidence may include many things (e.g., a description of a patient's reaction to prescribed treatment or evidence of recurrent hospitalizations), a primary piece of medical evidence to support a respiratory disability application is the result of one or more pulmonary function tests (PFTs). Monitoring pulmonary function is central to discussions about respiratory health for people with asthma, COPD, CF, and other respiratory diseases, and most people with respiratory concerns will have medical records that contain documentation of a PFT.

Table 8-1 outlines the various PFTs accepted under SSA disability criteria for Listings 3.02, 3.03, 3.04, 103.02, and 103.04, along with sex-specific criteria used for disability evaluation.

Questions around sex and gender identity become important for certain PFTs, given that SSA's respiratory disease Listings follow current medical guidelines by including sex-specific diagnostic criteria, as outlined in Table 8-1. This section examines spirometry and DLCO tests, sex-specific components of these tests, and whether modified or alternative approaches to spirometry and DLCO are appropriate for TGD people and people with VSTs.

Spirometry

Spirometry, the most common PFT, plays an important role in the diagnosis and management of chronic lung conditions (Graham et al., 2019). Spirometry tests assess how well a patient's lungs work by measuring how much air they can breathe in and out of their lungs and how efficiently they can exhale air from their lungs (ALA, 2023b). These results may be used to monitor the progression of lung disease and response to therapy.

Key spirometry measurements include the following:

- **Forced expiratory volume (FEV_1).** The volume of air a person exhales in the first second of the spirometry test. Lower FEV_1

TABLE 8-1 Disability Evaluation Under SSA Criteria: Pulmonary Function Tests Included Under Listings 3.02, 3.03, 3.04, 103.02, and 103.04

Listing	Pulmonary Function Test Included in Criteria	Sex-Specific Criteria
3.00 Respiratory Disorders—Adult		
3.02 Chronic respiratory disorders due to any cause except CF	Spirometry • Forced expiratory volume (FEV_1) reading under 3.02A • Forced vital capacity (FVC) reading under 3.02B	An adult claimant's FEV_1 or FVC value must be less than or equal to the value in the table for the claimant to meet disability criteria. • For adults aged 18 and older, FEV_1 and FVC values are calculated by gender and height without shoes.
	Diffusing capacity of the lungs for carbon monoxide (DLCO) (3.02C1)	Average of two unadjusted, single-breath DLCO measurements less than or equal to the table value. • For adults aged 18 and older, DLCO values are calculated by gender and height without shoes.
	Arterial blood gas (ABG) test (3.02C2)[a]	None
	Pulse oximetry (3.02C3)[b]	None
3.03 Asthma	Spirometry • FEV_1 reading under 3.03A	An adult claimant's FEV_1 value must be less than or equal to the value in the table for the claimant to meet disability criteria. • For adults aged 18 and older, FEV_1 values are calculated by gender and height without shoes.
3.04 Cystic fibrosis	Spirometry • FEV_1 reading under 3.04A	An adult claimant's FEV_1 value must be less than or equal to the value in the table for the claimant to meet disability criteria. • For adults aged 18 and older, FEV_1 values are calculated by gender and height without shoes.
	Pulse oximetry (3.04F)[b]	None

continued

TABLE 8-1 (Continued)

Listing	Pulmonary Function Test Included in Criteria	Sex-Specific Criteria
103.00 Respiratory Disorders—Childhood		
103.02 Chronic respiratory disorders due to any cause except CF	Spirometry • FEV_1 reading under 103.02A • FVC reading under 103.02B	A child claimant's FEV_1 or FVC value must be less than or equal to the value in the table for the claimant to meet disability criteria. • For children aged 13 to attainment of age 18, values are calculated by gender and height without shoes. • For children aged 6 to attainment of age 13, the values are not sex specific. (Spirometry values not included under SSA criteria for assessment of children younger than 6).
103.04 Cystic fibrosis	Spirometry • FEV_1 reading under 103.04A	

[a] An ABG test—which measures the oxygen and carbon dioxide levels in the blood, as well as the blood's acidity (pH)—is one of the tests used for COPD diagnosis. It does not have sex-specific criteria, meaning a provider does not interpret readings differently for male and female patients.
[b] Pulse oximetry measures arterial oxygen saturation levels (how much oxygen the hemoglobin in the blood is carrying) and is commonly used in the management of COPD, CF, and other lung conditions to check pulmonary function. A pulse oximetry reading can help a provider determine whether a patient requires supplemental oxygen or whether hospitalization may be appropriate. Pulse oximetry measurements do not have sex-specific criteria, meaning a provider does not interpret readings differently for male and female patients.
NOTE: CF = cystic fibrosis; COPD = chronic obstructive pulmonary disease; SSA = Social Security Administration.
SOURCES: SSA, n.d.-a., n.d.-b.

readings indicate greater severity of breathing problems and more significant obstruction. SSA uses an applicant's highest FEV_1 value to evaluate respiratory function under 3.02A/103.02A ("Chronic respiratory disorders due to any cause except CF"), 3.03A ("Asthma"),[7] and 3.04A/103.04A ("Cystic fibrosis").

- **Forced vital capacity (FVC).** The maximum amount of air a person can forcefully exhale after breathing as deeply as possible. An FVC reading lower than normal indicates restricted breathing. Under 3.02B/103.02B ("Chronic respiratory disorders due to any cause except CF"), SSA uses an applicant's highest FVC value to evaluate respiratory function.

Questions around sex and gender identity become important in spirometry testing because spirometry values are calculated based on age, height, and sex (Stanojevic et al., 2022).

Current recommendations from the European Respiratory Society/ American Thoracic Society (ERS/ATS) advise clinicians that "biological sex" is the appropriate reference sex for calculating percent predicted values and interpreting spirometry results (Graham et al., 2019; Stanojevic et al., 2022). While the guidelines acknowledge the importance of gender identity, they make clear that sex recorded at birth is the more accurate predictor of lung size. The 2022 ERS/ATS *Technical Standard on Interpretive Strategies for Routine Lung Function Tests* (ERS/ATS Technical Standard) states (Stanojevic et al., 2022):

> Sex is an important predictor of lung size, even after accounting for differences in height. Thus, while gender identity should be respected, use of biological sex will yield a more accurate prediction of lung function. (p. 6)

These guidelines echo the ERS/ATS *Standardization of Spirometry, 2019 Update,* which states (Graham et al., 2019):

> When requesting birth sex data, patients should be given the opportunity to provide their gender identity as well and should be informed that although their gender identity is respected, it is birth sex and not gender that is the determinant of predicted lung size. Inaccurate entry of birth sex may lead to incorrect diagnosis and treatment. (p. e75)

---

[7] SSA criteria do not ask for a spirometry test under the childhood Listing for asthma (103.03). A child applicant will meet criteria for disability due to asthma with evidence of exacerbations or complications requiring three hospitalizations (of at least 48 hours) within a 12-month period and at least 30 days apart (SSA, n.d-b).

Diffusing Capacity of the Lungs for Carbon Monoxide (DLCO)

DLCO is a measure used to assess the lungs' ability to transfer oxygen to the bloodstream upon inhalation (Modi and Cascella, 2024). SSA includes DLCO under disability evaluation criteria for Listing 3.02, "Chronic respiratory disorders due to any cause except CF."

The results of a DLCO test are given as a percentage of what a given patient's expected DLCO (predicted value) would be based on age, height, and sex. A low DLCO value means the lungs are not working efficiently to move oxygen from the air to the bloodstream. Table 8-2 shows the classification of DLCO, which is used to indicate the severity of respiratory disease.

The most recent ERS/ATS guidelines for DLCO, from 2017, call for the value of DLCO to vary with age, height, and sex (Graham et al., 2017). In contrast with spirometry, the DLCO guidelines do not mention whether and how gender identity should be assessed when interpreting DLCO tests.

PFT Interpretation for TGD People and People with VSTs

Given unclear evidence about how puberty-delaying medications and GAHT impact measurements of lung function, current spirometry guidelines do not call for modified spirometry measurements for TGD populations. However, the ERS/ATS Technical Standard recognizes that the impact of GAHT on lung function is not well understood and could be important for spirometry interpretation (Stanojevic et al., 2022):

> The effect of gender-affirming hormonal therapy on lung function is poorly understood, so the appropriate reference equation for transgender individuals is currently not known. Timing of gender reassignment, especially during adolescence, may impact lung growth and development and thus needs to be considered when interpreting results during adulthood. (p. 6)

For health care providers measuring lung function in TGD patients or patients with VSTs, it is not always clear which chart—male or female—is the more appropriate to use, and providers may get it wrong. Interpretation

TABLE 8-2 Results of Test for Diffusing Capacity of the Lungs for Carbon Monoxide (DLCO): Classification of DLCO

Normal DLCO	Lungs functioning at >75% of predicted value, up to 140%
Mildly reduced DLCO	60–75% of the lower limit of normal predicted value
Moderately reduced DLCO	40–60%
Severely reduced DLCO	<40%

SOURCE: Adapted from Modi and Cascella, 2024.

of PFTs using an inappropriate reference sex could lead to errors in either identifying a pulmonary abnormality that does not exist or failing to identify a pulmonary abnormality that does exist.

Part of the challenge in selecting the appropriate reference sex is that medical records may contain incorrect information (e.g., incorrect sex recorded in the patient chart), or providers may not ask questions that would provide a complete picture of patient characteristics (e.g., failing to ask about VSTs or about gender identity as separate from sex recorded at birth). Chapter 3 of this report describes these challenges in greater detail, but they are worth mentioning again here as the realities of medical record data collection can certainly impact interpretation of PFTs for TGD patients and patients with VSTs. Moreover, even when medical records contain a complete and accurate record of gender identity and sex recorded at birth such that providers are aware they are assessing a TGD patient or a patient with a VST, providers may lack familiarity with caring for these patients and may not know how or when TGD or VST lived experience impacts patient care and clinical decision making.

A few studies describe how choice of sex reference impacts PFT interpretation for TGD people. One study examining providers' reference sex choice for 15 TGD patients found that providers used female and male reference ranges inconsistently for these patients (Foer et al., 2021). Overall, providers predominantly selected a female reference range, independent of gender identity: a female reference was used to interpret PFTs for 60 percent of transgender men, 75 percent of transgender women, and 100 percent of gender nonbinary patients (Foer et al., 2021). The researchers found that use of the other gender reference range affected PFT interpretation, concluding that it may be appropriate to use both binary reference ranges for PFT interpretation to improve shared decision making with TGD patients.

Prior research has also described how reference choice impacts spirometry interpretation in particular, and how PFT interpretations based on the incorrect sex may place patients at risk for misdiagnosis and inappropriate treatment (Al-Hadidi and Baldwin, 2017; Haynes and Stumbo, 2018). Inaccurate medical tests, including misinterpretation of spirometry, can be especially harmful to TGD populations, as they already face stigma; discrimination; and systematic barriers, both institutional and structural.

Chest Binders and Pulmonary Function Tests

To obtain an estimate of lung function without restrictions in place, clinicians may ask patients to remove their chest binder or other restrictive clothing. As described above, however, for some TGD people, chest binders are worn daily and for extended periods of time as a critical component of gender-affirming care. Where a patient has removed their chest binder for the purposes of undergoing a PFT, that measurement of lung function may not take into account their daily lived experience. For this reason, it may be appropriate for some patients to continue wearing their binder during a PFT, and clinicians who are attuned to the needs of their TGD patients or patients with VSTs may engage them in decision making about the best approach to PFT measurement. However, medical records may not indicate whether a chest binder was worn during a PFT.

Alternative Measurements

To eliminate the error in selection of a reference sex for TGD and VST populations, using measures that are independent of sex may be preferable. Pulse oximetry and arterial blood gas tests (described in Table 8-1) are tests accepted by SSA that do not have sex-specific criteria and may be appropriate for measuring lung function in people with certain respiratory conditions, including COPD and CF.

In theory, it might be possible to devise alternative measures of lung function, such as calculating height along with chest circumference to predict the shape and size of a patient's thoracic cavity. As these kinds of measures are independent of sex or other variables (such as age), they could serve as a more accurate functional measure compared with a PFT (Fechter-Leggett, 2023). However, the currently available prediction equations include sex as a variable. While the ERS/ATS spirometry guidelines state that height may be a reasonable proxy for chest size, the authors state: "Sex is an important predictor of lung size, even after accounting for differences in height" (Stanojevic et al., 2022, p. 6).

Until guidelines shift to a sex-independent reference metric, providers will continue using reference sex in interpreting PFTs.

Dual Calculations

While current guidelines do not call for running PFT results against both reference sex ranges, some practitioners conducting spirometry for TGD patients use dual PFT calculations in practice to improve decision making for their patients (Foer, 2023). Guidelines in other clinical specialties—for example, measurements of bone mineral density (Rosen et al., 2019)—state that providers and patients may consider using both binary reference ranges as an option to improve clinical decision making. The strategy for running interpretations under both sex ranges has also been put forward for assessing body mass index in young TGD people (Kidd et al., 2019).

Terminology in SSA Criteria

As noted, current ERS/ATS recommendations advise that sex recorded at birth is the appropriate sex to use when interpreting spirometry and DLCO test results (Graham et al., 2017, 2019; Stanojevic et al., 2022). However, as displayed in Table 8-1, SSA's disability criteria use the term "gender" in reference to these measurements of lung function: "values are calculated by *gender* and height without shoes" [emphasis added]. This language may incorrectly indicate that it is "gender identity" that is determinative when interpreting lung function in Listings related to respiratory disease. The conflation of these terms throughout disability evaluation criteria can lead to confusion for both applicants and adjudicators. SSA might consider updating language under 3.02. 3.03, 3.04, 103.02, and 103.04 to reflect current guidelines. For example, under 3.02 (adult Listing for asthma), SSA criteria state:

> "For adults aged 18 and older, FEV_1 values are calculated by *gender* and height without shoes" [emphasis added].

This language would better reflect current guidelines if it read:

> "For adults aged 18 and older, FEV_1 values are calculated by *sex recorded at birth* and height without shoes."

SELECTING APPROPRIATE PULMONARY FUNCTION TEST REFERENCE SEX FOR TRANSGENDER ADULTS: AN INNOVATIVE APPROACH

The National Institute for Occupational Safety and Health (NIOSH) leads research on worker safety and health. As a research agency within CDC, NIOSH does not engage in regulation or enforce workplace safety regulations; these functions are within the purview of the Occupational Safety and Health Administration (OSHA, 2013) within the Department of Labor. Rather, NIOSH funds and conducts research, makes recommendations, provides technical assistance, and trains occupational safety and health professionals to ensure safe and healthful working conditions for all Americans. NIOSH's Respiratory Health Division focuses on researching, identifying, evaluating, and preventing work-related respiratory diseases, such as work-related asthma, COPD, and pneumoconiosis (NIOSH, 2018). Through field studies, it evaluates the frequency and severity of respiratory disease within various workplaces—for example, where workers are required to wear a respirator during work or perform jobs that cause exposure to possible lung hazards (e.g., asbestos)—and provides workplaces with appropriate recommendations for respiratory disease prevention (NIOSH, 2018).

The Respiratory Health Division uses spirometry testing as a primary means of surveilling respiratory health across the workforce. In 2019, NIOSH set out to develop better spirometry testing procedures and protocols for TGD workers (Fechter-Leggett et al., 2022). NIOSH's concern is that common PFT protocols—which state that to predict lung function, PFTs should be compared against a reference range corresponding to a person's sex recorded at birth—may not be appropriate for TGD workers, particularly those who were treated with puberty-delaying medications and began GAHT during puberty. These concerns are echoed by the ERS/ATS standards, which state: "Timing of gender reassignment, especially during adolescence, may impact lung growth and development and thus needs to be considered when interpreting results during adulthood" (Stanojevic et al., 2022, p. 6).

NIOSH Algorithm for Selection of Reference Sex

As noted above, if PFTs are interpreted with an inappropriate reference sex, the result could be either identifying a pulmonary abnormality that does not exist or failing to identify a pulmonary abnormality that does. To correct for these potential errors, NIOSH consulted with national experts in designing questions and an algorithm to inform the selection of a PFT reference sex for all adults, including TGD adults (Fechter-Leggett et al., 2022). The algorithm acknowledges that use of puberty-delaying medications (using the terminology "hormone blocking medications") and GAHT during puberty could impact PFT results. Therefore, instead of using "sex recorded at birth" as the metric for choosing the PFT reference sex, the algorithm uses "hormonal sex at puberty," or the hormone that was predominant during puberty (estrogen or testosterone) that influenced the shape and size of the thoracic cavity.

NIOSH's panel of experts reasoned that when people wait until adulthood to begin GAHT, their body completes the puberty of their sex recorded at birth. For these individuals, their body size and habitus, along with their thoracic cavity, can reasonably be expected to follow a pattern similar to that of peers of their same sex recorded at birth (Fechter-Leggett, 2023). For these individuals, the appropriate PFT reference sex may be their sex recorded at birth. However, the use of puberty-delaying medications and initiation of GAHT during puberty could promote the development of a body habitus similar to that of a person's affirmed gender. For this portion of the transgender population, affirmed gender—not sex recorded at birth— may be the more appropriate PFT reference sex.

NIOSH's algorithm starts with asking gender identity and sex recorded at birth (referred to as "sex assigned at birth" or "SAAB") in two separate questions, as shown in Figure 8-1. For most workers being tested for pulmonary function, their gender identity and sex recorded at birth will be

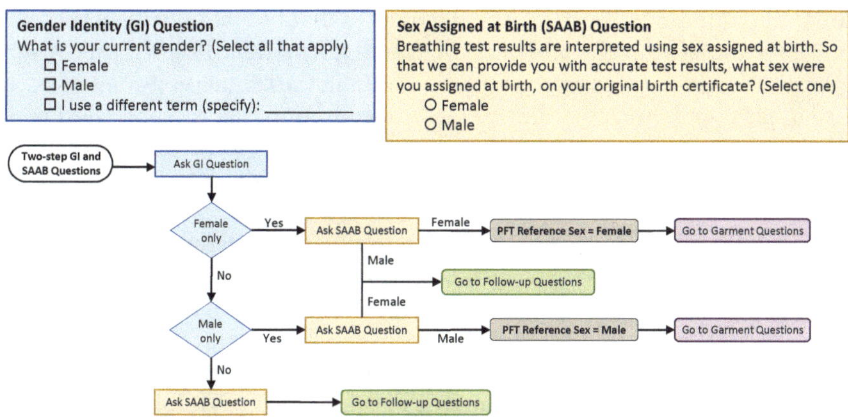

FIGURE 8-1 Selection of pulmonary function test (PFT) reference sex in adults: Questions about gender identity and sex recorded at birth.
SOURCE: Presented by Fechter-Leggett on September 14, 2023.

the same and determining the appropriate PFT reference sex requires only those two demographic questions. For people who have a different gender identity from their sex recorded at birth, the algorithm proceeds to a series of additional questions related to the use and timing of hormone therapy to determine the appropriate PFT reference sex (see Figure 8-2). Within these

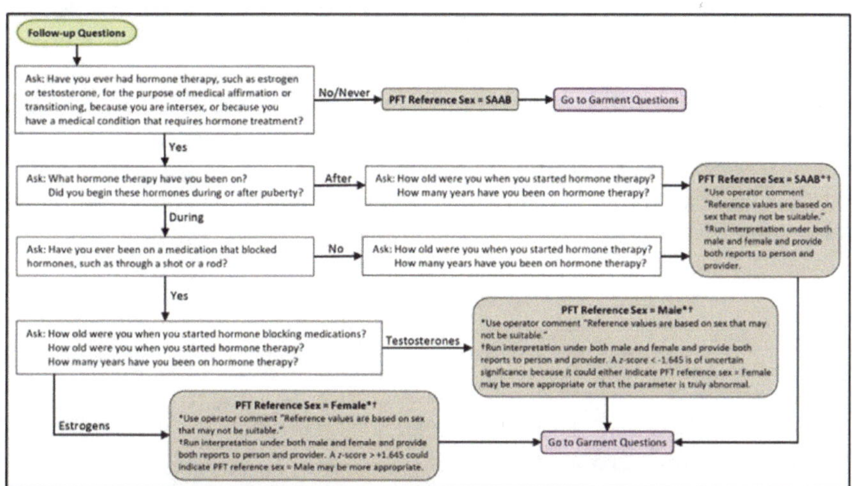

FIGURE 8-2 Selection of pulmonary function test (PFT) reference sex in adults: Follow-up questions.
SOURCE: Presented by Fechter-Leggett on September 14, 2023.

follow-up questions, the algorithm recognizes that not all individuals access hormone therapy for the purposes of gender affirmation. The first follow-up question encompasses persons with VSTs (using the terminology "intersex") and other populations that have a medical condition that requires hormone treatment. For all patients, there is a garment question to determine whether any garments are being worn that could interfere with PFT results, such as chest binders (Figure 8-3).

The algorithm guides providers in selecting the PFT reference sex most appropriate to the individual worker's gender identity and medical history. Ultimately, however, the available PFT reference ranges were constructed for a cisgender population. For individuals who have accessed hormone therapy, the reference values may be unsuitable regardless of which reference range is selected (male or female). For this reason, NIOSH's algorithm instructs providers to "run interpretation under both male and female and provide both reports to person and provider," and gives further instructions on interpreting these results (Figure 8-2). There is also a note at the bottom of the algorithm (shown in Figure 8-3) instructing clinicians to compare the current PFT results with those of previously recorded PFTs, where possible.

The algorithm distinguishes between individuals who began hormone therapy "during" and "after" puberty. Additional follow-up questions are included, such as "How old were you when you started hormone blocking medications?," "How old were you when you started hormone therapy?," and "How many years have you been on hormone therapy?" At this time, these questions do not impact decision making. For example, if two people began hormone therapy in adulthood, and one has been on hormone therapy for 2 years and the other on the same therapy for 25 years, the algorithm does not distinguish between these individuals. However, if future research determines that length of time on hormone therapy (or, e.g., age at onset of puberty-delaying medication) impacts lung function or severity of respiratory outcomes, then, by collecting these data today, providers can later reinterpret PFT results (Fechter-Leggett, 2023).

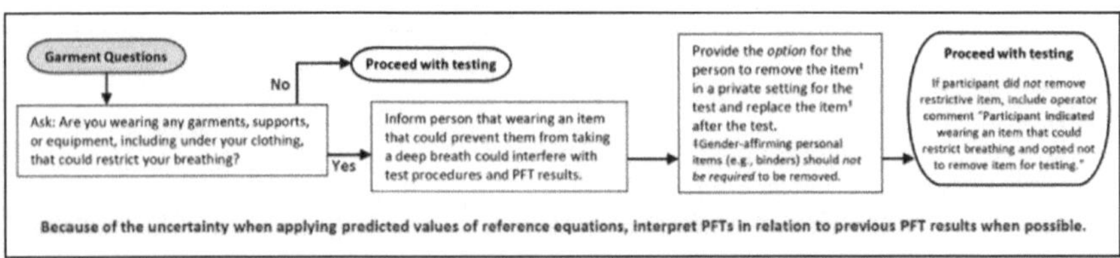

FIGURE 8-3 Selection of pulmonary function test (PFT) reference sex in adults: Garment questions.
SOURCE: Presented by Fechter-Leggett on September 14, 2023.

NIOSH is currently in the process of integrating the algorithm for selection of PFT reference sex into its work. The Respiratory Health Division expects to deploy, test, and evaluate the algorithm and its accompanying questions in field studies (Fechter-Leggett, 2023).

Sex Selection and Impact on Eligibility for SSDI

Dr. Ethan Fechter-Leggett, Research Epidemiologist, Field Studies Branch, NIOSH Respiratory Health Division, presented to the committee preliminary data on estimating the impact of decisions about reference sex on populations applying for SSDI (Fechter-Leggett, 2023). Using data from the 2007–2012 National Health and Nutrition Examination Survey (NHANES), Fechter-Leggett's team analyzed data on all adults over 18 who had acceptable spirometry documented (best-test FEV_1 and FVC estimates had quality ratings of A, B, or C as defined by the survey) and did not have missing height measurements (N = 13,589). Using SSA disability criteria under adult Listings 3.02, "Chronic respiratory disorders due to any cause except CF," and 3.03, "Asthma," the researchers analyzed how often the individuals included in the data set would meet SSA disability criteria using sex recorded at birth (sex in the NHANES data set is assumed to be sex recorded at birth) versus using the opposite sex. Tables 8-3 and 8-4 show preliminary results of this analysis.

As might be expected, most of the individuals in the data set (98 percent of those under criteria for 3.02 and 91.2 percent of individuals under criteria for 3.03) did not meet SSA disability criteria with either reference sex; for these individuals, changing the PFT reference sex would not ultimately change eligibility for SSDI. A small percentage (1.1 percent of individuals under criteria for 3.02 and 4.4 percent of those under criteria for 3.03)

TABLE 8-3 Listing 3.02A/B: FEV_1 or FVC Criteria for Chronic Respiratory Disorders, Any Cause except Cystic Fibrosis

	Opposite Sex		
Sex Recorded at Birth*	Does not meet 3.02A/B criteria	Meets 3.02A/B criteria	Total
Does not meet 3.02A/B criteria	13,314 (98%)	87 (0.6%)	13,401
Meets 3.02A/B criteria	41 (0.3%)	147 (1.1%)	188
Total	13,355	234	13,589

* Sex in the data set is assumed to be sex recorded at birth.
SOURCE: Fechter-Leggett, 2023.

TABLE 8-4 Listing 3.03A: FEV_1 Criteria for Asthma

	Opposite Sex		
Sex Recorded at Birth*	Does not meet 3.03A criteria	Meets 3.03A criteria	Total
Does not meet 3.03A criteria	12,399 (91.2%)	412 (3.0%)	12,811
Meets 3.03A criteria	185 (1.4%)	593 (4.4%)	778
Total	12,584	1,005	13,589

* Sex in the data set is assumed to be sex recorded at birth.
SOURCE: Fechter-Leggett, 2023.

met SSA disability criteria under both reference sexes; for these individuals, their lung function was poor enough that they would meet disability criteria under either scenario.

The remaining portion of the data set (0.9 percent of individuals under criteria for 3.02 and 4.4 percent of those under criteria for 3.03) had discordant results. For these individuals, if their spirometry test were interpreted with the opposite reference sex, they had a change in ability to meet SSDI disability criteria. All persons with sex recorded male at birth with discordant results (0.3 percent of those under criteria for 3.02 and 1.4 percent of those under criteria for 3.03) would no longer meet SSA disability criteria if evaluated with the opposite reference sex. All persons with sex recorded female at birth with discordant results (0.6 percent of those under criteria for 3.02 and 3.0 percent of those under criteria for 3.03) would meet disability criteria if evaluated with the opposite reference sex.

Overall, percent discordance differed by sex and was greater among persons with sex recorded female at birth. When breaking the data down by race/ethnicity, researchers found a larger percentage discordant results among non-Hispanic Black persons (both with sex recorded male at birth and sex recorded female at birth). Differences by race/ethnicity and sex highlight potentially disproportionately affected groups if an inappropriate reference sex is used for PFT interpretation.[8]

---

[8] The population in the NHANES data set is not the same as the population applying for disability benefits, so percentages of discordant results could be different among SSA disability benefit applicants. Still, patterns in the NHANES data of greater discordant results among females and non-Hispanic Black populations are worth noting and may indicate populations disproportionately impacted by choice of reference for PFT interpretation.

SUMMARY OF KEY POINTS

Chronic respiratory disorders can lead to significant impairment and disability. Although respiratory disorders in TGD populations and populations with VSTs are not well researched, existing data suggest that these populations may have a greater burden of respiratory disease.

Spirometry and DLCO are common PFTs that interpret lung function by comparing results against male and female reference ranges. For many applicants for disability benefits, PFTs can be appropriately compared against a reference range corresponding to a person's sex recorded at birth. However, SSA's disability criteria use the term "gender" in reference to PFTs, which may incorrectly indicate that "gender identity" is the determining factor in the interpretation of these measurements. SSA might consider changing the language in the respiratory disorder Listings to replace the word "gender" with "sex recorded at birth." Making this change would allow for clearer assessment for some TGD applicants and some applicants with VSTs.[9] Using the phrase "sex recorded at birth" rather than simply "sex" clarifies that sex as recorded at birth is the important patient characteristic for these specific assessments, not "sex" as may be recorded on other administrative records (e.g., driver's license, passport).

For other applicants, sex recorded at birth may *not* be the appropriate reference sex for assessing pulmonary function, particularly for populations who began puberty-delaying medications and GAHT during puberty. Here, research suggests that "hormonal sex at puberty"—the hormone that was predominant during puberty (estrogen or testosterone) and influenced the shape and size of the thoracic cavity—may be a more accurate metric for choosing the PFT reference sex. For this portion of the population, affirmed gender—not sex recorded at birth—may be the more appropriate PFT reference sex.

However, it may be appropriate for providers to interpret PFT results against both reference sex ranges ("dual calculations") to aid in clinical decision making for their patients, and SSA should be aware that it may receive medical records containing PFTs interpreted using both charts. SSA may also receive PFT calculations from both charts when providers were mistaken or lacked training and guidance on which chart to use. While considerable research is needed to determine best approaches, it is

---

[9] The committee stresses that even though sex recorded at birth is important for the assessments listed here, this does not negate the importance of gender identity for disability applicants in general or for other types of disability assessments. In addition, the committee acknowledges that for some people with VSTs, sex assignment at birth (which becomes the sex recorded on birth certificates and medical records) may not be straightforward and can change after the initial determination.

the consensus of the committee, based on its clinical expertise and professional judgment, that when the medical record contains PFTs interpreted using both charts, SSA would best serve applicants who receive GAHT by using the lowest recorded spirometry or DLCO reading to determine the presence of disability. Given the unknowns as to how GAHT impacts lung function, such an approach would ensure appropriate adjudication for TGD people and people with VSTs[10] who have not had access to providers trained to interpret their results thoughtfully and with consideration of their individual patient history.

Finally, use of chest binders is a common gender-affirming practice for TGD people assigned female sex at birth, as well as some people with VSTs. While minimal research exists on the impact of chest binders on pulmonary function, some patients may wear a chest binder during administration of a PFT. The medical record may not indicate whether a chest binder was worn during a PFT, but when the medical record contains different PFT values, SSA needs to be aware that those differences could be attributable to the fact that the patient wore a binder during one test but not another. For this reason and based on its clinical expertise and professional judgment, the committee concludes that SSA would best serve TGD applicants and applicants with VSTs by using the lowest recorded PFT value to determine disability under respiratory disorder Listings.

REFERENCES

Abid, S., S. K. Xie, M. Bose, P. W. Shaul, L. S. Terada, S. L. Brody, P. J. Thomas, J. A. Katzenellenbogen, S. H. Kim, D. E. Greenberg, and R. Jain. 2017. 17β-estradiol dysregulates innate immune responses to respiratory infection and is modulated by estrogen receptor antagonism. *Infection and Immunity* 85(10):e00422-17.

ALA (American Lung Association). 2023a. *Introduction to pulmonary fibrosis.* https://www.lung.org/lung-health-diseases/lung-disease-lookup/pulmonary-fibrosis/introduction#:~:text=What%20Is%20Pulmonary%20Fibrosis%3F,absorb%20oxygen%20into%20the%20bloodstream (accessed January 12, 2024).

ALA. 2023b. *What is spirometry and why it is done.* https://www.lung.org/lung-health-diseases/lung-procedures-and-tests/spirometry (accessed March 12, 2024).

ALA. 2023c. *Asthma-COPD overlap syndrome* (ACOS). https://www.lung.org/lung-health-diseases/lung-disease-lookup/asthma/learn-about-asthma/types/asthma-copd-overlap-syndrome (accessed May 21, 2024).

ALA. 2024. *Learn about bronchiectasis.* https://www.lung.org/lung-health-diseases/lung-disease-lookup/bronchiectasis/learn-about-bronchiectasis (accessed January 12, 2024).

Al-Hadidi, N., and J. L. Baldwin. 2017. Spirometry considerations in transgender patients. *Journal of Allergy and Clinical Immunology* 139(2):sAB198.

---

[10] Where people with VSTs take GAHT, the above approaches may be appropriate; however, research is limited on the impact of GAHT in populations with VSTs. The committee notes that people with VSTs take hormone therapy for a multitude of reasons beyond gender-affirming care and care is extremely individualized; the impact of various hormone therapies on sex-specific measurements is unknown.

Almqvist, C., M. Worm, and B. Leynaert. 2008. Impact of gender on asthma in childhood and adolescence: A GA2LEN review. *Allergy* 63(1):47–57.

Barnes, P. J. 2010. Chronic obstructive pulmonary disease: Effects beyond the lungs. *PLoS Medicine* 7(3):e1000220.

Barnes, P. J. 2016. Sex differences in chronic obstructive pulmonary disease mechanisms. *American Journal of Respiratory and Critical Care Medicine* 193(8):813–814.

Basile, M. J., L. Dhingra, S. DiFiglia, J. Polo, R. Portenoy, J. Wang, P. Walker, B. Middour-Oxler, R. W. Linnemann, C. Kier, D. Friedman, M. Berdella, R. Abdullah, L. M. Yonker, M. Markovitz, D. Hadjiliadis, M. Shiffman, F. Fischer, S. Pollinger, M. Hardcastle, N. Chaudhary, and A. M. Georgiopoulos. 2023. Development of a cystic fibrosis primary palliative care intervention: Qualitative analysis of patient and family caregiver preferences. *Journal of Patient Experience* 10:e23743735231161486.

Becerra-Diaz, M., M. Song, and N. Heller. 2020. Androgen and androgen receptors as regulators of monocyte and macrophage biology in the healthy and diseased lung. *Frontiers in Immunology* 11:1698.

Boers, E., M. Barrett, J. G. Su, A. V. Benjafield, S. Sinha, L. Kaye, H. J. Zar, V. Vuong, D. Tellez, R. Gondalia, M. B. Rice, C. M. Nunez, J. A. Wedzicha, and A. Malhotra. 2023. Global burden of chronic obstructive pulmonary disease through 2050. *JAMA Network Open* 6(12):e2346598–e2346598.

Bojesen, A., S. Juul, N. H. Birkebaek, and C. H. Gravholt. 2006. Morbidity in Klinefelter syndrome: A Danish register study based on hospital discharge diagnoses. *Journal of Clinical Endocrinology & Metabolism* 91(4):1254–1260.

Bønnelykke, K., O. Raaschou-Nielsen, A. Tjønneland, C. S. Ulrik, H. Bisgaard, and Z. J. Andersen. 2015. Postmenopausal hormone therapy and asthma-related hospital admission. *Journal of Allergy and Clinical Immunology* 135(3):813–816.

Bradley, J. M., S. W. Blume, M.-M. Balp, D. Honeybourne, and J. S. Elborn. 2013. Quality of life and healthcare utilisation in cystic fibrosis: A multicentre study. *European Respiratory Journal* 41(3):571–577.

Cairns, C., and K. Kang. 2021. *National hospital ambulatory medical care survey: 2021 Emergency department summary tables.* Hyattsville, MD: National Center for Health Statistics, Centers for Disease Control and Prevention. https://www.cdc.gov/nchs/data/nhamcs/web_tables/2021-nhamcs-ed-web-tables-508.pdf (accessed February 29, 2024).

Carlson, C. S., M. Cushman, P. L. Enright, J. A. Caule, and A. B. Newman. 2001. Hormone replacement therapy is associated with higher FEV1 in elderly women. *American Journal of Respiratory and Critical Care Medicine* 163(2):423–428.

CDC (Centers for Disease Control and Prevention). 2023a. *2020 healthcare use data.* https://www.cdc.gov/asthma/healthcare-use/2020/data.htm (accessed March 10, 2024).

CDC. 2023b. *2023 NHIS: National Health Interview Survey.* Hyattsville, MD: National Center for Health Statistics, Centers for Disease Control and Prevention. https://www.cdc.gov/nchs/nhis/2023nhis.htm (accessed March 10, 2024).

CFF (Cystic Fibrosis Foundation). n.d.-a. *About cystic fibrosis.* https://www.cff.org/intro-cf/about-cystic-fibrosis (accessed January 12, 2024).

CFF. n.d.-b. *Living with advanced CF lung disease.* https://www.cff.org/managing-cf/living-advanced-cf-lung-disease (accessed January 14, 2024).

Chalmers, J. D., A. B. Chang, S. H. Chotirmall, R. Dhar, and P. J. McShane. 2018. Bronchiectasis. *Nature Reviews Disease Primers* 4(1):45.

Chichester, C. H., A. R. Buckpitt, A. Chang, and C. G. Plopper. 1994. Metabolism and cytotoxicity of naphthalene and its metabolites in isolated murine Clara cells. *Molecular Pharmacology* 45(4):664–672.

Chotirmall, S. H., S. G. Smith, C. Gunaratnam, S. Cosgrove, B. D. Dimitrov, S. J. O'Neill, B. J. Harvey, C. M. Greene, and N. G. McElvaney. 2012. Effect of estrogen on pseudomonas mucoidy and exacerbations in cystic fibrosis. *New England Journal of Medicine* 366(21):1978–1986.

Coakley, R. D., H. Sun, L. A. Clunes, J. E. Rasmussen, J. R. Stackhouse, S. F. Okada, I. Fricks, S. L. Young, and R. Tarran. 2008. 17β-estradiol inhibits Ca2+-dependent homeostasis of airway surface liquid volume in human cystic fibrosis airway epithelia. *Journal of Clinical Investigation* 118(12):4025–4035.

Cortes-Puentes, G. A., C. J. Davidge-Pitts, C. A. Gonzalez, M. M. Dulohery Scrodin, C. C. Kennedy, and K. G. Lim. 2023. A 64-year-old patient assigned male at birth with COPD and worsening dyspnea while on estrogen and antiandrogen agents. *Respiratory Medicine Case Reports* 44:e101876.

de Marco, R., F. Locatelli, J. Sunyer, and P. Burney. 2000. Differences in incidence of reported asthma related to age in men and women. A retrospective analysis of the data of the European Respiratory Health Survey. *American Journal of Respiratory and Critical Care Medicine* 162(1):68–74.

de Marco, R., G. Pesce, A. Marcon, S. Accordini, L. Antonicelli, M. Bugiani, L. Casali, M. Ferrari, G. Nicolini, M. G. Panico, P. Pirina, M. E. Zanolin, I. Cerveri, and G. Verlato. 2013. The coexistence of asthma and chronic obstructive pulmonary disease (COPD): Prevalence and risk factors in young, middle-aged and elderly people from the general population. *PLoS ONE* 8(5):e62985.

de Souza, D. A. S., F. R. Faucz, L. Pereira-Ferrari, V. S. Sotomaior, and S. Raskin. 2018. Congenital bilateral absence of the vas deferens as an atypical form of cystic fibrosis: Reproductive implications and genetic counseling. *Andrology* 6(1):127–135.

DeBoer, M. D., B. R. Phillips, D. T. Mauger, J. Zein, S. C. Erzurum, A. M. Fitzpatrick, B. M. Gaston, R. Myers, K. R. Ross, J. Chmiel, M. J. Lee, J. V. Fahy, M. Peters, N. P. Ly, S. E. Wenzel, M. L. Fajt, F. Holguin, W. C. Moore, S. P. Peters, D. Meyers, E. R. Bleecker, M. Castro, A. M. Coverstone, L. B. Bacharier, N. N. Jarjour, R. L. Sorkness, S. Ramratnam, A. M. Irani, E. Israel, B. Levy, W. Phipatanakul, J. M. Gaffin, and W. Gerald Teague. 2018. Effects of endogenous sex hormones on lung function and symptom control in adolescents with asthma. *BMC Pulmonary Medicine* 18(1):58.

Demko, C. A., P. J. Byard, and P. B. Davis. 1995. Gender differences in cystic fibrosis: *Pseudomonas aeruginosa* infection. *Journal of Clinical Epidemiology* 48(8):1041–1049.

Dragon, C. N., P. Guerino, E. Ewald, and A. M. Laffan. 2017. Transgender Medicare beneficiaries and chronic conditions: Exploring fee-for-service claims data. *LGBT Health* 4(6):404–411.

Dutton, L., K. Koenig, and K. Fennie. 2008. Gynecologic care of the female-to-male transgender man. *Journal of Midwifery and Womens Health* 53(4):331–337.

Fechter-Leggett, E. 2023. *Selecting appropriate pulmonary function test reference sex for transgender and gender-diverse people.* Paper presented to the National Academies Committee on Sex and Gender Identification and Implications for Disability Evaluation: Meeting 3, Washington, DC.

Fechter-Leggett, E., B. R. Ansell, R. Harvey, K. M. Kidd, and D. Weissman. 2022. *Selecting appropriate pulmonary function test reference sex for transgender adults to address health disparities: Methods for data collection and interpretation.* Poster presented at the American Thoracic Society 2022 International Conference, San Francisco, CA.

Foer, D. 2023. *Selecting appropriate pulmonary function test reference sex for transgender and gender-diverse people.* Paper presented to the National Academies Committee on Sex and Gender Identification and Implications for Disability Evaluation: Meeting 3, Washington, DC.

Foer, D., D. Rubins, A. Almazan, P. G. Wickner, D. W. Bates, and O. R. Hamnvik. 2021. Gender reference use in spirometry for transgender patients. *Annals of the American Thoracic Society* 18(3):537–540.

Fu, L., R. J. Freishtat, H. Gordish-Dressman, S. J. Teach, L. Resca, E. P. Hoffman, and Z. Wang. 2014. Natural progression of childhood asthma symptoms and strong influence of sex and puberty. *Annals of the American Thoracic Society* 11(6):939–944.

Fuseini, H., and D. C. Newcomb. 2017. Mechanisms driving gender differences in asthma. *Current Allergy and Asthma Reports* 17(3):19.

Gaston, B., N. Marozkina, D. C. Newcomb, N. Sharifi, and J. Zein. 2021. Asthma risk among individuals with androgen receptor deficiency. *JAMA Pediatrics* 175(7):743–745.

Global Asthma Network. 2022. The global asthma report 2022. *International Journal of Tuberculosis and Lung Disease* 26(Supp 1):1–104.

Gómez Real, F., C. Svanes, E. H. Björnsson, K. A. Franklin, D. Gislason, T. Gislason, A. Gulsvik, C. Janson, R. Jögi, T. Kiserud, D. Norbäck, L. Nyström, K. Torén, T. Wentzel-Larsen, and E. Omenaas. 2006. Hormone replacement therapy, body mass index and asthma in perimenopausal women: A cross sectional survey. *Thorax* 61(1):34–40.

Graham, B. L., V. Brusasco, F. Burgos, B. G. Cooper, R. Jensen, A. Kendrick, N. R. MacIntyre, B. R. Thompson, and J. Wanger. 2017. 2017 ERS/ATS standards for single-breath carbon monoxide uptake in the lung. *European Respiratory Journal* 49(1):e1600016.

Graham, B. L., I. Steenbruggen, M. R. Miller, I. Z. Barjaktarevic, B. G. Cooper, G. L. Hall, T. S. Hallstrand, D. A. Kaminsky, K. McCarthy, M. C. McCormack, C. E. Oropez, M. Rosenfeld, S. Stanojevic, M. P. Swanney, and B. R. Thompson. 2019. Standardization of spirometry 2019 update: An official American Thoracic Society and European Respiratory Society technical statement. *American Journal of Respiratory and Critical Care Medicine* 200(8):e70–e88.

Guo, J., A. Garratt, and A. Hill. 2022. Worldwide rates of diagnosis and effective treatment for cystic fibrosis. *Journal of Cystic Fibrosis* 21(3):456–462.

Guta, M. T., T. Tekalign, N. Awoke, R. O. Fite, G. Dendir, and T. L. Lenjebo. 2021. Global burden of anxiety and depression among cystic fibrosis patient: Systematic review and meta-analysis. *International Journal of Chronic Diseases* 2021:e6708865.

Han, Y. Y., E. Forno, and J. C. Celedón. 2020. Sex steroid hormones and asthma in a nationwide study of U.S. Adults. *American Journal of Respiratory and Critical Care Medicine* 201(2):158–166.

Hannema, S. E., and I. A. Hughes. 2007. Regulation of Wolffian duct development. *Hormone Research* 67(3):142–151.

Harness-Brumley, C. L., A. C. Elliott, D. B. Rosenbluth, D. Raghavan, and R. Jain. 2014. Gender differences in outcomes of patients with cystic fibrosis. *Journal of Women's Health* 23(12):1012–1020.

Haynes, J. M., and R. W. Stumbo. 2018. The impact of using non-birth sex on the interpretation of spirometry data in subjects with air-flow obstruction. *Respiratory Care* 63(2):215–218.

Henderson, E. R., T. L. Boyer, H. L. Wolfe, and J. R. Blosnich. 2023. Causes of death of transgender and gender diverse veterans. *American Journal of Preventive Medicine* 66(4):664–671.

Henkle, E., B. Chan, J. R. Curtis, T. R. Aksamit, C. L. Daley, and K. L. Winthrop. 2018. Characteristics and health-care utilization history of patients with bronchiectasis in U.S. Medicare enrollees with prescription drug plans, 2006 to 2014. *Chest* 154(6):1311–1320.

Herman, J. L., and K. O'Neill. 2020. *Vulnerabilities to COVID-19 among transgender adults in the US.* Los Angeles, CA: UCLA School of Law Williams Institute. https://williamsinstitute.law.ucla.edu/wp-content/uploads/Trans-COVID19-Apr-2020.pdf (accessed February 29, 2024).

Holtrop, M., S. Heltshe, V. Shabanova, A. Keller, L. Schumacher, L. Fernandez, and R. Jain. 2021. A prospective study of the effects of sex hormones on lung function and inflammation in women with cystic fibrosis. *Annals of the American Thoracic Society* 18(7):1158–1166.

Hunninghake, G. M., M. E. Soto-Quirós, L. Avila, H. P. Kim, J. Lasky-Su, N. Rafaels, I. Ruczinski, T. H. Beaty, R. A. Mathias, K. C. Barnes, J. B. Wilk, G. T. O'Connor, W. J. Gauderman, H. Vora, J. W. Baurley, F. Gilliland, C. Liang, J. S. Sylvia, B. J. Klanderman, S. S. Sharma, B. E. Himes, C. J. Bossley, E. Israel, B. A. Raby, A. Bush, A. M. Choi, S. T. Weiss, and J. C. Celedón. 2010. TSLP polymorphisms are associated with asthma in a sex-specific fashion. *Allergy* 65(12):1566–1575.

Imam, J. S., and A. G. Duarte. 2020. Non-CF bronchiectasis: Orphan disease no longer. *Respiratory Medicine* 166:e105940.

Jarrett, B. A., A. L. Corbet, I. H. Gardner, J. D. Weinand, and S. M. Peitzmeier. 2018. Chest binding and care seeking among transmasculine adults: A cross-sectional study. *Transgender Health* 3(1):170–178.

Jo, H. E., I. Glaspole, C. Grainge, N. Goh, P. M. A. Hopkins, Y. Moodley, P. N. Reynolds, S. Chapman, E. H. Walters, C. Zappala, H. Allan, G. J. Keir, A. Hayen, W. A. Cooper, A. M. Mahar, S. Ellis, S. Macansh, and T. J. Corte. 2017. Baseline characteristics of idiopathic pulmonary fibrosis: Analysis from the Australian idiopathic pulmonary fibrosis registry. *European Respiratory Journal* 49(2):1601592.

Job, S. A., A. R. Kaniuka, K. M. Reeves, and B. D. Brooks. 2023. Interactions of sexual orientation and gender identity with race/ethnicity in prevalence of lifetime and current asthma diagnosis. *LGBT Health* 10(5):372–381.

Jones, T., A. Bolger, T. Dune, A. Lykins, and G. Hawkes. 2015. *Female-to-male (FTM) transgender people's experiences in Australia*. Cham, Switzerland: Springer Nature.

Julian, J. M., B. Salvetti, J. I. Held, P. M. Murray, L. Lara-Rojas, and J. Olson-Kennedy. 2021. The impact of chest binding in transgender and gender diverse youth and young adults. *Journal of Adolescent Health* 68(6):1129–1134.

Khan, F. N., K. Mason, A. H. Roe, and V. Tangpricha. 2022. CF and male health: Sexual and reproductive health, hypogonadism, and fertility. *Journal of Clinical & Translational Endocrinology* 27:e100288.

Kidd, K. M., G. M. Sequeira, C. P. Dhar, G. T. Montano, S. F. Witchel, and D. Rofey. 2019. Gendered body mass index percentile charts and transgender youth: Making the case to change charts. *Transgender Health* 4(1):297–299.

Ladias, S., and S. Katsenos. 2018. Klinefelter syndrome and bronchial asthma: Is there any relationship between the low testosterone levels and asthma exacerbations? *Lung India* 35(4):368–369.

Lam, G. Y., J. Goodwin, P. Wilcox, and B. S. Quon. 2020. Worsening pulmonary outcomes during sex reassignment therapy in a transgender female with cystic fibrosis (CF) and asthma/allergic bronchopulmonary aspergillosis: A case report. *BMC Pulmonary Medicine* 20(1):234.

Latchford, G., and A. J. Duff. 2013. Screening for depression in a single CF centre. *Journal of Cystic Fibrosis* 12(6):794–796.

Lee, A., P. Simpson, and B. Haire. 2019. The binding practices of transgender and gender-diverse adults in Sydney, Australia. *Culture, Health & Sexuality* 21(9):969–984.

Liu, Y., S. A. Carlson, K. B. Watson, F. Xu, and K. J. Greenlund. 2023. Trends in the prevalence of chronic obstructive pulmonary disease among adults aged >/=18 years: United States, 2011–2021. *MMWR: Morbidity and Mortality Weekly Report* 72(46):1250–1256.

Maher, T. M., E. Bendstrup, L. Dron, J. Langley, G. Smith, J. M. Khalid, H. Patel, and M. Kreuter. 2021. Global incidence and prevalence of idiopathic pulmonary fibrosis. *Respiratory Research* 22(1):197.

Malinczak, C. A., W. Fonseca, A. J. Rasky, C. Ptaschinski, S. Morris, S. F. Ziegler, and N. W. Lukacs. 2019. Sex-associated TSLP-induced immune alterations following early-life RSV infection leads to enhanced allergic disease. *Mucosal Immunology* 12(4):969–979.

Mall, M. A., and J. S. Elborn. 2014. *Cystic fibrosis*, edited by A. M. Marcus and J. S. Elborn. Lausanne, Switzerland: European Respiratory Society.

Mannino, D. M., and A. S. Buist. 2007. Global burden of COPD: Risk factors, prevalence, and future trends. *The Lancet* 370(9589):765–773.

Martinez-Garcia, M. A., and M. Miravitlles. 2017. Bronchiectasis in COPD patients: More than a comorbidity? *International Journal of Chronic Obstructive Pulmonary Disease* 12:1401–1411.

Maycock, L. B., and H. P. Kennedy. 2014. Breast care in the transgender individual. *Journal of Midwifery & Women's Health* 59(1):74–81.

McCleary, N., B. I. Nwaru, U. B. Nurmatov, H. Critchley, and A. Sheikh. 2018. Endogenous and exogenous sex steroid hormones in asthma and allergy in females: A systematic review and meta-analysis. *Journal of Allergy and Clinical Immunology* 141(4):1510–1513.

McManus, J. M., B. Gaston, J. Zein, and N. Sharifi. 2022. Association between asthma and reduced androgen receptor expression in airways. *Journal of the Endocrine Society* 6(5):bvac047.

Minnesota Department of Health. 2019. *Asthma among middle & high school students: Results from the 2019 Minnesota Student Survey (MSS)*. St. Paul, MN. https://www.health.state.mn.us/diseases/asthma/data/documents/asthmainmnschools.pdf (accessed March 13, 2024).

Miravitlles, M., and A. Ribera. 2017. Understanding the impact of symptoms on the burden of COPD. *Respiratory Research* 18(1):67.

Miravitlles, M., M. Bhutani, J. R. Hurst, F. M. E. Franssen, J. F. M. van Boven, E. M. Khoo, J. Zhang, S. Brunton, D. Stolz, T. Winders, K. Asai, and J. E. Scullion. 2023. Implementing an evidence-based COPD hospital discharge protocol: A narrative review and expert recommendations. *Advances in Therapy* 40(10):4236–4263.

Modi, P., and M. Cascella. 2024. *Diffusing capacity of the lungs for carbon monoxide*. [Updated 2023 March 13], Statpearls. Treasure Island, FL: StatPearls Publishing.

Mohan, S. S., M. W. Knuiman, M. L. Divitini, A. L. James, A. W. Musk, D. J. Handelsman, J. Beilin, M. Hunter, and B. B. Yeap. 2015. Higher serum testosterone and dihydrotestosterone, but not oestradiol, are independently associated with favourable indices of lung function in community-dwelling men. *Clinical Endocrinology* 83(2):268–276.

Morales-Estrella, J. L., M. Boyle, and J. G. Zein. 2018. Transgender status is associated with higher risk of lifetime asthma. *American Journal of Respiratory and Critical Care Medicine* 197:A1371.

Naeem, A., and P. Silveyra. 2019. Sex differences in paediatric and adult asthma. *European Medical Journal (Chelmsford, England)* 4(2):27–35.

Nan, H., Y. Zhang, and Z. Chen. 2013. A case of Klinefelter's syndrome with refractory asthma, diabetes mellitus and rib fracture. *Chinese Medical Journal* 126(1):196.

National Center for Environmental Health. 2023. *2021 National Health Interview Survey (NHIS) data: Most recent asthma data*. Atlanta, GA: Centers for Disease Control and Prevention. https://www.cdc.gov/asthma/most_recent_national_asthma_data.htm (accessed March 1, 2024).

NIOSH (National Institute for Occupational Safety and Health). 2018. *NIOSH Respiratory Health Division (RHD) fact sheet*. Publication No. 2018-142. Washington, DC. https://www.cdc.gov/niosh/docs/2018-142/default.html (accessed May 21, 2024).

OSHA (Occupational Safety and Health Administration). 2013. *Spirometry testing in occupational health programs: Best practices for health professionals*. Washington, DC: U.S. Department of Labor.

Pavey, H., M. I. Polkey, C. E. Bolton, J. Cheriyan, C. M. McEniery, I. Wilkinson, D. Mohan, R. Casaburi, B. E. Miller, R. Tal-Singer, and M. Fisk. 2023. Circulating testosterone levels and health outcomes in chronic obstructive pulmonary disease: Results from ECLIPSE and ERICA. *BMJ Open Respiratory Research* 10(1):e001601.

Peitzmeier, S., I. Gardner, J. Weinand, A. Corbet, and K. Acevedo. 2017. Health impact of chest binding among transgender adults: A community-engaged, cross-sectional study. *Culture, Health & Sexuality* 19(1):64–75.

Peitzmeier, S. M., I. H. Gardner, J. Weinand, A. Corbet, and K. Acevedo. 2022. Chest binding in context: Stigma, fear, and lack of information drive negative outcomes. *Culture, Health & Sexuality* 24(2):284–287.

Pergolizzi, J. V., Jr., J. A. LeQuang, M. Varrassi, F. Breve, P. Magnusson, and G. Varrassi. 2023. What do we need to know about rising rates of idiopathic pulmonary fibrosis? A narrative review and update. *Advances in Therapy* 40(4):1334–1346.

Pinart, M., T. Keller, A. Reich, M. Fröhlich, B. Cabieses, C. Hohmann, D. S. Postma, J. Bousquet, J. M. Antó, and T. Keil. 2017. Sex-related allergic rhinitis prevalen witch from childhood to adulthood: A systematic review and meta-analysis. *International Archives of Allergy and Immunology* 172(4):224–235.

Potera, C. 2019. Black lung disease resurges in Appalachian coal miners. *American Journal of Nursing* 119(4):14.

Ranjbar, M., M. Mojdeh, A. Mohammad-Ali, F. Morteza, S. Fatemeh, S. Saeed, and J. Leila. 2020. Association between two single nucleotide polymorphisms of thymic stromal lymphopoietin (TSLP) gene and asthma in Iranian population. *Iranian Journal of Allergy, Asthma and Immunology* 19(4):362–372.

Rea, J., J. T. Babek, R. M. Anderson, R. Bacani, J. Staggs, and M. Vassar. 2024. The current state of health inequities in COPD. *Respiratory Care* 69(2):238–249.

Riekert, K. A., S. J. Bartlett, M. P. Boyle, J. A. Krishnan, and C. S. Rand. 2007. The association between depression, lung function, and health-related quality of life among adults with cystic fibrosis. *Chest* 132(1):231–237.

Rosen, H. N., O. R. Hamnvik, U. Jaisamrarn, A. O. Malabanan, J. D. Safer, V. Tangpricha, L. Wattanachanya, and S. S. Yeap. 2019. Bone densitometry in transgender and gender non-conforming (TGNC) individuals: 2019 ISCD official position. *Journal of Clinical Densitometry* 22(4):544–553.

Rosenfeld, M., R. Davis, S. FitzSimmons, M. Pepe, and B. Ramsey. 1997. Gender gap in cystic fibrosis mortality. *American Journal of Epidemiology* 145(9):794–803.

Santo, L., and K. Kang. 2023. National hospital ambulatory medical care survey: 2019 National summary tables. Hyattsville, MD: National Center for Health Statistics, Centers for Disease Control and Prevention. https://www.cdc.gov/nchs/data/ahcd/namcs_summary/2019-namcs-web-tables-508.pdf (accessed March 12, 2024).

Sathish, V., Y. N. Martin, and Y. S. Prakash. 2015. Sex steroid signaling: Implications for lung diseases. *Pharmacology & Therapeutics* 150:94–108.

Sauleda, J., B. Núñez, E. Sala, and J. B. Soriano. 2018. Idiopathic pulmonary fibrosis: Epidemiology, natural history, phenotypes. *Medical Sciences* (Basel, Switzerland) 6(4):110.

Schatz, M., and C. A. Camargo, Jr. 2003. The relationship of sex to asthma prevalence, health care utilization, and medications in a large managed care organization. *Annals of Allergy, Asthma & Immunology* 91(6):553–558.

Seitz, A. E., K. N. Olivier, J. Adjemian, S. M. Holland, and D. R. Prevots. 2012. Trends in bronchiectasis among Medicare beneficiaries in the United States, 2000 to 2007. *Chest* 142(2):432–439.

Sesé, L., H. Nunes, V. Cottin, D. Israel-Biet, B. Crestani, S. Guillot-Dudoret, J. Cadranel, B. Wallaert, A. Tazi, B. Maître, G. Prévot, S. Marchand-Adam, S. Hirschi, S. Dury, V. Giraud, A. Gondouin, P. Bonniaud, J. Traclet, K. Juvin, R. Borie, Z. Carton, O. Freynet, T. Gille, C. Planès, D. Valeyre, and Y. Uzunhan. 2021. Gender differences in idiopathic pulmonary fibrosis: Are men and women equal? *Frontiers in Medicine* 8:e713698.

Shaffer, L., K. Bozkanat, M. Lau, P. Sharma, M. Sathe, X. Lopez, and R. Jain. 2021. Gender-affirming hormone therapy in cystic fibrosis: A case of new *Pseudomonas* infection. *Respiratory Medicine Case Reports* 32:e101353.

Shaffer, L. R., E. McCormack, G. S. Sawicki, A. Keller, and R. Jain. 2022. Understanding the intersection between gender transition and health outcomes in cystic fibrosis. *Annals of the American Thoracic Society* 19(3):504–506.

Shah, A. S., H. Tibble, R. Pillinger, and S. McLean. 2021. Hormone replacement therapy and asthma onset in menopausal women: National cohort study. *Journal of Allergy and Clinical Immunology* 147(5):1662–1670.

Shah, R., and D. C. Newcomb. 2018. Sex bias in asthma prevalence and pathogenesis. *Frontiers in Immunology* 9:2997.

Shi, P., X. Xing, S. Xi, H. Jing, J. Yuan, Z. Fu, and H. Zhao. 2020. Trends in global, regional and national incidence of pneumoconiosis caused by different aetiologies: An analysis from the global burden of disease study 2017. *Occupational and Environmental Medicine* 77(6):407–414.

Shriver, T. E., and A. Bodenhamer. 2018. The enduring legacy of black lung: Environmental health and contested illness in Appalachia. *Sociology of Health & Illness* 40(8):1361–1375.

Siroux, V., F. Curt, M. P. Oryszczyn, J. Maccario, and F. Kauffmann. 2004. Role of gender and hormone-related events on IgE, atopy, and eosinophils in the epidemiological study on the genetics and environment of asthma, bronchial hyperresponsiveness and atopy. *Journal of Allergy and Clinical Immunology* 114(3):491–498.

SSA (Social Security Administration). n.d.-a. *Disability evaluation under social security: Respiratory disorders, adult: 3.03, asthma.* https://www.ssa.gov/disability/professionals/bluebook/3.00-Respiratory-Adult.htm (accessed May 21, 2024).

SSA. n.d.-b. *Disability evaluation under social security: Respiratory Disorders, childhood: 103.03, asthma.* https://www.ssa.gov/disability/professionals/bluebook/103.00-Respiratory-Childhood.htm#103_03. (accessed May 21, 2024).

SSA. 2022. *SSI annual statistical report.* Washington, DC: Social Security Administration.

SSA. 2023. *Annual statistical report on the social security disability insurance program, 2022.* Washington, DC: Social Security Administration.

Stanojevic, S., D. A. Kaminsky, M. R. Miller, B. Thompson, A. Aliverti, I. Barjaktarevic, B. G. Cooper, B. Culver, E. Derom, G. L. Hall, T. S. Hallstrand, J. D. Leuppi, N. MacIntyre, M. McCormack, M. Rosenfeld, and E. R. Swenson. 2022. ERS/ATS technical standard on interpretive strategies for routine lung function tests. *European Respiratory Journal* 60(1)e2101499.

Tam, A., D. Morrish, S. Wadsworth, D. Dorscheid, S. F. P. Man, and D. D. Sin. 2011. The role of female hormones on lung function in chronic lung diseases. *BMC Women's Health* 11(1):24.

Tam, A., S. Wadsworth, D. Dorscheid, S.-F. P. Man, and D. D. Sin. 2014. Estradiol increases mucus synthesis in bronchial epithelial cells. *PLoS ONE* 9(6):e100633.

Troisi, R. J., F. E. Speizer, W. C. Willett, D. Trichopoulos, and B. Rosner. 1995. Menopause, postmenopausal estrogen preparations, and the risk of adult-onset asthma: A prospective cohort study. *American Journal of Respiratory and Critical Care Medicine* 152(4 Pt 1):1183–1188.

Turner, G. A., N. J. Amoura, and H. M. Strah. 2021. Care of the transgender patient with a pulmonary complaint. *Annals of the American Thoracic Society* 18(6):931–937.

Vadagam, P., and K. M. Kamal. 1995. Hospitalization costs of cystic fibrosis in the United States: A retrospective analysis. *Hospital Practice* 46(4):203–213.

Van Winkle, L. S., A. D. Gunderson, J. A. Shimizu, G. L. Baker, and C. D. Brown. 2002. Gender differences in naphthalene metabolism and naphthalene-induced acute lung injury. *American Journal of Physiology Lung Cellular and Molecular Physiology* 282(5):L1122–L1134.

Wu, M., T. Daley, and D. Fadoju. 2022. Case report of a Hispanic female with cystic fibrosis and short stature. *Respiratory Medicine Case Reports* 39:e101726.

Yoon, J. C., J. L. Casella, M. Litvin, and A. S. Dobs. 2019. Male reproductive health in cystic fibrosis. *Journal of Cystic Fibrosis* 18:S105–S110.

Yung, J. A., H. Fuseini, and D. C. Newcomb. 2018. Hormones, sex, and asthma. *Annals of Allergy, Asthma & Immunology* 120(5):488–494.

Zein, J. G., and S. C. Erzurum. 2015. Asthma is different in women. *Current Allergy and Asthma Reports* 15(6):28.

Zein, J. G., J. M. McManus, N. Sharifi, S. C. Erzurum, N. Marozkina, T. Lahm, O. Giddings, M. D. Davis, M. D. DeBoer, S. A. Comhair, P. Bazeley, H. J. Kim, W. Busse, W. Calhoun, M. Castro, K. F. Chung, J. V. Fahy, E. Israel, N. N. Jarjour, B. D. Levy, D. T. Mauger, W. C. Moore, V. E. Ortega, M. Peters, E. R. Bleecker, D. A. Meyers, Y. Zhao, S. E. Wenzel, and B. Gaston. 2021. Benefits of airway androgen receptor expression in human asthma. *American Journal of Respiratory and Critical Care Medicine* 204(3):285–293.

Zemp, E., T. Schikowski, J. Dratva, C. Schindler, and N. Probst-Hensch. 2012. Asthma and the menopause: A systematic review and meta-analysis. *Maturitas* 73(3):212–217.

Zhang, G., R. Basna, M. B. Mathur, C. Lässer, R. Mincheva, L. Ekerljung, G. Wennergren, M. Rådinger, B. Lundbäck, H. Kankaanranta, and B. I. Nwaru. 2023. Exogenous female sex steroid hormones and new-onset asthma in women: A matched case-control study. *BMC Medicine* 21(1):337.

9

Childhood Growth Failure

During infancy, childhood, and adolescence,[1] growth (increases in length or height and weight) represents the outcome of ongoing interactions among nutritional, genetic, hormonal, and environmental factors (Thompson, 2021). Linear growth velocities are programmed such that normal growth velocity is high during infancy, slows during the juvenile years, and increases with puberty. Even short-term interruptions during these critical growth periods may have long-term impact. Given recognition of subsequent growth impairment and, in some cases, impaired cognitive performance among infants with early growth failure, early identification and intervention are essential (Boddy et al., 2000; Cooke et al., 2023). Understanding of youth[2] growth trajectory is often limited when only a single measurement of height and weight is available, and documenting changes in height and/or weight over time is fundamental to clinical decision making. Growth is typically assessed by measuring increases (or the lack thereof) in three common measures: (1) length or height, (2) weight, and (3) head circumference. Other measurements may be obtained in specialty settings, including, for example, mid–upper arm circumference (Tang et al., 2021; WHO, 2009).

---

[1] The American Academy of Pediatrics defines "infancy" as the first 11 months of life, "childhood" as years 1–10, and "adolescence" as years 11–21 (Hagan et al., 2017).

[2] For the purposes of this chapter, when the committee uses the term "youth," it applies to childhood and adolescent age ranges.

Many pediatric illnesses, particularly chronic disorders, can result in growth failure. For example, many youth with chronic kidney disease are at risk for developing growth failure because damaged kidneys may be unable to perform functions necessary to regulate nutrients from food that are necessary for growth and may not effectively help the body metabolize growth hormones (NIDDK, 2022). In addition, some youth with chronic kidney disease may not feel hungry or may not have the energy to eat. For these reasons, growth failure due to any chronic renal disease has its own disability Listing under 106.08.

Growth failure may be due to many different chronic conditions, and the Social Security Administration's (SSA's) disability Listings include criteria for growth failure within several disease categories, as outlined in Box 9-1. SSA currently considers a child applicant to meet criteria for growth failure based on low weight-for-length (for young children from birth to attainment of age 2 years) or low body mass index (BMI) (for older children age 2 years to attainment of age 18), with additional criteria as displayed in Box 9-1.

Factors contributing to growth failure include inadequate caloric intake, mechanical feeding issues, insufficient gastrointestinal absorption of nutrients, chromosomal disorders, hormone deficiencies, and increased metabolic needs (due, e.g., to chronic inflammation or infection). Some or all of these factors may be present in certain illnesses (Kyle, 2015). Insufficient weight gain, regardless of etiology, may ultimately impair linear growth velocity (also known as "height velocity").

While the etiology for growth failure and needed treatments vary for specific chronic conditions, SSA's measure for determining whether a child applicant meets criteria for growth failure is currently the same across conditions:

- "For children from birth to attainment of age two, [Listings] use the pediatric *weight-for-length table* corresponding to the child's gender"
- "For children age two through attainment of age eighteen, [Listings] use the body mass index *(BMI)-for-age table* corresponding to the child's gender"[3]

As suggested by SSA's language, both weight-for-length and BMI-for-age (calculated as weight divided by height-squared) measures have sex-specific criteria (although, notably, the term "gender" rather than "sex" is used in the SSA criteria, the implications of which are discussed in further detail later in this chapter). Hence it is important to consider how best to use these measures for childhood disability applicants who are transgender or gender

---

[3] Listing of Impairments 100.05, 103.06, 104.02, 105.08, 106.08, and 114.11(I) [emphasis added].

BOX 9-1
SSA Childhood Disability Listings Related to Growth Failure

Childhood Listings
100.05 Failure to thrive in children from birth to attainment of age 3*
103.06 Growth failure due to any chronic respiratory disorder
104.02 Chronic heart failure
105.08 Growth failure due to any digestive disorder
106.08 Growth failure due to any chronic renal disease
114.11(I) Human immunodeficiency virus (HIV) infection; Immune
     suppression and growth failure

Growth Failure Measurements
Growth failure as required in 1 or 2:

(1) *For children from birth to attainment of age 2,* three weight-for-
length measurements that are: (a) within a consecutive 12-month
period; and (b) at least 60 days apart; and (c) less than the third
percentile on the appropriate weight-for-length Table I or II under
105.08B1

OR

(2) *For children age 2 to attainment of age 18,* three BMI-for-age
measurements that are: (a) within a consecutive 12-month period;
and (b) at least 60 days apart; and (c) less than the third percentile
on the appropriate BMI-for-age Table III or IV under 105.08B2.

** For Listing 100.05, "Failure to thrive in children from birth to attainment of age 3," the body
mass index (BMI) chart is used for children age 2 years to attainment of age 3 (rather than
age 18 years as is used in the other growth failure Listings). Otherwise, the criterion for this
Listing is the same as for all other childhood growth failure Listings.*

---

diverse (TGD) or have variations in sex traits (VSTs). For this reason, SSA
included these conditions for consideration by this committee. Regardless
of gender identity or biological sex (XX or XY), sole reliance on weight-
for-length and BMI-for-age may miss cases of growth failure. For example,
a child with a chronic illness who has both low weight and short stature
might have a normal BMI, resulting in a lost opportunity for beneficial
therapeutic intervention(s).

This chapter examines the pediatric weight-for-length and BMI-for-age
tables, considers the flaws in these measures, examines the impact of
gender-affirming hormone therapy on measurements of body composition,
reviews the use of weight-for-length and BMI-for-age in disability criteria

for pediatric populations, and describes other measures of body composition that may be appropriate for TGD populations and populations with VSTs.

NORMAL DIVERSITY IN BODY COMPOSITION

Normal linear growth follows a predictable pattern. Growth charts display this pattern as percentile trajectory curves showing the distribution of selected body measurements over time as children age. Normal growth typically follows a specific trajectory within the normative range (3rd–97th percentile). Figure 9-1 charts normal growth velocity from age 2 to 18. Growth velocity is most rapid during fetal life with an approximate length increase of 25 cm during the first year of life. Growth slows to 10–15 cm per year during the second year of life. From 4 years of age until the onset of puberty, linear growth velocity is approximately 5 cm per year. Growth velocity increases again during puberty.

Accurately interpreting growth parameters requires accurate measurements, and, particularly early in life, even small errors in measurement (e.g., by 1 or several centimeters) can result in large changes in the calculated percentile for age. Thus, obtaining multiple measurements over time is extremely helpful because those that are outliers may represent measurement errors that should not be considered in an assessment of growth. However, crossing two percentile lines (e.g., because of a sudden weight loss or failure to grow in height) is often concerning and deserving of closer scrutiny. Whereas crossing length centiles is concerning after 2 years of age, it is important to be cognizant that infants may cross length centiles as they transition from their prenatal to their postnatal linear growth trajectories (Jorge et al., 2021).

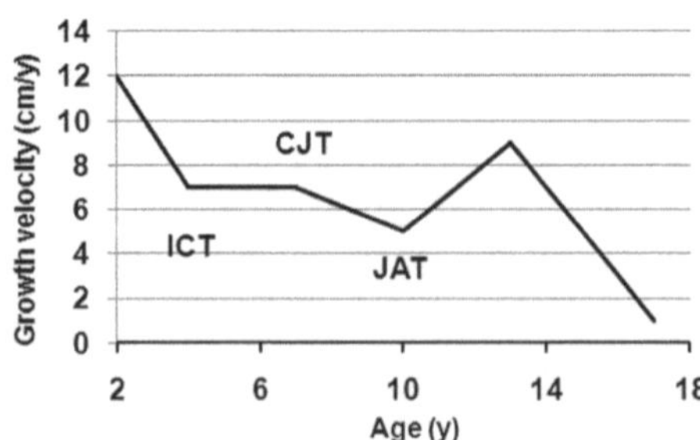

FIGURE 9-1 Growth during preadult life history stages.
NOTE: CJT = childhood–juvenility transition; ICT = infancy–childhood transition; JAT = juvenility–adolescence transition.
SOURCE: Hochberg, 2011. CC BY 4.0.

MEASUREMENTS OF GROWTH IN PEDIATRIC POPULATIONS

As part of routine health care, infants, young children, and adolescents are weighed and their length or height and head circumference are measured to assess growth. Deviations from standardized curves may indicate acute or chronic health issues needing additional evaluation to identify disorders associated with growth failure or impairment.

Although accuracy in such measurements is essential, height measurements are particularly prone to error due to technical issues. Height should be measured with a wall-mounted stadiometer with the patient positioned erect and with the lower margins of the orbits and the upper margins of the ear canals lying in the same horizontal plane. Hair ornaments that might affect height measurement should be removed. Flip-up floppy arms found on weighing scales are often inaccurate because of inconsistency in both the patient's posture and the angle of the horizontal bar. For infants, recumbent length is measured using a recumbent length board. Two people are required for accurate length measurement—one holding the infant's head and the other keeping the knees straight. When height cannot be measured accurately with a wall-mounted stadiometer, such as when measuring a nonambulatory person, measurement of arm span can approximate height. To assess for disproportionate short stature, such as a skeletal dysplasia, the ratio of sitting height to standing height can be helpful. However, age-, sex-, and population-specific reference data are needed to interpret these measurements (Hawkes et al., 2020).

Infants and children less than 2 years old should be weighed naked or with a clean diaper. Children more than 2 years old should be weighed with light clothing and no shoes. For those in whom accurate weight cannot readily be determined, measurement of mid–upper arm circumference can approximate nutritional status.

The Centers for Disease Control and Prevention (CDC) publishes five gender-specific anthropometric indices (measures combining weight, stature, length, or head circumference with age or length/stature) that are commonly used to assess size and growth in children (see Table 9-1).

Two of these assessments are currently used for assessing children at risk for growth failure: (1) weight-for-length and (2) BMI-for-age. The following sections describe these two measures and their utility in assessing growth for pediatric populations with chronic health needs.

Weight-for-Length Charts

CDC (2010) and the American Academy of Pediatrics (AAP, 2022) recommend that infants and children under 2 years of age be tracked using the weight-for-length growth standard charts published by the World

TABLE 9-1 Centers for Disease Control and Prevention: Clinical Growth Charts

Clinical Growth Chart	Age Ranges
BMI-for-age "is an anthropometric index of weight and height combined with age. BMI-for-age is used to classify children and adolescents as underweight, overweight, or at risk of overweight."	• Children and adolescents, 2–20 years
Stature/length-for-age "describes linear growth relative to age. Stature- or length-for-age is used to define shortness or tallness."	• Infants, birth–36 months • Children and adolescents, 2–20 years
Weight-for-age "reflects body weight relative to age and is influenced by recent changes in health or nutritional status. It is not used to classify infants, children and adolescents as under or overweight. However, it is important in early infancy for monitoring weight and helping explain changes in weight-for-length and BMI-for-age in older children."	• Infants, birth–36 months • Children and adolescents, 2–20 years
Weight-for-length/stature "reflects body weight relative to length and requires no knowledge of age. It is an indicator to classify infants and young children as overweight and underweight."	• Infants, birth–36 months • Preschoolers, 2–5 years[a]
Head circumference-for-age "is critical during infancy and can be charted up to 36 months of age. Head circumference measurements reflect brain size."	• Infants, birth–36 months

[a] The weight-for-stature charts are included as an option for assessing children primarily between 2 and 5 years of age as pediatric health care providers make the transition to the BMI-for-age chart.
NOTE: BMI = body mass index.
SOURCES: CDC, 2017, 2022b.

Health Organization (WHO). Using these charts involves measuring a child's weight and length and plotting them appropriately on the designated growth chart according to the child's clinician-identified sex. Weight-for-length is considered an appropriate way to track growth and development in early infancy. It also serves as a way to ascertain atypical growth, which could be an indicator of a larger health concern (AAP, 2022).

WHO's weight-for-length growth charts can offer clinicians a way to diagnose failure to thrive for children under age 2 years. Failure to thrive—also termed "weight faltering" or "growth failure"—is not a disease itself but a description of a growth pattern for children characterized by very low weight for age or height (Homan, 2016). Although there is no consensus on the definition of "failure to thrive," the term is often used to describe young children who fall below the 5th percentile for sex and age as measured by WHO's weight-for-length charts (Homan, 2016; Yoo et al., 2013). For the purposes of SSA's disability criteria, children under age 2 must be below the 3rd percentile for weight to qualify for disability, in addition to meeting other criteria described under each listing.

Weight-for-length has limitations as a growth measure. It is likely a poor approximation of adiposity (or body fat), especially in preterm infants (Nagel et al., 2021), and may not account for the normal variability in growth observed in infancy. Research shows that infant growth percentiles may decline during the first year of life. Tracking weight and length growth over time is essential to distinguish infants with clinically significant "faltering growth" from healthy infants with fluctuating growth velocities (Bennett et al., 2014).

BMI-for-Age Chart

CDC and AAP recommend that children and adolescents aged 2–20 years be tracked using the BMI growth reference charts published by CDC. Separate charts are available for boys and girls. BMI-for-age growth charts serve as a reference for monitoring growth and development among children and can be used as a screening tool to identify children who may be under- or overweight. BMI is calculated by dividing weight in kilograms by height in meters squared (BMI = weight [kg]/height [m]^2). Hence, BMI is easy to calculate and is considered appropriate for assessing weight in relation to stature in children and adolescents over age 2 years (CDC, 2022b; Hampl et al., 2023). For pediatric populations between 2 and 20 years old, given that body fat changes with age and may vary with sex, BMI measurements are compared with those of other youth of the same sex and similar age.[4] Figure 9-2 displays the BMI-for-age charts for boys and girls aged 2–20 years, published by CDC.

Despite its common use as an indicator of general health and a proxy for obesity in epidemiological studies, BMI's usefulness is limited. Historically, BMI is attributed to calculations performed by Adolphe Quetelet, who conducted a cross-sectional study of newborns and children based on height and weight in 1831–1832 (Jelliffe and Jelliffe, 1979). In an effort to account mathematically for differences in body build, the current BMI formula was adopted based on the concept that the body, particularly the trunk, could be considered a three-dimensional volume or mass. Thus, BMI is currently considered to reflect body composition as a measure of body adiposity. However, BMI is not a direct measure of body fat and does not distinguish between fat mass and fat-free mass (Vehrs et al., 2022); it simply assesses weight relative to height (Nevill et al., 2021; Nuttall, 2015). The increase in BMI typically seen in boys, especially with puberty, can be attributed to

---

[4] BMI is calculated the same way for adults and children, but the results are interpreted differently. For adults over age 20, BMI classifications no longer depend on age or sex (CDC, 2022b).

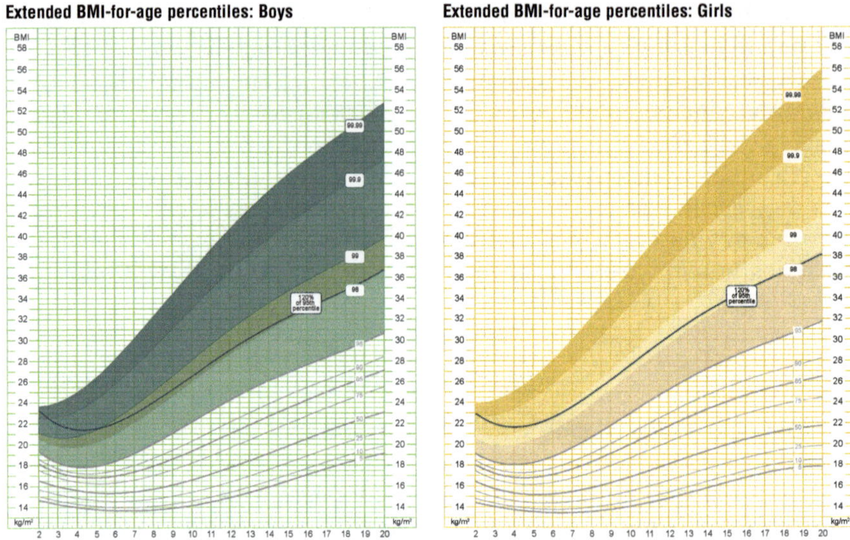

FIGURE 9-2 Body mass index for age, boys and girls, ages 2–20 years.
SOURCE: National Health Examination Survey and National Health and Nutrition Examination Survey. Developed by: National Center for Health Statistics in collaboration with National Center for Chronic Disease Prevention and Health Promotion, 2022.

an increase in fat-free mass, whereas girls typically show an increase in fat mass. High muscle mass, such as is seen in professional athletes, for example, can result in an elevated BMI even in the relative absence of adiposity.

At the same time, however, BMI measurements parallel measurements obtained by direct measures of body fat (such as underwater weighing and dual-energy X-ray absorptiometry), and for this reason can be considered a proxy for underlying adiposity (Hampl et al., 2023). Research fails to demonstrate that BMI is better at detecting under- and overweight youth as compared with weight-for-length measurements (Mei et al., 2002). Unlike other methods of body fat measurement that may require special equipment, BMI is a simple, inexpensive, and noninvasive tool. Thus, despite its limitations, advantages of using BMI include that it can easily be calculated and tracked into adulthood (Hampl et al., 2023; Simmonds et al., 2015).

On the other hand, although BMI is deeply integrated into clinical care and health systems, several flaws become apparent when it is used as a sole metric for evaluating an individual's health. In adults, there is a relatively poor correlation between percent body fat mass and BMI (Romero-Corral et al., 2008). Furthermore, BMI does not ascertain body fat distribution; does not, as noted above, differentiate between lean and fat body mass (a person can have a high BMI but still have a very low fat mass and vice versa); and does not provide insight into the origins of a person's weight status (Bray, 2023; Calcaterra, 2019; Flegal et al., 2009; Wellens et al., 1996). Calculation of BMI also depends on accurate height and weight measurements. These same limitations, found when using BMI in children and adolescents, may impact whether BMI can serve as an appropriate indicator of chronic disease status (Javed et al., 2015; Weber et al., 2013). For example, studies examining the utility of BMI for youth with asthma note that it paints an incomplete picture, as it does not examine adiposity indicators associated with asthma, asthma severity or control, atopy, and other factors relevant for lung function (den Dekker et al., 2016; Forno et al., 2014).

Additionally, an individual with a chronic disease and growth failure may have short stature and low weight and yet have a BMI that lies above the 3rd percentile. Indeed, BMI-for-age may not be a reliable indicator at the extremes of weight, as the accuracy of the predictive value of BMI declines in very lean and very overweight adolescents (Horlick, 2001). CDC BMI-for-age growth charts include percentiles between the 3rd and 97th, but may not give reliable percentage curves above the 97th or below the 3rd percentile (CDC, 2022a; Kuczmarski et al., 2002).

Finally, the BMI charts are based on the growth and development patterns of Caucasian youth. Therefore, BMI may under- or overdetect excess adiposity in youth with different genetic backgrounds (AMA, 2023a; Wagner and Heyward, 2000; WHO Expert Consultation, 2004).

For these reasons, in 2023 the American Medical Association (AMA, 2023a,b) adopted a new policy to recognize the significant limitations associated with the widespread use of BMI in clinical settings due to its inability to account for differing genetic factors.

Growth Measurement for Youth with Special Health Care Needs

Despite their limitations, the male and female WHO weight-for-length growth standards and CDC BMI-for-age growth standards published and updated by CDC and WHO continue to be used to assess growth in many populations. However, when youth have conditions that are known to interfere with growth, such as Turner syndrome or trisomy 21, more specific growth references may be available that better define growth patterns unique to these subpopulations when used along with guidelines for evaluating growth in youth with special health care needs (HRSA, 2014; Tang et al., 2021).[5]

Turner syndrome is a sex chromosome aneuploidy, a type of VST, due to loss or structural rearrangement of the second X chromosome.

---

[5] Children with Down syndrome (DS) often have lower birthweights and grow more slowly compared with children without DS, and growth charts specific to children with DS can help providers monitor growth and assess how well a child with DS is developing relative to peers with DS (CDC, 2022b; Zemel et al., 2015).

This condition, which affects 1 in 2,000–2,500 female liveborn infants, is associated with short stature, congenital heart disease, renal malformations, developmental delay, delayed puberty, and infertility, with potential implications for SSA disability determinations (Isojima and Yokoya, 2023). Comparing childhood growth against a well-defined reference population of people with Turner syndrome can help providers better assess individual growth for patients with this condition and aid in decision making about initiating growth hormone treatment (Isojima and Yokoya, 2023; Lyon et al., 1985; Turner Syndrome Society of the United States, n.d.). Although growth charts developed for specific pediatric populations have some limitations (e.g., old data, limited sample sizes, inconsistent measurement techniques used with initial data), they may offer better assessment of growth and inform appropriate intervention strategies for youth with special health care needs (HRSA, 2014).

On the other hand, specific growth charts do not exist for every condition—or indeed, for most conditions. Published growth charts for BMI-for-age assume that a patient's growth will be similar to that of typically developing (healthy) American youth, and do not account for atypical body and muscle development or physical challenges in measuring height (e.g., inability to stand, contractures, scoliosis, lack of head and trunk control) (HRSA, 2014; Polfuss et al., 2021). Studies examining youth with spina bifida, cerebral palsy, skeletal dysplasias, and muscular dystrophy raise concerns about the reliability of BMI as a measure for chronic conditions that are associated with atypical growth patterns or that impact bone and muscle development (Duran et al., 2019; Polfuss et al., 2021; Rempel, 2015; Whitney et al., 2019).

Because BMI is not an indicator of body composition and does not differentiate between lean mass and fat body mass, it may not adequately examine the important markers of malnutrition that impact chronic disease outcomes in patients of underweight status (Calcaterra, 2019; Nuttall, 2015). Best practices call for providers to offer continuous nutritional assessment and use BMI measurement along with additional methods of body growth (e.g., arm span and body composition assessments) (Calcaterra et al., 2019; Polfuss et al., 2021).

GROWTH MEASUREMENT IN TRANSGENDER AND GENDER DIVERSE YOUTH AND YOUTH WITH VARIATIONS IN SEX TRAITS

For providers measuring BMI-for-age in TGD youth or youth with VSTs, it is not always clear which chart—male or female—is the most appropriate to use. Pediatric BMI charts differ for males and females, and the female BMI chart has a wider span, including more extremes of weight (Kidd et al., 2019; Kuczmarski et al., 2002). Measuring TGD patients or patients with VSTs using the incorrect gendered BMI chart can place these patients in the wrong BMI percentiles, which can impact care and treatment recommendations (Kidd et al., 2019) and may impact ability to qualify for disability under SSA's listings. However, providers often lack adequate training regarding whether to use growth charts corresponding to sex recorded at birth or to gender identity.

Part of the challenge in selecting an appropriate BMI reference sex is that medical records may contain incorrect information (e.g., incorrect sex recorded in the patient chart) or lack documentation that would provide a complete picture of patient characteristics (e.g., failure to ask about gender identity or VSTs as separate from sex recorded at birth). Chapter 3 of this report describes these challenges in greater detail, but they are worth mentioning again here, as the realities of medical record data collection can impact interpretation of BMI for TGD youth and youth with VSTs. Moreover, even when medical records contain a complete and accurate record of patient sex and gender characteristics, such that providers are aware they are assessing a TGD patient or patient with a VST, providers may lack familiarity in caring for these patients and may not know how or when TGD or VST lived experience impacts patient care and clinical decision making. For these many reasons, selecting the appropriate BMI growth chart in these populations is challenging.

This section presents literature on how gender-affirming hormone therapy (GAHT) impacts youth body composition and how GAHT may impact BMI measurement and provider decision making.

Before proceeding, it should be noted that the literature does not contain research on the impact of GAHT on weight-for-length, as this measurement is intended for children aged 36 months (and is not used in SSA's disability determinations for children aged 2 and older), and GAHT is not provided to this age group. While providers assessing body composition in infants and very young children may face similar barriers to clinical decision making (e.g., medical records may record sex improperly), in general this measurement of growth and development is not impacted by decisions around gender-affirming care. For this reason, this section on the impact of GAHT on body composition does not address the weight-for-length measurement.

Impact of GAHT on Adolescent Body Composition

Given that BMI is calculated using the patient's weight and height, it is important to consider how GAHT may impact youth weight and body fat distribution, and height.[6]

---

[6] As described in Chapter 5, GAHT is not used until puberty. This section describes the impact of GAHT on youth only during and after puberty. For prepubescent children, hormone therapy, surgeries, and other gender-affirming treatment options are not appropriate, but psychosocial interventions may be beneficial.

Weight/Body Fat Distribution

Various studies of adult TGD populations have suggested exogenous sex hormones can lead to alterations in body composition, with testosterone administration resulting in more masculine body fat distribution (an increase in lean mass and a decrease in body fat percentage), and estrogen administration causing a more feminine body fat distribution (a decrease in lean mass and an increase in total body fat and fat accumulation) (Katznelson et al., 1996; Klaver et al., 2018; Van Caenegem et al., 2015).[7] However, body composition changes vary during hormone therapy; some people receiving GAHT will see no measurable change (van Velzen et al., 2020). Studies on the impact of GAHT on TGD youth are limited but show that body fat distribution shifts toward that of the affirmed sex, similar to what has been observed in the adult population (Boogers et al., 2023; Klaver et al., 2018). However, for TGD youth who receive these treatments, body composition is affected not only by GAHT but also by puberty-delaying medications—when individuals receive, for example, gonadotropin-releasing hormone (GnRH) agonists (e.g., leuprolide). Studies on body composition in TGD youth reveal an increase in fat percentage among both transgender boys and transgender girls during GnRH agonist treatment (Klaver et al., 2018; Nokoff et al., 2021; Schagen et al., 2016). The timing of GAHT and pubertal onset may also influence weight, as body composition trends among TGD youth who initiate pubertal delay differ between early and late pubertal starters (although these trends tend to level off after about 3 years) (Boogers et al., 2023).

Height

Very limited published literature provides guidance on how best to predict the impact on GnRH agonist treatment and GAHT during puberty on linear growth (height). Two recent studies found that TGD youth—both transgender males and transgender females—show a decrease in growth velocity when they begin receiving GnRH agonist treatment to pause puberty, followed by an increase during administration of GAHT (Boogers et al., 2022; Willemsen et al., 2023).

The large variation in treatment doses, protocols, and administration methods confound the generalization of the limited studies on GAHT and body composition. In addition, variable patient adherence may also influence outcome data. Available data regarding the pace of changes in body composition during GAHT are quite limited and likely affected by specific treatment protocols. Furthermore, because most available studies

---

[7] Appendix C explores differences in body composition among adult TGD populations in greater depth.

do not compare body mass changes in TGD youth relative to cisgender peers, these studies are difficult to interpret, as rapid growth in adolescence causes changes to body composition regardless of whether puberty-delaying medication or GAHT is received. It should also be noted that TGD populations may differ in body composition from cisgender peers at baseline even without receiving GAHT, which further complicates interpretation of the impact of GAHT on body composition (Ceolin et al., 2024; Van Caenegem et al., 2015).

Impact of GAHT on BMI Measurement

GnRH agonist treatment associated with pubertal delay and GAHT may alter weight, height, and other aspects of body composition. Hence, TGD youth who receive these treatments may experience a change in their BMI measurement. Available data on BMI trends in TGD youth are sparse, and the extent to which pubertal delay or GAHT in adolescence impacts BMI is unclear (Jarin et al., 2017; Olson et al., 2015; Sequeira et al., 2017). One retrospective study compared 42 transgender males (aged 14–21) with BMI-matched cisgender females, finding a significant increase in BMI for the transgender males after the initiation of testosterone therapy (Valentine et al., 2021). The transgender group had an increase in BMI of +3.29 percentiles from baseline through final follow-up (average length of time: 10.8 months), compared with a decrease of 1.77 percentiles for the cisgender group. A study by Klaver and colleagues (2020) similarly shows an increase in BMI (+2.3 kg/m^2; 95% confidence interval [CI] 1.7–2.9 kg/m^2) for 121 transgender males aged 15–22 receiving GAHT, while findings by Boogers and colleagues (2023) show a smaller increase in BMI among a cohort of 235 transgender males aged 18 years or younger (+1.0 kg/m^2; 95% CI 0.5–1.5 kg/m^2), remaining stable thereafter. Other studies report that transgender males see an increase in BMI after initiation of testosterone treatment but have not found these effects to be sustained over time.

For adolescent transgender females who receive estradiol, two studies found an increase in BMI: one study examining a cohort of 71 transgender females aged 15–22 found a significant increase in BMI (+3.0 kg/m^2; 95% CI 1.6–4.4 kg/m^2); the other found a smaller increase in BMI (+1.7 kg/m^2; 95% CI 1.0–2.3 kg/m^2) among 111 transgender girls aged 18 or younger (Klaver et al., 2020; Boogers et al., 2023). However, other studies have found no significant change in BMI among adolescent transgender females receiving GAHT.

The mixed reports on BMI among TGD youth echo similarly mixed results found in assessing BMI for adults receiving GAHT. Additional studies are needed to better understand the role of GAHT in BMI measurement for transgender youth.

While this area is insufficiently studied, providers need to consider TGD care experience when interpreting BMI. The literature calls on providers to recognize the importance of "prior patient history, pubertal stage, and any gender-affirming pharmacological interventions that may alter height/weight" when selecting the optimal BMI chart for TGD youth (Kidd et al., 2019, p. 299). While pubertal delay and GAHT administration may impact adolescent body composition, each patient may be different, and plotting changes over time is likely to be more useful than interpreting a single measurement.

Dual Calculations

As discussed previously in this report, dual calculations of BMI (trending the patient using both male and female charts) may aid in clinical decision making for some TGD patients (Kidd et al., 2019), as studies have found that TGD youth receiving GAHT (either testosterone or estradiol) show body composition values that fall between BMI-matched cisgender males and cisgender females (Bomberg et al., 2023). A dual calculation approach may also help providers navigate the use of gendered growth charts for some patients with VSTs.

Provider Decision Making for BMI Interpretation

Commonly, and potentially inaccurately, clinicians use the sex recorded in the medical record (whether or not recorded accurately) as the basis for BMI interpretation when using CDC growth reference charts. Some providers may take into account individual patient history related to gender-affirming care when measuring BMI, but without guidelines in place, providers may have to make difficult or arbitrary judgments about which chart is most appropriate for a given patient at a given time. Depending on which growth chart providers choose, they may diagnose growth failure when it does not exist or fail to diagnose it when it does—both outcomes impacting eligibility for SSA disability benefits.

Kidd and colleagues (2019) propose that providers consider dual calculations of BMI (trending the patient using both male and female charts) for all TGD youth to help "navigate the inherent limitations of using gendered growth charts" (p. 299). Kidd and colleagues (2019) state that dual calculations are most critical for individuals at the extremes of BMI. Bomberg and colleagues (2023) propose that sex-nonspecific growth charts and BMI curves be used for TGD youth. In their research on 39,119 youth, the authors developed new growth charts that "age smooth differences in pubertal timing between sexes to determine how youth are growing as 'children' versus 'girls or boys'" (see Figure 9-3; Bomberg et al., 2023, p. 1).

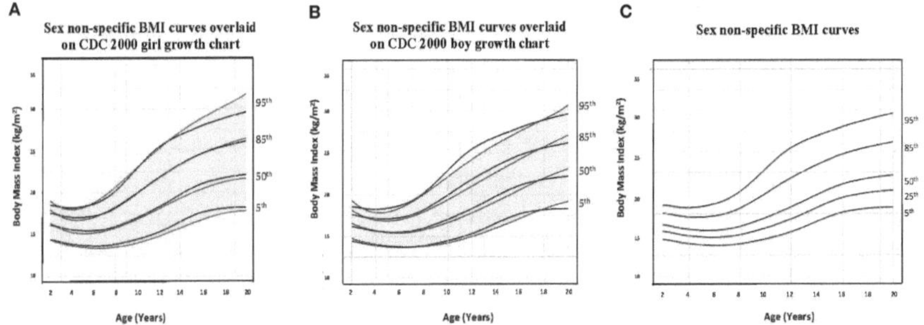

FIGURE 9-3 Comparison of age-adjusted, sex-nonspecific body mass index (BMI) curves with Centers for Disease Control and Prevention (CDC) 2000 age- and sex-adjusted BMI curves.
NOTE: Bomberg and colleagues (2023) provide the following explanation of the above figure: "(A) shows our age-adjusted sex non-specific BMI curves overlaid on the CDC 2000 girl age- and sex-adjusted BMI curves, highlighting the 5th, 50th, 85th, and 95th percentiles. (B) shows our age-adjusted sex non-specific BMI curves overlaid on the CDC 2000 boy age- and sex-adjusted weight curve, highlighting the 3rd, 50th, 85th, and 95th percentiles. (C) shows our age-adjusted sex non-specific BMI growth curves. Here, we highlight the 5th (underweight), 25th, 50th, 85th (overweight), and 95th (obesity) percentiles given their clinical utility." (p. 4)
SOURCE: Bomberg et al., 2023. Originally published by *Frontiers*. CC BY 4.0 DEED.

The committee found no research to indicate the extent to which the approaches proposed by Kidd and colleagues (2019) or Bomberg and colleagues (2023) are used among providers. In the committee's opinion, however, these approaches are not common and not yet validated.

Given considerable challenges involved in selecting the appropriate BMI reference chart for certain adolescent TGD patients and patients with VSTs, BMI may be a particularly unreliable measure for these populations. Coupling this reality with the fact that BMI is considered to be an unreliable indicator for underweight children below the 3rd percentile (and thus for identifying growth failure using SSA's criteria), BMI is likely to be particularly inaccurate in diagnosing growth failure in youth who undergo pubertal delay and/or receive GAHT.

GROWTH FAILURE AND SSA DISABILITY DETERMINATION

The various SSA growth failure categories listed in Box 9-1 all use the weight-for-length table (for children from birth to attainment of age 2 years) and the BMI-for-age table (for children age 2 years to attainment of age 18). As in other areas of the disability Listings, weight-for-length and

BMI-for-age measurements are just one component of the medical evidence accepted to demonstrate growth failure and disability. For example, for growth failure related to immune suppression (under 114.11[I]), the childhood applicant must also submit a CD4 count—the result of a laboratory test that measures the number of CD4 T cells and serves as an indicator of the effectiveness of the antiretroviral treatment. Likewise, for growth failure due to any chronic respiratory disorder (103.06), the childhood applicant must also submit medical evidence of hypoxemia (low levels of oxygen in the blood).

Still, BMI-for-age measurements are a key component of meeting disability criteria for children and adolescents over age 2 years. For TGD applicants and applicants with VSTs, if their health care provider has not selected the appropriate CDC growth chart to assess BMI-for-age, the BMI percentile recorded in the patients' medical records may not indicate their health status accurately, impacting their ability to qualify for disability benefits.

Given the many challenges described in this chapter, SSA might consider certain adjustments to its growth failure disability Listings to ensure that adjudicators have the appropriate tools for accurately assessing growth failure for TGD populations or populations with VSTs. The next sections review considerations for SSA with respect to terminology related to both the weight-for-length and BMI-for-age tables published under Listing 105.08B (SSA, n.d.-a). Most important, this section describes alternative measures for assessing growth failure and disability in TGD youth and youth with VSTs.

Terminology in SSA Criteria

For each of the listings in Box 9-1, SSA evaluates growth failure using either the weight-for-length table or BMI-for-age table provided under Listing 105.08B (SSA, n.d.-a). As is standard in growth charts used across pediatrics, weight-for-length and BMI-for-age tables use sex recorded at birth as the appropriate reference sex, meaning that a provider must compare weight-for-length or BMI-for-age against a male or female growth chart (CDC, 2022b). However, SSA's disability criteria use the term "gender" in reference to these growth measurements: "[W]e evaluate a child's growth failure by using the appropriate table for age and *gender*" [emphasis added] (SSA, n.d.-a). This language may incorrectly indicate that it is "gender identity" that is determinative when interpreting weight-for-length and BMI-for-age in Listings related to childhood growth failure.

The committee notes that BMI is also used as a measure of weight loss under the adult Listings to document weight loss related to digestive disorders (5.08); kidney disease (6.05B4); and HIV infection (14.11G).[8] While SSA follows clinical guidelines by not tying BMI to sex-specific criteria, SSA again uses the term "gender" here (SSA, n.d.-b). The conflation of these terms throughout disability evaluation criteria can lead to confusion for both applicants and adjudicators. SSA might consider updating this language to reflect current guidelines, differentiating sex recorded at birth from gender identity as defined in Chapter 2.

Growth Failure under SSA Criteria: Relevant Measures of Growth for Children Aged 2–18

Other than BMI-for-age, the various SSA Listings for which evidence of growth failure is required include no other available measurements of body composition. However, best practices call for providers to use BMI measurement along with additional methods of body composition assessment because of concerns about the utility of BMI as a sole indicator of appropriate weight and health. In 2023, AMA (2023a,b) adopted a new policy to support using BMI in conjunction with other valid measures, stating that additional appropriate body composition measures may include measurements of visceral fat, body adiposity index, body composition, relative fat mass, waist circumference, and genetic/metabolic factors.

Linear Growth Velocity

Chronic disease can result in a slowing of the normal rate of linear growth (i.e., attainment of height) in children and adolescents of all ages. As discussed previously, this rate of growth is referred to as linear growth velocity (or height velocity) and is equal to the difference in two length or height measurements taken at different points in time (at least 3–6 months apart), divided by the time between those two measurements in years. Appropriate linear growth indicates integrity of the hypothalamic-pituitary-growth axis, nutritional sufficiency, and a safe socioeconomic environment. Linear growth deceleration provides an indicator of potential nutritional inadequacy, deleterious genetic variants, hormone deficiencies, and/or chronic disease (Benjamin-Chung et al., 2023; De Sanctis et al., 2021). Linear growth velocity is therefore considered the single most relevant assessment of child health, especially from 2 years of age through achievement of adult height. According to Thompson (2021), "linear growth is considered the 'best overall indicator of child well-being'" (p. 2).

---

[8] This chapter does not examine adult Listings for BMI, as SSA's disability Listings make clear, under 5.00F2, that "calculation and interpretation of the BMI are independent of gender in adults" (SSD, n.d.-b).

A practical rule is that at any age, linear growth velocity of less than 4 centimeters per year is diagnostic of growth failure. What constitutes a normal linear growth velocity varies based on a child's age (e.g., children aged 1–4 years typically grow ~10–15 cm/year, but children and adolescents typically grow only ~5 cm/year before their pubertal growth spurt). Therefore, the most accurate approach is to plot growth on a height velocity chart. Notably, these charts are sex based, and thus careful consideration of sex and gender identity is essential in selecting the correct chart, as discussed earlier in this chapter. A height velocity below the 10th percentile for age and sex indicates growth failure. As with percentage weight loss, described below, the ideal time frame for assessing height velocity differs from SSA's usual windows of at least 60 days to under 12 months. The two or more measurements that go into calculating an individual's height velocity should be obtained at least 3–6 months apart (60 days would be insufficient), and often might be obtained beyond the 12-month maximum required under the SSA disability criteria, outlined in Box 9-1.

Percentage Weight Loss

Percentage weight loss is a measure used to identify malnutrition, a key risk factor for growth failure in the setting of chronic disease. When individuals with chronic medical conditions are unable to meet their nutritional needs, they can experience severe, clinically significant weight loss that may not necessarily result in a BMI low enough to qualify an individual for disability. In these cases, if two or more weight measurements are available, youth aged 2 years and older whose weight decreases by 10 percent or more of their usual body weight meet criteria for "severe" malnutrition. Such weight loss occurring in the setting of an already low BMI (i.e., <50th percentile for sex and age) in an individual with a chronic medical condition would be highly concerning, even if it does not lead to a BMI below the 3rd percentile. Documenting percentage weight loss can therefore be useful for assessing health for youth at risk of growth failure and could be worth including in SSA's disability criteria.

Other Measures

For pediatric populations at risk of poor nutritional status because of chronic disease and disability, other appropriate assessments of body composition include dual-energy X-ray absorptiometry, doubly labeled water, and bioelectrical impedance analysis (BIA) (Calcaterra et al., 2019; Pelizzo et al., 2017; Whitney et al., 2019). Such technology is not readily available in all settings but may be used in specialty settings. For example, BIA offers an accurate and reproducible method for assessing body composition.

Unlike BMI, BIA provides detailed information about the individual components of body composition, including the amount of body fat, muscle mass, and body water. Some literature suggests that BIA can provide a fast, simple, and low-cost alternative to BMI and that it may provide more accurate measurement of body composition for youth with chronic illness. However, no guidelines, normative ranges, or best practices have been clearly established for its use (Calcaterra et al, 2019).

These alternative measures deserve further study in youth with TGD or VST lived experience—particularly those who have received puberty-delaying medications or received GAHT—and can supplement BMI as commonly used clinical indicators of growth failure when SSA makes a disability determination.

Regardless of how body parameters are assessed, the medical literature points to the requirement for multiple assessments of growth and body composition. Multiple longitudinal measurements for ascertaining physical health are more accurate than single cross-sectional measurements in youth with chronic diseases, ultimately resulting in better decision making and selection of treatment options (Calcaterra et al., 2019).

SUMMARY OF KEY POINTS

This chapter has presented literature and guidelines that call for use of alternative measures of body composition along with BMI or instead of BMI, given concerns about the utility and accuracy of BMI-for-age as the sole measurement. BMI-for-age may be an especially poor measure for identifying growth failure, as it is not considered a reliable indicator for youth below the 3rd percentile of weight. In addition, because BMI does not differentiate between lean and fat body mass, it may not adequately account for the important elements of body composition that matter for youth who are experiencing growth failure related to underlying chronic disease.

BMI can be particularly inaccurate in identifying growth failure in youth receiving GAHT.[9] In this population, linear growth velocity may be a better indicator of growth failure. Percentage weight loss—a common measure for identifying malnutrition, a key risk factor for growth failure in the setting of chronic disease—is another useful metric for assessing health for children at risk of growth failure, and it may be worth including in SSA's

---

[9] Where people with VSTs take GAHT, the approaches described here may be appropriate; however, research is limited on the impact of GAHT in populations with VSTs. The committee notes that people with VSTs take hormone therapy for a multitude of reasons beyond gender-affirming care and care is extremely individualized; the impact of various hormone therapies on sex-specific measurements is unknown.

disability criteria. SSA may better serve pediatric populations by including these alternative measures in the 105.08B criteria and across various childhood growth failure Listings, as these measures may provide for more accurate assessment of not only TGD youth but all pediatric populations that apply for disability benefits.

However, as discussed previously, BMI-for-age is a common measure of childhood growth and is readily obtained in clinical settings. For this reason, it will continue to be present in medical records submitted to SSA. This chapter has presented the available literature on the impact of pubertal delay and GAHT on body composition and BMI measurement. While more research is needed in this area, the evidence available indicates that pubertal delay and GAHT matter for measuring body composition such that it is important for providers to take these experiences into account when interpreting BMI. It may be appropriate for providers to calculate BMI using both male and female charts ("dual calculations") to aid in clinical decision making for their patients, and SSA should be aware that it may receive medical records for TGD youth containing measurements of BMI using both charts. SSA may also receive BMI calculations from both charts if providers are mistaken or lack training and guidance on which chart to use.

It is the consensus of the committee, based on its clinical expertise and professional judgment, that in cases where the medical record contains BMI measurements from both charts, SSA would best serve TGD applicants and applicants with VSTs by using the lower percentile BMI value to determine disability. Given what remains unknown about how GAHT impacts body composition and the lack of guidance available for how BMI should be interpreted for TGD youth and youth with VSTs, such an approach would ensure fairness for youth with TGD or VST lived experience who have not had access to providers trained to interpret their results thoroughly and thoughtfully and with consideration of their individual patient history.

REFERENCES

AAP (American Academy of Pediatrics). 2022. *WHO growth charts for infants 0-24 months.* https://www.aap.org/en/patient-care/newborn-and-infant-nutrition/newborn-and-infant-nutrition-assessment-tools/term-infant-growth-tools/ (accessed April 2, 2024).

AMA (American Medical Association). 2023a. *Report 07 of the council on science and public health (A-23).* Chicago, IL. https://www.ama-assn.org/system/files/a23-csaph07.pdf (accessed March 9, 2024).

AMA. 2023b. *AMA adopts new policy clarifying role of BMI as a measure in medicine.* https://www.ama-assn.org/press-center/press-releases/ama-adopts-new-policy-clarifying-role-bmi-measure-medicine#:~:text=Jun%2014%2C%202023&text=The%20report%20also%20outlined%20the,genders%2C%20and%20age%2Dspan (accessed July 15, 2023).

Benjamin-Chung, J., A. Mertens, J. M. Colford, A. E. Hubbard, M. J. van der Laan, J. Coyle, O. Sofrygin, W. Cai, A. Nguyen, N. N. Pokpongkiat, S. Djajadi, A. Seth, W. Jilek, E. Jung, E. O. Chung, S. Rosete, N. Hejazi, I. Malenica, H. Li, R. Hafen, V. Subramoney, J. Häggström, T. Norman, K. H. Brown, P. Christian, B. F. Arnold, S. Abbeddou, L. S. Adair, T. Ahmed, A. Ali, H. Ali, P. Ashorn, R. Bahl, M. L. Barreto, F. Begín, P. O. Bessong, M. K. Bhan, N. Bhandari, S. K. Bhargava, Z. A. Bhutta, R. E. Black, L. Bodhidatta, D. Carba, I. Gonzalez Casanova, W. Checkley, J. E. Crabtree, K. G. Dewey, C. P. Duggan, C. H. D. Fall, A. S. G. Faruque, W. W. Fawzi, J. Q. da Silva Filho, R. H. Gilman, R. L. Guerrant, R. Haque, S. Y. Hess, E. R. Houpt, J. H. Humphrey, N. T. Iqbal, E. Y. Jimenez, J. John, S. M. John, G. Kang, M. Kosek, M. S. Kramer, A. Labrique, N. R. Lee, A. Â. M. Lima, M. Mahfuz, T. C. Mahopo, K. Maleta, D. S. Manandhar, K. P. Manji, R. Martorell, S. Mazumder, E. Mduma, V. R. Mohan, S. E. Moore, I. Mostafa, R. Ntozini, M. E. Nyathi, M. P. Olortegui, W. A. Petri, P. S. Premkumar, A. M. Prentice, N. Rahman, H. S. Sachdev, K. Sadiq, R. Sarkar, N. M. Saville, S. Shaikh, B. P. Shrestha, S. K. Shrestha, A. M. Soares, B. Sonko, A. D. Stein, E. Svensen, S. Syed, F. Umrani, H. D. Ward, K. P. West, L. S. F. Wu, S. Yang, P. P. Yori, and The Ki Child Growth Consortium. 2023. Early-childhood linear growth faltering in low- and middle-income countries. *Nature* 621(7979): 550–557.

Bennett, W. E., Jr., K. S. Hendrix, R. T. Thompson, A. E. Carroll, and S. M. Downs. 2014. The natural history of weight percentile changes in the first year of life. *JAMA Pediatrics* 168(7):681–682.

Boddy, J., D. Skuse, and B. Andrews. 2000. The developmental sequelae of nonorganic failure to thrive. *Journal of Child Psychology and Psychiatry* 41(8):1003–1014.

Bomberg, E. M., B. S., Miller, O. Y., Addo, A. D., Rogol, M. M., Jaber, and K. Sarafoglou. 2023. Sex non-specific growth charts and potential clinical implications in the care of transgender youth. *Frontiers in Endocrinology* 14:1227886.

Boogers, L. S., C. M. Wiepjes, D. T. Klink, I. Hellinga, A. S. P. van Trotsenburg, M. den Heijer, and S. E. Hannema. 2022. Transgender girls grow tall: Adult height is unaffected by GnRH analogue and estradiol treatment. *Journal of Clinical Endocrinology & Metabolism* 107(9):e3805–e3815.

Boogers, L. S., S. J. P. Reijtenbag, C. M. Wiepjes, A. S. P. van Trotsenburg, M. den Heijer, and S. E. Hannema. 2023. Time course of body composition changes in transgender adolescents during puberty suppression and sex hormone treatment. *Journal of Clinical Endocrinology & Metabolism* 109(8):e1593–e1601.

Bray, G. 2023. Beyond BMI. *Nutrients* 15(10):2254.

Calcaterra, V. P. 2019. BMI is a poor predictor of nutritional status in disabled children: What is the most recommended method for body composition assessment in this pediatric population? *Frontiers in Pediatrics* 226.

Calcaterra, V., H. Cena, M. Manuelli, L. Sacchi, V. Girgenti, C. Larizza, C., and G. Pelizzo. 2019. Body hydration assessment using bioelectrical impedance vector analysis in neurologically impaired children. *European Journal of Clinical Nutrition* 73(12): 1649–1652.

CDC (Centers for Disease Control and Prevention). 2010. *WHO growth standards are recommended for use in the U.S. For infants and children 0 to 2 years of age.* https://www.cdc. gov/growthcharts/who_charts.htm#print (accessed April 2, 2024).

CDC. 2017. *Clinical growth charts.* https://www.cdc.gov/growthcharts/clinical_charts.htm (accessed April, 2024).

CDC. 2022a. *Adult BMI calculator.* Division of Nutrition, Physical Activity, and Obesity, National Center for Chronic Disease Prevention and Health Promotion. https://www. cdc.gov/healthyweight/assessing/bmi/adult_bmi/english_bmi_calculator/bmi_calculator. html (accessed March 13, 2024).

CDC. 2022b. *Clinical growth charts.* National Center for Health Statistics. https://www.cdc.gov/growthcharts/clinical_charts.htm (accessed March 9, 2024).

Ceolin, C., A. Scala, M. Dall'Agnol, C. Ziliotto, A. Delbarba, P. Facondo, A. Citron, B. Vescovi, S. Pasqualini, S. Giannini, V. Camozzi, C. Cappelli, A. Bertocco, M. De Rui, A. Coin, G. Sergi, A. Ferlin, A. Garolla, and Gender Incongruence Interdisciplinary Group. 2024. Bone health and body composition in transgender adults before gender-affirming hormonal therapy: Data from the comet study. *Journal of Endocrinological Investigation* 47(2):401–410.

Cooke, R., O. Goulet, K. Huysentruyt, K. Joosten, A. V. Khadilkar, M. Mao, R. Meyer, A. M. Prentice, and A. Singhal. 2023. Catch-up growth in infants and young children with faltering growth: Expert opinion to guide general clinicians. *Journal of Pediatric Gastroenterology and Nutrition* 77(1):7–15.

De Sanctis, V., A. Soliman, N. Alaaraj, S. Ahmed, F. Alyafei, and N. Hamed. 2021. Early and long-term consequences of nutritional stunting: From childhood to adulthood. *Acta Biomedica: Atenai Parmensis* 92(1):e2021168.

den Dekker, H., K. Ros, J. de Jongste, I. Reiss, V. Jaddoe, and L. Duijts. 2016. Body fat mass distribution and interrupter resistance, fractional exhaled nitric oxide and asthma at school-age. *Journal of Allergy and Clinical Immunology* 139(3):810–818.

Duran, I., K. Martakis, M. Rehberg, O. Semler, and E. Schoenau. 2019. Anthropometric measurements to identify undernutrition in children with cerebral palsy. *Developmental Medicine and Child Neurology* 61:1168–1174.

Flegal, K. M., J. A. Shepherd, A. Looker, B. Graubard, L. Borrud, C. Ogden, T. Harris, J. Everhart, and N. Schenker. 2009. Comparisons of percentage body fat, body mass index, waist circumference, and waist-stature ratio in adults. *American Journal of Clinical Nutrition* 89(2):500–508.

Forno, E., E. Acosta-Perez, J. Brehm, Y. Han, M. Alvarez, A. Colon-Semidey, G. Canino, and J. Celedón. 2014. Obesity and adiposity indicators, asthma, and atopy in Puerto Rican children. *Journal of Allergy and Clinical Immunology* 133(5):1308–1314.

Hagan, J. F., J. S. Shaw, and P. M. Duncan (eds). 2017. *Bright futures: Guidelines for health supervision of infants, children, and adolescents.* Elk Grove Village, IL: American Academy of Pediatrics.

Hampl, S., S. Hassink, A. Skinner, S. Armstrong, S. Barlow, C. Bolling, K. Avila Edwards, I. Eneli, R. Hamre, M. Joseph, D. Lunsford, E. Mendonca, M. Michalsky, N. Mirza, E. Ochoa, M. Sharifi, A. Staiano, A. Weedn, S. Flinn, J. Lindros, and K. Okechukwu. 2023. Clinical practice guideline for the evaluation and treatment of children and adolescents with obesity. *Pediatrics* 151(2):e2022060640.

Hawkes, C. P., S. Mostoufi-Moab, S. E. McCormack, A. Grimberg, and B. S. Zemel. 2020. Sitting height to standing height ratio reference charts for children in the United States. *Journal of Pediatrics* 226:221–227.e15.

Hochberg, Z. 2011. Developmental plasticity in child growth and maturation. *Frontiers in Endocrinology* 2.

Homan, G. J. 2016. Failure to thrive: A practical guide. *American Family Physician* 94(4):295–299.

Horlick, M. 2001. Body mass index in childhood—measuring a moving target. *Journal of Clinical Endocrinology and Metabolism* 86:4059–4060.

HRSA (Health Resources and Services Administration). 2014. *CDC growth charts for children with special health care needs.* North Bethesda, MD. https://depts.washington.edu/growth/cshcn/text/page1a.htm (accessed March 9, 2024).

Isojima, T., and S. Yokoya. 2023. Growth in girls with Turner syndrome. *Frontiers in Endocrinology* 13.

Jarin, J., E. Pine-Twaddell, G. Trotman, J. Stevens, K. A. Conard, E. Tefera, and V. Gomez-Lobo. 2017. Cross-sex hormones and metabolic parameters in adolescents with gender dysphoria. *Pediatrics* 139(5).

Javed, A., M. Jumean, M. Murad, D. Okorodudu, S. Kumar, V. Somers, O. Sochor, and F. Lopez-Jimenez. 2015. Diagnostic performance of body mass index to identify obesity as defined by body adiposity in children and adolescents: A systematic review and meta-analysis. *Pediatric Obesity* 10(3):234–244.

Jelliffe, D. B., and E. F. Jelliffe. 1979. Underappreciated pioneers Quételet: Man and index. *American Journal of Clinical Nutrition* 32(12):2519–2521.

Jorge, A. A. L., A. Grimberg, M. T. Dattani, and J. Baron. 2021. Disorders of human growth. In *Sperling pediatric endocrinology*, 5th ed., edited by M. A. Sperling, J. A. Majzoub, R. K. Menon, and C. A. Stratakis. Amsterdam, Netherlands: Elsevier.

Katznelson, L., J. S. Finkelstein, D. A. Schoenfeld, D. I. Rosenthal, E. J. Anderson, and A. Klibanski. 1996. Increase in bone density and lean body mass during testosterone administration in men with acquired hypogonadism. *Journal of Clinical Endocrinology & Metabolism* 81(12):4358–4365.

Kidd, K. S., G. Sequeira, C. Dhar, G. montano, S. Feldman Witchel, and D. Rofey. 2019. Gendered body mass index percentile charts and transgender youth: Making the case to change charts. *Transgender Health* 4(1):297–299.

Klaver, M., R. de Mutsert, C. M. Wiepjes, J. Twisk, M. den Heijer, J. Rotteveel, and D. Klink. 2018. Early hormonal treatment affects body composition and body shape in young transgender adolescents. *Journal of Sexual Medicine* 15:251–260.

Klaver, M., R. de Mutsert, M. van der Loos, C. M. Wiepjes, J. W. R. Twisk, M. den Heijer, J. Rotteveel, and D. T. Klink. 2020. Hormonal treatment and cardiovascular risk profile in transgender adolescents. *Pediatrics* 145(3).

Kuczmarski, R. J., C. L. Ogden, S. S. Guo, L. M. Grummer-Strawn, K. M. Flegal, Z. Mei, R. Wei, L. Curtin, A. Roche, and C. Johnson. 2002. 2000 CDC growth charts for the United States: Methods and development. *Vital Health Statistics* 11:1–190.

Kyle, U. S.-B. 2015. Growth failure and nutrition considerations in chronic childhood wasting diseases. *Nutrition in Clinical Practice* 30(2):227–238.

Lyon, A. J., M. A. Preece, and D. B. Grant. 1985. Growth curve for girls with Turner syndrome. *Archives of Disease in Childhood* 60:932–935.

Mei, Z., L. M. Grummer-Strawn, A. Pietrobelli, A. Goulding, M. I. Goran, and W. H. Dietz. 2002. Validity of body mass index compared with other body-composition screening indexes for the assessment of body fatness in children and adolescents. *American Journal of Clinical Nutrition* 75(6):978–985.

Nagel, E., C. Desjardins, C. Earthman, S. Ramel, and E. Demerath. 2021. Weight for length measures may not accurately reflect adiposity in preterm infants born appropriate for gestational age during hospitalisation or after discharge from the neonatal intensive care unit. *Pediatric Obesity* 16(5):e12744.

NCHS (National Center for Health Statistics). 2022. Evaluation of alternative body mass index (BMI) metrics to monitor weight status in children and adolescents with extremely high BMI using CDC BMI-for-age growth charts: Data evaluation and methods research. *Vital and Health Statistics* 2(197). https://www.cdc.gov/nchs/data/series/sr_02/sr02-197.pdf (accessed March 9, 2024).

Nevill, A. M., C. P. Reuter, C. Brand, A. R. Gaya, J. Mota, J. D. P. Renner, and M. J. Duncan. 2021. BMI fails to reflect the developmental changes in body fatness between boys and girls during adolescence. *International Journal of Environmental Research and Public Health* 18(15):7833.

NIDDK (National Institute of Diabetes and Digestive and Kidney Diseases). 2022. *Growth failure in children with chronic kidney disease.* https://www.niddk.nih.gov/health-information/kidney-disease/children/helping-child-adapt-life-chronic-kidney-disease/growth-failure-chronic-kidney-disease (accessed March 9, 2024).

Nokoff, N. J., S. L. Scarbro, K. L. Moreau, P. Zeitler, K. Nadeau, D. Reirden, E. Juarez-Colunga, and M. Kelsey. 2021. Body composition and markers of cardiometabolic health in transgender youth on gonadotropin-releasing hormone agonists. *Transgender Health* 6(2):111–119.

Nuttall, F. 2015. Body mass index: Obesity, BMI, and health: A critical review. *Nutrition Today* 50:117–128.

Olson, J., S. Schrager, M. Belzer, L. Simons, and L. Clark. 2015. Baseline physiologic and psychosocial characteristics of transgender youth seeking care for gender dysphoria. *Journal of Adolescent Health* 57:374–380.

Pelizzo, G., V. Calcaterra, V. Carlini, M. Fusillo, M. Manuelli, C. Klersy, N. Pasqua, E. Luka, R. Albertini, M. De Amici, and H. Cena. 2017. Nutritional status and metabolic profile in neurologically impaired pediatric surgical patients. *Journal of Pediatric Endocrinology and Metabolism* 30:289–300.

Polfuss, M., B. Forseth, D. Schoeller, C. Huang, A. Moosreiner, P. Papanek, K. Sawin, K. Zvara, and L. Bandini. 2021. Accuracy of body mass index in categorizing weight status in children with intellectual and developmental disabilities. *Journal of Pediatric Rehabilitation Medicine* 14(4):621–629.

Rempel, G. 2015. The importance of good nutrition in children with cerebral palsy. *Physical Medicine and Rehabilitation Clinics of North America* 26(1):39–56.

Romero-Corral, A., V. K. Sommers, J. Sierra-Johnson, R. Thomas, M. Collazo-Clavell, J. Korinek, T. G. Allison, J. A. Batsis, F. Sert-Kuniyoshi, and F. Lopez-Jimenez. 2008. Accuracy of body mass index in diagnosing obesity in the adult general population. *International Journal of Obesity* 32(6):959–966.

Schagen, S. E., P. T. Cohen-Kettenis, H. A. Delemarre-van de Waal, and S. E. Hannema. 2016. Efficacy and safety of gonadotropin-releasing hormone agonist treatment to suppress puberty in gender dysphoric adolescents. *Journal of Sexual Medicine* 13(7):1125–1132.

Sequeira, G., E. Miller, H. McCauley, and K. Eckstrand. 2017. Impact of gender expression on disordered eating, body dissatisfaction and BMI in a cohort of transgender youth. *Journal of Adolescent Health* 60:S87.

Simmonds, M., J. Burch, A. Llewellyn, C. Griffiths, H. Yang, C. Owen, S. Duffy, and N. Woolacott. 2015. The use of measures of obesity in childhood for predicting obesity and the development of obesity-related diseases in adulthood: A systematic review and meta-analysis. *Health Technology Assessment* 19(43):1–336.

SSA (Social Security Administration). n.d.-a. *105.08 Growth failure due to any digestive disorder.* Baltimore, MD. https://www.ssa.gov/disability/professionals/bluebook/105.00-Digestive-Childhood.htm#105_08B (accessed March 9, 2024).

SSA. n.d.-b. *5.00F How do we evaluate weight loss due to any digestive disorder under 5.08?* Baltimore, MD. https://www.ssa.gov/disability/professionals/bluebook/5.00-Digestive-Adult.htm#5_00 (accessed March 9, 2024).

Tang, M. N., S. Adolphe, S. R. Rogers, and D. A. Frank. 2021. Failure to thrive or growth faltering: Medical, developmental/behavioral, nutritional, and social dimensions. *Pediatrics in Review* 42(11):590–603.

Thompson, A. L. 2021. What is normal, healthy growth? Global health, human biology, and parental perspectives. *American Journal of Human Biology* 33(5).

Turner Syndrome Society of the United States. n.d. *Physical health: Growth.* Houston, TX. https://www.turnersyndrome.org/growth (accessed March 9, 2024).

Valentine, A., N. Nokoff, A. Bonny, G. Chelvakumar, J. Indyk, S. Leibowitz, and L. Nahata. 2021. Cardiometabolic parameters among transgender adolescent males on testosterone therapy and body mass index-matched cisgender females. *Transgender Health* 6(6):369–373.

Van Caenegem, E., K. Wierckx, Y. Taes, T. Schreiner, S. Vandewalle, K. Toye, B. Lapauw, J.-M. Kaufman, and G. T'Sjoen. 2015. Body composition, bone turnover, and bone mass in trans men during testosterone treatment: 1-year follow-up data from a prospective case-controlled study (ENIGI). *European Journal of Endocrinology* 172(2):163–171.

van Velzen, D. M., N. M. Nota, S. Simsek, E. B. Conemans, G. T'Sjoen, and M. den Heijer. 2020. Variation in sensitivity and rate of change in body composition: steps toward individualizing transgender care. *European Journal of Endocrinology* 183(5):529–536.

Vehrs, P. R., G. W. Fellingham, A. McAferty, and L. Kelsey. 2022. Trends in BMI percentile and body fat percentage in children 12 to 17 years of age. *Children (Basel, Switzerland)* 9(5):744.

Wagner, D. R., and V. H. Heyward. 2000. Measures of body composition in black and whites: A comparative review. *American Journal of Clinical Nutrition* 71:1392–1402.

Weber, D., R. Moore, M. Leonard, and B. Zemel. 2013. Fat and lean BMI reference curves in children and adolescents and their utility in identifying excess adiposity compared with BMI and percentage body fat. *American Journal of Clinical Nutrition* 98(1):49–56.

Wellens, R. I., A. Roche, H. Khamis, A. Jackson, M. Pollock, and R. Siervogel. 1996. Relationships between the body mass index and body composition. *Obesity Research* 4(1):35–44.

Whitney, D., F. Miller, R. Pohlig, and C. Modlesky. 2019. BMI does not capture the high fat mass index and low fat-free mass index in children with cerebral palsy and proposed statistical models that improve this accuracy. *International Journal of Obesity* 43:82–90.

WHO (World Health Organization). 2009. *WHO child growth standards: Growth velocity based on weight, length and head circumference: Methods and development.* Geneva, Switzerland. https://www.who.int/publications/i/item/9789241547635 (accessed March 9, 2024).

WHO Expert Consultation. 2004. Appropriate body-mass index for Asian populations and its implications for policy and intervention strategies. *The Lancet* 363(9403):157–163.

Willemsen, L. A., L. S. Boogers, C. M. Wiepjes, D. T. Klink, A. S. P. van Trotsenburg, M. den Heijer, and S. E. Hannema. 2023. Just as tall on testosterone: A neutral to positive effect on adult height of GnRHa and testosterone in trans boys. *Journal of Clinical Endocrinology and Metabolism* 108(2):414–421.

Yoo, S. D., E. H. Hwang, Y. J. Lee, and J. H. Park. 2013. Clinical characteristics of failure to thrive in infant and toddler: Organic vs. nonorganic. *Pediatric Gastroenterology, Hepatology & Nutrition* 16(4):261–268.

Zemel, B. S., M. Pipan, V. A. Stallings, W. Hall, K. Schadt, D. S. Freedman, and P. Thorpe. 2015. Growth charts for children with Down syndrome in the United States. *Pediatrics* 136(5):e1204–e1211.

10

Chronic Kidney Disease

Chronic kidney disease (CKD) occurs when the kidneys can no longer properly manage the multiple complex and critical tasks necessary for maintaining balance, or homeostasis, in the body, including management and removal of waste products and toxins; management of excess fluid; blood filtering to manage key balances in vital electrolytes (e.g., including potassium, sodium, and calcium); and regulation of hormones that have a role in maintaining optimal blood pressure and red blood cell production. Early-stage kidney disease is not always symptomatic and may be managed with medications that slow its progression. As it progresses, kidney disease may cause painful and debilitating complications, and a person with CKD may require various forms of kidney replacement therapy—either dialysis treatments (home, in-center, or peritoneal), kidney transplant (using a kidney from either a deceased or a living donor), and sometimes conservative care. Patients experiencing kidney failure may find it difficult to continue working because of time-consuming dialysis treatments and the toll these treatments take on the body (Murtagh et al., 2007). For people who receive a kidney transplant, the recovery time required may also impact the ability to engage in substantial gainful activity and employment, as recovery from surgical complications may be substantial. In addition, advanced CKD may cause other complications—including severe bone pain, damaged nerves, muscle weakness, and vascular congestion and fluid overload syndromes—that cause significant impairment and disability. For these many reasons, some people with CKD seek disability benefits from the Social Security Administration (SSA).

While a person can meet SSA's disability criteria for kidney disease in multiple ways (as described in brief in this chapter), SSA asked the committee to examine criteria related to "chronic kidney disease with impairment of kidney function" under disability Listings 6.05 (adult) and 106.05 (childhood), as outlined in Box 10-1. Within these Listings, questions around sex and gender are important, specifically with regard to the estimated glomerular filtration rate (eGFR) measurement used in the disability criteria under Listings 6.05A3 and 106.05C. As described in this chapter, eGFR is commonly used in clinical practice to determine or estimate kidney function. It is calculated based on a set of factors that include a patient's sex. For this reason, it is important to understand how eGFR is calculated for transgender and gender diverse (TGD) populations and populations with variations in sex traits (VSTs), and whether there may be other appropriate

---

BOX 10-1
Disability Evaluation for Genitourinary Disorders with
Sex-Specific Diagnostic Criteria under
Listings 6.00 and 106.00

6.00 Genitourinary Disorders (Adult)
6.05 Chronic kidney disease, with impairment of kidney function, with A and B:

A. Reduced glomerular filtration evidenced by one of the following laboratory findings documented on at least two occasions at least 90 days apart during a consecutive 12-month period:

1. Serum creatinine of 4 mg/dL or greater; or
2. Creatinine clearance of 20 ml/min. or less; or
3. Estimated glomerular filtration rate (eGFR) of 20 ml/min/1.73m^2 or less.

AND

B. One of the following:

1. Renal osteodystrophy (see 6.00C3) with severe bone pain and imaging studies documenting bone abnormalities, such as osteitis fibrosa, osteomalacia, or pathologic fractures; or
2. Peripheral neuropathy (see 6.00C4); or

evaluation criteria for these populations, particularly for people who receive gender-affirming hormone therapy (GAHT). This chapter examines these questions.

CHRONIC KIDNEY DISEASE: PREVALENCE AMONG TRANSGENDER AND GENDER DIVERSE PEOPLE AND PEOPLE WITH VARIATIONS IN SEX TRAITS

In the United States, an estimated 35.5 million adults have CKD; prevalence is higher in older adults, cisgender women, and racial and ethnic minorities, and in adults with diabetes and hypertension (CDC, 2023; Kovesdy, 2022). Nearly 808,000 people in the United States are living with end-stage kidney disease (ESKD) (also known as end-stage renal disease or

---

3. Fluid overload syndrome (see 6.00C5) documented by one of the following:

   a. Diastolic hypertension greater than or equal to diastolic blood pressure of 110 mm Hg despite at least 90 consecutive days of prescribed therapy, documented by at least two measurements of diastolic blood pressure at least 90 days apart during a consecutive 12-month period; or
   b. Signs of vascular congestion or anasarca (see 6.00C6) despite at least 90 consecutive days of prescribed therapy, documented on at least two occasions at least 90 days apart during a consecutive 12-month period; or
4. Anorexia with weight loss (see 6.00C7) determined by body mass index (BMI) of 18.0 or less, calculated on at least two occasions at least 90 days apart during a consecutive 12-month period.

106.00 Genitourinary Disorders (Childhood)
106.05 Chronic kidney disease, with impairment of kidney function, with one of the following documented on at least two occasions at least 90 days apart during a consecutive 12-month period:

A. Serum creatinine of 3 mg/dL or greater; OR
B. Creatinine clearance of 30 ml/min/1.73m^2 or less; OR
C. Estimated glomerular filtration rate (eGFR) of 30 ml/min/1.73m^2 or less.

SOURCES: SSA, n.d.-a, b.

kidney failure), 69 percent of whom are on dialysis and 31 percent of whom have had a kidney transplant (NIDDK, 2022). The most common causes of CKD among adults in the United States include diabetes and hypertension. However, many individuals are unaware of the risk these conditions pose for kidney health and become aware of the presence of CKD only at its later stages (Plantinga et al., 2010; Schoolwerth et al., 2005).

Research has not described the causes of the greater prevalence of CKD among cisgender women and of kidney failure or ESKD among cisgender men (García et al., 2022). However, several factors have been proposed as potential contributors to these disparities, including longer life expectancy among cisgender women versus men and inaccurate and/or biased kidney function estimation using existing binary (male vs. female) estimation equations (Carrero et al., 2018). Further studies have also posited that gender-related differences in exposures, including less access to nephrology care and evidence-based therapy receipt among cisgender women versus men, contribute to these disparities (Jankowska et al., 2023).

CKD and TGD Populations

An estimated 0.5 percent of the U.S. population (Herman et al., 2022), or nearly 1.3 million adults, identifies as TGD, including growing proportions of the younger population (Collister et al., 2021; Mohottige and Lunn, 2020). Based on these estimates, and assuming that people with TGD experience have CKD at the same rate as the general population, nearly 176,000 TGD people in the United States may have CKD, and an estimated 4,000 TGD people may have ESKD. However, given the lack of robust and accurate collection of sexual orientation and gender identity (SOGI) data (described in detail in Chapter 3 of this report), these figures may reflect gross underestimation of the TGD population overall. Prior studies have suggested that nearly 30–50 percent of TGD people may not disclose their identity in their medical records as a result of bias and direct or vicarious experiences of discrimination (Sequeira et al., 2021). Therefore, figures estimating the prevalence of kidney disease among TGD people may be underestimates as well. The lack of systematic and accurate SOGI data collection in health surveys and medical records complicates adequate detection, surveillance, and management of kidney disease among TGD people (Ahmed et al., 2021; Sutha and Streed, 2023).

CKD is largely unexamined in TGD populations, but polled data from the Behavioral Risk Factor Surveillance System (which included 22,114 older adults) suggest that CKD prevalence is higher among older LGBTQ+ men, who were more likely than their non-LGBTQ+ counterparts to self-report having kidney disease (Chandra et., 2023). Notably, this study did not specifically examine the prevalence of CKD or acute kidney injury among TGD people alone, and it poorly captured considerations of sex and gender.

Findings of studies examining CKD among TGD are mixed. One single-center study found a CKD prevalence of 36 percent among transgender patients—a substantially higher prevalence than would be expected relative to cisgender data (Eckenrode et al., 2022b). On the other hand, a cross-sectional study of 30,763 sexual and gender minority (SGM) adults and 316,106 non-SGM adults enrolled in the National Institutes of Health–sponsored All of Us Research Program did not identify greater odds of kidney disease among TGD people, after adjustment for age, income, employment, and other factors (Tran et al., 2023). However, this study was limited by several factors, including that researchers did not have available data to link self-reported gender identity and sex recorded at birth to electronic health record data; therefore, records for TGD study participants were potentially incomplete (Tran et al., 2023). In addition, there is known underreporting and inadequate diagnosis of CKD in electronic health records (Owosela et al., 2024; Quartarolo et al., 2007).

CKD and People with VSTs

Up to 1.7 percent of the population may have VSTs (Blackless et al., 2000). Based on this estimate, and assuming people with VSTs experience CKD at the same rate as the general population, nearly 603,500 people with VSTs in the United States may have CKD, and an estimated 13,700 people with VSTs may have ESKD. Certain people with VSTs may be at elevated risk for CKD. Testosterone deficiency (hypogonadism) is associated with CKD (Romejko et al., 2022) and is common in patients receiving dialysis (Carrero and Stenvinkel, 2012; Edey, 2017). Research shows that testosterone levels decrease in parallel with reduction of kidney function and, in patients with progressive CKD, low testosterone levels have been linked with increased risk of mortality from cardiovascular events (Carrero et al., 2010; Yilmaz et al., 2011) and risk of other chronic illnesses (Iglesias et al., 2012). Development of chronic kidney insufficiency in puberty has been associated with several gonadal disorders, such as gonadal dysgenesis, Leydig cell hypoplasia, Turner syndrome, and Klinefelter syndrome (Benz et al., 2006).

Disparities in Care and Outcomes

CKD care and outcomes in the United States are emblematic of numerous long-standing disparities that cause specific populations to experience sociostructural barriers to care, including TGD people and people with VSTs. Although racial and ethnic disparities in kidney outcomes in the United States are well described (Crews et al., 2013; Mohottige et al., 2021; Nicholas et al., 2015; Norris and Nissenson, 2008; Norton et al., 2016), other factors that may impact kidney care for TGD people are poorly understood because of the lack of uniform SOGI data collection within medical records and across the health care system, along with limited clinician and health system capture of barriers to care and other care considerations for TGD people (Streed et al., 2023; Sutha and Streed, 2023). These data collection limitations notwithstanding, people who are both TGD and racially/ethnically minoritized may experience unique, multilevel, cascading barriers to kidney care. Common risk factors for CKD—including diabetes and hypertension—are also characterized by disparities in race, ethnicity, and socioeconomic status. To date, no studies have described differences in kidney disease risk factors among TGD individuals versus their cisgender counterparts.

The literature has also described the long-standing racial and ethnic disparities in kidney transplantation. For instance, Black Americans have a four-fold higher risk of developing ESKD compared with their White counterparts, yet they remain less likely than their White counterparts to be evaluated for kidney transplant, achieve waitlist status, and receive a preemptive or living donor transplant (Mohottige et al., 2021). Gender disparities have also been described, primarily between cisgender women and cisgender men.[1] While no known studies have examined disparities in access to and receipt of kidney transplants among TGD people, the literature has described numerous inequities faced by TGD people seeking transplantation in general. More research is needed to characterize disparities in transplant access and outcomes encountered by these populations (Leeies et al., 2023; Ramadan et al., 2020).

Several risk factors for kidney disease need to be considered carefully when evaluating kidney disease risk and associated sequelae among TGD people. These include increased cardiovascular events (e.g., myocardial infarction) associated with stress from marginalization and discrimination (Streed et al., 2021), and well-documented disparities between TGD

---

[1] For instance, cisgender women are less likely to be waitlisted for a kidney transplant and receive deceased and living donor kidneys compared with cisgender male counterparts, despite the fact that cisgender women are more likely than cisgender men to become living kidney donors (Katz-Greenberg and Shah, 2022).

and cisgender people in access to bias-free preventive and chronic disease care, which may impact care for predisposing risk factors for CKD, including hypertension, metabolic syndrome, and diabetes (Caceres et al., 2020).

PEDIATRIC CONSIDERATIONS FOR CHRONIC KIDNEY DISEASE

CKD is characterized by structural or functional abnormalities of the kidneys that often impact individuals from the time of birth through early adulthood. Estimating the incidence of CKD in children has been difficult, but based on registry data for U.S. children aged 0–17 the estimated incidence is 13.0 per million (Harada et al., 2022; Harambat et al., 2012).

Importantly, the etiologies of CKD and kidney failure differ between children and adults. Whereas the most common causes of CKD and ESKD among adults in the United States include diabetes and hypertension (followed by glomerular disease and cystic diseases of the kidney), the most common causes of kidney disease among pediatric populations include hereditary congenital diseases (accounting for 50 percent of cases of CKD diagnosed during the first three decades of life), glomerulonephritis, vasculitis, interstitial nephritis, and miscellaneous conditions (Harambat et al., 2012). In younger children, congenital anomalies of the kidneys and urinary tract (CAKUT) (including obstructive uropathy and renal hypodysplasia) are most common, and posterior urethral valves and prune belly syndrome more often occur among individuals with sex recorded as male at birth than as female (Lombel et al., 2022). Pediatric kidney disorders are often associated with deleterious genetic variants (Becherucci et al., 2016; Kolvenbach et al., 2023).[2] Renal dysplasia, which may include cystic disease as well as hypoplasia or small kidneys with reduced nephron volume, may result in functional kidney impairments as well (Lombel et al., 2022).

In children, kidney anomalies may be isolated or associated with other clinical manifestations (syndromic). Some disorders progress to kidney failure, necessitating kidney replacement therapy (dialysis or transplantation) within the first few years of life, during adolescence, or in young adulthood. Furthermore, some conditions, including forms of glomerular disease, may recur in adulthood or even after transplantation (Uffing et al., 2021; Vivarelli et al., 2017). Acute kidney injury in children can also lead to CKD as the result of a range of factors, including volume depletion or

---

[2] Some genetic variants associated with CAKUT are also associated with ocular phenotypes, including coloboma, microphthalmia, optic disc anomalies, refraction errors (astigmatism, myopia, and hypermetropia), and cataracts (Virth et al., 2024).

acute infection, chemotherapy for childhood cancer, and nephrotoxic drugs. Studies have shown variable decline in kidney function between individuals with CAKUT and those with hereditary diseases, such as polycystic kidney disease and Alport syndrome (Mong Hiep et al., 2010), that may progress particularly rapidly, requiring earlier initiation of kidney replacement therapy. Vigilance and early detection and diagnosis are essential for each of these conditions throughout an individual's life course.

Impact on Growth and Development

For youth with CKD, progressive kidney failure can lead to anemia, deceleration of linear growth velocity, delayed pubertal development, and impaired bone mineralization (Capossela et al., 2023; Haffner, 2020; Haffner and Zivicnjak, 2017; Silverstein, 2018). In addition to these physical manifestations, CKD extracts a psychological toll on growing youth: they are shorter than peers, have delayed pubertal development, and experience frequent school absences (Assadi, 2013). The quality-of-life and physiological changes related to CKD may require that a pediatric nephrologist and multidisciplinary care team pay careful attention to malnutrition, protein-calorie wasting, acidosis, growth hormone resistance, and metabolic derangements.

Impact on Education and Employment (Children and Caregivers)

Disease progression and intercurrent illnesses, as well as the need for dialysis and kidney transplants, which require significant time and effort to maintain a functional health status, can rapidly tip the health and quality-of-life balance for youth with CKD, impacting their ability to attend school or employment, and leading to other forms of disability. A systematic review including 34 studies concluded that children with CKD scored lower in cognition, executive function, and memory when compared with children without CKD (Chen et al., 2018). As is true for most chronic pediatric disorders, moreover, a child's illness significantly impacts daily life for caregivers (parents or guardians), who may have to limit participation in gainful employment to provide full-time care. Furthermore, clinical transitions between pediatric and adult care may be particularly challenging for these patients and may require concerted efforts to ensure appropriate trust building and understanding of complex care needs (Harada et al., 2022). Lapses in appropriate transition due to inadequate communication among pediatric and adult teams with respect to multidisciplinary care needs may result in anxiety, distress, and challenges with medication nonadherence, leading to poor outcomes (including exacerbation of disease states or even loss of transplant function if, e.g., immunosuppressive medications are missed) (Gold et al., 2015; Laederach-Hofmann and Bunzel, 2000; Raina et al., 2018).

CHRONIC KIDNEY DISEASE AND SSA DISABILITY DETERMINATIONS

As of December 2022, 1.8 percent of all Social Security Disability Income recipients (158,233 people) and 0.9 percent of Supplemental Security Income recipients (46,330 people) qualified for those benefits as a result of CKD, SSA's definition of disability under Listing 6.00 Genitourinary Disorders—Adult, or 106.00 Genitourinary Disorders—Childhood (SSA, 2022, 2023). In general, a person (child or adult) with CKD can meet SSA's definition of disability for CKD if they meet any of the following criteria:

- They require **dialysis** (ongoing dialysis must have lasted or be expected to last for a continuous period of at least 12 months).
- They received a **kidney transplant** (SSA considers a person disabled for 1 year from the date of transplant. After that, disability benefits can continue, but the recipient will need to medically qualify each year to have benefits renewed).[3]
- They have **chronic kidney disease with impairment of kidney function.** This Listing requires specific medical tests to demonstrate level of glomerular filtration, or how well (or poorly) the kidneys are removing waste products from the blood. Adult SSA applicants must also provide medical evidence of certain other conditions caused by a CKD, as outlined earlier in Box 10-1. SSA does not require child applicants to demonstrate these conditions.

---

[3] Transplant and related care are not within the purview of the present study. However, the committee notes that transplant care teams may consider altering the dose of or discontinuing feminizing GAHT (specifically estrogen therapies) in the context of transplantation because of possible perioperative risk of venous thromboembolism and other thromboembolic events (Getahun et al., 2018). However, there are no systematic reviews of risk associated with kidney transplantation, and there is no definitive evidence regarding risk for venous thromboembolism to suggest that low-risk individuals should stop estrogen before or after surgery (Arnold et al., 2016). Alternatives to complete discontinuation should be considered (e.g., dose reductions or transition to transdermal formulations), given the potential harm and psychological distress of GAHT discontinuation. TGD people receiving kidney transplant require comprehensive care to ensure that some side effects related to transplant medications are mitigated. All discussions regarding GAHT are essential for transplant teams to consider in consultation with a multidisciplinary team and, most notably, with an approach based on patient-centered shared and informed decision making (Collister et al., 2021; Eckenrode et al., 2022a; Jue et al., 2020; Katz-Greenberg and Shah, 2022).

- They have **nephrotic syndrome.**[4]
- They have **complications of chronic kidney disease** requiring hospitalization (at least three hospitalizations within a consecutive 12-month period and occurring at least 30 days apart).[5]

It is in the third category above, **chronic kidney disease with impairment of kidney function,** that questions around sex and gender identity become important. Under this category, applicants must demonstrate reduced glomerular filtration via one of three laboratory findings (following criteria outlined in Table 10-1):

- serum creatinine,
- creatinine clearance, or
- eGFR (SSA, n.d.-a,b).[6]

Among the different measures of kidney function, the eGFR is most commonly used in clinical practice. Clinicians and health care systems use eGFR because obtaining an accurate GFR through the measured GFR (mGFR)

---

[4] Nephrotic syndrome is a condition whereby specific quantities of protein and albumin are lost in the urine as a result of various forms of kidney disease. This condition is not within the purview of the present study. However, the committee notes that common measures of nephrotic syndrome may be influenced by the receipt of GAHT and the sex hormone configuration, but this connection has not been explicitly studied among TGD people. Although there are no consistently used sex-based equations for assessing urine proteinuria/albuminuria (and SSA criteria do not include sex-based measurement under Listing 6.06 and 106.06), several authors have suggested that sex-specific ranges be used to interpret spot urine creatinine measures (Marco Mayayo et al., 2016). Given the critical importance of albuminuria and proteinuria assessments among individuals with CKD risk and known kidney disease, it is essential that urine measures of proteinuria/albuminuria be carefully collected among TGD people. Guidance suggests that both male and female values be input into albumin- or protein-to-creatinine ratio conversions to assess 24-hour albuminuria/proteinuria based on spot measures. Ideally, when precision is needed, 24-hour measures of urinary protein or albumin excretion are used, as these represent common occurrences of intraindividual variability (Pierre et al., 2023). Furthermore, just as is done among cisgender populations with CKD and CKD risk factors, urine albumin and protein excretion need to be monitored carefully among TGD people to guide therapeutic and diagnostic decision making. Finally, adjudicators need to consider the potential bias introduced in 24-hour urine creatinine collections due to a range of factors, including inadequate collection techniques, as well as the potential influence of sex and gender and GAHT on these measures.

[5] Under SSA's childhood disability listings, in addition to the above, children can meet disability criteria based on eligibility under two additional categories: (1) "Congenital genitourinary disorder" and (2) "Growth failure due to any chronic renal disease" (Listing 106.00, Genitourinary Disorders—Childhood).

[6] There is no standard for the use of measures of serum creatinine or creatinine clearance on its own for clinical care purposes. For instance, two adult individuals with serum creatine measurements of 4 mg/dL could have widely variable clinical symptoms that might be disabling, and/or electrolyte imbalances or other condition requiring kidney replacement therapy. Serum creatinine is often used in equations to estimate GFR, as described in this chapter.

TABLE 10-1 Historical and Current Estimated Glomerular Filtration Rate (eGFR) Equations for Adults

Equation	Population Included	Race or Sex Coefficients for Adjustment
Cockcroft Gault (1973)[a]	Adult individuals aged 18–92 recruited from a Canadian hospital, presumed to be cisgender men.	**Multiply by 0.85 if female;** no race variable
MDRD (1999)[b]	Nondiabetic individuals with chronic kidney disease, aged 18–70, primarily White. **No explicit inclusion of transgender and gender diverse (TGD) individuals.**	**Multiply by 0.742 if female;** multiply by 1.21 if Black
CKD-EPI (2009)[c]	Adult cohort (43.7% identified as female). **No explicit inclusion of TGD individuals.**	**Multiply by 1.018 if female.** Equation includes a multiplying factor of 1.159 if Black. (According to the authors, "The predicted female-to-male ratio for estimated GFR varies from 0.83 to 0.92 when serum creatinine is between 44 to 71 µmol/L (0.5 and 0.8 mg/dL), and is 0.75 when serum creatinine is ≥80 µmol/L (≥0.9 mg/dL), whereas it is constant for the MDRD Study equation at 0.74 at all values for serum creatinine.")
CKD-EPI (2021)[d]	Adult cohort (38% identified as female). **No explicit inclusion of TGD individuals.**	**Multiply by 1.012 if female.** (This equation does not include race.)

[a] The Cockcroft–Gault (1973) equation is no longer in clinical use but may be used for drug research.
[b] Some clinical laboratories are still reporting GFR estimates using the MDRD Study equation.
[c] The National Institute of Diabetes and Digestive and Kidney Diseases (NIDDK) maintains use of the Chronic Kidney Disease Epidemiology Collaboration (CKD-EPI) 2009 equation during the transition to the updated 2021 equation.
[d] The CKD-EPI 2021 equation is the new equation recommended by the National Kidney Foundation (NKF), NIDDK, American Society of Nephrology, and others.
SOURCES: Cockcroft and Gault, 1976; Delgado et al., 2022; Levey et al., 1999, 2009.

test may be challenging (Delgado et al., 2022; Hsu et al., 2011; van Eeghen, 2023). mGFR measures directly how well the kidneys remove waste products from the blood, but the test requires complicated, lengthy, and expensive evaluation methods performed in specialized centers, along with multiple blood samples taken over several hours (Gounden et al., 2023; Hsu et al., 2011). For these reasons, eGFR, and its ability to provide an estimate of GFR, is the more practical and widely used test for assessing kidney function

(NKF, 2022a; Pierre et al., 2023). eGFR assessment may, directly or indirectly, influence clinical determination of patient care needs, including (1) initiation of dialysis, (2) referral to evaluation and waitlisting for kidney transplant, (3) management or detection of conditions such as uremia (buildup of toxic waste) due to impaired kidney function or CKD, (4) detection and further evaluation for causes of nephrotic syndrome, and (5) careful consideration for medication dosing and determination of contraindicated medications.

eGFR is calculated based on a blood test that measures either serum creatinine[7] levels or cystatin C[8] levels in the blood, together with the patient's age, sex, and body type. Given that normal GFR varies according to age, sex, and body size, the eGFR equation takes these factors into account (Delgado et al., 2022). The eGFR equation is different for adult versus pediatric and young adult populations.

Adult eGFR Equations

SSA criteria do not specify how eGFR submitted under Listing 6.05A3 should be calculated (see Box 10-1), and a number of different GFR estimating equations are in clinical use (see Table 10-1). However, the National Kidney Foundation (NKF), American Society of Nephrology, National Institute of Diabetes and Digestive and Kidney Diseases (NIDDK), and American Association for Clinical Chemistry (AACC) all recommend the Chronic Kidney Disease Epidemiology Collaboration (CKD-EPI 2021) eGFR equation for adults, which estimates GFR from creatinine and/or cystatin C, age, and sex; however, in a departure from earlier estimating equations, this eGFR estimating equation does not include race as a coefficient (Delgado et al., 2022; Inker et al., 2021; NIDDK, 2022; Pierre et al., 2023). Additional studies have demonstrated promise in additional equations, such as the European Kidney Function Consortium (EKFC)–developed eGFRcr and the EKFC eGFRcys, the latter of which uses age-based rescaling factors without sex or race coefficients (yet requires cystatin C for measurement); these equations have not been widely adopted in U.S. settings (Pottel et al., 2023).

Pediatric eGFR Equations

SSA criteria do not specify how eGFRs submitted for pediatric populations under Listing 106.05C should be calculated (see Box 10-1). While the 2009 Chronic Kidney Disease in Children (CKiD) "bedside" calculator

---

[7] Creatinine is a chemical waste product of creatine (a chemical made by the body to supply energy to muscles). Creatinine is removed from the body by the kidneys, and creatinine measurements provide some idea of how the kidneys are working.

[8] Cystatin C is a protein produced by body cells. If the level of cystatin C in the blood is too high, this may mean the kidneys are not working well.

is still used in routine clinical practice for measuring kidney function in children (NKF, n.d.-b; Schwartz et al., 2009), NIDDK prefers the 2021 CKiD U25 estimating equations, as they exhibit less bias across a broader age range (up to age 25) (NIDDK, 2022). The 2021 CKiD U25 estimating equations offer two formulas: one based on height and creatinine, the other based on cystatin C; both formulas require that age and sex be specified (Ng and Pierce, 2021; Pierce et al., 2021). If all necessary information is available—height, serum creatinine, and cystatin C—estimates are created using each formula, and an average of the two eGFR values is taken. For patients aged 18–25, NIDDK recommends comparing the estimates from both the pediatric 2021 CKiD U25 calculator and the adult CKD-EPI 2021 calculator, as doing so will provide a more informed assessment of kidney function as patients transition to adulthood (NIDDK, 2022). Just as in adults, eGFR equations in children are only estimates of kidney function and are subject to inaccuracy—even with optimal equations—notably overestimating eGFR in the setting of rapidly declining kidney function because of the time required for equilibration (den Bakker et al., 2022).

Variables Included in eGFR Equations for Adult and Pediatric Populations.

Both adult and pediatric eGFR equations use a binary definition of sex, and for this reason, SSA asked this committee to examine whether this measurement of kidney function is appropriate for TGD people and people with VSTs; whether modifications to these measures might be required for these populations; or whether alternative tests, evaluations, or laboratory values might be more appropriate for understanding kidney function—and level of disability—among TGD people and people with VSTs. Box 10-2 displays the variables included in eGFR equations for adult and pediatric populations.

The sections below examine evidence related to the impact of GAHT on measures of kidney function, the implications for measuring eGFR, and current guidelines from AACC/NKF on appropriate eGFR measurement for TGD people and people with VSTs.

Impact of GAHT on Measurements of Kidney Function

Creatinine—a key biomarker used to estimate GFR—is the most common marker for kidney function used in routine clinical practice. Creatinine may be influenced by non-GFR determinants, including skeletal muscle metabolism, muscle mass, body weight, diet, medications, and a range of other factors (Bartholomae et al., 2022; Baxmann et al., 2008; Inker et al., 2021)

BOX 10-2
Variables Included in Estimated Glomerular
Filtration Rate (eGFR) Calculation

Adult eGFR Variables

- ☐ Serum creatinine
- ☐ Serum cystatin C
- ☐ Age
- ☐ Gender (male/female)
- ☐ Standardized assays (yes/no/not sure)
- ☐ Adjust for body surface area (yes/no/not sure)

Pediatric eGFR Variables

- ☐ Serum creatinine
- ☐ Serum cystatin C
- ☐ Height
- ☐ Blood urea nitrogen
- ☐ Gender (male/female)

NOTE: Source documents male or female gender.
SOURCES: NKF, n.d.-a,b.

---

that can cause eGFR over- or underestimation.[9] Use of cystatin C (another kidney function biomarker) is less common in clinical practice, but national guidelines call for expanding its use as a confirmatory test, given its relative accuracy in eGFR equations when race is no longer a coefficient (Adingwupu et al., 2023; Baxmann et al., 2008; Inker et al., 2021; Lees et al., 2022; Pierre et al., 2023). Like creatinine, cystatin C is impacted by non-GFR determinants, including smoking, obesity, diabetes, inflammation, and thyroid disease

---

[9] eGFR may be overestimated because of decreased serum creatinine due to such factors as frailty syndromes, anorexia, sarcopenia, cirrhosis, thyroid disease, or a vegan diet (Pierre et al., 2023). Conversely, eGFR may be underestimated because of increased creatinine due to having greater muscle mass, obesity, rhabdomyolysis (muscle breakdown), higher meat consumption, or use of creatine/muscle-building formulations, as well as when a person takes medications that inhibit kidney tubule secretion of creatinine (including trimethoprim and multiple medications used to treat HIV and hepatitis) (Patel et al., 2012; Pierre et al., 2023).

(Anderson et al., 2012; Goede et al., 2009; Panaich et al., 2013; Rule et al., 2013).[10]

As GAHT may impact body composition (including muscle mass, body fat distribution, bone mass, and other measures of body composition, as described in Chapter 9 and Appendix C), it stands to reason that it may also impact serum creatinine (SCr), cystatin C, and other kidney function biomarkers that are influenced by body composition. However, evidence on the influence of GAHT on eGFR and SCr has been mixed (Collister et al., 2021), and data describing the impact of GAHT on cystatin C are lacking (Krupka et al., 2022).

A 2022 systematic review and meta-analysis by Krupka and colleagues (2022) aimed to characterize how GAHT changes SCr, other kidney function biomarkers, and GFR in adult TGD patients (Krupka et al., 2022). The review found that, at 12 months after initiating GAHT, SCr levels had increased in transgender men (SCr increased by 0.15 mg/dL; 95% confidence interval [CI] 0.00–0.29 mg/dL), but had not significantly changed in transgender women (SCr decreased by 0.05 mg/dL; 95% CI 0.16–0.05 mg/dL). The findings of this review are consistent with those of other studies that suggest that (1) masculinizing hormone therapies increase muscle mass, which results in increased SCr levels (Collister et al., 2021; Maheshwari et al., 2021, 2022; SoRelle et al., 2019), and (2) feminizing hormone therapies decrease muscle mass and increase fat mass, which results in variable changes in SCr over time (Allen et al., 2021; Maheshwari et al., 2022).

Although the seminal review of Krupka and colleagues (2022) provides important insights into the impact of GAHT on SCr, several noteworthy limitations reduce the generalizability and applicability of its findings. Further studies are needed to examine the long-term associations between GAHT and long-term kidney function and associated biochemical parameters. First, subjects across these studies may have used different GAHT doses, formulations (e.g., intramuscular, transdermal), durations, and combinations (e.g., spironolactone and estrogen). Chapter 5 describes the wide variability in gender-affirming care, and this factor may make it difficult to generalize about the impact of GAHT across TGD populations with CKD. Longer-term implications of

---

[10] Understanding discordance between eGFR creatinine- and cystatin C–based assessments often requires additional guidance, and recent findings from an observational study demonstrate that when eGFR based on cystatin C is lower than that based on creatinine, this may identify individuals at risk of poor outcomes, including acute kidney injury and the need for dialysis (Carrero et al., 2023). However, lack of published data across contexts and limited evolving familiarity with the use of cystatin C in U.S. settings has made its implementation and broad utilization challenging (Gottlieb et al., 2023).

GAHT exposure on measures of kidney function, including eGFR and albuminuria, are largely unknown, as are clear descriptions of the mechanisms through which GAHT influences kidney function. In addition, the review by Krupka and colleagues (2023) did not uncover any studies that reported the effect of GAHT on albuminuria, proteinuria, cystatin C, or measured GFR, precluding any conclusions on these important kidney function biomarkers. It is also unclear whether the changes observed only reflect changes in muscle mass or body distribution caused by GAHT or indicate actual changes in kidney function. Finally, available studies included only adult transgender populations, and these populations included were predominantly younger, healthier individuals without CKD. Therefore, it is unknown how GAHT affects kidney function biomarkers in pediatric, adolescent, or nonbinary populations or in populations with advanced kidney disease; it is also unknown how GAHT relates to the various causes of kidney disease (e.g., diabetic kidney disease, polycystic kidney disease, glomerulonephritis).

Additional reviews have demonstrated that, on average, creatinine increases by 5–10 µmol/L among transgender men receiving GAHT while decreasing 5–10 µmol/L among transgender women receiving GAHT. However, the clinical relevance of this finding and the true difference in actual GFR remain poorly understood, especially considering the lack of data on GAHT dose and formulation; achieved hormone levels; and non-GFR determinants of SCr, including medications and dietary intake (Collister et al., 2021). In addition, these studies may not take into account other factors related to TGD experience beyond GAHT. One single-center study of transgender individuals who had received GAHT had a lower prevalence of CKD and acute kidney injury versus counterparts who had not received GAHT, suggesting that the risk of CKD was not conferred by the use of GAHT, but unmeasured factors (Eckenrode et al., 2022a).

As for the impact of GAHT on cystatin C, because it is less influenced by muscle mass, relative to creatinine (Stevens et al., 2009), and is thought to be less influenced by sex hormones (Weinert et., 2010), cystatin C–based GFR estimates could, in theory, improve CKD monitoring in TGD people (Pierre et al., 2023). One recent study used data from the European Network for the Investigation of Gender Incongruence to examine changes in SCr and serum cystatin C during the first year of individual receipt of GAHT (van Eeghen et al., 2023). In this cohort, transgender women receiving estradiol and cyproterone acetate (n = 260) saw a decrease in cystatin C of 0.069 mg/L (CI 0.049–0.089 mg/L), corresponding to a 7 mL/min per 1.73 m^2 increase in eGFR; transgender men receiving testosterone (n = 285) saw an increase in cystatin C of 0.062 mg/dL (CI 0.310–0.072 mg/dL), corresponding to a 6 mL/ min per 1.73 m^2 decrease in eGFR (van Eeghen et al., 2023). Notably, creatinine-based eGFR varied depending on the sex coefficient used in the equations.

eGFR Determination, GAHT, and Pediatric Populations

Data are limited on the influence of GAHT in pediatric populations. However, the authors of one notable study calculated SCr changes among TGD youth in a cohort of patients recruited from the Trans Youth Care Study in the United States (Millington et al., 2022). The authors estimated GFR for study participants using both the CKiD U25 equation (Pierce et al., 2021) and the CKD-EPI 2021 equation (Inker et al., 2021). They found that among the total of 286 individuals, all had significant changes in SCr by 6 months of GAHT. Individuals with sex recorded male at birth who had been treated with estradiol (n = 92) had a decrease in SCr of 0.07 +/– 0.14 mg/dL over 6 months, and no changes beyond that point. Individuals with sex recorded female at birth who had been treated with testosterone (n = 194) had an increase in SCr of 0.11 +/– 0.1 mg/dL over the first 6 months of treatment and an additional increase between 6 and 12 months, for a total increase of 0.14 +/– 0.11 mg/dL over the first year. Although median doses of testosterone and estradiol were assessed in this study, the exact dose–response association between GAHT and creatinine-based eGFR is unclear. However, these results are consistent with those of studies in adult TGD populations that have found that feminizing GAHT tends to decrease SCr levels, while masculinizing GAHT tends to increase SCr levels. Additional research is needed to confirm these results and understand their impact on true kidney function and outcomes for pediatric patients.

Sex Coefficients in eGFR Determination: Evolving Guidelines

While the impact of exogenous hormones used for GAHT on SCr (and other kidney function biomarkers) remains unclear, sex differences in SCr levels form the basis of the eGFR equations. Existing eGFR equations include binary sex (male versus female) as a covariate because of findings that, on average, cisgender females generate less creatinine compared with cisgender males as the result of lower muscle mass and/or possible differences in creatinine production (Baxmann et al., 2008; Krupka et al., 2022; Malmgren and Grubb, 2023). For instance, several studies have demonstrated that serum and urine creatinine correlate significantly with lean mass and body weight (Baxmann et al., 2008).

While the CKD-EPI 2021 equation represents a substantial step forward in reassessing the inclusion of race in diagnosing CKD, it does not address potential problems with using sex as a coefficient in eGFR equations. Importantly, equations used to estimate eGFR in adults have varied over time, reflecting evolving views on the factors (including sex) hypothesized to influence muscle mass and thus SCr or other kidney function biomarkers. Since 1973, several creatinine-based GFR estimating equations have been used in clinical practice, and the evolution of their use is relevant to current practice (see Table 10-1). The female sex multiplier has changed multiple times over the years as understanding of sex differences in kidney function has evolved. Historically, efforts to develop the eGFR equations have not included TGD populations.

Given modern conceptions of sex and gender in medicine and the potential impact of GAHT on important kidney function biomarkers, some members of the nephrology community have called for recognition and reconsideration of what "sex" represents in the eGFR equations (Fadich et al., 2022; Inker et al., 2021; Levey et al., 2009, 2020; Mohottige and Tuot, 2022). To achieve greater precision in estimating kidney function for TGD people, experts have called for future estimating equations to include data from populations with a range of sexual and gender identities, including individuals receiving GAHT (Mohottige and Tuot, 2022).

Chronic Kidney Disease Guidelines and Gender-Affirming Hormone Therapy

Despite the limited research on GAHT and kidney function biomarkers presented above, no studies have described specific eGFR equations for TGD individuals based on GAHT or sex hormone configuration. However, prominent organizations have recently offered guidance on eGFR measurements for people with TGD or VST experience. According to 2023 guidance from AACC/NKF on the appropriate use of the 2021 CKD-EPI equation (Pierre et al., 2023):

> The authors did not find any literature whereby mGFR and eGFR were evaluated in transgender people, making it difficult to distinguish which sex-variable or alternate variable, if any, would allow for a more accurate estimation of GFR calculated by the currently available equations. Until additional data are available, regardless of hormone therapy or other intervention use, we recommend evaluating eGFR using both the male and female constants with the CKD-EPI 2021 equations in transgender, nonbinary, or intersex people. If either of these results crosses a clinical threshold a holistic approach should be taken to determine appropriate management anchored to the muscle mass of the individual based on their sex hormone configuration and gender identity. (p. 809)

Further, the AACC/NKF guidance states that the urine albumin–creatinine ratio (uACR)[11] and 24-hour urine creatinine clearance[12] may be a better measure than the 2021 CDK-EP1 equation for determining kidney function in TGD people. However, as urine creatinine itself may be influenced by sex hormone configurations (Forni Ogna et al., 2015), researchers have suggested that gender-specific ranges be used to improve interpretation of these measurements (Marco Mayayo et al., 2016; Yang et al., 2022). Further studies are needed to examine long-term changes in urine albuminuria/proteinuria related to GAHT.

The Kidney Disease Improving Global Outcomes also updated clinical practice guidelines for CKD evaluation and management; proposed guidelines ensure scientifically rigorous and equity-focused care for TGD patients (Stevens et al., 2024). The 2024 guidelines offer further insight into appropriate eGFR measurement for people with TGD experience, including considerations of CKD staging, as well as considerations of the circumstances in which using cystatin C may be beneficial (Stevens et al., 2024).

SUMMARY OF KEY POINTS

Inaccurate estimations of kidney function have numerous implications for health, including the potential to worsen disparities in care for TGD people, resulting, for example, in inappropriate GAHT dosing, delays in nephrology care and disease-modifying therapies, and delayed referrals for kidney transplant evaluation. To avoid exacerbating disparities in care delivery and outcomes among TGD people with imprecise eGFR measurements, clinical teams may need to consider the most precise methods for assessing kidney function among individuals with TGD or VST lived experience, including the use of 24-hour urine creatinine clearance or mGFR, where feasible. These measurements of kidney function are not currently

---

[11] The urine albumin-to-creatinine ratio (uACR) calculates the amount of albumin and creatinine in urine and is an important test for identifying kidney damage, in addition to the eGFR test. Healthy kidneys allow very little albumin (which is a type of protein normally found in the blood) to enter the urine, but damaged kidneys may allow albumin to leak out. When a patient has albumin in their urine, it is called albuminuria or proteinuria. Where a patient has a high amount of albumin in their urine, they may be at an increased risk of having CKD progress to kidney failure. uACR may be determined from a one-time "spot" urine sample or a 24-hour collection, and the spot specimen correlates well with 24-hour urine collections (NKF, n.d.-c).

[12] Creatinine clearance measurements examine creatinine in the urine (whereas serum creatine—used in most eGFR equations—is creatine in the blood). Creatinine clearance requires a timed urine sample (usually 24 hours), the result of which shows how much creatinine has passed through the kidneys into the urine. This indicates how well kidneys are removing waste from the blood (https://www.kidney.org/es/node/27522; accessed March 15, 2024).

included in SSA criteria under Listing 6.05 or 106.05. It is true that fewer patients are likely to have access to these measures relative to those more commonly used in clinical practice, given that they are not part of routine care and may not be covered by insurance. When used to clarify kidney function in patients (including those with TGD or VST lived experience), however, these more precise measures may help inform disability determination. Furthermore, when SSA sees evidence in the medical record that eGFR was estimated using an inappropriate sex reference (e.g., when providers are mistaken about patient sex and gender identity or lack training and guidance on which sex coefficient to use for TGD patients or patients with VSTs), it may be beneficial, where clinically appropriate, to order as part of a consultive exam a test that offers more precise measurement of kidney function (e.g., mGFR). However, individual applicants should always have the choice whether to submit to a consultive examination.

In addition, until further research is available to clarify the appropriate clinical approach for people who receive GAHT, current AACC/NKF guidelines recommend estimating eGFR using both the male and female constants with the 2021 CKD-EPI eGFR equation ("dual calculations"). The committee for the present study does not know how often providers use dual calculations for estimating eGFR, but believes that this is not yet part of common practice, especially considering that the AACC/NKF guidance on this subject was so recently issued (Pierre et al., 2023). Still, in contrast to dual calculations sometimes used for evaluation of pulmonary function (described in Chapter 8) and body mass index measurements (described in Chapter 9), areas in which there are no guidelines in place for providers, the issuance of this recent guidance may make dual calculations of eGFR more commonplace in kidney care.

For this reason, SSA may see dual eGFR calculations in medical records submitted for disability determination, especially as the AACC/NKF guidance works its way into clinical practice. When disability adjudicators receive medical records containing dual eGFR calculations, they may have to determine which eGFR measure to choose, male or female, to determine eligibility for disability benefits. It is the consensus of the committee, based on its clinical expertise and professional judgment, that SSA will best serve applicants who have used GAHT at some point in their care[13] by using the lowest eGFR value recorded to determine the presence of CKD and related conditions under Listings 6.05 and 106.05.

---

[13] The committee has evaluated the evidence base regarding factors—specifically receipt of GAHT—that may influence eGFR or other kidney function estimation among TGD individuals. There are no data to the committee's knowledge describing shifts in eGFR among individuals who are not utilizing GAHT; hence the committee's conclusion focuses on estimation among applicants who have used GAHT at some point in their care.

REFERENCES

Adingwupu, O. M., E. R. Barbosa, P. M. Palevsky, J. A. Vassalotti, A. S. Levey, and L. A. Inker. 2023. Cystatin C as a GFR estimation marker in acute and chronic illness: A systematic review. *Kidney Medicine* 5(12):100727.

Ahmed, S. B., N. Saad, and S. M. Dumanski. 2021. Gender and CKD: Beyond the binary. *Clinical Journal of the American Society of Nephrology* 16(1):141–143.

Allen, A. N., R. Jiao, P. Day, P. Pagels, N. Gimpel, and J. A. SoRelle. 2021. Dynamic impact of hormone therapy on laboratory values in transgender patients over time. *Journal of Applied Laboratory Medicine* 6(1):27–40.

Anderson, A. H., W. Yang, C. Y. Hsu, M. M. Joffe, M. B. Leonard, D. Xie, J. Chen, T. Greene, B. G. Jaar, P. Kao, J. W. Kusek, J. R. Landis, J. P. Lash, R. R. Townsend, M. R. Weir, H. I. Feldman, and CRIC Study Investigators. 2012. Estimating GFR among participants in the Chronic Renal Insufficiency Cohort (CRIC) study. *American Journal of Kidney Diseases* 60(2):250–261.

Arnold, J. D., E. P. Sarkodie, M. E. Coleman, and D. A. Goldstein. 2016. Incidence of venous thromboembolism in transgender women receiving oral estradiol. *Journal of Sexual Medicine* 13(11):1773–1777.

Assadi, F. 2013. Pediatric kidney transplantation: Kids are different. *Iranian Journal of Kidney Diseases* 7(6):429–431.

Bartholomae, E., J. Knurick, and C. S. Johnston. 2022. Serum creatinine as an indicator of lean body mass in vegetarians and omnivores. *Frontiers in Nutrition* 9:e996541.

Baxmann, A. C., M. S. Ahmed, N. C. Marques, V. B. Menon, A. B. Pereira, G. M. Kirsztajn, and I. P. Heilberg. 2008. Influence of muscle mass and physical activity on serum and urinary creatinine and serum cystatin C. *Clinical Journal of the American Society of Nephrology* 3(2):348–354.

Becherucci, F., R. M. Roperto, M. Materassi, and P. Romagnani. 2016. Chronic kidney disease in children. *Clinical Kidney Journal* 9(4):583–591.

Benz, K., C. Plank, K. Amann, B. Mucha, H. G. Dörr, W. Rascher, and J. Dötsch. 2006. Hypergonadotropic hypogonadism and renal failure due to WT1 mutation. *Nephrology Dialysis Transplantation* 21(6):1716–1718.

Blackless, M., A. Charuvastra, A. Derryck, A. Fausto-Sterling, K. Lauzanne, and E. Lee. 2000. How sexually dimorphic are we? Review and synthesis. *American Journal of Human Biology* 12(2):151–166.

Caceres, B. A., K. B. Jackman, D. Edmondson, and W. O. Bockting. 2020. Assessing gender identity differences in cardiovascular disease in us adults: An analysis of data from the 2014–2017 BRFSS. *Journal of Behavioral Medicine* 43(2):329–338.

Capossela, L., S. Ferretti, S. D'Alonzo, L. Di Sarno, V. Pansini, A. Curatola, A. Chiaretti, and A. Gatto. 2023. Bone disorders in pediatric chronic kidney disease: A literature review. *Biology* 12(11):1395.

Carrero, J. J., and P. Stenvinkel. 2012. The vulnerable man: Impact of testosterone deficiency on the uraemic phenotype. *Nephrology Dialysis Transplantation* 27(11):4030–4041.

Carrero, J. J., A. R. Qureshi, A. Nakashima, S. Arver, P. Parini, B. Lindholm, P. Bárány, O. Heimbürger, and P. Stenvinkel. 2010. Prevalence and clinical implications of testosterone deficiency in men with end-stage renal disease. *Nephrology Dialysis Transplantation* 26(1):184–190.

Carrero, J. J., M. Hecking, N. C. Chesnaye, and K. J. Jager. 2018. Sex and gender disparities in the epidemiology and outcomes of chronic kidney disease. *Nature Reviews Nephrology* 14(3):151–164.

Carrero J. J., E. L. Fu, Y. Sang, S. Ballew, M. Evans, C. G. Elinder, P. Barany, L. A. Inker, A. S. Levey, J. Coresh, and M. E. Grams. 2023. Discordances between creatinine- and cystatin C-based estimated GFR and adverse clinical outcomes in routine clinical practice. *American Journal of Kidney Diseases* 82(5):534–542.

CDC (Centers for Disease Control and Prevention). 2023. *Chronic kidney disease in the United States, 2023.* https://www.cdc.gov/kidney-disease/php/data-research/?CDC_AAref_Val=https://www.cdc.gov/kidneydisease/publications-resources/ckd-national-facts.html (accessed May 18, 2024).

Chandra, M., M. Hertel, S. Cahill, K. Sakaguchi, S. Khanna, S. Mitra, J. Luke, M. Khau, J. Mirabella, and A. Cropper. 2023. Prevalence of self-reported kidney disease in older adults by sexual orientation: Behavioral risk factor surveillance system analysis (2014–2019). *Journal of the American Society of Nephrology* 34(4):682–693.

Chen, K., M. Didsbury, A. van Zwieten, M. Howell, S. Kim, A. Tong, K. Howard, N. Nassar, B. Barton, S. Lah, J. Lorenzo, G. Strippoli, S. Palmer, A. Teixeira-Pinto, F. Mackie, S. McTaggart, A. Walker, T. Kara, J. C. Craig, and G. Wong. 2018. Neurocognitive and educational outcomes in children and adolescents with CKD: A systematic review and meta-analysis. *Clinical Journal of the American Society of Nephrology* 13(3):387–397.

Cockcroft, D. W., and M. H. Gault. 1976. Prediction of creatinine clearance from serum creatinine. *Nephron* 16(1):31–41.

Collister, D., N. Saad, E. Christie, and S. Ahmed. 2021. Providing care for transgender persons with kidney disease: A narrative review. *Canadian Journal of Kidney Health and Disease* 8:e2054358120985379.

Crews, D. C., T. Pfaff, and N. R. Powe. 2013. Socioeconomic factors and racial disparities in kidney disease outcomes. *Seminars in Nephrology* 33:468–475.

Delgado, C., M. Baweja, D. C. Crews, N. D. Eneanya, C. A. Gadegbeku, L. A. Inker, M. L. Mendu, W. G. Miller, M. M. Moxey-Mims, G. V. Roberts, W. L. St Peter, C. Warfield, and N. R. Powe. 2022. A unifying approach for GFR estimation: Recommendations of the NKF-ASN task force on reassessing the inclusion of race in diagnosing kidney disease. *American Journal of Kidney Disease* 79(2):268–288.e261.

den Bakker, E., A. Bökenkamp, and D. Haffner. 2022. Assessment of kidney function in children. *Pediatric Clinics* 69(6):1017–1035.

Eckenrode, H. E., J. C. Carwie, and L. M. Curtis. 2022a. Does gender affirming hormone therapy increase the risk of kidney disease? *Seminars in Nephrology* 42(3):e151284.

Eckenrode, H. E., O. M. Gutierrez, G. Osis, A. Agarwal, and L. M. Curtis. 2022b. Kidney disease prevalence in transgender individuals. *Clinical Journal of the American Society of Nephrology* 17(2):280–282.

Edey, M. M. 2017. Male sexual dysfunction and chronic kidney disease. *Frontiers in Medicine* 4:32.

Fadich, S. K., A. Kalayjian, D. N. Greene, and L. R. Cirrincione. 2022. A retrospective analysis of creatinine-based kidney function with and without sex assigned at birth among transgender adults. *Annals of Pharmacotherapy* 56(7):791–799.

Forni Ogna, V., A. Ogna, P. Vuistiner, M. Pruijm, B. Ponte, D. Ackermann, L. Gabutti, N. Vakilzadeh, M. Mohaupt, and P.-Y. Martin. 2015. New anthropometry-based age- and sex-specific reference values for urinary 24-hour creatinine excretion based on the adult Swiss population. *BMC Medicine* 13:40.

García, G. G., A. Iyengar, F. Kaze, C. Kierans, C. Padilla-Altamira, and V. A. Luyckx. 2022. Sex and gender differences in chronic kidney disease and access to care around the globe. *Seminars in Nephrology* 42(2):101–113.

Getahun, D., R. Nash, W. D. Flanders, T. C. Baird, T. A. Becerra-Culqui, L. Cromwell, E. Hunkeler, T. L. Lash, A. Millman, V. P. Quinn, B. Robinson, D. Roblin, M. J. Silverberg, J. Safer, J. Slovis, V. Tangpricha, and M. Goodman. 2018. Cross-sex hormones and acute cardiovascular events in transgender persons: A cohort study. *Annals of Internal Medicine* 169(4):205–213.

Goede, D. L., P. Wiesli, M. Brändle, L. Bestmann, R. L. Bernays, C. Zwimpfer, and C. Schmid. 2009. Effects of thyroxine replacement on serum creatinine and cystatin C in patients with primary and central hypothyroidism. *Swiss Medical Weekly* 139(23-24):339–344.

Gold, A., K. Martin, K. Breckbill, Y. Avitzur, and M. Kaufman. 2015. Transition to adult care in pediatric solid-organ transplant: Development of a practice guideline. *Progress in Transplantation* 25(2):131–138.

Gottlieb, E. R., C. Estiverne, N. V. Tolan, S. E. Melanson, and M. L. Mendu. 2023. Estimated GFR with cystatin-C and creatinine in clinical practice: A retrospective cohort study. *Kidney Medicine* 5(3):e100600.

Gounden, V., H. Bhatt, and I. Jialal. 2023. *Renal function tests*. [Updated 2023 July 17]. Treasure Island, FL: StatPearls Publishing.

Haffner, D. 2020. Strategies for optimizing growth in children with chronic kidney disease. *Frontiers in Pediatrics* 8:399.

Haffner, D., and M. Zivicnjak. 2017. Pubertal development in children with chronic kidney disease. *Pediatric Nephrology* 32(6):949–964.

Harada, R., Y. Hamasaki, Y. Okuda, R. Hamada, and K. Ishikura. 2022. Epidemiology of pediatric chronic kidney disease/kidney failure: Learning from registries and cohort studies. *Pediatric Nephrology* 37(6):1215–1229.

Harambat, J., K. J. van Stralen, J. J. Kim, and E. J. Tizard. 2012. Epidemiology of chronic kidney disease in children. *Pediatric Nephrology* 27(3):363–373.

Herman, J. L., A. R. Flores, and K. K. O'Neill. 2022. *How many adults and youth identify as transgender in the United States?* Los Angeles, CA: UCLA Williams Institute. https://williamsinstitute.law.ucla.edu/wp-content/uploads/Trans-Pop-Update-Jun-2022.pdf (accessed February 27, 2024).

Hsu, C. Y., K. Propert, D. Xie, L. Hamm, J. He, E. Miller, A. Ojo, M. Shlipak, V. Teal, R. Townsend, M. Weir, J. Wilson, and H. Feldman. 2011. Measured GFR does not outperform estimated GFR in predicting CKD-related complications. *Journal of the American Society of Nephrology* 22(10):1931–1937.

Iglesias, P., J. J. Carrero, and J. J. Díez. 2012. Gonadal dysfunction in men with chronic kidney disease: Clinical features, prognostic implications and therapeutic options. *Journal of Nephrology* 25(1):31.

Inker, L. A., N. Eneanya, J. Coresh, H. Tighiouart, D. Wang, Y. Sang, D. C. Crews, A. Doria, M. M. Estrella, M. Froissart, M. E. Grams, T. Greene, A. Grubb, V. Gudnason, O. M. Gutiérrez, R. Kalil, A. B. Karger, M. Mauer, G. Navis, R. G. Nelson, E. D.Poggio, R. Rodby, P. Rossing, A. D. Rule, E. Selvin, J. C. Seegmiller, M. G. Shlipak, V. E. Torres, W. Yang, S. H. Ballew, S. J. Couture, N. R. Powe, A. S. Levey, and the Chronic Kidney Disease Epidemiology Collaboration. 2021. New creatinine- and cystatin C–based equations to estimate GFR without race. *New England Journal of Medicine* 385(19):1737–1749.

Jankowska, M., M. J. Soler, K. I. Stevens, and R. Torra. 2023. Why do we keep ignoring sex in kidney disease? *Clinical Kidney Journal* 16(12):2327–2335.

Jue, J. S., M. Alameddine, and G. Ciancio. 2020. Kidney transplantation in transgender patients. *Current Urology Reports* 21(1):1.

Katz-Greenberg, G., and S. Shah. 2022. Sex and gender differences in kidney transplantation. *Seminars in Nephrology* 42(2):219–229.

Kolvenbach, C. M., S. Shril, and F. Hildebrandt. 2023. The genetics and pathogenesis of CAKUT. *Nature Reviews Nephrology* 19(11):709–720.

Kovesdy, C. P. 2022. Epidemiology of chronic kidney disease: An update 2022. *Kidney International Supplements* 12(1):7–11.

Krupka, E., S. Curtis, T. Ferguson, R. Whitlock, N. Askin, A. C. Millar, M. Dahl, R. Fung, S. B. Ahmed, N. Tangri, M. Walsh, and D. Collister. 2022. The effect of gender-affirming hormone therapy on measures of kidney function: A systematic review and meta-analysis. *Clinical Journal of the American Society of Nephrology* 17(9):1305–1315.

Laederach-Hofmann, K., and B. Bunzel. 2000. Noncompliance in organ transplant recipients: A literature review. *General Hospital Psychiatry* 22(6):412–424.

Leeies, M., D. Collister, J. Ho, A. Trachtenberg, J. Gruber, M. J. Weiss, J. A. Chandler, O. Mooney, T. Carta, B. Klassen, C. Draenos, K. Sutha, S. Randell, M. Strang, B. Partain, C. T. Whitley, S. Cuvelier, L. J. MacKenzie, S. D. Shemie, and C. Hrymak. 2023. Inequities in organ and tissue donation and transplantation for sexual orientation and gender identity diverse people: A scoping review. *American Journal of Transplantation* 23(6):707–726.

Lees, J. S., E. Rutherford, K. I. Stevens, D. C. Chen, R. Scherzer, M. M. Estrella, M. K. Sullivan, N. Ebert, P. B. Mark, and M. G. Shlipak. 2022. Assessment of cystatin C level for risk stratification in adults with chronic kidney disease. *JAMA Network Open* 5(10):e2238300.

Levey, A. S., J. P. Bosch, J. B. Lewis, T. Greene, N. Rogers, and D. Roth. 1999. A more accurate method to estimate glomerular filtration rate from serum creatinine: A new prediction equation. Modification of Diet in Renal Disease Study Group. *Annals of Internal Medicine* 130(6):461–470.

Levey, A. S., L. A. Stevens, C. H. Schmid, Y. L. Zhang, A. F. Castro, 3rd, H. I. Feldman, J. W. Kusek, P. Eggers, F. Van Lente, T. Greene, and J. Coresh. 2009. A new equation to estimate glomerular filtration rate. *Annals of Internal Medicine* 150(9):604–612.

Levey, A. S., R. T. Gansevoort, J. Coresh, L. A. Inker, H. L. Heerspink, M. E. Grams, T. Greene, H. Tighiouart, K. Matsushita, and S. H. Ballew. 2020. Change in albuminuria and GFR as end points for clinical trials in early stages of CKD: A scientific workshop sponsored by the National Kidney Foundation in collaboration with the U.S. Food and Drug Administration and European Medicines Agency. *American Journal of Kidney Diseases* 75(1):84–104.

Lombel, R. M., P. R. Brakeman, B. S. Sack, and L. Butani. 2022. Urologic considerations in pediatric chronic kidney disease. *Advances in Chronic Kidney Disease* 29(3):308–317.

Maheshwari, A., T. Nippoldt, and C. Davidge-Pitts. 2021. An approach to nonsuppressed testosterone in transgender women receiving gender-affirming feminizing hormonal therapy. *Journal of the Endocrine Society* 5(9):bvab068.

Maheshwari, A., V. Dines, D. Saul, T. Nippoldt, A. Kattah, and C. Davidge-Pitts. 2022. The effect of gender-affirming hormone therapy on serum creatinine in transgender individuals. *Endocrine Practice* 28(1):52–57.

Malmgren, L., and A. Grubb. 2023. Muscle mass, creatinine, cystatin C and selective glomerular hypofiltration syndromes. *Clinical Kidney Journal* 16(8):1206–1210.

Marco Mayayo, M. P., M. Martinez Alonso, J. M. Valdivielso Revilla, and E. Fernandez-Giraldez. 2016. A new gender-specific formula to estimate 24-hour urine protein from protein to creatinine ratio. *Nephron* 133(4):232–238.

Millington, K., E. Barrera, A. Daga, N. Mann, J. Olson-Kennedy, R. Garofalo, S. M. Rosenthal, and Y. M. Chan. 2022. The effect of gender-affirming hormone treatment on serum creatinine in transgender and gender-diverse youth: Implications for estimating GFR. *Pediatric Nephrology* 37(9):2141–2150.

Mohottige, D., and M. R. Lunn. 2020. Ensuring gender-affirming care in nephrology: Improving care for transgender and gender-expansive individuals. *Clinical Journal of the American Society of Nephrology* 15(8):1195–1197.

Mohottige, D., and D. S. Tuot. 2022. Advancing kidney health equity: Influences of gender-affirming hormone therapy on kidney function. *Clinical Journal of the American Society of Nephrology* 17(9):1281–1283.

Mohottige, D., L. M. McElroy, and L. E. Boulware. 2021. A cascade of structural barriers contributing to racial kidney transplant inequities. *Advances in Chronic Kidney Disease* 28(6):517–527.

Mong Hiep, T. T., K. Ismaili, F. Collart, R. Van Damme-Lombaerts, N. Godefroid, M.-S. Ghuysen, K. Van Hoeck, A. Raes, F. Janssen, and A. Robert. 2010. Clinical characteristics and outcomes of children with stage 3–5 chronic kidney disease. *Pediatric Nephrology* 25(5):935–940.

Murtagh, F. E., J. Addington-Hall, and I. J. Higginson. 2007. The prevalence of symptoms in end-stage renal disease: A systematic review. *Advances in Chronic Kidney Disease* 14(1):82–99.

Ng, D. K., and C. B. Pierce. 2021. Kidney disease progression in children and young adults with pediatric CKD: Epidemiologic perspectives and clinical applications. *Seminars in Nephrology* 41(5):405–415.

Nicholas, S. B., K. Kalantar-Zadeh, and K. C. Norris. 2015. Socioeconomic disparities in chronic kidney disease. *Advances in Chronic Kidney Disease* 22(1):6–15.

NIDDK (National Institute of Diabetes and Digestive and Kidney Diseases). 2022. *Recommended eGFR calculators.* https://www.niddk.nih.gov/health-information/professionals/clinical-tools-patient-management/kidney-disease/laboratory-evaluation/estimated-gfr-calculators (accessed May 16, 2024).

NKF (National Kidney Foundation). n.d.-a. *EGFR calculator.* https://www.kidney.org/professionals/kdoqi/gfr_calculator (accessed January 7, 2024).

NKF. n.d.-b. *Pediatric GFR calculator.* https://www.kidney.org/professionals/KDOQI/gfr_calculatorPed (accessed January 7, 2024).

NKF. n.d.-c. *Kidney failure risk factor: Urine albumin-creatinine ratio (uACR).* https://www.kidney.org/content/kidney-failure-risk-factor-urine-albumin-to-creatinine-ration-uacr (accessed July 5, 2024).

NKF. 2022. *Diagnostic tests & procedures: Estimated glomerular filtration rate.* https://www.kidney.org/sites/default/files/01-10-8374_2212_patflyer_egfr.pdf (accessed February 29, 2024).

Norris, K., and A. R. Nissenson. 2008. Race, gender, and socioeconomic disparities in CKD in the United States. *Journal of the American Society of Nephrology* 19(7):1261–1270.

Norton, J. M., M. M. Moxey-Mims, P. W. Eggers, A. S. Narva, R. A. Star, P. L. Kimmel, and G. P. Rodgers. 2016. Social determinants of racial disparities in CKD. *Journal of the American Society of Nephrology* 27(9):2576–2595.

Owosela, B. O., R. S. Steinberg, S. L. Leslie, L. A. Celi, S. Purkayastha, R. Shiradkar, J. M. Newsome, and J. W. Gichoya. 2024. Identifying and improving the "ground truth" of race in disparities research through improved EMR data reporting. A systematic review. *International Journal of Medical Informatics* 182:105303.

Panaich, S., V. Veeranna, S. Zalawadiya, A. Kottam, and L. Afonso. 2013. Association of cystatin C with measures of obesity and its impact on cardiovascular events among healthy U.S. adults. *Journal of the American College of Cardiology* 61(10S):e1420.

Patel, K., C. Diamantidis, M. Zhan, V. D. Hsu, L. D. Walker, J. Gardner, M. R. Weir, and J. C. Fink. 2012. Influence of creatinine versus glomerular filtration rate on non-steroidal anti-inflammatory drug prescriptions in chronic kidney disease. *American Journal of Nephrology* 36(1):19–26.

Pierce, C. B., A. Muñoz, D. K. Ng, B. A. Warady, S. L. Furth, and G. J. Schwartz. 2021. Age- and sex-dependent clinical equations to estimate glomerular filtration rates in children and young adults with chronic kidney disease. *Kidney International* 99(4):948–956.

Pierre, C. C., M. A. Marzinke, S. B. Ahmed, D. Collister, J. M. Colón-Franco, M. P. Hoenig, T. Lorey, P. M. Palevsky, O. P. Palmer, S. E. Rosas, J. Vassalotti, C. T. Whitley, and D. N. Greene. 2023. AACC/NKF guidance document on improving equity in chronic kidney disease care. *Journal of Applied Laboratory Medicine* 8(4):789–816.

Plantinga, L. C., D. S. Tuot, and N. R. Powe. 2010. Awareness of chronic kidney disease among patients and providers. *Advances in Chronic Kidney Disease* 17(3):225–236.

Pottel, H., J. Björk, A. D. Rule, N. Ebert, B. O. Eriksen, L. Dubourg, E. Vidal-Petiot, A. Grubb, M. Hansson, E. J. Lamb, K. Littmann, C. Mariat, T. Melsom, E. Schaeffner, P. O. Sundin, A. Åkesson, A. Larsson, E. Cavalier, J. B. Bukabau, E. K. Sumaili, E. Yayo, D. Monnet, M. Flamant, U. Nyman, and P. Delanaye. 2023. Cystatin C-based equation to estimate GFR without the inclusion of race and sex. *New England Journal of Medicine* 388(4):333–343.

Quartarolo, J. M., M. Thoelke, and S. J. Schafers. 2007. Reporting of estimated glomerular filtration rate: Effect on physician recognition of chronic kidney disease and prescribing practices for elderly hospitalized patients. *Journal of Hospital Medicine* 2(2):74–78.

Raina, R., G. A. Abusin, P. Vijayaraghavan, J. J. Auletta, L. Cabral, H. Hashem, B. A. Vogt, K. R. Cooke, and R. F. Abu-Arja. 2018. The role of continuous renal replacement therapy in the management of acute kidney injury associated with sinusoidal obstruction syndrome following hematopoietic cell transplantation. *Pediatric Transplantation* 22(2):e13139.

Ramadan, O. I., A. Naji, M. H. Levine, P. M. Porrett, T. B. Dunn, S. M. Nazarian, R. M. Weinrieb, M. Kaminski, D. Johnson, and J. Trofe-Clark. 2020. Kidney transplantation and donation in the transgender population: A single-institution case series. *American Journal of Transplantation* 20(10):2899–2904.

Romejko, K., A. Rymarz, H. Sadownik, and S. Niemczyk. 2022. Testosterone deficiency as one of the major endocrine disorders in chronic kidney disease. *Nutrients* 14(16):3438.

Rule, A. D., K. R. Bailey, J. C. Lieske, P. A. Peyser, and S. T. Turner. 2013. Estimating the glomerular filtration rate from serum creatinine is better than from cystatin C for evaluating risk factors associated with chronic kidney disease. *Kidney International* 83(6):1169–1176.

Schoolwerth, A. C., M. M. Engelgau, and T. H. Hostetter. 2005. A public health action plan is needed for chronic kidney disease. *Advances in Chronic Kidney Disease* 12(4):418–423.

Schwartz, G. J., A. Muñoz, M. Schneider, R. Mak, F. Kaskel, B. Wrady, and S. Furth. 2009. New equations to estimate GFR in children with CKD. *Journal of the American Society of Nephrology* 20(3):629–637.

Sequeira, G. M., K. M. Kidd, R. W. Coulter, E. Miller, D. Fortenberry, R. Garofalo, L. P. Richardson, and K. N. Ray. 2021. Transgender youths' perspectives on telehealth for delivery of gender-affirming care. *Journal of Adolescent Health* 68(6):1207–1210.

Silverstein, D. M. 2018. Growth and nutrition in pediatric chronic kidney disease. *Frontiers in Pediatrics* 6:205.

SoRelle, J. A., R. Jiao, E. Gao, J. Veazey, I. Frame, A. M. Quinn, P. Day, P. Pagels, N. Gimpel, and K. Patel. 2019. Impact of hormone therapy on laboratory values in transgender patients. *Clinical Chemistry* 65(1):170–179.

SSA (Social Security Administration). n.d.-a. *Listing of impairments—Adult Listings (Part A).* https://www.ssa.gov/disability/professionals/bluebook/AdultListings.htm (accessed February 29, 2024).

SSA. n.d.-b. *Listing of impairments—Childhood Listings (Part B).* https://www.ssa.gov/disability/professionals/bluebook/ChildhoodListings.htm (accessed February 29, 2024).

SSA. 2022. *SSI annual statistical report.* https://www.ssa.gov/policy/docs/statcomps/ssi_asr/index.html#:~:text=About%207.5%20million%20people%20received,in%20federally%20administered%20state%20supplementation (accessed February 29, 2024).

SSA. 2023. *Annual statistical report on the social security disability insurance program, 2022.* https://www.ssa.gov/policy/docs/statcomps/di_asr/index.html (accessed February 28, 2024).

Stevens, L. A., C. H. Schmid, T. Greene, L. Li, G. J. Beck, M. M. Joffe, M. Froissart, J. W. Kusek, Y. L. Zhang, and J. Coresh. 2009. Factors other than glomerular filtration rate affect serum cystatin C levels. *Kidney International* 75(6):652–660.

Stevens, P. E., S. B. Ahmed, J. J. Carrero, B. Foster, A. Francis, R. K. Hall, W. G. Herrington, G. Hill, L. A. Inker, R. Kazancıoğlu, E. Lamb, P. Lin, M. Madero, N. McIntyre, K. Morrow, G. Roberts, D. Sabanayagam, E. Schaeffner, M. Shlipak, R. Shroff, N. Tangri, T. Thanachayanont, I. Ulasi, G. Wong, C.-W. Yang, L. Zhang, and A. Levin. 2024. KDIGO 2024 clinical practice guideline for the evaluation and management of chronic kidney disease. *Kidney International* 105(4S):S117–S314.

Streed, C. G., L. B. Beach, B. A. Caceres, N. L. Dowshen, K. L. Moreau, M. Mukherjee, T. Poteat, A. Radix, S. L. Reisner, and V. Singh. 2021. Assessing and addressing cardiovascular health in people who are transgender and gender diverse: A scientific statement from the American Heart Association. *Circulation* 144(6):e136–e148.

Streed, C. G., J. E. Perlson, M. P. Abrams, and E. Lett. 2023. On, with, by—advancing transgender health research and clinical practice. *Health Equity* 7(1):161–165.

Sutha, K., and C. G. Streed, Jr. 2023. Including sexual orientation and gender identity data to advance nephrology care. *Nature Reviews Nephrology* 19(6):355–356.

Tran, N. K., M. R. Lunn, C. E. Schulkey, S. Tesfaye, S. Nambiar, S. Chatterjee, D. Kozlowski, P. Lozano, F. T. Randal, and Y. Mo. 2023. Prevalence of 12 common health conditions in sexual and gender minority participants in the All of Us Research Program. *JAMA Network Open* 6(7):e2324969.

Uffing, A., F. Hullekes, L. V. Riella, and J. J. Hogan. 2021. Recurrent glomerular disease after kidney transplantation: Diagnostic and management dilemmas. *Clinical Journal of the American Society of Nephrology* 16(11):1730–1742.

van Eeghen, S. A., C. M. Wiepjes, G. T'Sjoen, N. J. Nokoff, M. den Heijer, P. Bjornstad, and D. H. van Raalte. 2023. Cystatin C-based eGFR changes during gender-affirming hormone therapy in transgender individuals. *Clinical Journal of the American Society of Nephrology* 18(12):1545–1554.

Virth, J., H. G. Mack, D. Colville, E. Crockett, and J. Savige. 2024. Ocular manifestations of congenital anomalies of the kidney and urinary tract (CAKUT). *Pediatric Nephrology* 39(2):357–369.

Vivarelli, M., L. Massella, B. Ruggiero, and F. Emma. 2017. Minimal change disease. *Clinical Journal of the American Society of Nephrology* 12(2):332–345.

Weinert, L. S., A. B. Prates, F. B. do Amaral, M. Z. Vaccaro, J. L. Camargo, and S. P. Silveiro. 2010. Gender does not influence cystatin C concentrations in healthy volunteers. *Clinical Chemistry and Laboratory Medicine* 48(3):405–408.

Yang, F., J.-S. Shi, S.-W. Gong, X.-D. Xu, and W.-B. Le. 2022. An equation to estimate 24-hour total urine protein excretion rate in patients who underwent urine protein testing. *BMC Nephrology* 23(1):49.

Yilmaz, M. I., A. Sonmez, A. R. Qureshi, M. Saglam, P. Stenvinkel, H. Yaman, T. Eyileten, K. Caglar, Y. Oguz, and A. Taslipinar. 2011. Endogenous testosterone, endothelial dysfunction, and cardiovascular events in men with nondialysis chronic kidney disease. *Clinical Journal of the American Society of Nephrology* 6(7):1617–1625.

11

Cancers of the Reproductive System

According to the American Cancer Society, over 2 million people are diagnosed with cancer each year, and more than 600,000 deaths due to cancer are recorded (Siegel et al., 2024). Cancer treatments can take a toll on anyone, but for some people, cancer treatment can be so intense and cause such severe side effects—including pain, cancer-related fatigue, nausea and vomiting, appetite loss, weight loss, bone density loss, heart problems, delirium, nerve problems, memory problems, and others—that they can limit a person's ability to work or complete routine daily activities (NCI, n.d.). Pharmacological treatments available to address side effects can be costly and produce additional side effects (Devlin et al., 2017). Some people with cancer experience severe side effects that last for months or even years after treatment is completed (Stein et al., 2008). In addition, despite treatment, cancer may metastasize to other organs, causing additional complications and symptoms that further prevent cancer patients from engaging in substantial gainful activity. For these reasons, some people with cancer in advanced stages may apply for disability benefits through the Social Security Administration (SSA).

SSA's adult disability Listings for cancer include several reproductive system cancers often associated with either cisgender women (including cancers of the uterus, uterine cervix, vulva, vagina, fallopian tubes, and ovaries) or cisgender men (including cancers of the prostate gland, testicles, and penis). Because these cancers are traditionally associated with one sex, SSA asked this committee to examine appropriate evaluation of these cancers for transgender and gender diverse (TGD) people and people with variations in sex traits (VSTs) and to determine what changes in current disability criteria may be necessary for them to serve as medically appropriate indicators of severity for TGD applicants and applicants with VSTs.

This chapter examines the prevalence of cancer among TGD people and people with VSTs, describes the impact of gender-affirming care on people with cancer, presents current guidelines that aim to decouple gender from cancer, and offers a gender- and sex-inclusive approach to disability determination for people with reproductive cancers.

PREVALENCE OF AND SCREENING FOR REPRODUCTIVE CANCERS AMONG TRANSGENDER AND GENDER DIVERSE PEOPLE AND PEOPLE WITH VARIATIONS IN SEX TRAITS

Given that data on sexual orientation and gender identity are not (to date) routinely collected in prospective databases (see Chapter 4 of this report), it is difficult to determine the prevalence of cancer among TGD individuals and those with VSTs. One review estimates that cancer impacts fewer than 600 members of sexual or gender minority (SGM) groups (or 0.005 percent of the U.S. population) annually (Jackson et al., 2021), but this is likely a significant undercount. In addition, low cancer screening rates contribute to the difficulty of tracking cancer among SGM people, and many cases may go undiagnosed (Jackson et al., 2021). The literature shows that SGM people are less likely to participate in cancer screening relative to the general population. For example, Herriges and colleagues (2021) used the Health Information Network Trends Survey to determine the screening behaviors of lesbian, gay, and bisexual (LGB) people; they found that those with prostates were significantly less likely to undergo prostate-specific antigen blood testing compared with heterosexual men; likewise, LGB people with breasts and those with cervices were less likely to undergo mammography or Papanicolaou (Pap) tests, respectively, compared with heterosexual women (Herriges et al., 2021). Among TGD people, studies have found transgender men to be significantly less likely to be up to date on Pap testing compared with cisgender women (Oladeru et al., 2022; Peitzmeier et al., 2014a,b; Tabaac et al., 2018). Studies have also found lower rates of prostate-specific antigen screening among transgender women compared with cisgender men (Ma et al., 2021; Nik-Ahd et al., 2023; Tabaac et al., 2018).

Hostilities experienced by TGD people and people with VSTs in health care settings are a potentially important reason for these low cancer screening rates. For example, Mirza and Rooney (2018) found that among LGB or queer respondents to a survey from the Center for American Progress, 6 percent had been refused care, and 8 percent were refused being seen by a health care provider; among transgender respondents, these figures were between 12 and 29 percent. In addition, where TGD populations receive care, that care may be less adequate than care provided to cisgender peers: one study found that transgender men who did receive Pap tests were 10 times more likely than cisgender women to have inadequate tests (i.e., the cell sample taken was insufficient for laboratory testing) (Peitzmeier et al., 2014b). Another study found that transgender women were significantly less likely than cisgender men to have ever had a discussion with a health care provider about the risks and benefits of prostate-specific antigen screening (Ma et al., 2021).

In addition, compared with their heterosexual counterparts, people from sexual and gender minority groups are more likely to be living in poverty; less likely to have health insurance; and for older individuals, twice as likely to be living alone (Sachdeva et al., 2021). Taken together, low screening rates, hostile and inadequate health care, and other health disparities may mean that TGD people may have a greater likelihood of presenting with more advanced disease compared with cisgender people. One study found transgender patients to be more likely to be diagnosed at later stages for lung cancer, and being transgender was associated with lower odds of treatment for kidney and pancreatic cancer (Jackson et al., 2021). Whether these same trends are true for reproductive cancers is difficult to evaluate given the lack of uniform data collection on sexual orientation and gender identity. Moreover, the literature evaluating the incidence and experience of cancer among people with VSTs is exceptionally limited and precludes any conclusions.

IMPACT OF GENDER-AFFIRMING MEDICAL CARE ON PEOPLE WITH CANCER

While the assumption that gender-affirming hormone therapy (GAHT) will increase the risk of hormonally sensitive cancers, such as prostate or ovarian cancer, in transgender individuals is common, the data do not support this assumption. A 2018 systematic review concluded that, based on the available retrospective studies, there was no association between GAHT and hormone-dependent tumors (McFarlane et al., 2018).

A few studies have examined this question for prostate cancer. In one study of the National Cancer Database (11,776,699 persons with cancer in the database, 589 of whom were transgender), transgender people were found to have higher rates of certain cancers (including anal cancer, liver cancer, nonmelanoma skin cancers, and Hodgkins and non-Hodgkins lymphoma) compared with their cisgender counterparts, but lower rates of prostate cancer (Jackson et al., 2021). Other studies support this finding. A 2022 review of the existing literature attempted to define the prevalence of prostate cancer in transgender women and identified only 24 publications, 10 of which were case reports; this review found that the risk of prostate cancer among transgender women who have not undergone GAHT or any gender-affirming surgery is the same as for cisgender men; however, transgender women who have received GAHT or undergone gender-affirming surgery were found to have a lower incidence of prostate cancer compared to cisgender men (Bertoncelli Tanaka et al., 2022). A separate cohort study evaluated the incidence of prostate cancer in transgender females treated with antiandrogens, estrogen, and bilateral orchiectomy (N = 2,306) (Gooren and Morgentaler, 2014). Here, only one case of prostate cancer was detected, although the authors concluded this finding was likely due to a lack of prostate cancer screening in general and the overall younger age of the cohort studied. Another retrospective study including 2,281 transgender women found six cases of prostate cancer after a median of 17 years of hormone therapy (de Nie et al., 2020). The results of this study indicate that transgender women receiving GAHT have a substantially lower risk for prostate cancer compared with people assigned male at birth.

Given how much is unclear about cancer outcomes among transgender individuals, the question of how hormones interact with cancers is quite important. For example, there are now data indicating that cancer treatment–related toxicities are associated with gender. In a study that included more than 23,000 volunteers who participated in a Phase 2 or 3 trial over a nearly 20-year span, women had a 34 percent increased risk of a severe adverse event, regardless of treatment type (Unger et al., 2022). With regard to immunotherapy, women had a nearly 70 percent increased risk of a severe and symptomatic adverse event compared with men. These data point to potential biological differences between the sexes and the importance of dosing (often based on calculations that include gender) in drug metabolism and tolerance; they raise the question of what degree of risk a transgender person truly faces when exposed to cancer treatment.

In addition, there is a lack of evidence—and a lack of consensus— around the safety of GAHT with respect to cancer outcomes (e.g., recurrence or survival) in people diagnosed and subsequently treated for cancer. SSA adjudicators may see language from treating oncology specialists recommending against continuation or reinitiation of GAHT in cancer survivors. The committee points out that such recommendations are not based on data or guidelines and may reflect a paternalistic approach to TGD patients rather than reflect shared decision making that takes into account the patient's own goals and desires.[1]

---

[1] "Paternalistic decision making" refers to a unidirectional flow of information from doctor to patient, with subsequent recommendations being made without patient input (Kane et al., 2014). In shared decision making, recommendations are based on bidirectional communication, whereby a patient's values and preferences are solicited alongside the information needed to make decisions—a goal often referred to as patients' values-aligned care (Barry and Edgman-Levitan, 2012; Charles et al., 1997).

<hr>

Panelist Perspective

"There was only one doctor for a long time that would prescribe hormones to trans people. I finally got an appointment with her and got my prescription. I just had to pick it up, and through My Chart my gynecologist found out that I was going to start hormones and she called up my new primary care doctor and told her it was irresponsible prescribing hormones, hormones to someone that had cancer. And she was just sure that it would cause my cancer to come back and my primary care just panicked, and was like, "Oh!" And just canceled my prescription. I had to call my gynecologist . . . she was always very kind to me, and supportive, but not necessarily trans knowledgeable about trans people. But she was knowledgeable about cancer, and she talked my other doctors down . . . and so I got my [hormone] prescription, eventually. But my gynecologist, who I did not keep after this, but she lectured me. She wrote page long notes in My Chart about her disagreeing, and she made me sign an AMA.[a]"

—Statement from patient–provider panel,
presented to the committee on December 1, 2023.

<hr>

[a] "AMA" stands for "against medical advice" document. A patient may be asked to sign an AMA when they decline medical advice from their health care provider.

GUIDELINES: DECOUPLING GENDER FROM CANCER

There is consensus today that disease is not associated with gender, but with specified organs. For example, the American Society of Clinical Oncology's (2022) Center for Research and Analytics published guidance intended to ensure inclusion of SGM patients in clinical trials (ASCO, 2022). Among the recommendations of this guidance is decoupling gender, sex assigned at birth, and current anatomy by avoiding such phrases as "men with prostate cancer." The guidance also advises that people receiving GAHT should be eligible to volunteer for clinical trials unless a clear contraindication exists. Both the American College of Obstetricians and Gynecologists (2021) and American Society for Colposcopy and Cervical Pathology (Perkins et al., 2020) have published on the topic of health care for TGD people, both recommending screening based on anatomy regardless of gender. The decoupling of gender and cancers is also more inclusive of people with VSTs, who may have organs that do not correspond to the sex assigned to them at birth.

Other organizations have modified language to be more gender inclusive. Examples include the following:

- The **American Cancer Society** (ACS, 2021) modified its language to eliminate gender–cancer associations. For example, screening and interventions are recommended for all "people with a cervix." Likewise, ACS guidelines recommend that all "people with a uterus" receive appropriate endometrial cancer care and that all "people with a prostate" receive appropriate prostate cancer care.
- Instead of reserving prostate cancer screenings for males, the **American Urological Association** recommends screening for all people aged 45–50 and beginning at age 40 for "people at increased risk of developing prostate cancer" (Wei et al., 2023).
- **National Comprehensive Cancer Network** Guidelines for Prostate Cancer Early Detection follow a similar approach; updated in 2022, the guidelines specify that the recommendations are "for individuals with a prostate opting to participate" in an early detection program (Freedman-Cass et al., 2023).

Current U.S. Preventive Services Task Force Guidelines related to cancer screening are sex specific, but the task force has expressed a commitment to making its recommendations gender inclusive (Caughey et al., 2021).

CANCER AND SSA DISABILITY DETERMINATIONS

SSA asked the committee for this study to examine reproductive cancers under Listing 13.00, Cancer—Adult, as these cancers are traditionally associated with only one sex. Box 11-1 outlines the cancers examined in this chapter.

Similar to current guidelines that recommend screening based on anatomy rather than sex assigned at birth or gender identity, many of SSA's criteria under its reproductive cancer Listings use inclusive language based on anatomy. For example, the category under Listing 13.24 is cancer of the "prostate gland," rather than "men with prostate cancer." The same is true for cancer of the testicles under 13.25 and cancer of the penis under 13.26. In theory, the current language under Listings 13.24, 13.25, and 13.26 is inclusive of transgender women who have prostate, testicular, or penile cancer (as well as other gender diverse applicants or applicants with VSTs who have these cancers) given that, in accordance with the language of the disability Listing, it does not matter what sex or gender is included in the applicant's medical records, only that the applicant has the cancer at issue. While the applicant will still have to provide medical evidence to show the extent of their impairment in support of their disability application (which may include documentation of their treatment history, response

BOX 11-1
Reproductive Cancers Included Under
Listings 13.23, 13.24, 13.25, and 13.26

13.23. Cancers of the female genital tract—carcinoma or sarcoma (including primary peritoneal carcinoma)

13.23A. Uterus (corpus), as described in 1, 2, or 3: (1) Invading adjoining organs; (2) With metastases to or beyond the regional lymph nodes; or (3) Persistent or recurrent following initial anticancer therapy.

13.23B. Uterine cervix, as described in 1, 2 or 3: (1) Extending to the pelvic wall, lower portion of the vagina, or adjacent or distant organs; (2) Persistent or recurrent following initial anticancer therapy; or (3) With metastases to distant (for example, para-aortic or supraclavicular) lymph nodes.

13.23C. Vulva or vagina, as described in 1, 2, or 3: (1) Invading adjoining organs; (2) With metastases to or beyond the regional lymph nodes; or (3) Persistent or recurrent following initial anticancer therapy.

13.23D. Fallopian tubes, as described in 1 or 2: (1) Extending to the serosa or beyond; or (2) Persistent or recurrent following initial anticancer therapy.

13.23E. Ovaries, as described in 1 or 2: (1) All cancers except germ-cell cancers, with at least one of the following: (a) Extension beyond the pelvis; for example, implants on, or direct extension to, peritoneal, omental, or bowel surfaces; (b) Metastases to or beyond the regional lymph nodes; or (c) Recurrent following initial anticancer therapy; or (2) Germ-cell cancer—progressive or recurrent following initial anticancer therapy.
OR
13.23F. Small-cell (oat cell) carcinoma.

13.24. Prostate gland—carcinoma.

(A) Progressive or recurrent (not including biochemical recurrence) despite initial hormonal intervention;
OR
(B) With visceral metastases (metastases to internal organs);
OR
(C) Small-cell (oat cell) carcinoma.

13.25. Testicles—cancer with metastatic disease progressive or recurrent following initial chemotherapy.

13.26. Penis—carcinoma with metastases to or beyond the regional lymph nodes.

SOURCE: SSA, n.d.

to anticancer therapy, cancer recurrence, evidence of metastasis, or other documentation included under Listing 13.00 Cancer—Adult or under the specific cancer Listing), the applicant need not document anything in relation to their sex or gender to qualify for disability benefits.

In contrast, the disability Listing 13.23, "Cancers of the female genital tract—carcinoma or sarcoma," is not similarly inclusive of TGD people or people with VSTs who do not identify as female. While the specific cancers under 13.23 (cancers of the uterus, uterine cervix, vulva, vagina, fallopian tubes, and ovaries) are all listed by anatomy rather than sex or gender, the fact that these cancers fall under the category of "female" cancers may cause would-be applicants to assume that they cannot apply for benefits to which they would otherwise be entitled because their affirmed gender (or gender listed on medical or legal documents) is not female. Labeling these cancers as "female" could also cause professionals who may counsel would-be disability applicants (health care providers, social workers, disability lawyers, and others) to assume that one must be "female" to apply for disability under "cancers of the female genital tract." The committee does not know whether SSA has rejected applicants who do not identify as female from qualifying under 13.23, but it appears possible from the way the Listing is written that disability adjudicators could reasonably deny benefits to TGD people or people with VSTs.

Furthermore, the fact that one reproductive cancer Listing is labeled "female" creates the inference that the other reproductive cancer categories must be "male." This alone could dissuade people who do not identify as male from applying for disability under Listings 13.24, 13.25, and 13.26. Again, it appears possible to the committee that SSA adjudicators could deny benefits based on the assumption that these categories are reserved for people who identify as male.

A second portion of SSA's disability criteria reinforces the idea that at least the ovarian cancer Listing (13.23E) does not include men. Section 13.00K7 explains criteria for evaluating primary peritoneal carcinoma (PPC),[2] which is included under the Listing for 13.23 (SSA, n.d.):

> **Primary peritoneal carcinoma.** We use the criteria in 13.23E [cancer of the ovaries] to evaluate primary peritoneal carcinoma in **women** because this cancer is often indistinguishable from ovarian cancer and is generally treated the same way as ovarian cancer. We use the criteria in 13.15A [Pleura or mediastinum] to evaluate primary peritoneal carcinoma in **men** because many of these cases are similar to malignant mesothelioma. [emphasis added]

---

[2] PPC is cancer of the peritoneum (a thin layer of tissue that lines and protects the abdomen), with presentation similar to that of ovarian cancer. PPC affects mainly people assigned female at birth, with only a few cases in males being reported in the medical literature. PPC is rare, with an estimated incidence of 6.78 cases per 1 million; given this condition's rarity, this committee did not uncover research on PPC among TGD populations or populations with VSTs (Goodman and Shvetsov, 2009; Guellil, 2022).

Here, use of the terms "men" and "women" confers assignment of gender, as discussed in Chapter 2, and would appear to emphasize that it is only "women" who are eligible for disability under the ovarian cancer listing.

Furthermore, the language of Section 13.00K7 may create unnecessary boundaries—and confusion—for TGD disability applicants and applicants with VSTs, who do not fall neatly into the gendered categories of PPC. When these populations seek disability benefits based on a diagnosis of PPC, it is unclear what criteria should be used. Would transgender men be evaluated for PPC under Listing 13.23E because they were assigned female sex at birth or under 13.15A because their affirmed gender is male? The determining factor here may be the happenstance of how sex or gender is recorded in the person's medical record, which (as discussed in Chapter 3) may not be accurate with respect to an individual's sex, gender identity or anatomy. Being more intentional in the disability criteria for these Listings could make a real difference in terms of the medical evidence required to demonstrate disability. Box 11-2 compares SSA's requirements under Listings 13.15A and 13.23E.

BOX 11-2
Disability Evaluation Under Social Security:
Comparison of 13.15A and 13.23E

13.15. Pleura or mediastinum.
    A. Malignant mesothelioma of pleura.

13.23 Cancers of the female genital tract—carcinoma or sarcoma (including primary peritoneal carcinoma).

    E. Ovaries, as described in 1 or 2:

1. All cancers except germ-cell cancers, with at least one of the following: (a) Extension beyond the pelvis; for example, implants on, or direct extension to, peritoneal, omental, or bowel surfaces; (b) Metastases to or beyond the regional lymph nodes; or (c) Recurrent following initial anticancer therapy; or
2. Germ-cell cancer—progressive or recurrent following initial anticancer therapy.

NOTE: The pleura is a two-layered membrane that covers and cushions the lung. Malignant mesothelioma of pleura is typically caused from exposure to asbestos fibers.
SOURCES: Cleveland Clinic, 2022; SSA, n.d.

SSA would eliminate boundaries for TGD people and people with VSTs by removing differentiation of PPC in women versus men within the Listing and instead base disability determination on the histopathology.

The following suggested rewording under 13.00K7 emphasizes histology and uses inclusive language:

> **Primary peritoneal adenocarcinoma.** We use the criteria in 13.23 to evaluate adenocarcinoma of the peritoneal cavity because this cancer is often indistinguishable from epithelial ovarian or fallopian tube carcinoma.
> **Peritoneal mesothelioma.** We use the criteria in 13.15A to evaluate peritoneal mesothelioma in people of all sexes, because many of these cases are similar to malignant mesothelioma.

This approach would clarify for applicants that it is not gender that matters for PPC disability evaluation, but the histopathologic characterization of the cancer itself. This is consistent with current practice guidelines (Kindler et al., 2018). Such suggested language change under 13.00K7 recognizes that primary peritoneal mesothelioma can occur in all people regardless of the presence or absence of ovaries, while primary peritoneal adenocarcinoma is almost exclusively diagnosed in people with ovaries. Importantly, the committee prefers decoupling gender from the oncologic diagnosis by removing reference to "men" and "women" from the PPC Listing and referring instead to organs (e.g., ovaries, fallopian tube). Not only does this phrasing bring clarity for TGD people, but it acknowledges that people with VSTs—who may have ovaries and fallopian tubes but may have been assigned male sex at birth—could apply for disability with a PPC diagnosis.

Pertaining to the umbrella category "Cancers of the female genital tract" under 13.23, SSA might better serve TGD applicants and applicants with VSTs by choosing inclusive language that makes clear that these disability categories are open to anyone who has the cancer at issue, regardless of their gender identity or sex recorded at birth. A suggested way to reword 13.23 using inclusive language would be to call this category "Cancers of the uterus, uterine cervix, vulva, vagina, fallopian tubes, and ovaries." Alternatively, SSA could split these cancers into separate categories as it does for cancers of the prostate gland, testicles, and penis.

SUMMARY OF KEY POINTS

TGD people and people with VSTs participate in reproductive cancer screening programs less commonly than cisgender people as a result of multiple barriers, including hostilities experienced from medical providers and lack of screening access. Lack of uniform data collection on sexual orientation and gender identity in medical records makes it difficult to determine the prevalence of reproductive cancers and stage of presentation of these cancers among TGD people and people with VSTs. At this time, there are no data to indicate that GAHT increases the risk of a hormonally driven cancer. Whether GAHT has an impact on cancer survival is even less clear.

Organizations have begun to call for more gender-inclusive language in their cancer screening and treatment recommendations, language that moves away from an association between gender or sex recorded at birth and specific cancers to organ-specific considerations for malignancy. SSA might best serve TGD people and people with VSTs by being more intentional in its reproductive cancer Listings by not associating sex (e.g., woman or man; male or female) with any one cancer type.

REFERENCES

ACOG (American College of Obstetricians and Gynecologists). 2021. ACOG committee opinion: Health care for transgender and gender diverse individuals, Number 823. *Obstetrics & Gynecology* 137(3):e75–e88.

ACS (American Cancer Society). 2021. *Cancer care for transgender and gender nonconforming people: Fact sheet for health care providers.* https://www.cancer.org/content/dam/cancer-org/cancer-control/en/booklets-flyers/cancer-care-for-transgender-and-gender-non-conforming-people.pdf (accessed March 11, 2024).

ASCO (American Society of Clinical Oncology). 2022. *Sexual and gender minority (SGM) inclusion in clinical trials.* https://old-prod.asco.org/sites/new-www.asco.org/files/content-files/research-data/documents/2022-ASCO-CENTRA-SGM-Inclusion-Trials.pdf (accessed March 11, 2024).

Barry, M. J., and S. Edgman-Levitan. 2012. Shared decision making—pinnacle of patient-centered care. *New England Journal of Medicine* 366(9):780–781.

Bertoncelli Tanaka, M., K. Sahota, J. Burn, A. Falconer, M. Winkler, H. U. Ahmed, T. G. Rashid, and Gender Research Collaborative. 2022. Prostate cancer in transgender women: What does a urologist need to know? *BJU International* 129(1):113–122.

Caughey, A. B., A. H. Krist, T. A. Wolff, M. J. Barry, J. T. Henderson, D. K. Owens, K. W. Davidson, M. A. Simon, and C. M. Mangione. 2021. USPSTF approach to addressing sex and gender when making recommendations for clinical preventive services. *JAMA* 326(19):1953–1961.

Charles, C., A. Gafni, and T. Whelan. 1997. Shared decision-making in the medical encounter: What does it mean? (Or it takes at least two to tango). *Social Science & Medicine* 44(5):681–692.

The Cleveland Clinic. 2022. *Pleural mesothelioma.* https://my.clevelandclinic.org/health/diseases/15044-pleural-mesothelioma (accessed March 10, 2024).

de Nie, I., C. J. M. de Blok, T. M. van der Sluis, E. Barbé, G. L. S. Pigot, C. M. Wiepjes, N. M. Nota, N. M. van Mello, N. E. Valkenburg, J. Huirne, L. J. G. Gooren, R. J. A. van Moorselaar, K. M. A. Dreijerink, and M. den Heijer. 2020. Prostate cancer incidence under androgen deprivation: Nationwide cohort study in trans women receiving hormone treatment. *Journal of Clinical Endocrinology & Metabolism* 105(9):e3293–e3299.

Devlin, E. J., L. A. Denson, and H. S. Whitford. 2017. Cancer treatment side effects: A meta-analysis of the relationship between response expectancies and experience. *Journal of Pain and Symptom Management* 54(2):245–258.e242.

Freedman-Cass, D. A., T. Fischer, A. B. Alpert, J. Obedin-Maliver, P. L. Kunz, W. J. Koh, and R. W. Carlson. 2023. The value and process of inclusion: Using sensitive, respectful, and inclusive language and images in NCCN content. *Journal of the National Comprehensive Cancer Network* 21(5):434–441.

Goodman, M. T., and Y. B. Shvetsov. 2009. Incidence of ovarian, peritoneal, and fallopian tube carcinomas in the United States, 1995–2004. *Cancer Epidemiology, Biomarkers & Prevention* 18(1):132–139.

Gooren, L., and A. Morgentaler. 2014. Prostate cancer incidence in orchidectomised male-to-female transsexual persons treated with oestrogens. *Andrologia* 46(10):1156–1160.

Guellil, A. 2022. Primary peritoneal high-grade serous carcinoma in a man: A case report. *Annals of Medicine and Surgery* 77:e103605.

Herriges, M. J., R. Pinkhasov, K. Lehavot, O. Shapiro, J. M. Jacob, T. Sanford, N. Liu, G. Bratslavsky, and H. Goldberg. 2021. The association between sexual orientation and screening of prevalent gender-specific cancers. *Journal of Clinical Oncology* 39(Suppl 6):198–198.

Jackson, S. S., X. Han, Z. Mao, L. Nogueira, G. Suneja, A. Jemal, and M. S. Shiels. 2021. Cancer stage, treatment, and survival among transgender patients in the United States. *Journal of the National Cancer Institute* 113(9):1221–1227.

Kane, H. L., M. T. Halpern, L. B. Squiers, K. A. Treiman, and L. A. McCormack. 2014. Implementing and evaluating shared decision making in oncology practice. *CA: A Cancer Journal for Clinicians* 64(6):377–388.

Kindler, H. L., N. Ismaila, S. G. Armato 3rd, R. Bueno, M. Hesdorffer, T. Jahan, C. M. Jones, M. Miettinen, H. Pass, A. Rimner, V. Rusch, D. Sterman, A. Thomas, and R. Hassan. 2018. Treatment of malignant pleural mesothelioma: American Society of Clinical Oncology clinical practice guideline. *Journal of Clinical Oncology* 36(13):1343–1373.

Ma, S. J., O. T. Oladeru, K. Wang, K. Attwood, A. K. Singh, D. A. Haas-Kogan, and P. M. Neira. 2021. Prostate cancer screening patterns among sexual and gender minority individuals. *European Urology* 79(5):588–592.

McFarlane, T., J. D. Zajac, and A. S. Cheung. 2018. Gender-affirming hormone therapy and the risk of sex hormone-dependent tumours in transgender individuals: A systematic review. *Clinical Endocrinology* 89(6):700–711.

Mirza, S. A., and Rooney, C. 2018. *Discrimination prevents LGBTQ people from accessing health care*. https://www.americanprogress.org/article/discrimination-prevents-lgbtq-people-accessing-health-care (accessed December 12, 2023).

NCI (National Cancer Institute). n.d. *Side effects of cancer treatment*. https://www.cancer.gov/about-cancer/treatment/side-effects (accessed January 24, 2024).

Nik-Ahd, F., A. De Hoedt, C. Butler, J. T. Anger, P. R. Carroll, M. R. Cooperberg, and S. J. Freedland. 2023. Prostate cancer in transgender women in the Veterans Affairs health system, 2000–2022. *Journal of the American Medical Association* 329(21):1877–1879.

Oladeru, O. T., S. J. Ma, J. A. Miccio, K. Wang, K. Attwood, A. K. Singh, D. A. Haas-Kogan, and P. M. Neira. 2022. Breast and cervical cancer screening disparities in transgender people. *American Journal of Clinical Oncology* 45(3):116–121.

Peitzmeier, S. M., K. Khullar, S. L. Reisner, and J. Potter. 2014a. Pap test use is lower among female-to-male patients than non-transgender women. *American Journal of Preventive Medicine* 47(6):808–812.

Peitzmeier, S. M., S. L. Reisner, P. Harigopal, and J. Potter. 2014b. Female-to-male patients have high prevalence of unsatisfactory Paps compared to non-transgender females: Implications for cervical cancer screening. *Journal of General Internal Medicine* 29(5):778–784.

Perkins, R. B., R. S. Guido, P. E. Castle, D. Chelmow, M. H. Einstein, F. Garcia, W. K. Huh, J. J. Kim, A. B. Moscicki, R. Nayar, M. Saraiya, G. F. Sawaya, N. Wentzensen, M. Schiffman, and the ASCCP Risk-Based Management Consensus Guidelines Committee. 2020. 2019 ASCCP risk-based management consensus guidelines for abnormal cervical cancer screening tests and cancer precursors. *Journal of Lower Genital Tract Disease* 24(2):102–131.

Sachdeva, I., S. Aithal, W. Yu, P. Toor, and J. C. H. Tan. 2021. The disparities faced by the LGBTQ+ community in times of COVID-19. *Psychiatry Research* 297:e113725.

Siegel, R. L., A. N. Giaquinto, and A. Jemal. 2024. Cancer statistics, 2024. *CA: A Cancer Journal for Clinicians* 74(1):12–49.

SSA (Social Security Administration). n.d. *13.00 Cancer—Adult.* Disability Evaluation Under Social Security. https://www.ssa.gov/disability/professionals/bluebook/13.00-NeoplasticDiseases-Malignant-Adult.htm (accessed March 10, 2024).

Stein, K. D., K. L. Syrjala, and M. A. Andrykowski. 2008. Physical and psychological long-term and late effects of cancer. *Cancer* 112(Suppl 11):2577–2592.

Tabaac, A. R., M. E. Sutter, C. S. J. Wall, and K. E. Baker. 2018. Gender identity disparities in cancer screening behaviors. *American Journal of Preventive Medicine* 54(3):385–393.

Unger, J. M., R. Vaidya, K. S. Albain, M. LeBlanc, L. M. Minasian, C. C. Gotay, N. L. Henry, M. J. Fisch, S. M. Lee, C. D. Blanke, and D. L. Hershman. 2022. Sex differences in risk of severe adverse events in patients receiving immunotherapy, targeted therapy, or chemotherapy in cancer clinical trials. *Journal of Clinical Oncology* 40(13):1474–1486.

Wei, J. T., D. Barocas, S. Carlsson, F. Coakley, S. Eggener, R. Etzioni, S. W. Fine, M. Han, S. K. Kim, E. Kirkby, B. R. Konety, M. Miner, K. Moses, M. G. Nissenberg, P. A. Pinto, S. S. Salami, L. Souter, I. M. Thompson, and D. W. Lin. 2023. Early detection of prostate cancer: AUA/SUO guideline Part I: Prostate cancer screening. *Journal of Urology* 210(1):46–53.

12

Considerations for HIV Manifestations Specific to Women

While many people living with human immunodeficiency virus (HIV) lead healthy, active lives, for some, HIV may progress to the point at which their immune system is severely damaged, and they develop one or more opportunistic infections or other serious illnesses that significantly impact their health and ability to work or complete activities of daily living (NIH, 2021a,b). At this advanced stage of disease, individuals with HIV may be eligible for disability benefits from the Social Security Administration (SSA).

SSA's (n.d.) adult disability Listings for HIV (14.11)[1] include several HIV-related impairments or complications of HIV infection that are considered severe enough to hinder a person's ability to engage in substantial gainful activity. Most medical manifestations of HIV are not sex or gender specific. Kaposi sarcoma, for example, presents in all populations with HIV (Sung et al., 2021), and accordingly, SSA does not set any sex-specific criteria for this cancer under 14.11E. However, SSA includes within its HIV evaluation criteria certain gynecological conditions and cancers that are traditionally associated with cisgender women under a category titled "HIV manifestations specific to women" (14.00F7).

This chapter examines HIV among transgender and gender diverse (TGD) people and people with variations in sex traits (VSTs), describes the impact of gender-affirming care on populations with HIV, and assesses SSA's

---

[1] There is a childhood disability Listing for HIV under 114.11, but this chapter does not evaluate SSA's criteria for HIV in children, as it was not within the purview of the statement of task. Chapter 12 examines childhood growth failure, and in that chapter, the committee examines immune suppression and growth failure as caused by HIV infection (Listing 114.11I).

399

criteria for "HIV manifestations specific to women," offering a gender- and sex-inclusive approach to disability determination for people with gynecological conditions related to HIV infection.

HIV PREVALENCE AMONG TRANSGENDER AND GENDER DIVERSE PEOPLE AND PEOPLE WITH VARIATIONS IN SEX TRAITS

Based on the most recent data from the Centers for Disease Control and Prevention (2024b), in 2022 approximately 1.2 million people in the United States were living with HIV. Approximately 38,000 people in the United States acquire HIV annually, and about 2 percent of new HIV diagnoses each year are among transgender people (CDC, 2024a). The burden of HIV among TGD people is disproportionately borne by transgender women. The most recent meta-analysis of laboratory-confirmed HIV among transgender people in the United States found a prevalence of 14.1 percent (95% confidence interval [CI] 8.7–22.2 percent) among transgender women and 3.2 percent (95% CI 1.4–7.1 percent) among transgender men (Becasen et al., 2019). No laboratory-confirmed data are available for individuals with a nonbinary gender identity. This review did not uncover research (beyond a handful of case studies) examining the epidemiology of HIV among people with VSTs, so the burden on HIV in this population is not known.

Engagement in care, adherence to antiretroviral therapy, and viral suppression are key to achieving and maintaining wellness among people living with HIV. Existing data from CDC (2024b) indicate that transgender individuals who are engaged in care achieve rates of viral suppression similar to those of cisgender individuals. However, these data also indicate that transgender people are more likely than cisgender people to miss medical appointments (31 vs. 20 percent) and to miss doses of their antiretroviral medications (65 vs. 38 percent). These differences in care engagement and adherence are driven largely by greater stigma, higher rates of poverty and homelessness, higher rates of depression, and greater unmet ancillary service needs among transgender people living with HIV compared with cisgender counterparts (CDC, 2023). While the literature does not examine HIV care and treatment among people with VSTs, this population also faces stigma and discrimination in their health care in general, and these factors may also impact their HIV management (Jones, 2016; Thyen et al., 2014; Zeeman et al., 2019).

The most recently available nationally representative data indicate that 44.5 percent (95% CI 42.7–46.4 percent) of people with HIV self-reported having a disability. The most frequently reported disabilities were related to mobility (24.8 percent) and cognition (23.9 percent) (Chowdhury et al., 2021). Data were disaggregated by male and female "gender" only, with no indication for sex assigned at birth; therefore, the proportion of TGD people with HIV who experience disability is unknown. The odds of disability were higher among people with lower education, household income below the poverty level, food insecurity, and at least one unmet ancillary service need. Since TGD people with HIV are more likely to experience each of these social determinants of health compared with cisgender people with HIV (Fletcher et al., 2014; Lee et al., 2022; Marcus et al., 2024), it may be reasonable to expect them to have a higher prevalence of disability.

IMPACT OF GENDER-AFFIRMING MEDICAL AND SURGICAL CARE ON HIV

Available data indicate no clinically significant drug–drug interactions between gender-affirming hormone therapy (GAHT) and recommended first-line antiretroviral treatment regimens. However, some antiretroviral medications may have pharmacokinetic interactions with GAHT; therefore, HIV treatment guidelines recommend routine monitoring with appropriate titrations of estradiol, testosterone, or androgen blockers, as needed (HHS, 2023). Despite these guidelines, some TGD people may fear that HIV medications could interfere with their GAHT, causing some to forgo HIV medication in favor of hormone therapy (Braun et al., 2017; Sevelius et al., 2016).

However, there are data to indicate that transgender adults with HIV who receive GAHT are more likely to remain engaged in HIV care and achieve viral suppression on antiretroviral therapy relative to those who do not receive GAHT (Summers et al., 2021). A large study of people with HIV enrolled in Medicaid found that, overall, transgender people with HIV were less likely than cisgender people to experience viral suppression (Rodriguez-Hart et al., 2023). But transgender people who underwent gender-affirming surgery were more likely than cisgender people to achieve viral suppression. Viral suppression rates increased just prior to surgery and remained high for up to 2 years thereafter (Rodriguez-Hart et al., 2023).

Guidelines

The World Professional Association of Transgender Care Standards of Care Version 8 recommend following existing guidelines for HIV prevention and treatment, counseling TGD people that the use of antiretroviral medications is not a contraindication to GAHT, and addressing concerns about potential interactions between antiretroviral medications and hormones (Coleman et al., 2022). The U.S. Department of Health and Human Services (HHS, 2023) Guidelines for the Use of Antiretroviral Agents in Adults and Adolescents with HIV include recommendations regarding transgender people with HIV. These recommendations include antiretroviral therapy for all transgender people with HIV and provision of HIV care within a gender-affirmative model. HHS (2023) recommends pregnancy testing for transgender people with HIV of childbearing potential prior to initiation of antiretroviral therapy. Because some gender-affirming medications have been associated with hyperlipidemia, elevated cardiovascular risk, and osteopenia, HIV treatment guidelines recommend choosing antiretroviral regimens that do not elevate these risks (HHS, 2023).

HIV MANIFESTATIONS SPECIFIC TO WOMEN AND SSA DISABILITY

SSA Listing 14.11I includes a general category for other manifestations of HIV infection that do not meet the criteria for other portions of the HIV Listings. Among the many conditions listed here are "gynecologic conditions," including cervical cancer, pelvic inflammatory disease, and other conditions as described under "HIV manifestations specific to women" (14.00F7). Box 12-1 presents the description under 14.00F7 explaining how SSA documents and evaluates this category.

The gender-specific language in 14.00F7 was included in the SSA disability Listing in 1993 after CDC updated its 1987 case definition for AIDS to include gynecological conditions commonly found among cisgender women with advanced HIV (Castro et al., 1992). More than 20 years later, proposals to remove this gender-specific language were met with resistance because of concern that disability adjudicators might not recognize that certain signs and symptoms were related to HIV infection in women unless they were given specific instructions to take these signs and symptoms into account when making disability determinations (SSA, 2016).

While this concern was certainly not unreasonable, it was flawed by the assumption that only women could manifest conditions such as vulvovaginal candidiasis, pelvic inflammatory disease, and cervical cancer[2] (ACS, 2021; Perkins et al., 2020). Transgender men and gender nonbinary individuals assigned female sex at birth may manifest these conditions, as well as associated symptoms such as chronic pelvic pain. Emerging data indicate that chronic pelvic pain is common among transgender men receiving gender-affirming testosterone. Such symptoms may be exacerbated by gynecological manifestations of HIV (Moulder et al., 2020; Zwickl et al., 2023). While the committee's review did not uncover specific research examining the epidemiology or presentation of HIV among people with VSTs, people with VSTs who do not identify as female could certainly experience these conditions as well. Therefore, limiting adjudicators to considering these conditions only in "women" unfairly excludes people with HIV who have TGD or VST lived experience and may present with the same disabling conditions.

There have been numerous recent efforts across the health care system to update language and criteria using a gender-inclusive approach. For example, as most cervical cancer screening guidelines call for TGD patients to receive

---

[2] Chapter 11 examines various disability listings for reproductive cancers, including cervical cancer.

BOX 12-1
HIV Manifestations Specific to Women Under Listing 14.00F7

14.00F7: HIV infection manifestations specific to women.

   a. General. Most women with severe immunosuppression secondary to HIV infection exhibit the typical opportunistic infections and other conditions, such as PCP, Candida esophagitis, wasting syndrome, cryptococcosis, and toxoplasmosis. However, HIV infection may have different manifestations in women than in men. Adjudicators must carefully scrutinize the medical evidence and be alert to the variety of medical conditions specific to, or common in, women with HIV infection that may affect their ability to function in the workplace.

   b. Additional considerations for evaluating HIV infection in women. Many of these manifestations (for example, vulvovaginal candidiasis or pelvic inflammatory disease) occur in women with or without HIV infection, but can be more severe or resistant to treatment, or occur more frequently in a woman whose immune system is suppressed. Therefore, when evaluating the claim of a woman with HIV infection, it is important to consider gynecologic and other problems specific to women, including any associated symptoms (for example, pelvic pain), in assessing the severity of the impairment and resulting functional limitations. We may evaluate manifestations of HIV infection in women under 14.11H-I, or under the criteria for the appropriate body system (for example, cervical cancer under 13.23[a]).

---

[a] *Chapter 11 of this report describes the SSA disability Listing for cervical cancer.*

NOTE: PCP = pneumocystis pneumonia.
SOURCE: SSA, n.d.

---

the same standard of care as cisgender patients (Perkins et al., 2020), the National Committee for Quality Assurance expanded its Healthcare Effectiveness Data and Information Set quality measure on cervical cancer screening to include TGD people and people with VSTs. Rather than reserving cervical cancer screening for "women," the new measure, effective August 2023, recommends cervical cancer screening for "all people with a cervix" (NCQA, 2023). Likewise, the U.S. Preventive Services Task Force (USPSTF) is currently reviewing recommendations on cervical cancer screening with the aim of adopting gender-neutral language "to communicate that recommendations are inclusive of people of any gender" (Caughey et al., 2021, p. 1953). Populations included in the USPSTF research approach for the recommendation update are "persons who have a cervix" (USPSTF, 2021). Chapter 13 describes other efforts under way to decouple gender from cancer by using organ-specific rather than gender-specific language in screening and treatment recommendations (ACS, 2021; ASCO, 2022; Wei et al., 2023).

These inclusive approaches promote equitable care for TGD people and people with VSTs by recognizing that traditional gender representations in screening and treatment may misidentify patient care needs. SSA could remove boundaries for TGD people and people with VSTs by removing gendered language from its HIV Listings. A suggested way to reword 14.00F7 using inclusive language would be to change the title to "Gynecologic manifestations of HIV" and to remove gender-specific language, as depicted in Box 12-2.

BOX 12-2
An Example of Gender-Inclusive Language
Under Listing 14.00F7

14.00F7: ~~HIV infection manifestations specific to women.~~ ***Gynecologic manifestations of HIV.***

    a.   General. Most ~~women~~ ***people*** with severe immunosuppression secondary to HIV infection exhibit the typical opportunistic infections and other conditions, such as PCP, Candida esophagitis, wasting syndrome, cryptococcosis, and toxoplasmosis. However, HIV infection may have ~~different manifestations in women than in men~~ ***specific gynecological manifestations***. Adjudicators must carefully scrutinize the medical evidence and be alert to the variety of medical conditions specific to, or common in, ~~women~~ ***individuals with reproductive anatomy that includes a vulva, vagina, cervix, and/or uterus*** with HIV infection that may affect their ability to function in the workplace.

    b.   Additional considerations for ~~evaluating HIV infection in women~~ ***gynecological manifestations of HIV***. Many of these manifestations (for example, vulvovaginal candidiasis or pelvic inflammatory disease) occur in ~~women~~ ***people*** with or without HIV infection, but can be more severe or resistant to treatment, or occur more frequently in ~~a woman~~ ***people*** whose immune system is suppressed. Therefore, when evaluating the claim of ~~a woman~~ ***someone*** with HIV infection, it is important to consider gynecologic ~~and other~~ problems ~~specific to women~~, including any associated symptoms (for example, pelvic pain), in assessing the severity of the impairment and resulting functional limitations. We may evaluate ***gynecological*** manifestations of HIV ~~infection in women~~ under 14.11H-I, or under the criteria for the appropriate body system (for example, cervical cancer under 13.23).

SUMMARY OF KEY POINTS

The burden of HIV is high among TGD people but unknown for people with VSTs. Intersecting social factors rooted in stigma and discrimination faced by TGD people and people with VSTs may serve as barriers to engagement in HIV care and adherence to antiretroviral medication. The same social factors are associated with increased odds of disabling conditions among people with HIV. Social programs that aim to support people with HIV need to be cognizant of the needs of TGD people and people with VSTs.

Increasingly, national organizations are moving away from using gendered language that restricts gynecological conditions and cancers to "women." Simple updates to language—for example, changing "women with cervical cancer" to "people with cervical cancer"—serve to include all populations that may have or may be at risk of developing these conditions regardless of sex assigned at birth or gender identity. Using more inclusive language within SSA's HIV disability criteria would reduce some barriers to appropriate disability adjudication for TGD people and people with VSTs.

REFERENCES

ACS (American Cancer Society). 2021. *Cancer care for transgender and gender nonconforming people for health care professionals.* https://www.cancer.org/content/dam/cancer-org/cancer-control/en/booklets-flyers/cancer-care-for-transgender-and-gender-nonconforming-people.pdf (accessed March 15, 2024).

ASCO (American Society of Clinical Oncology). 2022. *Sexual and gender minority (SGM) inclusion in clinical trials.* https://old-prod.asco.org/sites/new-www.asco.org/files/content-files/research-data/documents/2022-ASCO-CENTRA-SGM-Inclusion-Trials.pdf (accessed February 10, 2024).

Becasen, J. S., C. L. Denard, M. M. Mullins, D. H. Higa, and T. A. Sipe. 2019. Estimating the prevalence of HIV and sexual behaviors among the U.S. transgender population: A systematic review and meta-analysis, 2006–2017. *American Journal of Public Health* 109(1):e1–e8.

Braun, H. M., J. Candelario, C. L. Hanlon, E. R. Segura, J. L. Clark, J. S. Currier, and J. E. Lake. 2017. Transgender women living with HIV frequently take antiretroviral therapy and/or feminizing hormone therapy differently than prescribed due to drug-drug interaction concerns. *LGBT Health* 4(5):371–375.

Castro, K. G., J. W. Ward, L. Slutsker, J. W. Buehler, H. W. Jaffe, and R. L. Berkelman. 1992. 1993 Revised classification system for HIV infection and expanded surveillance case definition for AIDS among adolescents and adults. *Morbidity & Mortality Weekly Report: Recommendations & Reports* 41(RR-17):1–19.

Caughey, A. B., A. H. Krist, T. A. Wolff, M. J. Barry, J. T. Henderson, D. K. Owens, K. W. Davidson, M. A. Simon, and C. M. Mangione. 2021. USPSTF approach to addressing sex and gender when making recommendations for clinical preventive services. *Journal of the American Medical Association* 326(19):1953–1961.

CDC (Centers for Disease Control and Prevention). 2023. Behavioral and clinical characteristics of persons with diagnosed HIV infection: Medical monitoring project, United States, 2021 cycle (June 2021–May 2022). *HIV Surveillance Report* 32. https://www.cdc.gov/hiv-data/mmp/behavioral-clinical-characteristics-pwh.html (accessed November 5, 2023).

CDC. 2024a. Diagnoses, deaths, and prevalence of HIV in the United States and 6 territories and freely associated states, 2022. *HIV Surveillance Supplemental Report* 35. https://stacks.cdc.gov/view/cdc/156509 (accessed July 15, 2024).

CDC. 2024b. Monitoring selected national HIV prevention and care objectives by using HIV surveillance data: United States and 6 territories and freely associated states, 2022. *HIV Surveillance Supplemental Report, 2023* 29(2). https://stacks.cdc.gov/view/cdc/156511 (accessed July 15, 2024).

Chowdhury, P. P., L. Beer, F. Shu, J. Fagan, and R. Luke Shouse. 2021. Disability among adults with diagnosed HIV in the United States, 2017. *AIDS Care* 33(12):1611–1615.

Coleman, E., A. E. Radix, W. P. Bouman, G. R. Brown, A. L. C. De Vries, M. B. Deutsch, R. Ettner, L. Fraser, M. Goodman, J. Green, A. B. Hancock, T. W. Johnson, D. H. Karasic, G. A. Knudson, S. F. Leibowitz, H. F. L. Meyer-Bahlburg, S. J. Monstrey, J. Motmans, L. Nahata, T. O. Nieder, S. L. Reisner, C. Richards, L. S. Schechter, V. Tangpricha, A. C. Tishelman, M. A. A. Van Trotsenburg, S. Winter, K. Ducheny, N. J. Adams, T. M. Adrián, L. R. Allen, D. Azul, H. Bagga, K. Başar, D. S. Bathory, J. J. Belinky, D. R. Berg, J. U. Berli, R. O. Bluebond-Langner, M. B. Bouman, M. L. Bowers, P. J. Brassard, J. Byrne, L. Capitán, C. J. Cargill, J. M. Carswell, S. C. Chang, G. Chelvakumar, T. Corneil, K. B. Dalke, G. De Cuypere, E. De Vries, M. Den Heijer, A. H. Devor, C. Dhejne, A. D'Marco, E. K. Edmiston, L. Edwards-Leeper, R. Ehrbar, D. Ehrensaft, J. Eisfeld, E. Elaut, L. Erickson-Schroth, J. L. Feldman, A. D. Fisher, M. M. Garcia, L. Gijs, S. E. Green, B. P. Hall, T. L. D. Hardy, M. S. Irwig, L. A. Jacobs, A. C. Janssen, K. Johnson, D. T. Klink, B. P. C. Kreukels, L. E. Kuper, E. J. Kvach, M. A. Malouf, R. Massey, T. Mazur, C. McLachlan, S. D. Morrison, S. W. Mosser, P. M. Neira, U. Nygren, J. M. Oates, J. Obedin-Maliver, G. Pagkalos, J. Patton, N. Phanuphak, K. Rachlin, T. Reed, G. N. Rider, J. Ristori, S. Robbins-Cherry, S. A. Roberts, K. A. Rodriguez-Wallberg, S. M. Rosenthal, K. Sabir, J. D. Safer, A. I. Scheim, L. J. Seal, T. J. Sehoole, K. Spencer, C. St. Amand, T. D. Steensma, J. F. Strang, G. B. Taylor, K. Tilleman, G. G. T'Sjoen, L. N. Vala, N. M. Van Mello, J. F. Veale, J. A. Vencill, B. Vincent, L. M. Wesp, M. A. West, and J. Arcelus. 2022. Standards of care for the health of transgender and gender diverse people: Version 8. *International Journal of Transgender Health* 23(Suppl 1):S1–S259.

Fletcher J. B., K. A. Kisler, and C. J. Reback. 2014. Housing status and HIV risk behaviors among transgender women in Los Angeles. *Archives of Sexual Behavior* 43(8):1651–1661.

HHS (U.S. Department of Health and Human Services). 2023. *Guidelines for the use of antiretroviral agents in adults and adolescents with HIV: What's new in the guidelines.* https://clinicalinfo.hiv.gov/en/guidelines/hiv-clinical-guidelines-adult-and-adolescent-arv/whats-new (accessed December 13, 2023).

Jones, T. 2016. The needs of students with intersex variations. *Sex Education* 16(6):602–618.

Lee, K., L. Trujillo, E. Olansky, T. Robbins, C. Agnew Brune, E. Morris, T. Finlayson, D. Kanny, and C. Wejnert. 2022. Factors associated with use of HIV prevention and health care among transgender women—seven urban areas, 2019–2020. *Morbidity and Mortality Weekly Report* 71:673–679.

Marcus, R., L. Trujillo, E. Olansky, S. Cha, R. B. Hershow, A. R. Baugher, C. Sionean, and K. Lee. 2024. Transgender women experiencing homelessness—National HIV behavioral surveillance among transgender women, seven urban areas, United States, 2019–2020. *Morbidity and Mortality Weekly Report* 73(Suppl 1):40–50.

Moulder, J. K., J. Carrillo, and E. T. Carey. 2020. Pelvic pain in the transgender man. *Current Obstetrics and Gynecology Reports* 9(3):138–145.

NCQA (National Committee for Quality Assurance). 2023. *Cervical and breast cancer screening: Evidence and guidelines to support inclusive quality measures.* https://www.ncqa.org/wp-content/uploads/Cervical-and-Breast-Cancer-Screening-Evidence-and-Guidelines-to-Support-Inclusive-Quality-Measures.pdf (accessed March 1, 2024).

NIH (National Institutes of Health). 2021a. *HIV and opportunistic infections, coinfections, and conditions.* https://hivinfo.nih.gov/understanding-hiv/fact-sheets/what-opportunistic-infection (accessed July 15, 2024).

NIH. 2021b. *HIV overview: The stages of HIV infection.* https://hivinfo.nih.gov/understanding-hiv/fact-sheets/stages-hiv-infection (accessed July 15, 2024).

Perkins, R. B., R. S. Guido, P. E. Castle, D. Chelmow, M. H. Einstein, F. Garcia, W. K. Huh, J. J. Kim, A. B. Moscicki, R. Nayar, M. Saraiya, G. F. Sawaya, N. Wentzensen, M. Schiffman, and the 2019 ASCCP Risk-Based Management Consensus Guidelines Committee. 2020. 2019 ASCCP Risk-Based Management Consensus Guidelines for abnormal cervical cancer screening tests and cancer precursors. *Journal of Lower Genital Tract Disease* 24(2):102–131.

Rodriguez-Hart, C., G. Zhao, Z. Goldstein, A. Radix, and L. Torian. 2023. An exploratory study to describe transgender people with HIV who accessed Medicaid and their viral suppression over time in New York City, 2013–2017. *Transgender Health* 8(5):429–436.

Sevelius, J. M., J. Keatley, N. Calma, and E. Arnold. 2016. "I am not a man": Trans-specific barriers and facilitators to PrEP acceptability among transgender women. *Global Public Health* 11(7-8):1060–1075.

SSA (Social Security Administration). n.d. *Disability evaluation under social security.* https://www.ssa.gov/disability/professionals/bluebook/14.00-Immune-Adult.htm#14_11 (accessed December 13, 2023).

SSA. 2016. Revised medical criteria for evaluating human immunodeficiency virus (HIV) infection and for evaluating functional limitations in immune system disorders: Final rule. *Federal Register* 81(232):86915–86928.

Summers, N. A., T. T. Huynh, R. C. Dunn, S. L. Cross, and C. J. Fuchs. 2021. Effects of gender-affirming hormone therapy on progression along the HIV care continuum in transgender women. *Open Forum Infectious Diseases* 8(9):ofab404.

Sung, H., J. Ferlay, R. L. Siegel, M. Laversanne, I. Soerjomataram, A. Jemal, and F. Bray. 2021. Global cancer statistics 2020: GLOBOCAN estimates of incidence and mortality worldwide for 36 cancers in 185 countries. *CA: A Cancer Journal for Clinicians* 71(3):209–249.

Thyen, U., A. Lux, M. Jürgensen, O. Hiort, and B. Köhler. 2014. Utilization of health care services and satisfaction with care in adults affected by disorders of sex development (DSD). *Journal of General Internal Medicine* 29(Suppl 3):S752–S759.

USPSTF (U.S. Preventive Services Task Force). 2021. *Cervical cancer: Screening.* https://www.uspreventiveservicestaskforce.org/uspstf/document/draft-research-plan/cervical-cancer-screening-adults-adolescents (accessed December 13, 2023).

Wei, J. T., D. Barocas, S. Carlsson, F. Coakley, S. Eggener, R. Etzioni, S. W. Fine, M. Han, S. K. Kim, E. Kirkby, B. R. Konety, M. Miner, K. Moses, M. G. Nissenberg, P. A. Pinto, S. S. Salami, L. Souter, I. M. Thompson, and D. W. Lin. 2023. Early detection of prostate cancer: AUA/SUO guideline Part I: Prostate cancer screening. *Journal of Urology* 210(1):46–53.

Zeeman, L., N. Sherriff, K. Browne, N. McGlynn, M. Mirandola, L. Gios, R. Davis, J. Sanchez-Lambert, S. Aujean, N. Pinto, F. Farinella, V. Donisi, M. Niedźwiedzka-Stadnik, M. Rosińska, A. Pierson, F. Amaddeo, and H. L. Network. 2019. A review of lesbian, gay, bisexual, trans and intersex (LGBTI) health and healthcare inequalities. *European Journal of Public Health* 29(5):974–980.

Zwickl, S., L. Burchill, A. F. Q. Wong, S. Y. Leemaqz, T. Cook, L. M. Angus, K. Eshin, C. V. Elder, S. R. Grover, J. D. Zajac, and A. S. Cheung. 2023. Pelvic pain in transgender people using testosterone therapy. *LGBT Health* 10(3):179–190.

13

Considerations for Disability Adjudication for Transgender and Gender Diverse Applicants and Applicants with Variations in Sex Traits

This report has presented research on the importance of understanding an individual's gender identity and sex recorded at birth for proper evaluation of function and disability for people who suffer from various respiratory disorders, growth failure, kidney disorders, cancers of the reproductive system, and certain gynecological manifestations of HIV (see Chapters 8–12). In an ideal world, accurate information on a patient's gender identity, sex recorded at birth, and variations in sex traits (VSTs) would be collected, recorded, and updated frequently in medical records. Electronic health record systems have the capacity to collect the patient demographic data that are fundamental to understanding the lived experience of transgender and gender diverse (TGD) patients and patients with VSTs, including the capacity to collect sexual orientation and gender identity (SOGI) data by asking a sequence of questions about a patient's gender identity and sex recorded at birth (the "two-step" gender identity question, described in Chapter 3). Yet there is no guarantee that these data will be included in a given patient's medical record, or if they are, that they will be accurate. As discussed in Chapters 3 and 4, health systems and insurers are improving SOGI data policies and practices, but there remain substantial roadblocks to the collection of these data across the health care system, including a lack of collection or reporting mandates, provider misconceptions about the utility and purpose of SOGI data collection, a lack of appropriate training for providers on the importance of SOGI data for clinical use and patient care, and complex institutional and systemic barriers.

For these reasons, the typical individual applying for Social Security disability benefits is not likely to have SOGI data documented (or documented accurately) in their medical record. This reality has left the experts on this committee concerned about the following question: How will the Social Security Administration (SSA) know when TGD people and people with VSTs have applied for disability benefits?

One answer might be that SSA could use various techniques for identifying TGD applicants and applicants with VSTs by combing the medical records submitted as part of a disability application for other data that might serve to indicate or confirm gender identity or sex recorded at birth. For example, as described in Chapter 3, certain codes from the International Classification of Diseases, 10th revision (ICD-10) indicate a VST diagnosis or are related to care for TGD people; pharmacy data may indicate hormone therapy (e.g., testosterone or estrogen) that could indicate gender-affirming care; and certain keywords in narrative clinical notes might describe those with TGD or VST lived experience. While these data have their own limitations, they can help fill the gaps where patients' SOGI data are missing or incomplete. Therefore, it could be useful for SSA to examine these other data points in the medical records of some applicants for disability benefits.[1]

To implement this approach, however, SSA must first have medical records that contain these data. Consider an applicant with asthma, chronic obstructive pulmonary disease, cystic fibrosis, or other respiratory disorders under SSA's disability Listings.[2] Chapter 8 describes the importance of understanding a patient's gender identity, sex recorded at birth, and history and timing of gender-affirming hormone therapy (GAHT) to aid in clinical decision making around the interpretation of common pulmonary function tests, such as spirometry. Some respiratory health care providers may engage their TGD patients and patients with VSTs in robust discussion about what gender identity and sex recorded at birth may mean for evaluation of lung function. In these circumstances, SOGI data may be recorded in patient data fields, and narrative clinical notes or ICD codes may further describe important patient characteristics and the impact that gender-affirming care or care related to VSTs may have on clinical decision making. In turn, this information may be included in the medical records submitted to SSA as part of a disability application.

On the other hand, when a patient with a respiratory health complaint does not have access to a provider who understands the complexities and nuances of care for TGD people and people with VSTs, clinical notes (or

---

[1] The committee notes that it would not be appropriate or necessary for SSA to conduct a broad search of applicant records (through algorithm-type methods) for the sake of determining TGD/VST status as labeling disability files as "TGD" or VST" is neither respectful of applicants nor beneficial for disability determinations overall. However, on a case-by-case basis, it may still be important for SSA's adjudicators to examine narrative notes or ICD codes, as this information may be helpful for certain disability determinations.

[2] 20 C.F.R. § 404.1525 (2017), Listing of Impairments in Appendix 1; 20 C.F.R. § 416.925 (2017), Listing of Impairments in Appendix 1 of subpart P of Part 404.

other data in the medical record) may contain no information about TGD or VST lived experience. In these circumstances, how is SSA to know that it is adjudicating applications from TGD people or people with VSTs?

Moreover, providers' implicit or explicit biases with regard to these patients may call into question the accuracy of any narrative descriptions related to sex or gender identity (these significant considerations are discussed in Chapter 3). But how is SSA to know from the applicant's medical records where these biases exist, how they may have impacted the care provided, how they may have influenced the accuracy of various tests or measurements of function, and how all these factors may impact disability evaluation?

Perhaps additional medical records would contain pertinent clinical information. For example, suppose the disability applicant with a respiratory disorder also received gender-affirming care from a specialty clinic. If so, are such medical records likely to be submitted to SSA if they do not evaluate the disability at hand (in this case, a respiratory disorder)? How is SSA to know to obtain any such additional medical records if the records submitted to SSA—those that describe the applicant's lung function and related disability—offer no information about gender identity or VSTs?

These are important questions for SSA as it attempts to adjudicate disability accurately for TGD applicants and applicants with VSTs. For the several disability Listings examined in this report, sex and gender identity data in the medical record that are incorrect or incomplete introduce error into SSA's adjudication process by leading to identification of a disability that does not exist or failure to identify a disability that does exist.

The systemic, complicated, and stubborn gaps in SOGI data collection across the U.S. health care system cannot be resolved by SSA alone. However, SSA does have some tools at its disposal with which to address gaps in information for TGD applicants and applicants with VSTs. Chapters 3 and 4 describe how SSA could add SOGI data questions to disability application forms to help fill the gaps that result when health care providers, insurers, and institutions do not collect the patient data that SSA may need to adjudicate appropriately the applications for disability benefits of TGD people and people with VSTs. In addition, SSA can work to ensure the disability adjudication process—from the medical records it gathers, to the guidance it provides adjudicators, to the information it offers to applicants—results in an accurate and complete record that offers SSA the clearest picture of an applicant's disability.

This chapter provides an overview of the various experts involved in disability determinations at different points in the process, their training and qualifications, and the information they gather or provide to support adjudication of disability applications. The chapter examines current SSA policies and opportunities for SSA, within its current structure and authority, to ensure that it obtains the appropriate medical documentation needed to make disability determinations for TGD applicants and applicants with VSTs.

OVERVIEW OF EXPERTS INVOLVED IN DISABILITY DETERMINATION

Throughout the disability determination process, many experts may be involved in examining an applicant's impairment or reviewing an applicant's medical record to help determine whether they meet SSA disability criteria. Table 13-1 outlines the five major categories of experts involved in various stages of the disability determination process.

One avenue for supporting these different experts in adjudicating applications for disability filed by TGD people and people with VSTs is for

TABLE 13-1 Experts Involved in the Social Security Administration's Disability Determination Process

Expert	Description
Disability Examiners (DE)	• During initial disability determination or continuing disability review, the DE gathers all the records needed from the applicant and medical providers, requests additional medical evidence if needed, and prepares the case for review by medical and/or psychological consultants. • The DE works with medical/psychological consultants as part of an adjudicative team to make disability determinations.
Medical Consultants (MC) and Psychological Consultants (PC)	• During initial disability determination or continuing disability review, MCs and/or PCs examine the medical record provided to them by the DE to assess whether an applicant meets the medical criteria for qualifying for disability benefits. • MCs and PCs do not themselves examine the applicant but draw their conclusions from information present in the medical record.
Medical Source Statement from Treating Provider(s)	• The DE may request that the applicant's treating provider(s) write a statement on the applicant's condition for inclusion in the medical record. • The medical source statement describes the applicant's condition, the effects of the condition on the applicant's ability to function, and an explanation of how the assessment is supported by evidence in the medical record.
Consultative Examiners	• During initial disability determination or continuing disability review, the DE or MC/PC may order an additional consultative examination for various reasons—for example, if there is not enough evidence in the applicant's medical records to make a disability determination, or if there is a need to resolve inconsistency in the medical record.
Medical Experts	• When applicants have been denied disability benefits and appeal their case, they have a right to a hearing before an Administrative Law Judge (ALJ). The ALJ may ask a medical expert to review an applicant's case file and provide an impartial medical opinion about whether the applicant's condition meets disability criteria.

SSA to ensure that experts have appropriate training to recognize these applications when they are received, to determine how TGD or VST lived experience may impact various disability applications (if at all), and to know when to obtain or provide additional information to aid in accurate adjudication. Before examining training needs for various experts who contribute to disability determinations, it is first helpful to understand current SSA requirements for training and qualifications. The following sections walk through the basic role of each expert, their required qualifications, and training expectations for participating as experts in the disability determination process.

Disability Examiners

The disability examiner (DE) works with one or more medical and/or psychological consultants as an adjudicative team to make disability determinations.[3] The DE is an employee of the state Disability Determination Services (DDS) office,[4] which supports medical and psychological consultants by gathering all the evidence needed from the applicant and an applicant's medical providers, requesting additional medical evidence if needed, and preparing the case for review.

SSA requires the DE to develop a complete medical history for each applicant for at least a 12-month period prior to the application.[5] SSA (2023a) rules direct DEs to request records from all providers who have treated or evaluated the applicant during this period, except those who treated only ailments "clearly unrelated" to the claimed impairment. DEs request laboratory reports, X-rays, doctors' notes, and other information used in assessing the applicant's health and functional capacity from many types of providers, including physicians or psychologists; hospitals; community health centers; schools (for child applicants); and Department of Veterans Affairs, military, or prison health care facilities.

Training and Qualifications

The DE is a lay person without a medical degree or specialized medical knowledge. SSA does not set specific qualifications for DEs. State DDSs may set additional qualification criteria, such as requiring a bachelor's or master's degree.

---

[3] 20 C.F.R. § 404.1615 (2017).

[4] As with many federal programs, SSA funds state-level entities—including DDS offices—to operate its programs across 54 jurisdictions (50 states plus the District of Columbia, Puerto Rico, Guam, and the Virgin Islands). While DDS offices must adhere to SSA standards and policies, each DDS has leeway to operate individually to meet the needs of applicants in their jurisdiction.

[5] 20 C.F.R. § 404.1512 (2017).

SSA requires that DEs fully understand SSA disability criteria. At the federal level, SSA provides manuals, videos, case adjudication techniques, and other training materials through its Disability Examiner Basic Training Program. Many of these materials are available through the Program Operations Manual System (POMS)—the primary source of information DEs use to process applications for Social Security benefits (SSA, n.d.-a). The public version of the POMS resource is available online and provides a wealth of information about the factors DEs consider when making a disability determination.

While these federal-level resources form the basis of DE training materials, SSA itself does not generally conduct or identify specific training for state DDS offices. SSA regulations give "maximum management flexibility" to the DDS to manage the training and staff development process, and training requirements may vary across DDS offices (SSA, 2002).

Medical Consultants and Psychological Consultants

Physicians and psychologists or psychiatrists—known as medical consultants (MCs) or psychological consultants (PCs), respectively—work with the DE to review medical documentation collected as part of the disability application. State-level DDS offices may employ MCs and PCs internally as staff, may contract with outside consultants (who are often retired), or use a mix of both.

Using the case file prepared by the DE (with all medical records therein), the MC and/or PC follows SSA's five-step sequential evaluation process (described in Chapter 1) to assess whether applicants meet the medical criteria for qualifying for disability benefits.[6] MCs and PCs evaluate the evidence in the medical record; determine whether further medical testing is needed; assess the existence and severity of the applicant's impairment(s); determine whether the applicant's impairment(s) meets or medically equals a disability Listing (or, in the case of child applicants, whether the impairment(s) results in limitations that functionally equal the Listings); and in adult cases, perform a "residual functional capacity" assessment of the impairment.[7]

Training and Qualifications

An MC must be a licensed physician; a PC must be either a licensed psychologist or psychiatrist.[8] If the disability application involves cognitive or mental impairments, SSA rules state that the consultant must be a psychiatrist or psychologist.[9] SSA has no strict rules about which type of physician should

---

[6] 20 C.F.R. § 404.1520 (2012).

[7] "Functional capacity" is the maximum level of physical or mental performance that the applicant can achieve given the functional residual limitations resulting from their medical impairment(s). 20 C.F.R. §§ 416.1016 (2017), 404.1616 (2017).

[8] 20 C.F.R. §§ 416.1016 (2017), 404.1616 (2017), 404.1502(a)(1) (2017), 416.902 (2018).

[9] 20 C.F.R. §§ 416.1016 (2017), 404.1616 (2017).

review adult applications that involve physical impairments, but for children who apply based on physical impairments, SSA will make a reasonable effort to find an MC who is a pediatrician or who specializes in a field of medicine appropriate to the child's impairment(s). Many MCs work in the field of family or internal medicine, but individual DDS offices may employ or contract with physicians in specialty fields. The committee uncovered no statements from DDS offices that they employ or contract with MCs or PCs who have expertise in TGD health or in the health of people with VSTs.

MCs and PCs must fully understand SSA's requirements for disability claims documentation so they can assess the adequacy of medical evidence in relation to SSA regulations and disability Listing criteria. As for DEs, there are numerous federal-level training resources for MCs and PCs, including the POMS (described above). SSA also issues the "Blue Book"— a comprehensive online resource providing health professionals with an understanding of the disability programs administered by SSA (n.d.-b). SSA does not conduct training for MCs and PCs at the state level; each DDS has flexibility to design training programs for MCs and PCs, and training may vary across states.

Medical Source Statement from Treating Provider(s)

As described above, the DE prepares the applicant's case file for review by gathering relevant records related to the applicant's medical history. One important piece of information the DE gathers is a "medical source statement"—an opinion from the applicant's treating provider(s) regarding the nature and severity of the applicant's condition, including how the applicant's condition impacts their functional abilities (e.g., ability to work or engage in substantial gainful activity).[10] Because neither the DE nor the MC or PC examines the patient in person, SSA regards the opinions of treating providers as a prominent source of information in the applicant's record. The applicant's treating sources are often best able to provide a detailed picture of the applicant's medical impairment(s) and "may bring a unique perspective to the medical evidence that cannot be obtained from the objective medical findings alone."[11] So long as the treating providers' opinion in the medical source statement is not inconsistent with other evidence in the record and is well supported by medically acceptable clinical and laboratory diagnostic techniques, SSA regulations require disability examiners to consider the treating providers' opinion along with all other evidence in the file.[12]

---

[10] 20 C.F.R. §§ 404.1513 (2017), 416.913 (2017).

[11] 20 C.F.R. § 416.927(c)(2) (2017).

[12] This paragraph was edited after release of the prepublication report to more accurately describe SSA processes and regulations.

Training and Qualifications

SSA regulations list qualifications for providers submitting a medical source statement (e.g., licensed physicians, licensed psychologists).[13] While treating providers have access to all publicly available SSA training materials (such as the Blue Book and POMS), they are not SSA employees and may not have specific training in understanding how their patient's condition(s) may qualify them for disability benefits.

Consultative Examiners

When the gathered medical evidence in a disability application is insufficient to support a disability determination, DDS offices may order a consultative examination (CE).[14] The need for a CE may arise in several situations; for example, the medical record may be missing important tests or evaluations, or these may have been conducted 6 or more months ago.[15] Also, there may be inconsistency in the medical record, and having an additional examination would help clarify the applicant's case. Ultimately, it is within the discretion of the adjudicator team (consisting of the DE and MC or PC) to order a CE for any given disability applicant.

Training and Qualifications

The experts who perform a CE are independent clinicians who have contracted with the DDS office to perform CEs for a fee. SSA regulations require that consultative examiners be licensed and have the training and expertise necessary to perform the test or examination required.[16] An applicant's own medical source may perform the CE if that provider meets SSA's qualifications; indeed, SSA regulations state a preference for this arrangement because that provider is most familiar with the applicant's condition(s).[17,18] The "Green Book" is an online resource for health professionals who may serve as consultative examiners (SSA, n.d.-c). It explains SSA's disability programs and policies, what to look for in reviewing a case as a consultative examiner, and the essential elements of CE reports.

---

[13] 20 C.F.R. §§ 404.1502(a) (2017), 416.902(a) (2018).

[14] 20 C.F.R. § 404.1519 (2000).

[15] 20 C.F.R. § 404.1519a (2012).

[16] 20 C.F.R. § 404.1519g (2017).

[17] 20 C.F.R. § 404.1519h (2017).

[18] When the DDS is unable to obtain a CE from the applicant's provider, the DDS will select a qualified provider to perform the CE. If the applicant is not satisfied with the selected consultative examiner, SSA rules allow them to object on a number of grounds (including the presence of a language barrier, travel restrictions, or the applicant's previous negative experience with that provider). 20 C.F.R § 404.1519j (2000).

Medical Experts (at Appeals Stage)

If denied benefits after their initial application, applicants may request a reconsideration[19] within 60 days of initial determination; the DDS's DE, MC, and/or PC team (described above) makes the disability determination at the reconsideration stage. If reconsideration again results in a denial of disability benefits, the applicant can appeal for a hearing with an Administrative Law Judge (ALJ). The ALJ may ask an outside medical expert to review the medical record and provide an impartial medical opinion about whether an applicant's impairment(s) meets or medically equals a disability Listing (SSA, 2020). The ALJ will consider the medical expert's opinion when making a ruling.

The medical expert gives an opinion on the applicant's impairment(s) based on the evidence provided in the case record. Unlike the DE, the medical expert does not solicit additional records from providers (e.g., they cannot order a CE or request medical source statements), but they do review any additional information submitted by the applicant in connection with the appeal. For example, the applicant might submit additional medical records that were not part of the original case file. If, after reviewing the applicant's case, the medical expert requires additional information, they may prepare a written list of questions for the ALJ. The ALJ will then decide whether the requested information is pertinent to making a disability determination and if so, how that additional information should be obtained.

Training and Qualifications

Medical experts must understand Social Security disability policies in addition to having relevant medical knowledge of the applicant's health issues. The *Medical Expert Handbook* provides guidelines for medical experts who review disability cases (SSA, 2017). An applicant cannot get their own treating provider to testify on their behalf during the administrative hearing; the medical expert must be someone who meets SSA criteria and is invited to testify by the ALJ.

Summary of Various Experts Involved in the Disability Determination Process

Figure 13-1 shows the major experts described above, where they fall in the various stages of the disability determination process, and what information is compiled in the applicant's case file upon disability determination and upon appeal.

---

[19] SSA policy requires programs and activities to be conducted in a way that does not discriminate on the basis of "race, color, national origin, religion sex (including sexual orientation and gender identity), disability, age, or parental status" (SSA, 2023b, p. 1). There is a process for applicants to file a complaint of discrimination if applicants believe an SSA employee or administrative law judge "acted upon [the] claim based on bias or discrimination instead of the facts of [the] case" (SSA, 2023b, p. 1).

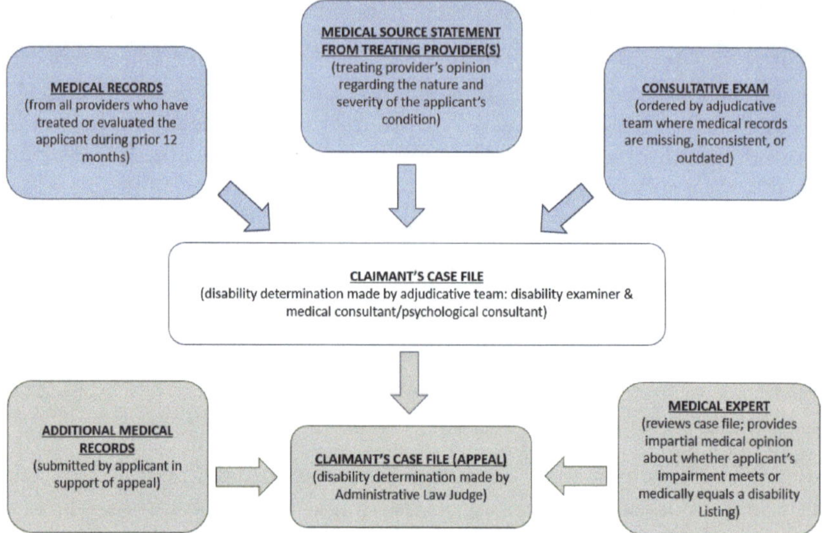

FIGURE 13-1 Diagram of experts involved in disability determinations. SSA also considers evidence from experts in their given fields as well as other nonmedical sources.[20]

GUIDANCE FOR EXPERTS INVOLVED IN DISABILITY DETERMINATIONS

Given the complexities of the disability determination process for some TGD applicants and applicants with VSTs, DEs, MCs, and PCs, as well as other experts, may need training and guidance on how aspects of gender-affirming care or other aspects of health, treatment, and care described in this report impact disability determinations. Areas of training and guidance may include (1) understanding how gender-affirming care and care related to VSTs may impact measurements of function related to various disability Listings; (2) identifying TGD applicants and applicants with VSTs from medical records; (3) knowing when additional medical records may be needed to describe gender-affirming care or care related to VSTs and how this additional information may impact disability adjudication; (4) knowing when an applicant's medical record does not fairly or accurately assess the applicant's condition such that it may be appropriate to order a CE; and (5) understanding biases often present in the medical records of TGD people and people with VSTs and how these biases may have impacted care and treatment received or recorded in the medical record (including in medical source statements by the treating provider).

These are complex issues related to health and disability. As discussed throughout this report, chronic disease among TGD people and people with

---

[20] This note was added after release of the prepublication report to clarify SSA processes.

VSTs has not been well studied, and this committee uncovered few experts with knowledge on these issues. Therefore, it may not be practicable for individual DDS offices to obtain the local expertise needed to guide robust training for DEs, MCs, and PCs on these topics. The following sections offer considerations for where, within the current disability determination process, SSA might be able to offer guidance to adjudicators on these complex issues.

Panelist Perspective

"[I]t's pretty darn near impossible, actually, for adults in most parts of the country to be able to access adult providers who know anything about variations in sex traits. You create the situation in which people are experiencing health disparities and are not able to access care . . . and what we see in the community is those health problems become increasingly disabling over time for people."

*—Statement from patient–provider panel,
presented to the committee on November 30, 2023.*

Training Conducted by Federal-Level SSA
(or Regional Offices) for Complex Issues

While SSA policies give state-level DDS offices flexibility and discretion in conducting staff trainings, SSA rules state:

> SSA will conduct or specify training if: (a) a State agency's performance approaches unacceptable levels; or (b) *the material required for the training is complex or the capacity of the State to deliver the training is in doubt* and uniformity of the training is essential [emphasis added].[21]

The intersection of TGD and VST lived experience with disability is arguably complex, and geographic differences or lack of local expertise may mean that individual DDS offices are not equipped to deliver training on these topics. Therefore, this is an area in which SSA could consider offering federal-level trainings and other resources. This approach would ensure consistency in the training on these issues across the 54 DDS jurisdictions and would support jurisdictions that have limited local-level expertise. Consistent training can also help offset the fact that most MCs and PCs

---

[21] 20 C.F.R. §§ 404.1622 (2012), 416.1022 (2012).

who work to adjudicate disability applications are unlikely to have a specialty (or perhaps, any medical training at all, as described in Chapter 3) in gender-affirming care or in care for people with VSTs. The Veterans Health Administration (VHA) (n.d.), the Sexual and Gender Minority Research Office (n.d.), and the National Center for HIV, Viral Hepatitis, STD, and TB Prevention (CDC, 2024a,b) offer evidence-based trainings and materials that could inform SSA's trainings, along with information provided in this report.

Hotline for Applications Related to TGD Health or the Health of People with VSTs

While training DEs, MCs, and PCs to understand the complex needs of TGD applicants and applicants with VSTs is important, the committee discussed at length how difficult these cases are and the reality that medical data to support decision making for these applicants is not always available. Thus, training may go only so far in improving disability adjudications.

SSA might better support its adjudicators in addressing these challenging questions by creating a hotline for DEs, MCs, and PCs to call when reviewing applications from people who are or may be TGD or who have or may have VSTs. One model worth considering is the National Transgender and Gender Diverse E-Consultation (e-consult) service operated by the VHA (Blosnich et al., 2019). Through the e-consult, VHA providers of any discipline can contact experts in TGD health to obtain a second opinion on appropriate care and treatment. The VHA operates two expert interdisciplinary teams (one located in Minneapolis, Minnesota, and the other in Tucson, Arizona) that receive and review e-consult requests from VHA providers. The e-consult team conducts an extensive and comprehensive chart review and consults the literature on best practices before providing an answer to the VHA provider with recommendations for the patient's care and treatment (Matza and McConnell, 2023). The VHA's e-consult program is meant to promote high-quality care for TGD veterans and increase competence among providers who may not have had specific training in transgender health during their graduate medical school education or other formal training (Matza and McConnell, 2023).

SSA could consider developing a similar national or regional specialty consultation service for the various experts that contribute to disability determinations (for the purposes of this discussion, the committee labels this team of experts the "TGD/VST specialist team"). Where feasible, hiring experts as part of the TGD/VST specialist team who have lived experience as being TGD or having a VST is important. Among other areas, the TGD/VST specialist team might consult on (1) whether there are gaps in the case file (and additional records need to be obtained); (2) whether ordering a CE is appropriate; (3) whether treating providers have assessed the applicant using appropriate criteria; (4) whether and how hormone or other gender-affirming therapy impacts the applicant's case; (5) how best to adjudicate medical records that use both male and female reference ranges for interpreting function[22]; (6) whether the applicant had "good cause" not to follow prescribed treatment (see further discussion below); (7) the extent to which co-occurring conditions need to be considered; and (8) whether stigmatizing language found in medical records signals suboptimal care delivery and the need for additional records or information (such as the opportunity for a CE). Similar to the VHA system, the TGD/VST specialist team would help to equalize access to accurate adjudication, especially in regions where area providers may be less knowledgeable about or accepting of TGD health or the health or persons with VSTs. Treating providers (who prepare medical source statements for the applicant's file), consultative examiners (who provide additional physical exams to help clarify the applicant's case), and medical experts (who review the case file on appeal) might also find it helpful to have a specialist to consult to better understand how questions around TGD and VST health, care, and treatment impact disability evaluation; SSA could consider making the TGD/VST specialist team available to these experts as well.

While the committee sees a system similar to the VHA e-consult system as potentially beneficial for the various experts who support disability adjudication, committee members expressed concern about reducing access for TGD applicants and applicants with VSTs if only one regional or national team can review applications for all of these populations. In many instances, being TGD or having VSTs may have no bearing on the documentation of disability under SSA criteria, and instituting requirements that the TGD/VST specialist team be consulted in every circumstance could introduce artificial problems into the system (e.g., unnecessary delays in applications being processed or the introduction of biases). At the same time, the committee would not want to limit access to the TGD/VST specialist team to only certain applicants (e.g., only those with the health conditions explored in this report), as there could be reasonable questions related to TGD/VST health in connection to other disability Listings. Therefore, SSA might develop guidance for when to consult the TGD/VST specialist team, such as in connection with the specific health conditions discussed in this report or with other aspects of affirming care and its impact on disability and health as discussed in general terms in this report.

---

[22] As discussed in Chapters 8–10, where there are calculations of lung function, kidney function, or growth failure using both male and female reference ranges, SSA adjudicators may best serve TGD applicants who receive gender-affirming hormone therapy by selecting the lowest recorded value to determine presence of disability.

Requirements for Collecting Medical Evidence Related to Gender-Affirming Care and Care for People with VSTs

As described above, DEs, MCs, and PCs have a role in shaping the outcome of disability adjudications because they determine what medical records and other information are to be collected for the case file. The case file forms the fundamental materials available for the medical expert to examine upon appeal as well, so compiling a complete case file from the beginning is important for accurate disability adjudication.

Training and specialty resources (such as a TGD/VST specialist team as suggested above) can support DEs, MCs, and PCs in knowing where and when to obtain additional medical records for TGD applicants and applicants with VSTs. Nonetheless, given the complexity of the issues involved, it may be helpful to have clear standards in place for obtaining such medical records when they are needed to adjudicate a disability application. Clear standards can reduce difficult decision making for adjudicators and ensure that all similarly situated applicants have the same opportunity to have complete medical records in their case file.

In the case of TGD applicants and applicants with VSTs, the adjudicator team makes at least four important decisions that may impact the level of information present in the medical record: (1) whether to obtain medical records beyond 12 months, (2) whether records documenting gender-affirming care or care for VSTs are "related" to the claimed impairment(s), (3) whether specialists involved in gender-affirming care or care for VSTs can be considered "treating providers" for purposes of a medical source statement, and (4) whether to order a CE. Decisions about what medical records to collect may also impact (5) whether medical records show "good cause" for failure to follow prescribed treatment. These issues are discussed in the sections below.

(1) Whether to Obtain Medical Records beyond 12 Months

SSA regulations require that the DE collect medical records for at least a 12-month period prior to the disability application. DEs must use their judgment as to whether information is needed beyond that period, and SSA regulations provide various reasons why obtaining such additional records may be necessary (e.g., to establish severity of condition or symptoms, to determine the date the applicant became unable to work because of their medical condition) (SSA, 2023a).

For purposes of this study, the important question to consider is whether evidence of gender-affirming care or care related to VSTs will be present in medical records for the prior 12-month period. For some applicants, the answer may be yes. But for applicants who received care many years ago, this information may not be present in the most recent medical records, especially if their providers do not take a detailed history or understand the need to ask about gender identity and sex recorded at birth for purposes of clinical decision making.

Suppose, for example, an adult transgender applicant with chronic kidney disease accessed GAHT for many years but stopped this therapy 2 years ago (this could be for any number of reasons—individual preference, change in economic circumstances, change in health insurance, etc.). Would evidence of GAHT from 2 years ago be present in this applicant's medical records if the records cover only the prior 12 months? Suppose the medical records for the past 12 months do not otherwise indicate that the applicant is transgender or mention anything about prior gender-affirming care. How is the DE to know to request any further documentation? If no additional records are requested, the MC and/or PC will not have potentially pertinent information about the applicant (e.g., that GAHT could have impacted kidney function, as described in Chapter 10).

POMS DI 22505.010, Developing Longitudinal Medical Evidence (SSA, 2001), lists certain situations in which medical evidence beyond the standard 12-month period may be required to make a fair and accurate disability finding. SSA might consider including within DI 22505.010 the example of obtaining gender-affirming care records beyond 12 months for TGD applicants and care records related to VST care beyond 12 months for applicants with VSTs.

(2) Whether Records Documenting Gender-Affirming Care or Care for VSTs Are "Related" to the Claimed Impairment

SSA guidance states that the disability examiner need not request records from providers who have treated ailments "clearly unrelated to the impairment(s)" at issue for the disability determination, offering "routine dental records" as an example of a record unrelated to an impairment (SSA, 2023a). This limitation makes sense. SSA does not want to slow down the adjudication process by having the DE pursue unnecessary records that will not be helpful in making a determination about disability.

However, subjectivity is involved here, as the DE makes the judgment call as to whether care provided is "related" to the disability claim at issue. Suppose records from an applicant's treating pulmonologist make no mention of gender-affirming care but state that the applicant removed a chest binder prior to a spirometry test (a test used to assess lung function, as described in Chapter 8). Suppose other medical records, if obtained, would show that the applicant currently accesses GAHT and uses a chest binder daily for 10 or more hours. If the DE does not draw a connection between the pulmonologist's chest binder statement and the possibility of other records describing gender-affirming care, the DE will not have obtained pertinent information about the applicant's lung health, and the case file will not paint a full picture of the applicant's circumstances. Depending on the specifics of the applicant's case, this lack of information could lead to an incorrect disability determination.

There are many scenarios in which the DE might fail to acquire records documenting gender-affirming care, as these records may seem unrelated to the impairment at issue. Therefore, SSA could consider including a statement under POMS DI 22505.006, Requesting Evidence—General (SSA, 2023a), that records related to gender-affirming care and care for VSTs may be related to certain impairments, including those examined in this report. SSA might also consider communicating to disability applicants that medical records related to gender-affirming care and care for VSTs may be relevant to certain disability applications and that it may be appropriate to use the additional "remarks" section on disability applications to describe how TGD or VST lived experience has impacted their health or opportunity to receive appropriate care for their impairment(s). Applicants should always have the choice to submit such records.

(3) Whether Specialists Involved in Gender-Affirming Care or Care for VSTs Can Be Considered "Treating Providers" for Purposes of a Medical Source Statement

The medical source statement from an applicant's treating provider is important in disability determinations.[23] The questions for purposes of this study are: Who is the "treating provider" writing the medical source statement, and what is their knowledge of gender-affirming care or care for VSTs and how this care impacts chronic disease and health?

Suppose a transgender individual applies to SSA based on a claim of disability related to reproductive cancer. Suppose that individual receives cancer treatment from an oncologist but also regularly sees specialists who assist with GAHT. Whom does SSA consider to be the "treating provider"?

It seems likely that the disability examiner would view the oncologist as the "treating provider" because that provider has presumably been heavily involved with cancer treatment decisions and understands various side effects of the treatment or the cancer itself that may be impacting function. A medical source statement from the treating oncologist would therefore be important information to include in the applicant's record.

An argument can be made, however, that the gender-affirming care specialist whom the patient sees regularly is also a "treating provider." Might the endocrinologist (or other specialists involved in gender-affirming

---

[23] This sentence was edited after release of the prepublication report to clarify SSA processes.

care) also have insight into the applicant's ability to work or engage in substantial gainful activity? After all, these providers might better understand co-occurring conditions or other factors that impact the applicant's overall health and are likely to be more attuned to the circumstances the applicant could be facing (e.g., challenges in obtaining appropriate health care that may contribute to poor health). Providers who offer gender-affirming care may also have different insight from that of other treating providers should there be a question as to whether an applicant failed to follow prescribed cancer treatment by continuing with gender-affirming care (see below).

SSA could consider including a statement in POMS DI 24503.005, Categories of Evidence (SSA, 2021), that specialists involved in gender-affirming care or in the care of people with VSTs may serve as acceptable medical sources. SSA might also consider communicating to potential disability applicants that medical source statements from providers engaged in gender-affirming care and care for VSTs may be relevant to certain disability applications. Applicants should always have the choice to submit such records.

Panelist Perspective

"I'm going to need SSDI [Social Security Disability Insurance] and Medicare for the rest of my life. Every month I go to a clinic for an IV infusion that is an immunosuppressant that sustains the life of my kidney. I need all of these medications. I see specialists every year, like it's a lifelong condition. And coming out [as transgender] is also a lifelong experience, and those things sort of happen in tandem."

—Statement from patient–provider panel,
presented to the committee on November 30, 2023.

(4) Whether to Order a Consultative Exam

The committee discussed at length the relative value of a CE in disability adjudications for TGD applicants and applicants with VSTs. Like anybody else, these applicants should have access to the CE where there are gaps in their records (e.g., a spirometry test was not given or was given more than 6 months ago). But suppose the adjudicator team is concerned that the treating provider of a TGD applicant or an applicant with a VST did not issue appropriate tests or that the tests performed were not interpreted correctly, such that the evidence in the medical record may be unreliable. Would ordering a CE be appropriate?

On one hand, the CE is a potentially important tool for correcting inaccurate or missing information in the medical record. As TGD people and people with VSTs face significant challenges in accessing quality health care by providers who are competent to understand their health care needs, the CE could be an opportunity to get things right. For example, as explained in Chapter 8, current guidelines state that spirometry should be interpreted on the basis of sex recorded at birth (Graham et al., 2019; Stanojevic et al., 2022). If the MC reviewing the case file of a transgender male saw that the treating provider had incorrectly used the male reference range rather than female (the applicant's sex recorded at birth), perhaps calling for a new spirometry test via a CE would be appropriate to correct the medical record.

On the other hand, the committee recognizes the challenges here: the science on how TGD and VST lived experience impacts chronic disease, function, and disability is limited, and experts working in these areas do not always agree on the best approach. In the case of spirometry interpretation, some pulmonologists who are accustomed to interpreting spirometry for TGD patients may run spirometry results against both reference sex ranges ("dual calculations") to improve decision making (Fechter-Leggett and Foer, 2023), and it may be appropriate to use affirmed gender, rather than sex recorded at birth, to interpret spirometry for patients who accessed GAHT during puberty (Fechter-Leggett et al., 2022). Here, the case file of a transgender male could show spirometry interpretation using the male reference range rather than the female (the applicant's sex recoded at birth), but this decision could have been made carefully in concert with the patient and with information about the patient's history of gender-affirming care in mind.

It may be difficult for MCs to know by reading medical records whether spirometry results have been interpreted inaccurately, or purposefully and thoughtfully. Therefore, it may be difficult to know when a CE is warranted. Furthermore, if a CE is ordered, is a given DDS office likely to be able to engage a provider who is highly trained to interpret spirometry for TGD people or people with VSTs?

While the above example centers around spirometry, similar scenarios are likely for interpretation of kidney function or growth failure measurements. Certainly, having more information in the case file can be useful, but the committee is wary of policies that might force TGD applicants or applicants with VSTs to submit to additional testing from medical providers, especially where many of these individuals have already faced discrimination in health care settings, and especially when available providers may be no more competent than providers already seen to assess their function.

For these reasons, the committee does not conclude that there is any need to order a CE as a general matter for TGD applicants or applicants with VSTs. In cases where interpreting the medical record is challenging, the

TGD/VST specialist team (discussed above) could provide useful consultation in determining when a CE is appropriate.

On the other hand, the CE could provide an opportunity to run test results/measurements against both reference sex ranges, if appropriate, or to administer appropriate alternative tests that have not been administered previously but could aid in determination of function. For some conditions within the committee's statement of task, the SSA disability Listing criteria include alternative tests. Under the adult Listing for cystic fibrosis (3.04), for example, SSA criteria allow for two different tests to show lung function: spirometry and pulse oximetry (SSA, n.d.-d). Of these, only spirometry includes sex-specific interpretation; questions around sex recorded at birth or gender identity are not relevant for interpretation of a pulse oximetry test. Ordering a CE to obtain a pulse oximetry measurement, therefore, could be appropriate for the applicant and helpful to SSA, as providers administering the CE need not understand the complicated science around the impact of gender-affirming care on lung function to administer and interpret a pulse oximetry test.

(5) Whether Records Show "Good Cause" for Failure to Follow Prescribed Treatment

SSA regulations state that an individual who otherwise meets the requirements for receiving disability benefits will not be entitled to benefits if "the individual fails, without good cause, to follow prescribed treatment that we expect would restore his or her ability to engage in substantial gainful activity" (SSA, 2018, paragraph A).[24] Evidence of "prescribed treatment"[25] must come from the applicant's own medical records; while the MC or PC may have the opinion that certain treatment should have been prescribed, the expectation to follow prescribed treatment applies only to treatment that was actually prescribed, as evidenced by the medical record. The medical source statement from the treating provider may also describe prescribed treatments and clarify whether the applicant followed treatment advice.

If an applicant did not follow prescribed treatment, SSA rules require adjudicators to determine whether the individual had "good cause" for

---

[24] 20 C.F.R. § 404.1530 (2017).

[25] Under the regulations, "prescribed treatment" means "any medication, surgery, therapy, use of durable medical equipment, or use of assistive devices. Prescribed treatment does not include lifestyle modifications (e.g., dieting, exercise, or smoking cessation)" (SSA, 2018, paragraph B, condition 2). If there is evidence in the medical record that an applicant did not follow prescribed treatment, the MC or PC must assess whether the prescribed treatment, if followed, would have restored the individual's ability to engage in substantial gainful activity (thus rendering them ineligible for disability benefits) (SSA, 2018).

not following that treatment. SSA regulations offer several examples of what could be considered good cause, including religious objection to the treatment, inability to afford the treatment, and the treatment's posing a high risk of loss of life or limb. "Medical disagreement" is another acceptable good cause for not following prescribed treatment (SSA, 2018):

> Medical disagreement: When the individual's own medical sources disagree about whether the individual should follow a prescribed treatment, the individual has good cause to not follow the prescribed treatment. Similarly, when an individual chooses to follow one kind of treatment prescribed by one medical source to the simultaneous exclusion of an alternate treatment prescribed by another medical source, the individual has good cause not to follow the alternate treatment. (paragraph C(2)(4))

Panelist Perspective

"I faced dilemmas receiving care because of responses to both my cancer and my transness. Panic at the 'C' word barred me from access to transition-related care. Once they learned I had cancer, some providers suggested discontinuing my hormones without offering any medical justification to explain how this would support my health. One provider told me I needed to start taking antidepressants because I was 'emotional,' and that if I did not, they would stop prescribing my hormone therapy. As a result, I was coerced into taking psychiatric medication I did not want. All of this led me to plead with these providers to understand that my health needs outside of cancer were just as important as those directly related to cancer. Other providers who were familiar and comfortable treating cancer had no idea how to interact with me as a transgender patient. The discomfort and hostility came from not just doctors but also nurses and other health professionals who participated in my care, such as technicians for my MRI and CT [computed tomography] scans. The dehumanizing discrimination I dealt with included having my clothes tugged and being told I was dressing inappropriately for wearing a skirt. Health care systems promote the image of equality without acknowledging that discrimination and unfairness are still rampant, including in oncology. This is especially dangerous for time-sensitive treatment—such as the radiation I needed—and when patients do not have a choice in who controls and facilitates their care, as is often the case with cancer."

—Statement from patient–provider panel,
presented to the committee on December 1, 2023.

> **Panelist Quote**
>
> "One thing that I want to stress is that we all know how serious cancer is, but trans people know how serious dysphoria is. I do not want to have a doctor who isn't patient centered and who believes that one ailment is higher than the other, and that was what I was experiencing. People were telling me that I need to wait. That this wasn't in my best interest, things like that. But internally I was not only battling cancer. I was also battling dysphoria, and not feeling comfortable with myself was one of the huge drivers in my mental health, which is a huge driver in physical health, which you know creates bad outcomes. So, I just need it to be known that dysphoria is equally as important and equally as devastating as any other ailment that somebody else is facing."
>
> *—Statement from patient–provider panel,*
> *presented to the committee on December 1, 2023.*

TGD patients may sometimes be advised to forgo gender-affirming care to improve outcomes for chronic care treatment. For example, an oncologist might advise a patient with cervical cancer to stop receiving GAHT before starting chemotherapy. Likewise, a pulmonologist might advise a patient with cystic fibrosis to cease GAHT or chest binding to improve lung function. Of course, the decision to stop receiving gender-affirming care is not an easy one given the significant benefits this treatment may have for the patient's mental health and well-being (see Chapter 5). Other providers may advocate for the patient to continue with gender-affirming care despite chronic care needs. If one provider thinks a patient should continue GAHT and another thinks they should stop, this situation arguably falls under the "medical disagreement" category for good cause.

SSA could consider including the decision to continue gender-affirming care and treatment as an example of good cause under the POMS DI 23010.011, How to Make a Failure to Follow Prescribed Treatment (FTFPT) Determination (SSA, 2019).[26]

---

[26] The committee notes that in June 2023, SSA (2023d) included "risk of addiction to opioid medication" as a suitable "good cause" for a person with inflammatory bowel disease to refuse to take prescribed narcotic medication to control pain. The need to weigh the benefits of chronic disease management against the risks of substance use can be considered a corollary to the similar need to balance the mental health risks of forgoing gender-affirming care against the benefits of chronic disease treatment.

However, MCs reviewing the case file can find such "medical disagreement" surrounding gender-affirming care in the record only if the DE has first obtained records related to gender-affirming care or asked for a medical source statement from providers of such care. Thus, it is important for DEs to have clear standards for requesting this additional medical information. In addition, it may be appropriate for TGD applicants and applicants with VSTs to use the "remarks" section on disability applications to describe additional factors weighing into a decision to forgo prescribed treatment in support of gender-affirming care (e.g., lack of access to knowledgeable providers or exposure to discriminatory care practices). SSA might consider communicating to disability applicants that such information could be relevant to their application.

SUMMARY OF KEY POINTS

Given the complexities of the disability determination process for some TGD applicants and applicants with VSTs, experts involved in the disability determination process may need guidance. As presented in this chapter, the current structure of the SSA adjudication system provides opportunities to offer such guidance. First, adjudicators may need training on the intersection of TGD/VST lived experience with disability (including the structural disadvantages facing many TGD people and people with VSTs and how these disadvantages may impact disability), and federal- or regional-level trainings on these topics could support DDS jurisdictions that lack local expertise. A hotline similar to the VHA's e-consult might support adjudicators who need consultation when issues concerning TGD health or the health of people with VSTs are complex, and medical records have gaps or inconsistencies. SSA might consider using its authority under 20 Code of Federal Regulations §§ 404.1622 and 416.1022 to deliver trainings and consultative services at the national level in recognition of the complex nature of these issues.

In addition, a statement within POMS that medical records related to gender-affirming care and care for people with VSTs may be relevant for disability evaluation is important for reducing difficult decision making among adjudicators. Inclusion of such a statement would help ensure that all similarly situated applicants have the same opportunity to have complete medical records in their case files. Finally, communicating to potential disability applicants that medical records related to gender-affirming care and care for VSTs may be relevant to their disability application would assist applicants in gathering medical documentation that provides the clearest picture of their health.

The statement of task asks the committee to focus on medical criteria within SSA's Listing of Impairments and, therefore, this chapter focuses on aspects of the disability determination process related to assessing medical impairment under SSA's Listings. As this report has highlighted, assessing disability for TGD people and people with VSTs is not easily done within the rubric of the Listings; this chapter has highlighted how difficult these disability determinations may be and the need for training experts involved in the adjudication process to make fair and accurate determinations where questions of sex and gender identity arise.

The committee notes that whether an applicant meets (or medically equals) the criteria for one of SSA's Listings is only one step in the disability determination process. Chapter 1 (Box 1-1) explains other steps in the process, including assessing an applicant's "residual functional capacity" or the maximum level of physical or mental performance that the applicant can achieve given the functional limitations resulting from their medical impairment(s). In other words, does the adult applicant have the functional capacity to work (perform substantial gainful activity) given their impairment(s)? Does the child applicant's impairment(s) prevent them from functioning at their expected level of development?

These function-related questions can be answered for the individual without making difficult clinical interpretations around sex or gender identity. Certainly, TGD or VST lived experience will factor into the assessment of functional capacity, but the report has not focused on these areas as they are outside of the statement of task and areas of expertise among committee members. However, the complexities raised by sex and gender identity reveal problems with relying heavily on measures of impairment severity as measured by laboratory tests or other evaluations. After all, impairment severity—ability to meet or medically equal criteria under the Listings—may not be a proxy for functional capacity for all applicants. The committee highlights for SSA the importance of evaluating functional capacity for TGD applicants and applicants with VSTs as a critical component of determining disability. The training and guidance mechanisms suggested by the committee in this chapter may apply to these other important aspects of disability determination as well.

REFERENCES

Blosnich, J. R., K. L. Rodriguez, K. L. Hruska, D. Kavalieratos, A. J. Gordon, A. Matza, S. M. Mejia, J. C. Shipherd, and M. R. Kauth. 2019. Utilization of the Veterans Affairs' Transgender e-Consultation Program by health care providers: Mixed-methods study. *JMIR Medical Informatics* 7(1):e11695.
CDC (Centers for Disease Control and Prevention). 2024a. *Issue brief: HIV and transgender communities.* Division of HIV Prevention, National Center for HIV, Viral Hepatitis, STD, and TB Prevention, Centers for Disease Control and Prevention. https://www.cdc.gov/hiv/policies/data/transgender-issue-brief.html#cdc-support (accessed July 16, 2024).

CDC. 2024b. *HIV Nexus: CDC resources for clinicians.* https://www.cdc.gov/hivnexus/hcp/index.html (accessed July 16, 2024).

Fechter-Leggett, E., and D. Foer. 2023. *Selecting appropriate pulmonary function test reference sex for transgender and gender-diverse patients.* Presentation to the National Academies of Science, Engineering and Medicine's Consensus Committee on Sex and Gender Identification and Implications for Disability Evaluation, Washington, DC.

Fechter-Leggett, E., B. R. Ansell, R. Harvey, K. M. Kidd, and D. Weissman. 2022. *Selecting appropriate pulmonary function test reference sex for transgender adults to address health disparities: Methods for data collection and interpretation.* Poster presented at the American Thoracic Society 2022 International Conference, San Francisco, CA.

Graham, B. L., I. Steenbruggen, M. R. Miller, I. Z. Barjaktarevic, B. G. Cooper, G. L. Hall, T. S. Hallstrand, D. A. Kaminsky, K. McCarthy, M. C. McCormack, C. E. Oropez, M. Rosenfeld, S. Stanojevic, M. P. Swanney, and B. R. Thompson. 2019. Standardization of Spirometry 2019 update: An official American Thoracic Society and European Respiratory Society technical statement. *American Journal of Respiratory and Critical Care Medicine* 200(8):e70–e88.

Matza, L., and A. McConnell. 2023. *Gender identity data collection & care decision making within the Veterans' Health Administration.* Presentation to the National Academies of Science, Engineering & Medicine's Consensus Committee on Sex and Gender Identification and Implications for Disability Evaluation, Washington, DC.

Sexual and Gender Minority Research Office. n.d. *Sexual and Gender Minority Research Office homepage.* Bethesda, MD: National Institute of Health, Department of Health and Human Services. https://dpcpsi.nih.gov/sgmro (accessed March 11, 2024).

SSA (Social Security Administration). n.d.-a. *POMS home.* https://secure.ssa.gov/apps10/poms.nsf/Home?readform (accessed March 11, 2024).

SSA. n.d.-b. *Medical/professional relations: Disability evaluation under social security.* https://www.ssa.gov/disability/professionals/bluebook (accessed March 12, 2024).

SSA. n.d.-c. *Consultative examinations: A guide for health professionals.* https://www.ssa.gov/disability/professionals/greenbook/ce-general.htm (accessed March 12, 2024).

SSA. n.d.-d. *3.00 Respiratory disorders—adult: 3.04 Cystic fibrosis.* https://www.ssa.gov/disability/professionals/bluebook/3.00-Respiratory-Adult.htm#3_04 (accessed March 12, 2024).

SSA. 2001. *DI 22505.010: Developing longitudinal medical evidence.* https://secure.ssa.gov/poms.nsf/lnx/0422505010 (accessed March 12, 2024).

SSA. 2002. *DI 39521.100: Training and staff development—general.* https://secure.ssa.gov/poms.nsf/lnx/0439521100 (accessed March 12, 2024).

SSA. 2017. *Medical expert handbook.* Baltimore, MD: Office of Hearings Operations. https://www.ssa.gov/appeals/public_experts/Medical_Experts_(ME)_Handbook-508.pdf (accessed March 12, 2024).

SSA. 2018. SSR 18-3p: Titles II and XVI: Failure to follow prescribed treatment. Policy interpretation ruling. *Federal Register* 83(191):49616. https://www.ssa.gov/OP_Home/rulings/di/02/SSR2018-03-di-02.html (accessed July 9, 2024).

SSA. 2019. *DI 23010.011: How to make a failure to follow prescribed treatment (FTFPT) determination.* https://secure.ssa.gov/poms.NSF/lnx/0423010011 (accessed March 12, 2024).

SSA. 2020. *I-2-5-34: When to obtain medical expert opinion.* https://www.ssa.gov/OP_Home/hallex/I-02/I-2-5-34.html (accessed March 12, 2024).

SSA. 2021. *DI 24503.005: Categories of evidence.* https://secure.ssa.gov/poms.nsf/lnx/0424503005 (accessed March 12, 2024).

SSA. 2023a. *DI 22505.006: Requesting evidence—general.* https://secure.ssa.gov/poms.nsf/lnx/0422505006 (accessed March 12, 2024).

SSA. 2023b. *Civil rights complaint form for allegations of program discrimination by the Social Security Administration; SSA-437-BK.* https://www.ssa.gov/forms/ssa-437.pdf (accessed May 15, 2024).

SSA. 2023d. Revised medical criteria for evaluating digestive disorders and skin disorders. *Federal Register* 88(110):37704–37731. https://www.govinfo.gov/content/pkg/FR-2023-06-08/pdf/2023-11771.pdf (accessed July 9, 2024).

Stanojevic, S., D. A. Kaminksy, M. R. Miller, B. Thompson, A. Alivert, I. Barjaktarevic, B. G. Cooper, B. Culver, E. Derom, G. L. Hall, T. S. Hallstrand, J. D. Leuppi, N. MacIntyre, M. McCormack, M. Rosenfeld, and E. R. Swenson. 2022. ERS/ATS technical standard on interpretive strategies for routine lung function tests. *European Respiratory Journal* 60(1):e2101499.

VHA (Veterans Health Administration). n.d. *VHA LGBTQ+ health trainings*. Washington, DC: Department of Veterans Affairs. https://www.patientcare.va.gov/LGBT/LGBT_Veteran_Training.asp (accessed March 12, 2024).

14

Overall Conclusions

This chapter presents thirteen overall conclusions derived by the committee from evidence presented throughout the report, along with narrative summaries of evidence supporting these conclusions. Each chapter (Chapters 2–13) ends with a summary of key points based on the evidence presented in that chapter. The overall conclusions presented in this chapter cut across those previous chapters and reflect the committee's assessment of the full body of evidence as it relates to the Social Security Administration's (SSA's) disability determinations. The committee formulated thirteen overall conclusions in seven categories: (1) collection of data on sex and gender identity, (2) variability of documentation for transgender and gender diverse (TGD) people and people with variations in sex traits (VSTs) in medical records, (3) Listings with sex-specific diagnostic criteria, (4) chest binders and considerations for pulmonary function tests, (5) alternative growth failure measurements, (6) inclusive language in Listings, and (7) guidance for adjudicators on assessing disability for TGD applicants and applicants with VSTs. In accordance with its statement of task, the committee offers conclusions but not recommendations.

Conclusions presented below are based on best available data. The committee acknowledges that clinical decisions need to be made—and are being made—even when evolving scientific data are limited, and that SSA needs a reasonable approach for adjudicating claims for TGD applicants and applicants with VSTs. The conclusions presented here represent the consensus of committee experts based on their clinical expertise and professional judgment.

Collection of Data on Sex and Gender Identity

Recent advances in electronic health records and health information technology provide opportunities to increase the visibility of TGD patients and patients with VSTs through the routine collection of sexual orientation and gender identity (SOGI) data. SOGI data collection—which allows for health care providers and patients to record sexual orientation, gender identity, sex recorded at birth, information about VSTs, and similar information within individual patient charts—is a key strategy for reducing the many health disparities faced by TGD people and people with VSTs. For TGD patients and patients with VSTs, robust SOGI data collection can enhance meaningful dialogue during clinical encounters, promote appropriate preventive screenings based on anatomy, reduce unequal and discriminatory health care practices, and foster respectful and patient-centered long-term care. Furthermore, comprehensive SOGI data collection enables accurate interpretation of common sex-specific measurements that are important for disability evaluations. Yet despite the importance of collecting these data and the capacity for medical records to facilitate that process, SOGI data collection and documentation by health care providers remains highly variable. Medical records therefore cannot be relied upon to capture accurately all patients with TGD or VST identity or lived experience.

Conclusion 1. Medical records alone may fail to identify the gender diversity of TGD applicants or appropriately capture biological characteristics relevant to applicants with VSTs. SSA application forms do not ask applicants about gender identity or sex recorded at birth. Because these patient characteristics matter for disability determination, the committee concludes giving applicants the option to enter their own gender identity and sex recorded at birth information when submitting a disability application would enable a more accurate assessment.

This approach would help fill the gaps that result when health care providers and institutions do not collect the patient data that SSA may need to adjudicate accurately the applications for disability benefits of TGD people and people with VSTs. Best practices include allowing people to enter gender identity separately from sex recorded at birth, offering a range of appropriate response options and providing a free-text response option, such as "I use something else." It is also important to include either separate questions about VSTs or free-text options that allow people with VSTs to share their individual experience. SSA forms give prompts to applicants to "explain in remarks" additional details about various questions on the application (e.g., citizenship status, military service), and similar prompts could be appropriate for applicants to describe additional information related to gender identity or sex recorded at birth. SSA might also benefit from including such optional questions in its National Beneficiary Survey to help it better understand the lived experience of those people it serves who are TGD or have VSTs. It is important to provide information to applicants and survey respondents on why these questions are being asked and how these data may impact disability determinations. In addition, best practices call upon health care providers and institutions to consistently refer to patients by their correct name (i.e., their chosen and presently used name) and pronouns in all records. SSA could conduct a review of its processes to ensure they meet this standard.

Variability of Documentation for Transgender and Gender Diverse People and People with Variations in Sex Traits in Medical Records

Gender-affirming care comprises an array of services for TGD people that may include medical, surgical, mental health, and nonmedical care. There is no "one size fits all" approach to gender-affirming care: health care services provided to TGD people may differ based on when the care was provided (both historically and across the lifespan), differences in access to care, and tailoring of care to the needs of individual patients. Likewise, appropriate care and treatment for people with VSTs is highly variable and condition and patient specific. Medical records specific to care for chronic conditions may not fully describe gender-affirming care or care related to VSTs. In addition, some TGD people and people with VSTs do not seek or are not able to access medical intervention, so one should not assume that TGD or VST identity or lived experience confers any particular type or amount of care.

Conclusion 2. There is considerable observed variability in gender-affirming care across the country for TGD people. This variability may impact documentation in medical records submitted to SSA for disability applications. The committee concludes that SSA would best serve TGD applicants by communicating to them that medical records related to gender-affirming care are likely relevant to certain disability determinations.

Having a sufficiently complete medical record of gender-affirming care is important for disability evaluations, as understanding the nature of any such care (along with its timing and duration) may be important to improve understanding of functional assessment and eligibility for disability benefits.

Conclusion 3. Individuals with VSTs are a heterogeneous group that includes persons with genetic, anatomical, and hormonal variations and/or variations in genitourinary system development affecting the genitourinary tract and reproduction system. The diverse VST diagnoses may differ as to the extent and type of impact they have on chronic disease and disability. Hence, care and treatment for these diagnoses is variable and patient specific, and medical records that merely list a VST diagnosis may fail to provide sufficient historical information for evaluating the need for disability benefits. The committee concludes that SSA would best serve applicants with VSTs by communicating to them that medical records related to VST care may be relevant to disability applications and their submission is greatly encouraged whenever possible.

Some people with VSTs experience lifelong and ongoing disability, whereas others experience sporadic severe health crises (e.g., experiencing sudden needs for lengthy hospitalization followed by periods of stability) or mental health and/or neurodiversity disabilities associated with VST-related stressors. To provide thorough disability adjudication, SSA needs to have medical records that sufficiently document care related to the management of VSTs. Given that a VST diagnosis is often made during early childhood and adolescence, records from many years ago may be relevant to the adjudication process; however, the committee acknowledges that old records may be very difficult to obtain, and an undue burden should not be placed on applicants to locate such records.

Listings with Sex-Specific Diagnostic Criteria

Listings for respiratory disease, childhood growth failure, and chronic kidney disease include sex-specific diagnostic criteria. Clinicians interpreting tests and measurements for these conditions must select an appropriate reference sex—male or female—to predict lung function, growth failure, or kidney function, respectively. For many applicants for disability benefits, sex recorded at birth is the appropriate reference sex. However, selecting the reference sex for TGD people or people with VSTs is often difficult, and it is not always clear which sex is the most appropriate to use.

Errors in the selection of reference sex may happen for a number of reasons, including incorrect sex recorded in the patient chart (especially when the medical record does not ask for gender identity separately from sex recorded at birth), failure to ask patients about VSTs, failure to ask patients about relevant gender-affirming care (e.g., timing of any hormone therapy), biases held by providers that negatively influence patient care, and the absence of guidelines for interpreting relevant tests and measurements for TGD patients and patients with VSTs. Moreover, even when medical records contain a complete and accurate accounting of patient sex and gender identity characteristics such that providers are aware they are assessing TGD patients or patients with VSTs, providers may lack training and experience in caring for these patients and may not know how or when TGD or VST lived experience impacts patient care and clinical decision making. Thus, providers may have to make difficult or arbitrary judgment calls about which reference sex is most appropriate for a given patient at a given time.

Gender-affirming hormone therapy (GAHT) further complicates this picture. In the case of pulmonary function, some research suggests that "hormonal sex at puberty"—the hormone that was predominant during puberty (estrogen or testosterone) and that influenced the shape and size of the thoracic cavity—may be a more accurate metric for choosing a reference sex for a pulmonary function test for individuals who initiated pubertal delay and began GAHT during puberty. For this portion of the population, affirmed gender—not sex recorded at birth—may be the more appropriate reference sex for this test. Similarly, some researchers propose, for the purposes of calculating body mass index (BMI), continuing to use the growth chart corresponding to sex recorded at birth during pubertal delay but switching to the affirmed-sex growth chart once GAHT has been initiated. In the case of assessing chronic kidney disease, the receipt of GAHT at any time (not just during puberty) is an important consideration for assessing kidney function, but conclusions cannot be drawn regarding the accuracy of either the male or female gender-based estimating equations for estimated glomerular filtration rate (eGFR) in populations receiving GAHT. To aid in clinical decision making for patients receiving GAHT, it may be appropriate for providers to interpret lung function, adolescent growth, and kidney function in comparison with both reference sex ranges ("dual calculations") or use measurements that are independent of sex, when available. However, these approaches to patient care have yet to be prospectively validated for clinical use. Where people with VSTs take GAHT, the above approaches may be appropriate, however, research is limited on the impact of GAHT in populations with VSTs. The committee notes that people with VSTs take hormone therapy for a multitude of reasons beyond gender-affirming care and care is extremely individualized; the impact of various hormone therapies on sex-specific measurements is unknown.

Conclusion 4. Sex recorded at birth may be the appropriate reference sex to use for some—but not all—TGD applicants and applicants with VSTs who apply for disability benefits by submitting medical records with sex-specific measurements of pulmonary function (i.e., spirometry and diffusion capacity of the lungs for carbon monoxide [DLCO] measurements), growth failure (i.e., weight-for-length and BMI-for-age measurements), or kidney function (i.e., estimated glomerular filtration rate [eGFR]). However, SSA's disability criteria use the term "gender" in reference to pulmonary function and growth failure measurements, which may incorrectly indicate that "gender identity" is the determining factor in the interpretation of these measurements.

SSA might consider changing the language in the respiratory disorder Listings[1] and Listings related to childhood growth failure[2] to replace the word "gender" with "sex recorded at birth." Making this change would allow for clearer assessments for some TGD applicants and some applicants with VSTs. Using the phrase "sex recorded at birth" rather than simply "sex" clarifies that sex as recorded at birth is the important patient characteristic for these specific assessments, not "sex" as may be recorded on other administrative records (e.g., driver's license, passport). The current SSA Listings for chronic kidney disease[3] do not use gender- or sex-specific language, and language changes are not necessary. The committee stresses that even though sex recorded at birth is important for the assessments listed here, this does not negate the importance of gender identity for disability applicants in general or for other types of disability assessments. In addition, the committee acknowledges that for some people with VSTs, sex assignment at birth (which becomes the sex recorded on birth certificates and medical records) may not be straightforward and can change after the initial determination.

> *Conclusion 5. Sex recorded at birth may <u>not</u> be the appropriate reference sex for assessing pulmonary function or growth failure for some TGD people or people with VSTs, particularly for those who began pubertal delay and GAHT during puberty. While considerable research is needed to determine best approaches, the committee concludes that SSA would best serve applicants who receive GAHT by using the lowest value recorded (e.g., lower percentile for BMI-for-age and weight-for-length/lower spirometry or DLCO reading) to determine the presence of disability.*

Some providers use "dual calculations" (e.g., interpreting spirometry using both male and female reference ranges) to enhance decision making for patients receiving GAHT, but use of this approach is not universal, and most assessments are likely to use whatever sex is listed in the medical record (even if this information is inaccurate). Medical records may also contain calculations from both charts because providers were mistaken or lacked training on which chart to use. Given these challenges, the committee concludes that when a disability applicant's medical record contains

---

[1] Listing of Impairments 3.02, 3.03, 3.04, 103.02, and 103.04.

[2] Listing of Impairments 105.08B, as applied across 100.05, 103.06, 104.02, 105.08, 106.08, and 114.11(I).

[3] Listing of Impairments 6.05A3 and 106.05C.

calculations from both reference ranges, SSA will best serve applicants who receive GAHT by using the *lowest recorded value* to determine disability under respiratory and childhood growth failure Listings.

> *Conclusion 6. Medical records submitted to SSA may provide an inaccurate estimation of kidney function in people who receive GAHT. The committee concludes that where medical records contain GFR measurements based on both the male and female coefficients, SSA would best serve applicants who receive GAHT by using measured GFR (when available) or the lowest eGFR value recorded to determine the presence of disability.*

Comprehensive data are lacking regarding the bias introduced by using binary sex coefficients in eGFR calculations for TGD people and people with VSTs, and clear conclusions cannot be drawn regarding the accuracy of either the male or female sex-based estimating equations for eGFR in populations receiving GAHT. Until further research clarifies the influence of GAHT on biomarkers that are important for calculating eGFR and determining kidney function, existing eGFR measurements for people who receive GAHT may be inaccurate and may overestimate kidney function. Given these challenges, SSA might consider using the *lowest eGFR value recorded* in the medical record for applicants receiving GAHT to determine disability under chronic kidney disease Listings.

> *Conclusion 7. In order to improve access to an accurate interpretation of pulmonary function, kidney function, or growth percentile, SSA may offer a consultative exam to TGD applicants and applicants with VSTs where SSA sees evidence in the medical record that measurements were or may have been calculated using an incorrect reference sex or where dual calculations were not provided but may be appropriate.*

In such cases, it may be beneficial, where clinically appropriate, to order a test that does not contain sex-specific criteria (e.g., pulse oximetry for evaluation of cystic fibrosis) or that offers more precise measurement of function (e.g., measured GFR to assess kidney function). Where more specific tests are not available or clinically appropriate, SSA could instruct the consultative examiner to interpret results using both male and female reference ranges. This approach would ensure fairness for TGD people and people with VSTs who have lacked access to providers trained to interpret their results thoughtfully and with specific consideration of individual patient histories (e.g., duration and timing of GAHT). It is essential that individual applicants always have the choice of whether to submit to a consultative examination without any detriment to their application if declined.

Chest Binders and Considerations for Pulmonary Function Tests

Chest binders are a common gender-affirming practice for transgender men and other TGD individuals. Some people with VSTs also use chest binders. Chest binding is not merely an elective activity to enhance appearance, but an essential daily practice for reducing chest dysphoria (i.e., distress from unwanted breast development) and improving mental health outcomes. While minimal research exists on the impact of chest binders on pulmonary function, some patients may wear a chest binder during administration of a pulmonary function test (PFT). The committee strongly believes providers should not require TGD people to remove chest binders prior to undergoing a PFT.

Conclusion 8. Evidence that an individual applying for disability benefits wore a chest binder during a PFT should not disadvantage their application.

As many people who bind do so daily and for extended periods of time (often exceeding 10 hours each day), SSA needs to be aware that when a chest binder has been removed for the purposes of undergoing a PFT, that measurement of lung function may not reflect daily lived experience. The medical record may not indicate whether a chest binder was worn during a PFT, but when the medical record contains different PFT values, SSA needs to be aware that those differences could be attributable to the fact that the patient wore a binder during one test but not another. For this reason, the committee concludes that SSA would best serve TGD applicants and applicants with VSTs by using the lowest recorded PFT value to determine disability under respiratory disorder Listings.

Alternative Growth Failure Measurements

Literature and guidelines call for the use of alternative measures of body composition along with BMI-for-age, given concerns about the utility and accuracy of BMI-for-age as the sole measure. BMI-for-age may be an especially poor measure for identifying growth failure in children, as it is not considered a reliable indicator for children below the third percentile of weight. In addition, because BMI does not differentiate between lean body mass and body fat, it may not adequately measure elements of body composition that matter for children who are experiencing growth failure related to underlying chronic disease.

Conclusion 9. Studies clearly show that for many children, BMI is a suboptimal measure for identifying growth failure. BMI can be particularly inaccurate in identifying growth failure in TGD adolescents receiving GAHT, which may affect linear growth and fat distribution.

In these adolescents, linear growth velocity may be a better indicator of growth failure. Similarly, a large-percentage weight loss strongly indicates malnutrition that places an individual at very high risk for growth failure. SSA might consider including alternative measures across various childhood growth failure Listings, as well as changing the window of time during which measurements must be taken. This approach might provide for more accurate assessment of not just TGD youth but all pediatric populations applying for disability benefits.

Inclusive Language in Listings

Increasingly, national organizations are moving away from using gendered language that restricts cancers and gynecological conditions to one's gender or sex recorded at birth. Simple updates to language—for example, changing "women with cervical cancer" to "people with cervical cancer"—serve to include all populations that may have or may be at risk of developing these conditions, regardless of gender identity or sex recorded at birth.

Conclusion 10: National organizations, such as the American Cancer Society and the American Society of Clinical Oncology, have begun to call for a more gender-inclusive approach to cancer screening, treatment, and care, whereby cancer terms reflect the organ in which they arise instead of being tied to gender. SSA might best serve disability applicants by removing gendered language from its cancer Listings.

The current SSA Listings for cancers of the prostate gland, testicles, and penis[4] exemplify this approach and are consistent with how the field is shifting toward inclusiveness in cancer language. SSA might consider changing the Listing for "Cancers of the female genital tract"[5] to "Cancers of the uterus, uterine cervix, vulva, vagina, fallopian tubes, and ovaries," which would align this Listing with organs rather than gender. Such a change would clarify that this Listing can apply to anyone who can meet the SSA criteria, regardless of their sex recorded at birth or gender identity. Similarly, SSA might consider removing the differentiation of women versus men within criteria under primary peritoneal carcinoma[6] and instead base

---

[4] Listing of Impairments 13.24, 13.25, and 13.26.
[5] Listing of Impairments 13.23.
[6] Listing of Impairments 13.00K7.

this condition on the histopathology. This approach recognizes that primary peritoneal mesothelioma can occur in all people regardless of the presence or absence of ovaries, while primary peritoneal adenocarcinoma is almost exclusively diagnosed in people born with ovaries.

> *Conclusion 11. Using more inclusive language in Listings would help achieve appropriate disability adjudication for TGD people and people with VSTs living with HIV. The committee concludes that SSA might best serve applicants with HIV by removing sex-specific language from its HIV disability criteria.*

SSA might consider changing the Listing category from "HIV infection manifestations specific to women"[7] to "Gynecologic manifestations of HIV," to make this Listing inclusive of and appropriate for all people with HIV who exhibit these medical conditions. Such an inclusive approach promotes equitable care by recognizing that gendered representations in HIV screening and treatment may misidentify patient care needs.

Guidance for Adjudicators on Assessing Disability for Transgender and Gender Diverse Applicants and Applicants with Variations in Sex Traits

Similar to health care providers who make difficult choices about appropriate chronic disease management for TGD patients and patients with VSTs, experts involved in the disability determination process must determine how TGD or VST lived experience may impact various disability applications (if at all) and whether additional information is needed to aid in accurate adjudication. In addition, these experts must understand how the multiple social determinants of health that disproportionately impact TGD applicants and applicants with VSTs intersect with chronic disease and disability.

> *Conclusion 12. Given the complexities of the disability determination process for some TGD applicants and some applicants with VSTs, experts involved in the disability adjudication process may need guidance on how aspects of gender-affirming care or other aspects of health, treatment, and care impact disability determinations. SSA might consider supporting adjudicators in these complex disability determinations by delivering national-level trainings and consultive services.*

Guidance to adjudicators can take many forms, including (1) training on the intersection of disability with TGD/VST lived experience; (2) access to national- or regional-level medical and mental health experts who can

---

[7] Listing of Impairments 14.00F7.

consult on disability applications submitted by TGD applicants and applicants with VSTs (the Veteran Health Administration's e-consult might serve as a model); (3) clear statements within the Program Operations Manual System that medical records related to gender-affirming care and care for people with VSTs may be relevant for accurate disability evaluation; and (4) communications to applicants that medical records related to gender-affirming care and care for VSTs may be relevant to certain disability applications and that it may be appropriate to use the "remarks" section on disability applications to describe how TGD or VST lived experience has impacted their health or opportunity to receive appropriate care for their impairment(s). Consistent training and guidance across the 54 Disability Determination Services offices is important, as geographic variability or lack of local expertise may mean that individual offices are not equipped to deliver trainings or provide consultation on these topics.

> *Conclusion 13. Multilevel obstacles to optimal health occur across the life course of TGD people and people with VSTs. These barriers contribute to a greater burden of co-occurring physical and mental health conditions and poorer overall health outcomes compared with the general population. SSA might consider supporting adjudicators in making determinations for TGD applicants and applicants with VSTs by including in guidance and trainings content on the structural disadvantages faced by these populations and how they may impact disability.*

While many applicants for disability benefits experience challenges with their health, TGD applicants and applicants with VSTs face significant and well-described structural disadvantages, including intrapersonal factors (internalized transphobia due to stigma and stress), interpersonal factors (e.g., lack of access to knowledgeable providers, exposure to discriminatory and suboptimal health care, consequences of implicit bias), and structural factors (e.g., lack of access to health insurance, inequitable access to employment opportunities). In addition, TGD people and people with VSTs are members of multiple diverse communities and may experience concomitant barriers to optimal health due to additional dimensions (e.g., race, ethnicity, age, socioeconomic status, and other domains) that influence their experiences with health care and the social drivers of health.

Thus, TGD people and people with VSTs may have systematically experienced delayed preventive screenings, late detection of chronic disease (and the predisposing conditions that contribute to chronic disease), and inadequate care to address chronic health concerns. These barriers coalesce, leading to poorer self-care, inadequate management of chronic disease, and poorer quality of life. These factors may ultimately result in delayed and/or inadequate care for multiple impairments that form the basis of a disability application. It is essential that disability adjudicators remain attuned to the structural and social-contextual factors that shape the applications of TGD people and people with VSTs. For example, adjudicators might receive guidance and training to consider, as part of a disability evaluation, potential stigmatizing language found in medical records that signals suboptimal care delivery.

Appendix A

Public Meeting Agendas

**COMMITTEE ON SEX AND GENDER IDENTIFICATION
AND IMPLICATIONS FOR DISABILITY EVALUATION**

MEETING 1

**MAY 30, 2023
VIRTUAL**

3:30 p.m.   **Welcome and Introductions**
Hortensia Amaro (she/her), *Committee Chair*
Steve Rollins, Acting Associate Commissioner,
U.S. Social Security Administration (SSA)

3:40 p.m.   **Social Security Administration Overview**
Vincent Nibali, Technical Expert, Office of Medical Policy,
Office of Disability Policy, SSA
- Sponsor perspective/motivations for the study
- Overview of SSA disability determination process

4:05 p.m.   **Questions and Discussion**
Committee Members and SSA Staff

4:35 p.m.   **Adjourn Public Session**

MEETING 2

JULY 19, 2023
NATIONAL ACADEMY OF SCIENCES BOARD ROOM

The National Academy of Sciences
2101 Constitution Ave NW
Washington, DC 20418

1:30 p.m.	**Welcome** Hortensia Amaro (she/her), *Committee Chair*
1:35 p.m.	**Presentation and Discussion: Chronic Kidney Disease: Sex Differences, Impact of Gender-Affirming Care, and Appropriate Evaluation Criteria** Sofia Ahmed, M.D., MMSc, FRCPC (she/her), Professor, Cumming School of Medicine, University of Calgary; Nephrologist, Alberta Health Services—Calgary Zone David Collister, M.D., Ph.D., FRCPC (he/him), Assistant Professor, Faculty of Medicine & Dentistry—Medicine Dept, University of Alberta
2:25 p.m.	**Presentation and Discussion: Breaking the Gender–Cancer Association: Lessons from Quality Measurement for Preventive Screenings** Rachel Harrington, Ph.D. (she/her), Senior Research Scientist, Health Equity, National Committee for Quality Assurance
3:15 p.m.	**Statement of Task Q&A**
3:20 p.m.	**Closing Remarks** Hortensia Amaro (she/her), *Committee Chair*
3:20 p.m.	**Adjourn Public Session**

MEETING 3

SEPTEMBER 14, 2023
KECK 209

The Keck Center,
500 Fifth Street, NW
Washington, DC 20001

1:30 p.m. **Welcome and Opening Remarks**
Hortensia Amaro (she/her), *Committee Chair*

1:35 p.m. **Presentation and Discussion: Gender Identity Data Collection and Care Decision Making within the Veterans Health Administration**

Lexi Matza, Ph.D. (they/them/theirs), Associate Director for Data & Analytics, LGBTQ+ Health Program, Patient Care Services, Veterans Health Administration

2:35 p.m. **Presentation and Discussion: Selecting Appropriate Pulmonary Function Test Reference Sex for Transgender and Gender Diverse Patients**

Ethan Fechter-Leggett, D.V.M., M.P.V.M. (he/him), Research Epidemiologist, Field Studies Branch, Respiratory Health Division, National Institute for Occupational Safety and Health, Centers for Disease Control and Prevention

Dinah Foer, M.D. (she/her), Assistant Professor, Harvard Medical School, Associate Physician, Division of Allergy and Clinical Immunology, Brigham and Women's Hospital

3:30 p.m. **Presentation and Discussion: Sexual Orientation and Gender Identity Data Collection in Electronic Medical Records**

Carl Streed Jr., M.D., M.P.H., FACP (he/him/his), Assistant Professor of Medicine, Section of General Internal Medicine, Boston University Aram V. Chobanian & Edward Avedisian School of Medicine; Research Lead, GenderCare Center, Boston Medical Center

4:25 p.m.   **Closing Remarks**
               Hortensia Amaro (she/her), *Committee Chair*

4:30 p.m.   **Adjourn Public Session**

MEETING 4

NOVEMBER 30, 2023, AND DECEMBER 1, 2023
KECK 201

The National Academy of Sciences
2101 Constitution Ave NW
Washington, DC 20418

DAY 1: November 30, 2023

9:15 a.m.   **Welcome and Opening Remarks**
               Hortensia Amaro (she/her), *Committee Chair*

9:20 a.m.   **Expert Panel: Variations in Sex Traits and Implications
               for Disability**

               Moderators:
               Amy Tishelman, Ph.D. (she/her), Research Associate
                   Professor, Psychology Department, Boston College

               Selma Feldman Witchel, M.D. (she/her), Professor Emerita,
                   University of Pittsburgh School of Medicine; University
                   of Pittsburgh Medical Center, Children's Hospital of
                   Pittsburgh

               Panelists:
               Katharine Dalke, Ph.D. (she/her, they/them), Associate
                   Professor of Clinical Psychiatry at University of
                   Pennsylvania Perelman School of Medicine

               Veronica Gomez-Lobo, M.D. (she/her), Division Chief of
                   Gynecology, Children's National Medical Center; and
                   Director, Positive Reevaluation of Urogenital Differences
                   (PROUD) Clinic

Louise Fleming, Ph.D., M.S.N.-E.D., RN (she/her),
Professor and Associate Dean, Undergraduate Programs,
The University of North Carolina at Chapel Hill
School of Nursing; Immediate Past Chair of the CARES
Foundation

Noi Liang, M.B.A., BCPA (she/her), Patient Advocate,
Children's Hospital Colorado; Member, SOAR Clinic
(an interdisciplinary differences of sexual development/
intersex care team)

Justin Tsang (he/him), Disability Rights Advocate;
Advocate for Intersex People; Board Member,
American Association for People with Disabilities

10:45 a.m.   **Patient Panel: Chronic Disease and Disability for
Transgender and Gender Diverse People**

Moderators:
Raksha Jain, M.D. (she/her/hers), Professor, Department
of Medicine, Division of Pulmonary and Critical Care
Medicine, University of Texas Southwestern Medical
Center; Medical Director, Adult Cystic Fibrosis Program

Dinushika Mohottige, M.D., M.P.H. (she/her/hers), Assistant
Professor, Institute of Health Equity Research at the
Icahn School of Medicine at Mount Sinai; Mount Sinai
Barbara T. Murphy Division of Nephrology

Panelists:
Jess Walters (they/them): Disability Justice Advocate;
Health Equity & Justice Fellow at the Center for Health
Humanities and Ethics, University of Virginia

Anonymous Panelist 2

11:30 a.m.   **Closing Remarks**
Hortensia Amaro (she/her), *Committee Chair*

11:35 a.m.   **Adjourn Public Session**

Day 2: December 1, 2023

9:15 a.m.   **Introduction to Public Meeting**
Hortensia Amaro (she/her), *Committee Chair*

9:20 a.m.   **Patient and Provider Panel—Transgender and Gender Diverse People with Cancer: Cancer Treatment, Care, and Implications for Disability**

Moderator:
Ash Alpert, M.D., M.F.A. (they/them/theirs), Instructor of Medicine (Hematology), Yale University School of Medicine

Panelists:
Yee Won Chong (he/they/dia), Filmmaker: *Trans Dudes with Lady Cancer*

Roman Ruddick (they/them), Cofounder, Transgender Cancer Patient Project

Charlie Manzano (he/him), Cofounder, Transgender Cancer Patient Project

10:20 a.m.   **Closing Remarks**
Hortensia Amaro (she/her), *Committee Chair*

10:25 a.m.   **Adjourn Public Session**

Appendix B

Committee Member Biosketches

Hortensia de los Angeles Amaro, Ph.D. (*Chair*), is distinguished university professor and senior scholar on community health at the Wertheim College of Medicine and Stempel College of Public Health and Social Work at Florida International University. Previously, Dr. Amaro served as associate vice-provost and dean's professor of public health and social work at the University of Southern California. Before that, she was distinguished professor and associate dean at the Northeastern University College of Health Sciences, where she founded the Institute on Urban Health Research, and professor at the Boston University School of Public Health, where she was the first to introduce courses on gender health disparities and on race and ethnicity health disparities in the early 1990s. Dr. Amaro's scholarship has focused on advancing the understanding of gender and ethnoracial inequities in health, particularly in treatment for substance use disorders and co-occurring disorders in women, HIV prevention, and other urgent public health challenges. She has authored more than 200 scholarly publications and has made landmark contributions to improving behavioral health care in community-based organizations by launching and informing addiction treatment programs around the world. In her distinguished career, Dr. Amaro has received more than 50 national and community awards, including two honorary doctoral degrees in humane letters from Simmons College in 1994 and the Massachusetts School of Professional Psychology in 2012. She has served on advisory committees to the National Institutes of Health, the National Institute on Drug Abuse, the Substance Abuse and Mental Health Services Administration, the Centers for Disease Control and Prevention, the Health Research and Services Administration, and the U.S. State Department's Latin America programs in Costa Rica and Venezuela. Dr. Amaro is a member of the National Academy of Medicine and has served on more than ten National Academies of Sciences, Engineering, and Medicine consensus studies, workshop committees, and boards. She is president-elect of the ASEM Florida. She received her Ph.D. in psychology from the University of California, Los Angeles.

Heidi Allen, Ph.D., is associate professor at Columbia School of Social Work. Her research focuses on eliminating health disparities through evidence-based health policy, an interest that evolved from her clinical practice in mental health and emergency department social work. She spent several years working in state health policy, focusing on delivery system redesign and coverage expansion. Dr. Allen is currently involved in research examining access and quality of health care for gender and sexual minorities, particularly those enrolled in public insurance. She is a commissioner on the Medicaid and CHIP Payment and Access Commission (MACPAC), a nonresident fellow at the Urban Institute, and a contributing writer at *The Milbank Quarterly*. Her recent research is funded by the National Institute on Minority Health and Health Disparities, National Institutes of Health; the Steven & Alexandra Cohen Foundation; and Columbia World Projects. Dr. Allen is a Columbia provost faculty teaching scholar and a Columbia University provost leadership fellow; she was awarded the 2019 Society for Social Work Research Social Policy Researcher Award. She holds an M.S.W. and Ph.D. in social work.

Walter Bockting, Ph.D., LP, is professor of medical psychology (in psychiatry and nursing) at Columbia University and a research scientist with the New York State Psychiatric Institute (NYSPI). He is area leader of gender, sexuality, and health at NYSPI/Columbia Psychiatry; director of the Program for the Study of LGBTQ+ Health at Columbia University Irving Medical Center; and director of Columbia Doctor's Gender and Sexuality Program. Previously, Dr. Bockting led the Transgender Health Services at the University of Minnesota Medical School (1991–2012) and cofounded the school's Leo Fung Center for Adrenal Hyperplasia and Disorders of Sex Development (2004). He is currently principal investigator for several National Institutes of Health–funded research studies on trans/nonbinary identity development across the lifespan and risk for behavioral cardiovascular disease; quality of life after gender-affirming surgery; and the role of social connectedness in the development of cognitive reserve and resilience among LGBTQ+ adults and their cisgender, heterosexual counterpart; and social connectedness and healthy aging among gender minority people of color. Dr. Bockting is currently serving on a task force for the World Health Organization formulating guidelines for gender-affirming care among adults. He served on the Institute of Medicine Committee on LGBT Health Issues and Research Gaps and Opportunities (2010–2011); is past president and fellow of the Society for the Scientific Study of Sexuality; and served as the 2009–2011 president of the World Professional Association for Transgender Health. Dr. Bockting received his Ph.D. in medical psychology from the Vrije Universiteit in Amsterdam, the Netherlands (1998), and trained extensively in psychology and human sexuality at Utrecht University (1987–1988) and the University of Minnesota (1988–1990).

Don S. Dizon, M.D., is professor of medicine and professor of surgery at Brown University and vice chair of diversity, equity, inclusion, and professional integrity at the SWOG Cancer Research Network, a member of the National Cancer Institute's National Clinical Trials Network. He also serves as editor-in-chief of *CA: A Cancer Journal for Clinicians,* the flagship journal of the American Cancer Society. Dr. Dizon is a medical oncologist specializing in ovarian, cervical, and uterine cancer; prevention, particularly as it relates to the human papilloma virus vaccine; sexuality after cancer for men and women; and professional use of social media. He is director of the Pelvic Malignancies Program, Brown University Health; director of medical oncology, Rhode Island Hospital; and associate director of community outreach and engagement, Legorreta Cancer Center at Brown University. Dr. Dizon is also a board member for multiple nonprofits, including the Hope Foundation for Cancer Research and the LGBTQ Cancer Network. He is a founding member of the Collaboration for Outcomes Using Social Media in Oncology. Dr. Dizon received his M.D. from the University of Rochester School of Medicine and Dentistry.

Scott Hadland, M.D., M.P.H., M.S., is chief of adolescent and young adult medicine at Massachusetts General Hospital and associate professor of pediatrics at Harvard Medical School. His clinical and research interests focus on the health and well-being of adolescents and young adults and, in particular, on mental health and substance use. As part of this work, he has carefully examined health outcomes among lesbian, gay, bisexual, transgender and gender diverse, and queer/questioning youth. Dr. Hadland's research has been funded by the National Institute on Drug Abuse, Patient-Centered Outcomes Research Institute, Centers for Disease Control and Prevention, and numerous foundations. He was the 2020 recipient of the Emerging Leader Award in Adolescent Health from the American Academy of Pediatrics. In 2023, Dr. Hadland was selected to the Presidential Leadership Scholars program, which brings together national leaders committed to facing critical challenges in partnership with the Clinton Presidential Center and George W. Bush Presidential Center. Dr. Hadland holds triple board certification in general pediatrics, adolescent medicine, and addiction medicine.

He received an M.D. from Washington University in St. Louis, M.P.H. in epidemiology and biostatistics from the Johns Hopkins Bloomberg School of Public Health, and M.S. in health policy and management from the Harvard T. H. Chan School of Public Health. He completed his pediatrics residency and chief residency at the Boston Combined Residency Program before pursuing fellowship training in adolescent medicine at Boston Children's Hospital and completing the Pediatric Health Services Research Fellowship at Harvard Medical School.

Raksha Jain, M.D., is professor of medicine and pulmonary critical care at the University of Texas Southwestern Medical Center. She is director of the Cystic Fibrosis and Bronchiectasis Program and leads of a number of multicenter clinical trials for therapeutic drug development for people with cystic fibrosis. Her area of interest focuses on sex and gender disparities in people with cystic fibrosis and bronchiectasis and the role of sex/gonadal hormones in immune response to infection. Dr. Jain is active in the respiratory research community and a fellow of the American Thoracic Society. She completed her B.S. at the Massachusetts Institute of Technology, M.D. at the University of Texas Houston Health Science Center, internal medicine training at the University of Texas Southwestern, and fellowship training in pulmonary and critical care and M.S. in clinical investigation at Washington University in St. Louis.

Dinushika Mohottige, M.D., M.P.H., is assistant professor in the Institute for Health Equity Research at the Icahn School of Medicine at Mount Sinai and the Barbara T. Murphy Division of Nephrology, and a general nephrologist. Dr. Mohottige engages in patient- and community-centered, inequity-focused research around the impact of sociostructural factors and racialized medicine on kidney health and kidney transplantation. As part of this work, she has interrogated the role of race and other sociopolitical variables in clinical algorithms, including kidney function estimation, and considered the role of racism and related sociostructural factors on kidney disease. She has also contributed to multiple perspective pieces regarding considerations for gender-affirming kidney care and inclusive care practices for the LGBTQ+ community, and she has partnered with experts in the application of an intersectional lens to kidney health research. Dr. Mohottige is a member of the National Kidney Foundation Health Equity Taskforce, the National Kidney Foundation Transplant Advisory Committee, the 2022 National Institutes of Health PhenX Social Determinants of Health Committee, the New York City Coalition to end Racism in Clinical Algorithms, and the End-Stage Renal Disease National Coordinating Center Health Equity Committee. She received a B.A. in public policy and a health policy certificate from Duke University in 2006, where she was a Robertson scholar. Dr. Mohottige then earned an M.P.H. in health behavior/health education from the University of North Carolina Gillings School of Global Public Health and a medical degree from The University of North Carolina at Chapel Hill School of Medicine, followed by internal medicine/chief residency and nephrology training at Duke University.

Tonia Poteat, Ph.D., is professor in the Duke University School of Nursing, Division of Healthcare in Adult Populations and codirector of the Duke Sexual and Gender Minority Health Program. Her research, teaching, and clinical practice attend to health equity with a specific focus on populations minoritized on the bases of gender, sexual orientation, and/or race. Dr. Poteat is associate editor of the journal *LGBT Health*, member of the World Professional Association for Transgender Health, member of the research committee for the U.S. Professional Association for Transgender Health, and former vice president for education for GLMA: Health Professionals Advancing LGBTQ Equality. She served on the National Academies of Sciences, Engineering, and Medicine committee that authored the report *Understanding the Well-Being of LGBTQI+ Populations*, published in 2020. Dr. Poteat completed a Ph.D. in international health at the Bloomberg School of Public Health, an M.P.H. in behavioral science from Rollins School of Public Health, a master's in medical science from Emory University, and a bachelor's in biology from Yale University.

Asa Radix, M.D., Ph.D., M.P.H., FACP, is Executive Vice President at the Callen-Lorde Community Health Center and clinical associate professor of medicine at the New York University Grossman School of Medicine, both in New York City. He has more than two decades of clinical experience with transgender and gender diverse individuals and has coauthored national and international guidelines in transgender health. Dr. Radix's research focuses predominately on access to care and health outcomes for transgender individuals. He serves on the New York State AIDS Institute's Medical Clinical Care Committee and the U.S. Department of Health and Human Services Panel on Antiretroviral Guidelines for Adults and Adolescents; he was also co-chair of the World Professional Association of Transgender Health (WPATH) Standards of Care 8 Revision Committee. In 2022, Dr. Radix was awarded the 2022 WPATH Gold Medal for major contributions to global trans health. He is associate editor of *Transgender Health* and the *International Journal of Transgender Health*. Dr. Radix is board certified in internal medicine and infectious disease and holds a Ph.D. in epidemiology from Columbia University.

Joshua D. Safer, M.D., FACP, FACE, is executive director of the Mount Sinai Center for Transgender Medicine and Surgery in New York City and professor of medicine at the Icahn School of Medicine at Mount Sinai. He is coauthor of the Endocrine Society guidelines for the medical care of transgender patients, the World Professional Association for Transgender Health (WPATH) *Standards of Care Version 8*, the gender-affirming hormone treatment sections for *UpToDate*, the transgender medical care review in the *New England Journal of Medicine*, and the review of transgender medical care in *Annals of Internal Medicine*. Dr. Safer was inaugural president of the U.S. Professional Association for Transgender Health (USPATH) and is currently a WPATH board member. He also serves on the Global Education Institute for WPATH and has been a scientific co-chair for multiple WPATH international meetings. Dr. Safer is associate editor of *Transgender Health* and serves on the editorial board for *Endocrine Practice*. He also chairs the DSD/Intersex and Transgender Athlete Panel of Experts for World Athletics. Dr. Safer has served as a paid consultant to the American Civil Liberties Union in cases related to transgender athletes in Connecticut, Idaho, Tennessee, West Virginia, and Florida. He received his medical degree from the University of Wisconsin School of Medicine.

Loren Schechter, M.D., is professor of surgery and urology and chief of gender-affirmation surgery at Rush University Medical Center in Chicago, Illinois. He serves on the executive committee of the World Professional Association for Transgender Health (WPATH), coauthored the WPATH *Standards of Care Version 7* (SOC-7), and served as co-lead for the Surgery and Post-Operative Care section of SOC-8. Dr. Schechter authored the first surgical atlas on gender-affirming surgery, *Surgical Management of Transgender Individuals*, and is a founding member and president-elect of the Society of Gender Surgeons. He is past president of the Illinois Society of Plastic Surgeons and the Chicago chapter of the American College of Surgeons. Dr. Schechter is associate editor for the *International Journal of Transgender Health* and serves on the editorial board for *Transgender Health*. He has served as an expert witness in federal lawsuits in states such as Florida, Idaho, North Carolina, and Washington where he has provided testimony on appropriate gender-affirming surgical interventions. He also often serves as an expert witness in medical malpractice cases providing testimony related to medical liability. Dr. Schechter received the 2013 Illinois State Bar Association Community Service Award for his advocacy efforts for the transgender community, was an invited discussant to the Pentagon in 2017 to discuss military service by transgender individuals and was named a Distinguished Sexual and Gender Health Revolutionary by the University of Minnesota Program in Human Sexuality. Dr. Schechter received his medical degree, with honors, from the University of Chicago Pritzker School of Medicine, where he was elected to the Alpha Omega Alpha honor society and graduated as The Outstanding Student in Surgery. He completed his residency in general and plastic surgery and a fellowship in reconstructive microsurgery at the University of Chicago Hospitals.

Amy Tishelman, Ph.D., is clinical and research psychologist and research associate professor at Boston College in the Department of Psychology and Neuroscience. She, along with colleagues, currently has funding from the National Institutes of Health (NIH) to co-develop a self-advocacy tool for youth and emerging adults with intersex variations, an effort that includes a large and diverse research network of stakeholders throughout the United States. She previously worked at Boston Children's Hospital (BCH) for close to three decades, where she last held the position as director of clinical research in the Behavioral Health, Endocrinology, and Urology Program and Gender Multispecialty Service. These programs provide clinical care to youth, young adults, and families related to differences of sex development, intersex variations. She was featured for her work by the Sexual and Gender Minority (SGM) office of the NIH in 2022. Dr. Tishelman was also senior attending psychologist at BCH and assistant professor at Harvard Medical School. She previously worked extensively in the areas of child maltreatment and trauma. She has been awarded several National Institutes of Health grants as a multiple-principal investigator or coinvestigator, investigating well-being and/or gender development in children and adolescents, and youth/young adults with intersex variations (also referred to with alternative terminology, such as Differences of Sex Development or Variations of Sex Traits). Dr. Tishelman coauthored a clinical report for the American Academy of Pediatrics, which was published in *Pediatrics*, on fertility and sexual function counseling for at-risk pediatric patients. She was selected by the World Professional Association of Transgender Health to be the international leader in developing new global standards of care for prepubescent children, and by the American Psychological Association to co-chair a national task force on DSD. Dr. Tishelman is on several journal editorial boards and speaks and publishes frequently in her areas of expertise. Dr. Tishelman has also served as an expert witness in lawsuits where she has provided testimony on transgender youth and variations in sex traits. She received her Ph.D. from West Virginia University.

Kathryn Whetten, Ph.D., is professor of public policy and global health at Duke University. They are also director of the Center for Health Policy and Inequalities Research, codirector of Duke's Sexual and Gender Minority (SGM) Wellness Program, and the research director of the Hart Fellows Program. As co-lead of the SGM Wellness Program, they work with clinician researchers to understand variations in gender-related laboratory test results when the patient is transgender or nonbinary. As a health policy and population health researcher, Dr. Whetten has devoted the majority of their research, practice, and training career to understanding how life-course events influence beliefs and behaviors that can put one at risk for HIV and other infectious and chronic diseases, and how these factors influence interactions with health care providers. They examine U.S. and international policies that influence access to health and other care services, including Medicaid and Medicare. The combination of being a health policy expert and population health scientist allows Dr. Whetten a unique view into how national and state-level policies influence health care reception and well-being of those who receive, or could receive, these services. As such, they have worked with legislators in both North Carolina and Washington, DC, to provide evidence-based research and findings to inform and change policies, such as eligibility for Medicaid and for Ryan White funds and services. The vast majority of Dr. Whetten's work has been funded by the National Institutes of Health and the Sexual and Gender Minority Research Office. They previously served on the Institute of Medicine committee dedicated to reviewing the impact and future of the U.S. President's Emergency Plan for AIDS Relief. Dr. Whetten received their Ph.D. in health policy and administration and population health sciences from The University of North Carolina at Chapel Hill.

Selma Feldman Witchel, M.D., is tenured professor emerita of pediatrics at the University of Pittsburgh Medical Center (UPMC) Children's Hospital of Pittsburgh and the University of Pittsburgh School of Medicine. She chairs the Differences in Sex Development Committee and is immediate past program director for the pediatric endocrinology fellowship training program at UPMC Children's Hospital of Pittsburgh. Dr. Witchel is primarily interested in the physiology and genetics of the hypothalamic-pituitary-gonadal and hypothalamic-pituitary-adrenal axes. Her research elucidated the concept of the "manifesting heterozygote" in patients with disorders of steroidogenesis, and her interests extend to the care of patients with variations in sex development and polycystic ovary syndrome and to health care for gender diverse youth. She participates in studies regarding fertility preservation in these patient groups. Dr. Witchel participated the 2018 publication of the *International Evidence-Based Guideline for the Assessment and Management of Polycystic Ovary Syndrome*, and she contributed to the 2023 update of these evidence-based guidelines. She is past chair of the Pediatric Endocrine Society Education subcommittee; she served as co-chair of the 50th-year anniversary annual meeting of the Pediatric Endocrine Society and was elected to its board of directors in 2022. Dr. Witchel is an active member of the Endocrine Society Annual Meeting Steering Committee. She served as the Clinical Program Chair for the 2024 Endocrine Society Annual Meeting. She is also a member of the American Academy of Pediatrics. Dr. Witchel is currently an Associate Editor for the *Journal of the Endocrine Society* and past president of the Androgen Excess-Polycystic Ovary Society. She has published more than 200 articles, reviews, and chapters. Dr. Witchel received her B.A. from Oberlin College and M.D. at the University of Pittsburgh, graduating as a member of Alpha Omega Alpha. She completed her pediatric residency at the Children's Hospital Medical Center, University of Cincinnati, and her pediatric endocrinology fellowship at the Children's Hospital of Pittsburgh, University of Pittsburgh.

Nancy Fugate Woods, Ph.D., RN, FAAN, is emerita professor of nursing at the University of Washington. She has served as an educator and researcher in women's symptom science and as a leader of initiatives in women's health, including the National Institutes of Health (NIH) Advisory Committee on Women's Health. Dr. Woods led the development of the first NIH-funded Center for Women's Health Research, established at the University of Washington in 1989. She has conducted NIH-funded research on menstrual cycle–related symptoms, the menopausal transition, and older women's health since the 1970s. Dr. Woods led the Seattle Midlife Women's Health Study, a longitudinal study of the menopausal transition, with up to 25 years of follow-up. Her early efforts focusing on sex and gender included publication of the text *Human Sexuality in Health and Illness* to ensure that health professionals caring for patients were adequately informed about current research about sexuality (1975); she has continued this effort by editing textbooks about women's health, such as *Women's Health Care in Advanced Practice Nursing*. Dr. Woods was elected to the American Academy of Nursing in 1980 and the National Academy of Medicine in 1993 and was awarded the Trailblazer Award by the U.S. Public Health Service. She has served on National Academy of Medicine committees on the health consequences of Gulf War service and environmental health in women. Dr. Woods received her Ph.D. in epidemiology and public health from The University of North Carolina at Chapel Hill.

STUDY CONSULTANTS

Patricia M. Owens, M.P.A., is senior disability expert for the U.S. Government Accountability Office (GAO). She has more than 30 years of experience in health- and disability-related programs and policy, and has held executive, policy development, and administrative positions in both the public and private disability sectors. Her experience serves as the basis for in-depth understanding of the multidimensional and interactive nature of health and disability in terms of social policy and risk management. Ms. Owens has consulted with both private- and public-sector organizations on health and disability issues, programs, and products. In addition to GAO, she has consulted for the Social Security Administration (SSA), the Veterans Health Administration, the Urban Institute, the National Academy of Social Insurance (board member), and the Rutgers Disability Income Studies. She helped UNUM, UK (an insurance company in Great Britain) launch a study of the cost of disability in 2000–2001. Ms. Owens is a member of the board of directors of Village Care of New York, a multimillion-dollar AIDS treatment network and community nursing and rehabilitation services provider for persons with impairment. She was a member of the National Research Council/Institute of Medicine Committee on Veterans' Compensation for Posttraumatic Stress Disorder. Ms. Owens serves on the National Academy of Medicine Standing Committee of Medical and Vocational Experts for SSA's Disability Programs. She earned an M.P.A. from the University of Missouri.

David Wittenburg, Ph.D., is director of health research at Mathematica Policy Research, Inc. An expert in interventions to promote employment for people with disabilities, particularly interventions that serve youth as they transition into adulthood, Dr. Wittenburg has two decades of experience in evaluation design and program evaluation for several federal agencies. He leads business development activities related to disability projects and recently worked in senior leadership roles on three Social Security Administration demonstration projects, helping to design and implement experimental and nonexperimental approaches to assess the efficacy of return-to-work interventions for people with disabilities. Dr. Wittenburg, who joined Mathematica in 2005, presents his findings to diverse research and policy audiences, including in congressional testimony, conference presentations, reports, and journal publications. He edited two special journal volumes on employment topics related to people with disabilities for the *IZA Journal of Labor Policy* and the *Journal of Disability Policy Studies*. A member of the National Academy of Social Insurance and formerly a senior associate at the Urban Institute and the Lewin Group, Dr. Wittenburg holds a Ph.D. in economics from Syracuse University.

Appendix C

Commissioned Paper: Physiological Sex Differences and the Effect of Gender-Affirming Hormone Therapy

Daniel J. Slack,[1] Jiby Yohannan,[1] Derek Chen,[2] Nithya Krishnamurthy,[2] Joshua D. Safer[1,3]
[1]Division of Endocrinology, Department of Medicine, Icahn School of Medicine at Mount Sinai, [2]Icahn School of Medicine at Mount Sinai, [3]Center for Transgender Medicine and Surgery, Mount Sinai Health System

Prepared for the National Academies of Sciences, Engineering, and Medicine Committee on Sex and Gender Identification and Implications for Disability Evaluation

Correspondence: Dr. Daniel J. Slack, Icahn School of Medicine at Mount Sinai, One Gustave L. Levy Place, New York, NY, USA 10029-6574; TEL: 212-241-6500; Daniel.slack@mssm.edu

Sex differences in normal physiology and disease pathophysiology are widespread throughout the human body. These differences range from readily apparent anatomical dimorphisms to subtle variations in signal transduction at the molecular level. They may have implications regarding the interpretation of serologic biomarkers and imaging, the diagnosis of disease, and the appropriate selection of therapeutics. Circulating endogenous sex hormones, particularly estrogen and testosterone, are the main driving factor behind some, but not all, of these differences. The study of human disease associated with states of sex hormone excess and deficiency provides a crucial window into the differential effect of sex hormones between the sexes.

Examining the clinical benefits and risks associated with the use of exogenous hormone therapy to replace hormone deficiencies or treat disease has been similarly informative.

Transgender and gender diverse (TGD) individuals have a gender identity that differs from the sex recorded at their birth based on observation of external genitalia. They may seek gender-affirming therapies, particularly gender-affirming surgery (GAS) and gender-affirming hormone therapy (GAHT).

Feminizing GAHT generally involves the use of exogenous estrogens, with or without adjunctive agents that also have antiandrogenic properties, to develop female secondary sex characteristics while suppressing or minimizing male secondary sex characteristics. Conversely, masculinizing GAHT generally involves the use of exogenous testosterone to develop male secondary sex characteristics. This narrative review takes a systems-based approach to synthesize the extant literature on physiologic sex differences, how gender-affirming care for TGD individuals may affect those sex differences, and the potential clinical implications of those changes.

BONE HEALTH AND BODY COMPOSITION

Sex Differences in Bone Health and Body Composition

An individual's bone mass at any point in adulthood is representative of their peak bone mass minus that which has been subsequently lost. Peak bone mass is achieved, on average, in the late teenage years and early twenties in cisgender females and by the second decade in cisgender males. Peak bone mass is primarily determined by heredity, with nutritional factors, physical activity, and circulating hormones playing a secondary role (Cosman et al., 2014). Adolescence is crucial for skeletal development, as the bone gained during adolescence accounts for up to 60 percent of peak bone mass (Wojtys, 2020). Estrogen and growth hormone (GH) are essential in the pubertal growth spurt, irrespective of sex. Estrogen stimulates insulin-like growth factor 1 (IGF-1) production by increasing the secretion of GH. IGF-1 is the most critical factor in promoting the maturation of chondrocytes and osteoblasts, which leads to epiphysial fusion (Finlayson et al., 2016). This is clinically evident in individuals with estrogen-receptor deficiency or aromatase deficiency, the latter a condition resulting in impaired conversion of testosterone to estrogen. These individuals exhibit diminished bone age, decreased bone density, and continued growth into the third decade. In those with aromatase deficiency, exogenous estrogen administration has been shown to advance bone age and increase bone density (Bilezikian et al., 1998).

There is less consensus regarding testosterone's role in achieving peak bone mass and maintaining bone health. Although puberty starts earlier in cisgender females, it lasts longer in cisgender males who exhibit increased periosteal bone formation and more significant marrow cavity enlargement, resulting in larger bones and greater bending strength (Duan et al., 2003; Rothman and Iwamoto, 2019). It is difficult to say how much of this observed dimorphism is due to a direct effect of testosterone on the bone, partly because the data from animal models do not agree with that from human studies. For example, while androgen-receptor knockout mice have reduced periosteal bone formation, patients with complete androgen insensitivity syndrome with nonfunctional androgen receptors have mostly normal bone mineral density (BMD) (Vanderschueren et al., 2014). Indirectly, testosterone contributes to observed sex differences in BMD through its effects on body composition. Whereas prepubertal individuals start with equal lean body mass, skeletal mass, and body fat, at maturity, cisgender males have approximately 1.5 times the lean body mass, skeletal mass, and muscle mass of cisgender females. In contrast, cisgender females have twice as much body fat as cisgender males (Loomba-Albrecht and Styne, 2009). Androgens, including testosterone, are known to increase muscle mass and decrease body fat, thus contributing to the observed sexual differentiation in body composition throughout puberty (Almeida et al., 2017).

In addition to attaining peak bone mass, estrogens also play a crucial role in maintaining bone health throughout adulthood. It is thought that, at least in part, this is due to estrogen suppression of interleukin 6 (IL-6) secretion, a cytokine that stimulates the proliferation of osteoclast precursors, thus accelerating bone turnover (Florencio-Silva et al., 2015). The impact of the loss of endogenous estrogen on bone health is demonstrated in cisgender females experiencing menopause, whereby an increase in daily calcium loss, reflecting an increase in bone resorption over formation, results in, on average, a loss of one standard deviation of BMD and a two-to-threefold increase in fracture risk after 10 years (Black and Rosen, 2016). Hormone replacement therapy (HRT) using conjugated equine estrogens has been shown to increase BMD and reduce the risk of hip and vertebral fractures by about 35 percent (Karim et al., 2011). Low-dose conjugated estrogens and estradiol also increase BMD, although their antifracture effect remains unknown (Tella and Gallagher, 2014).

In the adult cisgender male population, too, estrogen is critical to maintaining bone health. This was examined in a study in which goserelin acetate, a gonadotropin-releasing hormone (GnRH) agonist, was administered to cause hypogonadism. Then, exogenous testosterone was added back to one group in varying doses. At the same time, a second group received add-back testosterone in the same doses with the addition of an aromatase inhibitor. In the group with add-back testosterone only, BMD trended down with lower testosterone levels but did not differ significantly from controls, whereas in the group that also received aromatase inhibition, BMD declined by 1–2 percent in all groups, independent of the testosterone level (Finkelstein et al., 2016).

Our understanding of the differential impact of sex steroids on cortical versus trabecular bone continues to evolve. It was previously thought that the effect of estrogen was predominately on trabecular bone. Still, more recent data reveal that trabecular bone loss occurs in the third decade, before sex steroid deficiency in most individuals (Khosla et al., 2011). Cortical bone, on the other hand, maintains relative stability throughout adulthood before decreasing linearly in older adults. However, cortical bone is lower in postmenopausal cisgender females compared with age-matched cisgender males; this is potentially because of the rapid period of bone loss during menopause (Drake and Khosla, 2013). It seems likely that varying concentrations of estrogens and androgens in aging adults play a key role in apparent sex differences in bone density (Rothman and Iwamoto, 2019). When studying bone loss in later life, it is vital to consider and control for the progressive deficits in renal and intestinal function that occur in normal aging and may impair calcium homeostasis, irrespective of the effects of sex hormones.

GAHT, Bone Health, and Body Composition

Low bone mass has been observed with relatively high prevalence in transfeminine individuals (Fighera et al., 2018; T'Sjoen et al., 2009). These findings were previously thought to be related to inadequate estrogen treatment in the context of suppressed or absent gonadal sex hormone secretion, but multiple studies have now shown that transfeminine individuals tend to have lower bone mass and lower Z-scores compared with age-matched cisgender males even before any GAHT or GAS (Van Caenegem et al., 2013, 2015a). In addition to reproducing these findings, a more recent study found that transmasculine individuals also had low bone mass before GAHT, particularly at the femur, compared with cisgender female controls, but without significant differences in BMD Z-scores as determined by dual-energy X-ray absorptiometry (DEXA) (Ceolin et al., 2023). In that study, researchers aimed to investigate driving factors of low bone mass before treatment in TGD individuals, finding that TGD individuals had lower vitamin D values compared with their cisgender counterparts, that transfeminine individuals had more total fat mass while transmasculine individuals had more total lean mass, and that transfeminine individuals were more likely to be active smokers and to spend time indoors. Thus, it appears likely that body composition and lifestyle factors contribute to low BMD in TGD adults before initiation of GAHT.

Many studies report a positive change in BMD as early as 1 year following initiation of estrogen in transfeminine individuals (Singh-Ospina et al., 2017; Wiepjes et al., 2017). Long-term studies are sparse, but in a cohort study of transfeminine individuals followed for over 10 years, reassessment of bone density following 10 years of GAHT found a significant increase in Z-score despite no change in BMD at the lumbar spine (Wiepjes et al., 2019). In this study, a positive association between serum estradiol and lumbar spine BMD was noted such that those in the highest tertile of estradiol (mean 121 pg/mL) had a significant increase in lumbar spine BMD while those in the lowest tertile (mean 32 pg/mL) had a significant decrease in lumbar spine BMD. No relationship between level of luteinizing hormone (LH) or degree of testosterone suppression was observed. Only one study appears to have been powered to evaluate fracture outcomes in TGD individuals. In this study, fracture risk was found to be higher in older transfeminine individuals (age ≥50 years) than in age-matched reference cisgender males but not cisgender females. In contrast, in younger transfeminine individuals, fracture risk was increased compared with age-matched reference cisgender females but not cisgender males (Wiepjes et al., 2020). In a prospective cohort study of TGD adults newly initiated on GAHT, including both masculinizing and feminizing regimens, serum bone turnover markers (BTMs) decreased after a year of treatment, with modest negative correlations between changes in BTMs and changes in BMD noted (Vlot et al., 2019). Taken together, these data support the concept that the administration of exogenous estrogen in transfeminine individuals can increase bone density and potentially decrease fracture risk, even in the setting of testosterone suppression.

It is also essential to consider the impact of body composition changes that occur with GAHT and may influence bone health. Before GAHT, transfeminine individuals differ from age-matched cisgender males on measures of body composition, with lower muscle mass, strength, and lean body mass (Van Caenegem et al., 2015a). Feminizing GAHT increases fat mass and decreases lean mass, shifting body composition to mirror the average natal female body more closely (Alvares et al., 2021). It appears probable, then, that the high prevalence of low bone mass observed in transfeminine individuals may be due, in part, to low lean body mass and that some of the improvement in BMD seen with initiation of feminizing GAHT may be related to the appreciable increase in fat mass that occurs. Indeed, in a study of transfeminine individuals on feminizing GAHT for variable amounts of time, investigators found a positive correlation between appendicular lean mass and total fat mass with BMD, explaining 14.9 percent of the observed variation on lumbar spine BMD and 20.6 percent of the variation in total femur BMD (Fighera et al., 2018).

Recent data show that transmasculine individuals may have low bone mass at baseline compared with age-matched cisgender women before initiation of GAHT, mirroring trends seen in transfeminine individuals (Ceolin et al., 2023). Importantly, however, consensus has not been reached on this point; prior, smaller studies have reported similar BMD and body composition measures between transmasculine individuals and age-matched cisgender females (Van Caenegem et al., 2012, 2015b). Unlike transfeminine individuals receiving exogenous estrogen as part of feminizing GAHT, gains in BMD with testosterone treatment in transmasculine individuals are reported with less consistency. In one study, BMD measures did not change after a year of testosterone treatment, despite increases in bone formation and resorption markers; the authors proposed that the latter effect may reflect an anabolic effect of testosterone treatment rather than bone loss (Van Caenegem et al., 2015b). In a similar, more extensive cohort study assessing transmasculine individuals at baseline and following 1 year of testosterone therapy, increases in the total hip and lumbar spine but not femoral neck BMD were observed, with the increase in lumbar spine BMD found to be much more prominent in those who initiated treatment at an older age (≥50 years) (Wiepjes et al., 2017).

Longer-term data have become available more recently, showing that BMD was similar but that the lumbar spine Z-score had increased after 10 years of testosterone treatment. Again, this change was driven by those in the oldest age group when they initiated treatment (≥40 years) (Wiepjes et al., 2019). Similarly, in a study examining trends in BTMs in individuals newly initiated on GAHT, a difference was noted between younger transmasculine individuals (≤50 years), who experienced an increase in BTMs, whereas the older individuals did not (Vlot et al., 2019). This apparent divergence has led the authors to postulate a role for increased estradiol action via aromatization. However, a definitive relationship between serum estrogen or testosterone and BMD in transmasculine individuals has not been elucidated. Despite the lack of consensus regarding increases in BMD in transmasculine individuals with the use of GAHT, it is reassuring that there does not appear to be an appreciable decline in BMD despite a relative reduction in estrogen levels. Additionally, more recent data powered to evaluate fracture outcomes do not point to an increased risk of fracture in younger transmasculine individuals, although the risk in older transmasculine individuals remains unknown (Wiepjes et al., 2020).

As with estrogen, it is essential to consider the effects of testosterone use as masculinizing GAHT on measures of body composition that may influence BMD. As previously noted, prior to GAHT, transmasculine individuals have similar bone and body composition compared with age-matched cisgender female controls (Van Caenegem et al., 2015b). Several studies have reported changes in body composition following the initiation of testosterone treatment, including an increase in muscle mass and grip strength, a higher waist-to-hip ratio, and a decrease in fat mass, having the net effect of shifting the composition and contour of the body toward that of the average natal male body (Van Caenegem et al., 2012, 2015b). It seems then that acquiring lean mass in place of fat mass with testosterone helps stabilize BMD in transmasculine individuals. It remains unclear how much of the effect of testosterone on BMD is via such indirect mechanisms versus via a potential direct effect on the bone. In one of the studies, statistical models were used to compare transmasculine individuals before and after GAHT with cisgender female controls. They found a positive association with bone size and endosteal circumference at the radius after adjusting for grip strength, suggesting a direct effect of testosterone on the bone (Van Caenegem et al., 2012).

Research investigating the potential differential impact of various hormonal preparations and routes of administration (ROAs) of GAHT on bone health in TGD individuals has been limited. While data are mixed, it seems unlikely there is an actual differential impact of various sex hormone ROAs on BMD (Cirrincione and Narla, 2021). Further longitudinal research will help reach consensus and may stratify BTMs by ROA to investigate whether there are differences in how various preparations influence bone metabolism. Additionally, there is a need to investigate whether the use of adjunctive antiandrogens influences bone health in transfeminine individuals, as there are currently no data in this area.

Puberty is a critical period for the growth and development of the musculoskeletal system, regulated in part by circulating endogenous sex hormones. In TGD adolescents, GnRH agonists may be used to delay puberty to allow time to determine gender-affirming treatment goals without the development of unwanted secondary sexual characteristics. Through continuous stimulation, GnRH agonists inhibit the pulsatile secretion of gonadotropin, which markedly reduces the production of gonadal sex hormones and results in the cessation of pubertal development (Panagiotakopoulos, 2018). Absence of sex hormones may result in harmful effects on the bone that may be reversible. Experience using these medications to care for individuals with conditions such as central precocious puberty (CPP) and prostate cancer has been informative in elucidating potential effects on bone in TGD youth. Individuals with CPP experience early pubertal development resulting from premature hypothalamic-pituitary-gonadal axis activation. In these individuals, GnRH agonists are administered to delay puberty, generally for several years, to allow the adolescents to go through puberty at a more typical age. Studies investigating the long-term impact on BMD in patients with CPP treated with GnRH agonists have found that, while BMD levels decrease during GnRH agonist treatment, the effects are reversible and bone mass was sufficiently preserved after treatment (De Sanctis et al., 2019). Additionally, BTMs were found to be elevated before treatment, decreased while on GnRH agonists, and stabilized after treatment (van der Sluis et al., 2002). GnRH agonists are also used as a form of androgen deprivation therapy (ADT) for the treatment of prostate cancer. In this population, ADT is associated with a substantial decrease in BMD throughout the skeletal system at multiple sites, with the magnitude of BMD loss increasing with the duration of therapy and significantly increasing one's risk of fragility fracture (Pietzak and Mucksavage, 2016). Reassuringly, there does appear to be some reversibility in ADT-induced bone loss for those who discontinue the medication (Wang et al., 2017). Additionally, higher levels of BTMs were observed on ADT and normalized when treatment was withdrawn, in line with the observations pertaining to BMD.

The extant literature examining the effect of GnRH agonist use on bone health in TGD youth is more limited in scope, particularly regarding long-term outcomes and fracture risk, owing to the relatively recent introduction of pediatric GAHT. Before treatment with GnRH agonists or GAHT, TGD youth tend to have lower BMD compared with reference standards for sex designated at birth, mirroring observations in TGD adults (Lee et al., 2020). As with other conditions, TGD youth have been shown to experience a decrease in BMD Z-scores after initiation of GnRH agonists (Lee et al., 2020). Recently, reassuring longitudinal data have become available. In a cohort study of TGD individuals treated with GnRH agonists during adolescence followed by GAHT with an average follow-up duration of 15 years, Z-scores caught up with pretreatment levels on all accounts except for the lumbar spine in transfeminine individuals, which may have been related to low estradiol concentrations in this group (van der Loos et al., 2023). It appears, then, that the effect of pubertal suppression on peak bone mass is more delayed attainment rather than attenuation.

Previously, only one study was cited widely, wherein a small number of TGD youth treated with GnRH agonists (average age of initiation: 15 years) followed by GAHT (average age of initiation: 16.5 years) were evaluated. Individuals had not entirely made up their bone loss by age 22, as Z-scores were still lower than baseline despite a slight increase in BMD (Klink et al., 2015). The findings correlated with trends in BTMs, which were shown to decrease while using a GnRH agonist, in line with the observations in patients with CPP, and continued to decrease despite initiation of GAHT (Vlot et al., 2017). The study was criticized because treatment occurred later than would now be standard and with lower doses of GAHT.

It is important to note that some TGD youth are now starting puberty blockade at earlier ages than in years past, and it will be essential to delineate how the timing of pubertal blockade can impact skeletal development differentially. This concept was examined in a prospective study in which the investigators considered the timing of GnRH agonist initiation (i.e., early vs. late puberty) in their analysis, finding that, during GAHT, the increase in bone mineral apparent density Z-scores was most pronounced for the early pubertal TGD youth (Schagen et al., 2020). In that study, BTMs decreased on GnRH agonists in all but the late-pubertal transmasculine individuals who started with lower BTMs that did not change. BTMs were again shown to decrease on GAHT for all groups except, interestingly, in the early-pubertal transfeminine individuals who had an initial increase in BTMs in the first year of treatment before they began to decline, possibly because this group had the most growth potential.

DEXA is the most frequently employed imaging technique to measure BMD and diagnose low bone mass and osteoporosis. In its 2019 guidance on the interpretation of DEXA in TGD adults, the International Society of Clinical Densitometry (ISCD) recommended using BMD Z-scores concordant with gender identity in transgender adults and Z-scores concordant with sex recorded at birth in nonbinary adults (Rosen et al., 2019). Although the Endocrine Society Clinical Practice Guidelines recommend assessment of BMD by DEXA for TGD youth treated with GnRH agonist monotherapy and following BMD by DEXA until peak bone mass is attained, there is no official guidance regarding the interpretation of BMD by DEXA in TGD youth (Hembree et al., 2017).

There is now literature showing that hip bone geometry matches gender identity curves in TGD individuals who initiated GnRH agonists in early puberty. In contrast, those who initiated GnRH agonists in mid- to late puberty had skeletal trajectories that more closely mirrored the reference curve of their sex recorded at birth (van der Loos et al., 2021). In a recent prospective study investigating different methods of interpreting BMD Z-scores by DEXA in early pubertal TGD youth, the authors concluded that it might be helpful to utilize skeletal age in addition to both sex reference standards to interpret BMD before and during GnRH agonist monotherapy and to utilize reference standards of the affirmed gender when GnRH agonist therapy is stopped and either GAHT is started or endogenous puberty is allowed to proceed (Lee et al., 2022).

Key Points:
1. Endogenous estrogen is crucial in attaining peak bone mass and maintaining bone health throughout adulthood. Endogenous testosterone contributes to sex differences in BMD primarily through its effects on body composition.
2. Low bone mass has been observed with relatively high prevalence in TGD individuals, both transfeminine and transmasculine, before GAHT, in part because of body composition and lifestyle factors.
3. BMD increases, and fracture risk likely decreases, with exogenous estrogen use in transfeminine individuals. BMD does not appear to increase, but does not appreciably decline, with exogenous testosterone use in transmasculine individuals.
4. Feminizing GAHT increases fat mass and decreases lean mass, shifting body composition and contour toward that of the natal female body. Masculinizing GAHT increases lean mass and reduces fat mass, moving body composition and contour toward that of the natal male body.

5. Differences in ROA and dose of GAHT do not appear to affect BMD.
6. TGD youth may exhibit a decrease in BMD and levels of BTMs with the initiation of GnRH agonists. BMD then increases with initiation of GAHT, particularly in early pubertal TGD youth, although whether peak bone mass is attenuated is not entirely clear.
7. TGD youth who initiate GnRH agonists in early puberty may have skeletal trajectories that match their gender identity curves, whereas those who start GnRH agonists later in puberty more closely match the reference curve of cisgender individuals with the same sex recorded at birth.
8. For interpretation of DEXA in TGD adults, the ISCD recommends using BMD Z-scores concordant with gender identity in transgender adults and Z-scores concordant with sex recorded at birth in non-binary adults.
9. While limited data are available to guide the interpretation of DEXA in TGD youth, it may be helpful to utilize skeletal age in addition to both sex reference standards before and during GnRH agonist monotherapy and then to use reference standards for their affirmed gender once GnRH agonists are stopped and GAHT is started, or endogenous puberty is allowed to resume.

CARDIOVASCULAR SYSTEM

Sex Differences in the Cardiovascular System

The cardiovascular system serves as the channel through which blood is circulated throughout the body. Physiologic differences in the cardiovascular system between cisgender males and cisgender females have been well studied. While the size of the heart between the two sexes before puberty is similar, after puberty, the hearts of cisgender males have a greater degree of myocyte hypertrophy than the hearts of cisgender females (Prabhavathi et al., 2014). When adjusted for exercise ability, the hearts of cisgender females tend to beat faster than those of cisgender males, which is thought to be a compensatory mechanism resulting in equivalent cardiac output between the sexes (Ramaekers et al., 1998). Cardiovascular disease generally occurs later in cisgender females, and some studies suggest that cisgender females have a better prognosis than their cisgender male counterparts for diseases such as heart failure, myocardial ischemia, and hypertrophic cardiomyopathy (Deswal and Bozkurt, 2006; Vaccarino et al., 1999). Cisgender females also have lower blood pressure, on average, than that of cisgender males (St Pierre et al., 2022).

Sex hormones play a vital role in the physiology of the cardiovascular system. Circulating estrogen is cardioprotective. This is evidenced by premenopausal cisgender females having a decreased incidence of cardiovascular disease compared with cisgender males. In contrast, postmenopausal cisgender females, who have relative estrogen deficiency, tend to have similar or even higher rates of cardiovascular disease compared with cisgender males (Armeni and Lambrinoudaki, 2022). This may partly be due to estrogen's vasodilatory effects on endothelial cells lining the blood vessels (Chakrabarti et al., 2014). The estrogen receptor is present in estrogen receptor (ER)α, ERβ, and G-protein-coupled estrogen receptor (GPER) forms. These receptors are present in both sexes and found throughout the body, including the cardiovascular system. Stimulation of ERα results in the activation of the endothelial nitric oxide synthase (eNOS) pathway, leading to vasodilation and prevention of smooth muscle proliferation. ERβ stimulation helps prevent cardiac fibrosis (dos Santos et al., 2014). Murine models have shown that mice without ERβ receptors experience systolic and diastolic blood pressure elevations (Zhu et al., 2002). GPER regulates vascular tone and protects the heart from reperfusion injury (dos Santos et al., 2014). Estrogen also has protective effects on myocardial contractility, likely related to estrogen's role in modulating calcium homeostasis in the heart (Jiao et al., 2020). Indeed, a separate study using female rats found that gonadectomy was associated with decreased myocardial contractility, effects that were partially reversible with administration of exogenous estrogen (Scheuer et al., 1987).

Testosterone receptors are also present throughout the cardiovascular system in both sexes. While some studies have linked testosterone to adverse effects on myocardial remodeling following infarction, several studies have shown that physiologic levels of testosterone may inhibit the formation of atherosclerosis, prevent dyslipidemia, and decrease overall inflammation (Herring et al., 2013; Nahrendorf et al., 2003). Testosterone's effects on the vasculature are concentration dependent. At lower concentrations, testosterone exhibits vasorelaxation effects by modulating the calcium and potassium channels of smooth muscle cells as well as interacting with the eNOS, cyclic guanosine monophosphate, and cyclic adenosine monophosphate pathways (Deenadayalu et al., 2012; English et al., 2002; Jones et al., 2003; Montano et al., 2008). An antiarrhythmic effect of testosterone has also been observed in a study that showed a lower incidence of early afterdepolarizations of cardiac myocytes in rabbits with physiologic testosterone levels compared with those with testosterone deficiency (Pham et al., 2002). Additionally, testosterone has been shown to shorten the length of the QTc interval and thereby decrease the duration of the cardiac myocyte action potential, likely because of the modulation of potassium channels (Brouillette et al., 2005; Herring et al., 2013).

Given the known effects of endogenous sex hormones on the function of the cardiovascular system, it is essential to identify the impact that exogenous sex hormones may have on this system. In the cisgender population, the use of exogenous estrogen as HRT has been associated with increases in blood pressure and the risk of venous thromboembolism (VTE) (Harvey et al., 2015; Martinez et al., 2020). The Women's Health Initiative, the first and largest randomized controlled trial examining the risk of VTE with the use of exogenous estrogen in cisgender female individuals, started a larger conversation on the cardiovascular risks posed by HRT, particularly in postmenopausal cisgender females over the age of 60 (Howard and Rossouw, 2013). In this study, researchers found evidence of an increased risk in peri- and postmenopausal cisgender females using combined estrogen and progesterone HRT. The VTE risk was about twice as high for those taking HRT compared with those on placebo (Cushman et al., 2004). A retrospective analysis of cisgender women in the United Kingdom who had a history of VTE also found the use of HRT to increase one's risk of VTE, with those on combined estrogen/progesterone preparations being at higher risk than those on conjugated equine estrogen preparations (Vinogradova et al., 2019). Several studies have found no increased risk of VTE with transdermal preparations of exogenous estrogen (Mohammed et al., 2015; Olié et al., 2010). In a large study of exogenous estrogen and thromboembolic risk in a cohort of postmenopausal cisgender female individuals aged 45–70, those using oral preparations of estrogen had an approximately four-fold increased risk of VTE. In contrast, those on transdermal preparations did not have an increased risk (Scarabin et al., 2003).

On the other hand, testosterone replacement therapy (TRT) for hypogonadal cisgender male individuals does not appear to increase the risk of major adverse cardiovascular events when used appropriately and with routine monitoring (Jones et al., 2011; Lincoff et al., 2023). Supraphysiologic levels of testosterone resulting from overreplacement, however, do increase the risk of cardiovascular morbidity by decreasing high-density lipoprotein (HDL) levels and reducing insulin sensitivity (Bhasin and Herbst, 2003). The use of GnRH agonists as ADT in cisgender male individuals for the treatment of prostate cancer has been associated with an increase in adverse cardiovascular outcomes, including stroke, VTE, and myocardial infarction (MI) (Greiman and Keane, 2017; Zhao et al., 2014). It should be noted that spironolactone, a commonly used mineralocorticoid antagonist with antiandrogen properties, has known cardiac remodeling and blood pressure effects and is regularly used in the treatment of hypertension and heart failure (Kosmas et al., 2018).

GAHT and the Cardiovascular System

While extensive literature examines the effects of HRT on the cardiovascular system in cisgender individuals, available data examining these effects with the use of GAHT in the TGD population remain sparse. A recent study that included 2,671 TGD individuals detected an increased risk of cardiovascular disease compared with cisgender controls; the investigators speculated that GAHT may contribute to some of this elevated risk (Glintborg et al., 2022). More specifically, when analyzing the cohort of TGD individuals on GAHT, transmasculine individuals were found to have higher rates of cardiovascular disease than cisgender males, but this effect was not seen when comparing transfeminine individuals with cisgender females. This increased risk was attributed, in part, to the changes in one's lipid profile that may occur with masculinizing GAHT. Socioeconomic status, known to be a social determinant of health, was not found to be a confounding risk factor in this study (Glintborg et al., 2022; Harper and Lynch, 2007).

Some studies examining cardiovascular risk in transfeminine individuals on GAHT, however, have also detected higher rates of cardiovascular disease compared with their cisgender counterparts. In a large Dutch study, transfeminine individuals died more frequently of cardiovascular disease than did cisgender individuals (de Blok et el., 2021). Of note, the study did not attribute this finding to the use of feminizing GAHT because the highest risk for mortality was determined to be from non-hormone-related causes of death. In a separate U.S.-based study, transfeminine individuals receiving feminizing GAHT were found to have an increased incidence of MI (Getahun et al., 2018). Despite the favorable changes that feminizing GAHT may have on one's lipid profile, some researchers have noted that trans women still have a higher cardiovascular risk than cisgender controls (Cocchetti et al., 2021; Masumori and Nakatsuka, 2023). It is therefore essential to better understand the mechanisms by which GAHT may confer these risks.

Cardiovascular disease is intimately linked to metabolic dysregulation, with dyslipidemia being a validated biomarker for cardiovascular morbidity and mortality. As previously noted, most studies have shown that feminizing GAHT may lead to a more favorable lipid profile, raising HDL, although it is sometimes accompanied by a rise in triglycerides (Leemaqz et al., 2023; Maraka et al., 2017; Streed et al., 2021). The literature surrounding the effect of GAHT on lipids is explored in greater detail in the metabolism section of this review. In terms of blood pressure, studies have suggested that feminizing GAHT may decrease systemic blood pressure, mirroring findings in the cisgender population (Sharula et al., 2012; Streed et al., 2021).

Another primary cardiovascular clinical outcome that has been studied in patients receiving feminizing GAHT has been that of VTE. Feminizing GAHT has been associated with a shift toward a more procoagulable serologic milieu (Cocchetti et al., 2022; Scheres et al., 2021). A large study in the United States showed an increased incidence of VTE and ischemic stroke in transfeminine individuals receiving feminizing GAHT compared with cisgender men and women (Getahun et al., 2018). The effect of the ROA of exogenous estrogen on VTE risk has been explored, with studies finding that transdermal preparations may not increase one's risk of VTE, possibly because of bypassing the first-pass effect through the liver (Ott et al., 2010; Slack and Safer, 2021). Thus, the risks and benefits of providing feminizing GAHT should be considered in the context of the individual's overall cardiometabolic health, and there is a need for more concrete scoring tools to help assess risk in these patients (Arrington-Sanders et al., 2023).

Compared with feminizing GAHT, there is less consensus regarding the effect of masculinizing GAHT on measures of cardiovascular health. Exogenous testosterone, like estrogen, may influence one's lipid profile, thereby potentially modulating one's risk of cardiovascular disease. Unlike estrogen, however, testosterone may result in a shift toward a less favorable lipid profile, increasing triglyceride and low-density lipoprotein (LDL) levels while decreasing HDL levels (Leemaqz et al., 2023; Maraka et al., 2017; van Velzen et al., 2019). These changes do not appear to be affected by variations in the ROA of testosterone. A meta-analysis has also shown that testosterone therapy can increase blood pressure (Masumori and Nakatsuka, 2023). However, consistent replication of this finding is lacking, and the clinical significance of this increase, if present, remains unknown (Elamin et al., 2010; Emi et al., 2008). The literature is conflicting concerning the effect of masculinizing GAHT on adverse cardiovascular outcomes (Martinez et al., 2020). Both a U.S.-based study and a Belgian study showed no significant difference in the risk of ischemic stroke or MI in transmasculine individuals compared with cisgender controls (Getahun et al., 2018; Wierckx et al., 2013). Other studies have reported higher rates of MI in transmasculine individuals compared with cisgender controls (Alzahrani et al., 2019; Nota et al., 2019).

Testosterone's association with erythrocytosis and the prevalence of adverse outcomes associated with erythrocytosis are explored further in the hematology section of this review. Despite these hematologic changes, studies have not shown an increased incidence of VTE in transmasculine individuals receiving masculinizing GAHT (Getahun et al., 2018; Nota et al., 2019; Wierckx et al., 2013).

Few studies have investigated the effect of GnRH agonist therapy on the cardiovascular system. The use of GnRH agonists in TGD youth may increase overall fat mass and decrease lean body mass, potentially impacting overall cardiovascular risk (Schagen et al., 2016). Given the rising use of these agents and their use at younger ages than in the past, more research is needed to determine whether there is an effect on long-term cardiovascular outcomes.

Adjunct antiandrogens, including cyproterone acetate (CPA) and spironolactone, and their effects on lipid profiles have been studied in TGD individuals. In a Canadian study comparing the effects of these two agents on transfeminine individuals' lipid profiles, spironolactone was associated with a higher HDL than CPA (Fung et al., 2016). This study did not find a significant difference in the total cholesterol, LDL, or triglyceride levels between these two agents. Other studies have shown that CPA may decrease HDL levels compared with baseline (Ott et al., 2011; Wierckx et al., 2014a).

Key Points:
1. Cisgender females have lower blood pressure, on average, and generally experience cardiovascular disease later than cisgender males.
2. Estrogen appears to have a cardioprotective role, exhibiting vasodilatory effects on the vascular system and protective effects on myocardial contractility.
3. Physiologic testosterone levels may be cardioprotective, inhibiting atherosclerosis, decreasing inflammation, and causing vasorelaxation.
4. Feminizing GAHT appears to decrease systemic blood pressure, whereas masculinizing GAHT may increase blood pressure.
5. The association between GAHT and cardiovascular morbidity and mortality remains unclear. Transfeminine individuals using exogenous estrogen may have an increased incidence of MI and ischemic stroke, although other cardiometabolic risk factors may cloud the effect of GAHT. There is even less consensus regarding the risk associated with exogenous testosterone use in transmasculine individuals, with most studies failing to demonstrate increased risk.
6. Differences in the ROA, preparation, and dose of both feminizing and masculinizing GAHT do not appear to affect biochemical or clinical measures of cardiovascular health, except transdermal estrogen, which does not seem to portend an increased risk of VTE.

HEMATOLOGIC SYSTEM

Sex Differences in the Hematologic System

The hematologic system consists of blood and bone marrow—the tissue found in the center of bones involved in the production of the cellular elements of blood, including red blood cells, white blood cells, and platelets. Sex differences in the proportions of the cellular components of blood have been established (Bain and England, 1975; Murphy et al., 2010; Segal and Moliterno, 2006). For example, many studies have noted that iron-replete cisgender females have a 12 percent lower mean hemoglobin level than age- and race-matched cisgender males (Murphy, 2014). There are multiple theories to explain this sexual dimorphism, with some proposing a variable effect of erythropoietin, a hormone that stimulates red blood cell production; other studies suggest that there are no differences in serum erythropoietin concentrations between the sexes (Tilling et al., 2013). Instead, this variation may be explained by the contrasting effects of estrogen and testosterone on the kidney vasculature, which affects the red cell mass (Murphy, 2014). Other studies have examined polymorphisms of the erythropoietin gene or its receptor (EPOR) as the cause of the dimorphism. EPOR alleles EPORA1 and EPORA10 were noted more often in cisgender females than in cisgender males, while the EPOR5 allele was more frequent in cisgender males (Zeng et al., 2001).

Recently, Cui and colleagues (2023) postulated that the latexin/microRNA-Thrombospondin 1 (Thbs1) signaling pathway may account for sexual dimorphism in the hematopoietic system. In a murine model of male hematopoietic stem cells (HSCs), the researchers found downregulation of Thbs1, which decreases latexin's ability to enhance apoptosis and thus decreases self-renewal of HSCs (Cui et al., 2023). Furthermore, testosterone is associated with the inhibition of hepcidin, an iron-regulating molecule produced in the liver. In turn, this reduces the inhibitory hold of hepcidin on the incorporation of iron into red blood cells, thereby promoting hematopoiesis (Bachman et al., 2010; Guo et al., 2013).

Sexual dimorphism is also seen in white blood cells and platelets (Bain, 1996). Regarding leukocytes, cisgender males of all ages have a higher white blood cell count than cisgender females (Chen et al., 2017). Cross-sectional data from 46,879 individuals revealed that premenopausal cisgender females have higher neutrophil percentages, lower lymphocyte percentages, and a higher neutrophil-to-lymphocyte ratio than cisgender males; however, this is reversed after the age of 50 (Chen et al., 2017). Studies suggest that estradiol decreases lymphocyte production in the bone marrow while increasing the time for neutrophil apoptosis, accounting for the variation with age (Medina et al., 2000; Molloy et al., 2003). Additionally, cisgender females have higher cluster of differentiation (CD)4 T cells and higher CD4-to-CD8 T cell ratios and mount a stronger adaptive immune response than do cisgender males (Klein and Flanagan, 2016). Castrated male mice show a similar CD4-to-CD8 pattern as female mice, suggesting this may be an androgen-mediated effect (Roden et al., 2004). The clinical implications of these observations are explored in greater detail in the immunology section of this review. Concerning platelets, there are differences between the sexes, with cisgender females having higher platelet counts than cisgender males and showing increased sensitivity to platelet agonists (Godwin et al., 2022; Segal and Moliterno, 2006; Sloan et al., 2015).

GAHT and the Hematologic System

GAHT can influence platelet numbers and activation. One study found that platelet levels increased in transfeminine individuals significantly after

1 year of GAHT and continued to increase through the fifth year of therapy (Allen et al., 2021). Another study, looking at 48 transfeminine individuals on estradiol patches and CPA and 47 transmasculine individuals on testosterone gel, showed a significant increase at 1 year in platelet activation factors in transfeminine individuals compared with baseline. At the same time, there were no changes in transmasculine individuals (Schutte et al., 2022). Another study confirmed that there is a shift toward a more hypercoagulable serologic milieu in transfeminine individuals after a year of GAHT. Again, there was no change for transmasculine individuals (Scheres et al., 2021).

The clinical significance of GAHT's effects on the hematologic system is mainly due to the concern for erythrocytosis in transmasculine individuals on testosterone and concern for thrombosis with both masculinizing and feminizing GAHT (Hembree et al., 2017; Safer and Tangpricha, 2019). A recent study of 6,670 transmasculine individuals, the largest to date to examine the prevalence of erythrocytosis in this population, found that only 8.4 percent had a hematocrit level of greater than 50 percent and less than 1 percent had a hematocrit level greater than 54 percent, a level at which therapy would be discontinued and phlebotomy considered (Krishnamurthy et al., 2023). Historically, smaller studies reported significant variation in the incidence of erythrocytosis, although the majority of studies did not demonstrate a higher risk of thromboembolic events for transmasculine individuals (Bunderen et al., 2022; Irwig, 2017; Madsen et al., 2021; Scheres et al., 2021). A longitudinal study by Madsen and colleagues (2021) involving 1,073 TGD individuals on masculinizing GAHT found that 11 percent experienced erythrocytosis, defined as a hematocrit level greater than 50 percent on at least two laboratory assessments. Additionally, 2.2 percent of the cohort had at least one hematocrit level greater than 54 percent, the level at which it is recommended that phlebotomy be initiated (Madsen et al., 2021). In a separate study of 519 transmasculine individuals receiving testosterone therapy, the authors found a 20 percent incidence of erythrocytosis, with 42 percent requiring a dosage reduction and 4.8 percent requiring phlebotomy (Oakes et al., 2021). A 0.9 percent incidence of thromboembolic events, including one ischemic stroke, was also reported. Notably, 80 percent of those with a thromboembolic event had erythrocytosis at any time; however, none had erythrocytosis at the time of diagnosis (Oakes et al., 2021). Other studies have reported a rate of erythrocytosis in transmasculine individuals seven times greater than that of matched cisgender males and 83 times higher than that of matched cisgender females (Antun et al., 2020).

Reports on the effect of the ROA of testosterone, as it portends to the risk of erythrocytosis, are conflicting. In the study of 6,670 individuals previously mentioned, investigators found a lower mean hematocrit level in those treated with transdermal testosterone than in those treated with intramuscular (IM) formulations but concluded that the levels of increase in hematocrit were unlikely to be clinically meaningful (Krishnamurthy et al., 2023). Earlier studies have had varied results. In one study, transmasculine individuals on testosterone undecanoate had a lower incidence of erythrocytosis than those on testosterone esters or gel (DeLoughery, 2022). In another, those on injectable testosterone enanthate had a 25 percent incidence of erythrocytosis, while those on testosterone undecanoate had a 17 percent incidence, and those on transdermal testosterone had no incidence at all (Nolan et al., 2021). In contrast, a study including 140 trans men found no variations in testosterone formulations, but there was a notable 10 percent phlebotomy rate and a high prevalence of 33 percent for erythrocytosis (Perez-Luis et al., 2019).

The contrasting effects of estrogen and testosterone on the hematologic system are seen in a study comparing 424 transmasculine and 559 transfeminine individuals with matched cisgender controls at three large integrated U.S. health care centers. Transmasculine individuals had increased hematocrit levels, closer to reference ranges for cisgender males, while transfeminine individuals had a drop in hematocrit levels, moving closer to reference ranges for cisgender females (Antun et al., 2020). Similarly, the European Network for the Investigation of Gender Incongruence cohort studied 340 transfeminine individuals treated with oral estradiol and adjunct androgen blockers and 265 transmasculine individuals treated with testosterone formulations. At year 1 of the 3-year follow-up, the average hematocrit levels in transmasculine individuals had increased from 41 to 46 percent. Conversely, at 3 months follow-up, the hematocrit of transfeminine individuals had decreased from 45 to 41 percent and remained stable after that (Defreyne et al., 2018). Studies in adolescents and young adults have also shown similar changes to hematocrit on GAHT (Olson-Kennedy et al., 2018). Of note, these studies show a low incidence of erythrocytosis in those on testosterone therapy, ranging from 7 to 11 percent (Antun et al., 2020; Defreyne et al., 2018; Krishnamurthy et al., 2023).

While prospective longitudinal studies are needed to confirm the relative safety of GAHT concerning hematologic parameters, it is important to note that the effects of estrogen on hematocrit, white blood cells, and platelets, while affected in the short term, soon stabilize at a new baseline. Similarly, novel research including thousands of transmasculine individuals shows a relatively low rate of erythrocytosis and an even smaller rate of clinically significant elevations in hematocrit at the level where intervention would be recommended.

Key Points:
1. Sex hormones contribute to sexual differentiation of the hematology system, resulting in cisgender males having a higher red cell mass and cisgender females having higher platelet counts and altered white blood cell concentrations, leading to a more robust adaptive immune response.

2. Exogenous testosterone use increases red cell mass, resulting in hematocrit levels in transmasculine individuals that are closer to the normal range of cisgender males. In contrast, exogenous estrogen use, through its suppression of testosterone, shifts the hematocrit of transfeminine individuals closer to levels of cisgender females.
3. The risk of erythrocytosis with the use of exogenous testosterone in transmasculine individuals remains low. It is further decreased with the use of transdermal compared with injectable testosterone, with most studies failing to observe an increased risk of thromboembolic events.
4. Exogenous estrogen may increase platelet activation factors and lead to a more prothrombotic serologic milieu in transfeminine individuals.

IMMUNE SYSTEM

Sex Differences in the Immune System

The immune system is the body's mechanism for eliminating foreign material, pathogens, and aberrant cell bodies. It is divided into two parts—innate and adaptive—that contain different cell types. The innate immune system is the body's first-line defense mechanism and consists of monocytes, which differentiate into dendritic cells and macrophages, natural killer cells, neutrophils, basophils, and eosinophils. The adaptive immune system provides "memory" immunity. It consists of T and B lymphocytes that differentiate after exposure to new pathogens. These pathogen-specific lymphocytes can mount more rapid responses during repeat infections. While these two systems are common to both sexes, differences in their function and efficiency exist between the sexes, suggesting sexual dimorphism in immunity. It is well established that cisgender females have more robust innate and adaptive immune systems than cisgender males, thereby mounting stronger responses to bacterial and viral infections (Dias et al., 2022; Jacobsen and Klein, 2021; Shepherd et al., 2021). Indeed, in murine models of the H1N1 virus, female mice showed higher levels of antigen-specific B cells and higher titers of antibodies (Fink et al., 2018; Wilkinson et al., 2022). This difference in immunity may explain why, among HIV-positive patients, viral loads are usually lower in cisgender females than in cisgender males (Klein and Flanagan, 2016; Ziegler and Altfeld, 2016). However, more robust immune responses also predispose cisgender females to autoimmune conditions such as systemic lupus erythematosus and multiple sclerosis (Angum et al., 2020; Jacobsen and Klein, 2021). Conversely, while cisgender males experience lower rates of autoimmune conditions, they are more susceptible to pathogenic infections and have higher rates of cancer (Shepherd et al., 2021; Trigunaite et al., 2015). The biological basis for these differences is multifaceted, attributable to genetic and hormonal differences between the sexes (Klein and Flanagan, 2016). This review will focus on how sex steroid hormones modulate the immune system.

Estrogen is found in both sexes but is generally higher in cisgender females, particularly during pregnancy and the days preceding ovulation. It acts on several types of estrogen receptors—most notably ERα and ERβ—that are expressed differentially according to age and sex (Dias et al., 2022). Therefore, immunological differences related to estrogen are attributed to variations in hormone and receptor levels (Klein and Flanagan, 2016). Extant studies suggest that estrogen has bipotential effects on immune cells. Physiological levels of estrogen are associated with increased production of proinflammatory cytokines and a Th1-type response. Supraphysiological levels are associated with anti-inflammatory responses, such as increased production of anti-inflammatory cytokines and a shift toward a Th2-type response (Kovats, 2015; Straub, 2007). Indeed, an in vitro experiment with human-derived monocytes showed maximal and decreased IL-1 activity with physiological and supraphysiological estrogen levels, respectively (Polan et al., 1988). The effects of estrogen vary according to its concentration, but a complete lack of the hormone leads to dampened immune responses. This was observed in a murine model wherein ovariectomized mice experienced increased mortality from *Helicobacter pylori* infection, and estrogen replacement in these mice was associated with improved outcomes (Ohtani et al., 2007). In addition to conferring protection against infections, estrogen may increase the risk of developing autoimmune conditions (Klein and Flanagan, 2016). One explanation for this is the inverse association between estrogen signaling and the expression of regulatory T cells (Treg), which are important for preventing autoimmunity. Prior research has shown that deletion of ERα in T cells is associated with higher levels of Tregs (Mohammad et al., 2018).

Circulating testosterone is also present in both sexes, generally in much higher concentrations in cisgender males. It exerts its effect on the immune system through androgen receptors. Testosterone is associated with anti-inflammatory effects, observed in both animal experiments and clinical settings. In vivo exposure of mice to testosterone has been associated with decreased natural killer (NK) cell activity and lowered macrophage expression of toll-like receptor 4 (TLR4) (Hou and Zheng, 1988; Rettew et al., 2008). In female mice, exposure to testosterone has been associated with decreased secretion of interferon-gamma (IFNγ) by NK cells (Lotter et al., 2013). Clinically, cisgender male individuals who have rheumatoid arthritis, an autoimmune condition, have lower amounts of serum testosterone, and those who have androgen deficiencies have higher levels of proinflammatory cytokines (Liu et al., 2023; Malkin et al., 2004). It is notable, however, that androgens have differential effects on immune cells depending on sex. For example, in an in vitro study examining the effects of dihydrotestosterone (DHT) on human monocytes, DHT was associated with diminished IL-6 and tumor necrosis factor alpha (TNFα) responses in male-derived monocytes, but this effect was not seen in female-derived monocytes (de Bree et al., 2018). Finally, testosterone has also been shown to increase the expression of the FOXP3 transcription factor, which is a positive regulator of Tregs (Walecki et al., 2015). This partially explains the lower rates of autoimmune diseases found among cisgender males. While much is known about the biological underpinnings of sexual dimorphism in immunity, less is known about how hormone therapy used for gender affirmation among TGD individuals affects their immune systems. It is reassuring, however, that existing literature suggests hormone therapy among TGD individuals likely has similar immunological effects as do endogenous hormones among cisgender individuals.

GAHT and the Immune System

Extant literature on immunity in TGD individuals suggests that exogenous estrogen and gender-affirming procedures that affect androgen-producing organs may have proinflammatory effects. For example, oral estrogen has been associated with increased inflammatory markers among transfeminine individuals (Wilson et al., 2009). However, the hormone's proinflammatory effects were absent in individuals utilizing transdermal estrogen. It is unclear whether this difference is attributed to the ROA, differences in hormone levels, or both. It is also unclear whether this difference has any clinical significance. In a case report of new-onset lupus nephritis in a transfeminine individual who received a gonadectomy, the authors reported that the patient—who had been on exogenous estrogen and antiandrogen therapy for 9 years before their surgery—developed symptoms suggestive of an autoimmune pathology approximately 1 year after their surgery (Pontes et al., 2018). After further workup, they were confirmed to have lupus nephritis. The authors noted that this case echoed results from a study on systemic lupus erythematosus in murine models. Specifically, male mice that were castrated before estrogen administration developed more severe disease outcomes than those not castrated (Roubinian et al., 1978). This is likely attributable to decreased testosterone levels in the former group. In all, these studies suggest that the effects of gender-affirming estrogen therapy on a TGD individual's immune system depend on its dosage, ROA, and whether the patient has undergone any surgical procedure that affects androgen production.

Current studies on gender-affirming testosterone therapy and immunity suggest that the hormone may also have immunosuppressive effects on TGD individuals. One study showed that transmasculine individuals on testosterone had significantly higher levels of Treg cells than those of cisgender females (Robinson et al., 2022). Upon further investigation, the authors noted significant transcriptome changes related to Treg cell expression. These results suggest that, in theory, TGD individuals using testosterone may have dampened immune systems. However, the clinical significance of these results is unclear, as more research is needed to understand whether this differential Treg cell expression among TGD individuals will necessarily lead to adverse immunological outcomes.

The impact of hormone therapy on TGD patients' immune systems necessitates more attention. Based on the current literature, clinicians prescribing estrogen therapy for TGD patients may wish to monitor for autoimmune diseases, especially if the patients have had their gonads removed. Similarly, clinicians may want to watch for signs of immunosuppression among TGD patients receiving testosterone therapy. However, given the lack of data on this topic and the profound known mental and physical benefits of gender-affirming hormone therapy, immunological considerations should not preclude clinicians from prescribing these medications to TGD patients.

Key Points:
1. Sexual differentiation of the immune system results in cisgender females having more robust innate and adaptive immune systems, leading to decreased susceptibility to pathogenic infections and a greater propensity for autoimmunity compared with cisgender males.
2. Estrogen's effect on immune cells depends on its concentration, with deficiency leading to dampened immune response, physiologic levels associated with a proinflammatory state, and supraphysiologic levels associated with anti-inflammatory responses. Conversely, testosterone is associated with anti-inflammatory effects irrespective of concentration.
3. Exogenous estrogen is associated with increased markers of inflammation in transfeminine individuals. However, this may depend on the first-pass effect through the liver, as these changes are not seen with transdermal estrogen.
4. Exogenous testosterone use in transmasculine individuals may result in a dampened immune response, although an association with adverse clinical outcomes has yet to be observed.

METABOLISM

Sex Differences in Metabolism

Metabolism refers to the chemical reactions in the body that allow for energy production. Carbohydrates and lipids are the primary sources of energy in the body, with protein serving as a source of energy during states of starvation. Sexual dimorphism in metabolism begins at conception, as male and female reproductive cells differ vastly in their use of energy. The male gamete, sperm, requires energy for motility to reach the female gamete, the oocyte, which dedicates its mitochondria to the zygote to nurture life after fertilization (Mauvais-Jarvis, 2015). Sex differences in the production and use of energy continue throughout development and into adulthood.

Glucose, a carbohydrate, serves as the primary source of energy in the human body, and complex mechanisms are in place to maintain glucose homeostasis. There is evidence that sexual dimorphism exists in this fundamental process. For example, a study showed that fasting and postprandial glucose were higher in elderly cisgender females than in elderly cisgender males, despite endogenous glucose production rates not differing between the two groups (Basu et al., 2006). This differentiation may be due, in part, to the direct effects of both sex hormones on glucose metabolism. ERα-deficient mice are more insulin resistant, as evidenced by their higher hepatic glucose production (Mauvais-Jarvis et al., 2013). Additionally, estrogen has been shown to affect glucose uptake in skeletal cells by modulating the level of GLUT4, a transporter that regulates insulin-stimulated glucose uptake (Campbell and Febbraio, 2022; Mauvais-Jarvis et al., 2013). Similarly, testosterone increases GLUT4-mediated glucose uptake and decreases insulin resistance by increasing lipolysis and stimulating mitochondrial function (Grossmann, 2014; Mitsuhashi et al., 2016). States of impaired glucose metabolism, such as diabetes mellitus, provide an opportunity to explore the potential clinical effects of sex hormones on glycemic control.

Type 2 diabetes mellitus (T2DM) is particularly important from an epidemiologic standpoint as the prevalence of this already common disease is expected to increase over the next decade (Saeedi et al., 2019). Differences in the rate of diagnoses, complications, and even response to diabetes medications exist between the sexes (Kautzky-Willer et al., 2023). Estrogen is thought to be protective against T2DM, as demonstrated by the increased risk of T2DM in cisgender females who have primary ovarian insufficiency and the apparent ability to delay or prevent the development of T2DM when exogenous estrogen is given as HRT for postmenopausal cisgender females (Anagnostis et al., 2019; Mauvais-Javis et al., 2017). Testosterone deficiency in cisgender males is also a risk factor for T2DM, while testosterone excess is reported to be associated with the development of T2DM in cisgender females (Kautzky-Willer et al., 2023). It should be noted, however, that the latter conclusions were drawn from studies including cisgender females with polycystic ovarian syndrome (PCOS), individuals who are at higher risk for metabolic syndrome at baseline.

In addition to carbohydrate metabolism, there are known sex differences in fat metabolism and distribution. Cisgender males tend to distribute fat in the abdominal region (android distribution), while cisgender females generally distribute fat in the gluteal-femoral region (gynoid distribution). Generally, cisgender females tend to have higher amounts of body fat compared with cisgender males throughout their lifespans, but cisgender males have higher amounts of visceral adipose tissue (Blaak, 2001; Karastergiou et al., 2012). These differences become prominent during puberty, suggesting that the pubertal surge of sex hormones contributes to this observed dimorphism (Hattori et al., 2004; Maynard et al., 2001). Indeed, adipocytes have estrogen and androgen receptors, and sex hormones likely play a role in lipolysis, lipoprotein lipase expression, and leptin secretion (Karastergiou et al., 2012). Additionally, conditions that result in variations in the concentration of sex hormones have also been shown to modify fat distribution patterns. For example, menopause and PCOS, conditions of estrogen deficiency and androgen excess, respectively, often result in a shift toward a more android fat distribution in cisgender females (Carmina et al., 2007; Toth et al., 2000).

Notably, the sexual dimorphism of fat distribution may also have clinical implications. The gynoid distribution has been found to be protective for diabetes, cardiovascular risk, and overall mortality (Carey et al., 1997; Folsom et al., 1993; Lapidus et al., 1984). It has also been shown that if cisgender females develop a more android distribution of fat, they may develop metabolic complications at a rate similar to that of cisgender males (Jensen, 2008). The increased visceral adiposity seen in cisgender males has been linked to abnormal metabolic parameters, including elevated triglyceride and postprandial insulin levels (Muscogiuri et al., 2023).

Obesity, a chronic disease resulting in excessive body fat and associated with a wide variety of cardiometabolic complications, is a global epidemic that manifests differently between the sexes. Globally, obesity rates are higher in cisgender females than in cisgender males (Cooper et al., 2021). Animal models and clinical research explain why this might be. In addition to shifting body fat toward a more android distribution, states of estrogen deficiency, such as in cisgender females experiencing menopause, are associated with increased body weight and adiposity (Lovejoy et al., 2009). Mechanistically, this may be due to modifications in one's central regulation of hunger and baseline energy expenditure (Clegg et al., 2007; Lovejoy et al., 2008). In contrast, murine models have shown that when exposed to a high-fat diet, male mice generate more proinflammatory markers than female mice (Singer et al., 2015).

Carbohydrate Metabolism

Several studies have found differences in the prevalence of T2DM in TGD individuals compared with their cisgender counterparts. These include a Belgian study that observed a higher prevalence of T2DM in TGD individuals irrespective of gender and a U.S.-based study that observed a higher prevalence of T2DM in transfeminine compared with cisgender female but not cisgender male individuals (Islam et al., 2022; Wierckx et al., 2014a). In the latter study, no differences were observed between transmasculine and cisgender individuals, whether cisgender males or cisgender females. Importantly, investigators did not attribute these findings solely to GAHT use, given the complex and multifactorial pathogenesis of T2DM. It is also important to note that the differences between studies may be attributed, in part, to differences in baseline population prevalence. Indeed, other studies, including a Dutch study comparing the prevalence of T2DM in the TGD population with that of the cisgender population, have not observed any differences (van Velzen et al., 2022). Importantly, these studies did not conduct a subgroup analysis to determine if there is a difference in T2DM prevalence based on ROA, preparation, or dosage of GAHT.

Given the potential for confounders when studying T2DM at the population level, translational science can be informative. Several studies have investigated the relationship between GAHT and biochemical markers of insulin resistance. An early study of 31 TGD individuals suggested that GAHT for both transfeminine and transmasculine individuals leads to insulin resistance by demonstrating decreased glucose utilization during a hyperinsulinemic–euglycemic clamp after 4 months of GAHT (Polderman et al., 1994). Another study of 37 TGD individuals showed increased fasting insulin and insulin resistance as measured by glucose utilization in transfeminine subjects but not in transmasculine individuals (Elbers et al., 2003). These findings were confirmed in a more recent study in which transfeminine individuals were noted to have higher fasting insulin levels than their cisgender counterparts, suggesting a propensity for insulin resistance in transfeminine individuals (Deischinger et al., 2022). The Homeostatic Model Assessment for Insulin Resistance (HOMA-IR), a method of assessing beta cell function and insulin resistance using fasting glucose and insulin levels, has also been studied in the TGD population. A higher HOMA-IR is indicative of more insulin resistance (Bonora et al., 2002). More recent studies have not shown that masculinizing GAHT causes a significant difference in the HOMA-IR when compared with cisgender males (Gava et al., 2018; Shadid et al., 2019). In contrast, patients receiving feminizing GAHT have been shown to have higher HOMA-IR indices and fasting insulin levels compared with cisgender females (Colizzi et al., 2015; Shadid et al., 2020). Taken together, the extant literature suggests that feminizing GAHT may impair glucose metabolism, as indicated by trends in qualified biomarkers. However, available data are in discordance, and the clinical implications of these trends remain unknown.

Lipid Metabolism

In a meta-analysis of 26 studies investigating the effect of GAHT on body composition and fat distribution, individuals on masculinizing GAHT gained lean mass and lost fat mass. In contrast, those on feminizing GAHT gained fat mass and lost lean mass (Spanos et al., 2020). Importantly, while overall fat mass is lost with masculinizing GAHT, an increase in visceral abdominal fat has been observed (Elbers et al., 1997). A U.S.-based study also found that among those receiving GAHT, body mass index (BMI) increased in transfeminine individuals but not in transmasculine individuals. However, psychosocial and lifestyle factors likely contributed to this finding (Suppakitjanusant et al., 2020). More recent studies have noted that the size of adipose cells increases in transfeminine individuals and decreases in transmasculine individuals (Shah et al., 2022).

GAHT-driven changes in body composition are explored in more detail in the bone and body composition section of this review, but it is important to note here that these changes appear to occur in tandem with changes to the lipid profile. Both feminizing and masculinizing GAHT have been associated with changes in lipid profiles. While feminizing GAHT has been linked to an increase in HDL, masculinizing GAHT has shown the opposite effect, and both regimens have been linked to a rise in triglyceride levels (Elbers et al., 2003; Leemaqz et al., 2023; Maraka et al., 2017). For feminizing GAHT, this effect may be modified by the ROA, as a meta-analysis showed that oral estrogen increased triglyceride levels, while transdermal estrogen decreased triglyceride levels (Maraka et al., 2017). There were no comparisons made between ROAs for masculinizing GAHT. Notably, some researchers have observed that changes in lipid profiles were not associated with changes in markers of insulin resistance (Elbers et al., 2003). While the cardiovascular implications of GAHT are explored elsewhere in this review, more research is needed to investigate whether the observed changes in lipid profile and fat distribution are associated with cardiovascular morbidity and mortality rates and whether the ROA, preparation, or dosage of GAHT affects lipid parameters.

Key Points:

1. Sex hormones play a central role in the sexual dimorphism observed in human metabolism, with estrogen being linked to modulating energy expenditure and central control of food intake, and both estrogen and testosterone contributing to insulin sensitivity and glucose uptake.

2. Estrogen deficiency in cisgender females and testosterone deficiency in cisgender males have been associated with increased rates of T2DM. Conversely, syndromes of testosterone excess in cisgender females are associated with increased rates of T2DM.

3. Sex hormones contribute to sex differences in body fat distribution, with the gynoid distribution in cisgender females being protective against cardiometabolic disease.

4. Biomarkers of impaired glucose metabolism may increase with feminizing GAHT, and T2DM may be more common in transfeminine individuals compared with cisgender females. However, the explanation is likely multifactorial, and the contribution of feminizing GAHT remains unknown.

5. Masculinizing GAHT results in a gain of lean mass and loss of fat mass, whereas feminizing GAHT results in a loss of lean mass and an increase of fat mass.

6. Exogenous estrogen use in transfeminine individuals may contribute to a more favorable lipid profile by raising HDL. In contrast, exogenous testosterone use in transmasculine individuals may contribute to a less favorable lipid profile by raising triglycerides and LDL while decreasing HDL. Importantly, given the discordance in the literature, consensus has not been reached in this area.

GASTROINTENSTINAL SYSTEM

Sex Differences in the Gastrointestinal System

The gastrointestinal (GI) system consists of the alimentary tract and the accessory organs necessary to break down and absorb nutrients. The alimentary tract starts at the mouth; includes the esophagus, stomach, small intestine, and large intestine; and ends at the anus. The accessory organs of the GI system include the salivary glands, gallbladder, pancreas, and liver. There are noted sexual dimorphisms of the GI system. For example, cisgender males and cisgender females have different gut microbiomes, and differences in the microbiome are thought to occur during puberty (Sisk-Hackworth, 2023). Sexual dimorphisms are also found in the pancreas. For example, glucose-stimulated insulin secretion is higher in cisgender females than in cisgender males, which may be attributed to sex-specific regulation of pancreatic beta cells (McEwan et al., 2021).

The liver is a vital target organ for both sex hormones. Estrogen and testosterone are thought to have a role in fat and glucose metabolism in the liver. For example, lower levels of both testosterone and estrogen are risk factors for nonalcoholic fatty liver disease (NAFLD) (Kasarinaite et al., 2023). As such, HRT may play a role in improving NAFLD. Indeed, one study demonstrated that postmenopausal cisgender females receiving exogenous estrogen had lower levels of detectable liver enzymes in the blood. These changes were attributed to a reduction in fat content in the liver (McKenzie et al., 2006). Similarly, cisgender males receiving exogenous IM testosterone experienced a reduction in hepatic fat as measured by MRI (Apostolov et al., 2022).

Exogenous estrogen affects the production of liver proteins, such as angiotensinogen and coagulation factors (von Schoultz, 2009). The increase in production of procoagulant factors is one of the reasons that exogenous oral estrogen, which undergoes first-pass metabolism in the liver, is associated with VTE (Abou-Ismail et al., 2020). Oral estrogen and the use of anabolic androgenic steroids have also been associated with hepatic neoplasms, such as hepatic adenomas and hepatocellular carcinoma (Khalid et al., 2023; Lizardi-Cervera et al., 2006). CPA, an antiandrogen agent, is also associated with hepatotoxicity (Chitturi and Farrell, 2013).

Exogenous estrogen is a risk factor for gallstone formation. Studies have found that cisgender females using exogenous estrogen, both oral and transdermal, had higher rates of gallbladder disease, including cholelithiasis and cholecystitis (Cirillo et al., 2005; Uhler et al., 1998). This may be due to estrogen slowing gallbladder motility and increasing the formation of cholesterol crystals (Uhler et al., 1998). Exogenous testosterone has been shown to decrease gallbladder motility in animal models, although the clinical significance of this has yet to be determined (Kline and Karpinski, 2008). In a large Swedish study, estrogen used as HRT in cisgender females was associated with an increased risk of pancreatitis, possibly due to estrogen's effect of increasing triglyceride production in the liver and decreasing pancreatic enzyme secretion (Oskarsson et al., 2014). This risk was not further stratified by ROA, dosage, or preparation.

GAHT and the Gastrointestinal System

Several studies have investigated the effects of GAHT on liver enzymes with discordant findings. A U.S.-based study found that masculinizing GAHT increased the levels of alanine aminotransferase (ALT) and aspartate aminotransferase (AST), enzymes found in high levels in the liver that can serve as surrogates for liver damage; feminizing GAHT had no apparent effect on liver enzyme levels (Hashemi et al., 2021). This study controlled for factors such as BMI and alcohol use. A large Dutch study found that feminizing GAHT decreased ALT and AST levels, while masculinizing GAHT increased ALT and AST levels (Boekhout-Berends et al., 2023). However, a limitation of both studies was that the findings were not further stratified by hormone ROA, preparation, or dosage. Another Belgian study found that IM testosterone increased ALT and AST levels, oral estrogen decreased ALT and AST levels, and transdermal estrogen decreased AST levels but had no significant impact on ALT levels (Wierckx et al., 2014a). A smaller study found that both masculinizing and feminizing GAHT did not have any significant effect on liver enzyme levels (Fernandez and Tannock, 2016). A sizeable European-based study noted no substantial evidence of liver injury in TGD individuals on either masculinizing or feminizing GAHT, despite reported changes in liver enzyme levels (Stangl et al., 2021). The clinical significance of these biochemical changes therefore remains unknown.

In a case report of a transfeminine individual on oral estrogen who developed gallstone-induced pancreatitis, the authors proposed that the use of estrogen for feminizing GAHT was linked to gallstone development (Freirer et al., 2021). Several reports have associated the use of estrogen for feminizing GAHT with hypertriglyceridemia-induced pancreatitis as well (Shipley et al., 2020; Tirthani et al., 2021). There is a need for more extensive clinical studies investigating whether transfeminine individuals using feminizing GAHT experience higher rates of pancreatic and gallbladder disease. In the extant literature, case studies report the use of testosterone for masculinizing GAHT and hepatobiliary malignancies, namely hepatocellular carcinoma and cholangiocarcinoma (Pothuri et al., 2023). Larger studies are needed to better understand whether there is a casual association between masculinizing GAHT and hepatobiliary malignancies.

Key Points:
1. Sex differences are present throughout the GI system, particularly regarding the gut microbiome and the liver.
2. Estrogen deficiency in cisgender females and testosterone deficiency in cisgender males are associated with increased risk of NAFLD, findings that are potentially reversible with hormone replacement.
3. Exogenous estrogen has been associated with gallbladder disease and pancreatitis, and both exogenous estrogen and testosterone have been associated with hepatic neoplasms in the cisgender population, findings that, outside of case reports, have not been demonstrated in the TGD population.
4. Masculinizing GAHT may increase levels of hepatocellular liver enzymes in transmasculine individuals, whereas feminizing GAHT may either decrease these levels or have a neutral effect in transfeminine individuals. The clinical significance of these changes is unknown.

ENDOCRINE SYSTEM

Sex Differences in the Endocrine System

The endocrine system comprises glands that produce hormones to influence various bodily functions and is regulated by a complex series of hormonal feedback mechanisms. Aside from the hypothalamic-pituitary-gonadal (HPG) axis, which is most obviously influenced by sex hormones being that they are predominately produced in the gonads, estrogen and testosterone are also known to affect the GH, thyroid, and adrenal axes.

Pituitary

The pituitary gland, often referred to as the "master" gland, produces various hormones that primarily regulate the activity of other hormone-secreting glands throughout the body.

Pituitary glands tend to be larger in cisgender females than in cisgender males (Pecina et al., 2017). This may be due to differences in the hormonal milieu throughout adolescence that influence the growth of the pituitary gland itself (MacMaster et al., 2007). Sex hormones have well-known, suppressive effects on gonadotropic cells in the pituitary gland by providing feedback inhibition to the HPG axis.

Research has shown that sex hormones may also impact other pituitary cell types differentially. Somatotrophs, which produce GH, are stimulated by testosterone, thought to be via the local aromatization of estrogen (Birzniece et al., 2010). In one case report, a patient with Klinefelter syndrome who was receiving exogenous testosterone was found to have a somatotrophinoma (Fang et al., 2016). While these observations are provocative, further research is needed to delineate the association between a commonly used therapy and an exceedingly rare disease. Estrogen has also been associated with pituitary cell proliferation. In one study, estrogen treatment was found to have a suppressive effect on ERβ, a receptor that inhibits pituitary cell proliferation. This downregulation of ERβ subsequently reduced the expression of *PTEN*, a tumor-suppressor gene, in pituitary cells (Perez et al., 2018). Similarly, estrogen can stimulate the production and secretion of prolactin, in part by causing lactotroph cells to proliferate, while also inhibiting dopamine-releasing cells, which typically downregulate the production of prolactin (Cunha et al., 2015).

Growth Hormone

In concert with the sex hormones, GH is critical to normal growth, development, and metabolism. Regarding metabolism, GH can increase lipolysis, circulating glucose levels, and protein synthesis (Møller and Jørgensen, 2009). Deficiencies in either GH, estrogen, or testosterone all result in a similar phenotype of insulin resistance, low muscle mass, and fat deposition in the liver (Fernández-Pérez et al., 2016). There is sexual dimorphism in the secretion of GH itself that is influenced by the presence of estrogen and testosterone. Male rats have been found to have more infrequent pulses of GH with higher amplitudes than female rats, and females tend to have a higher baseline level of GH than males (Mode and Gustafsson, 2006). This influences the downstream pathways of IGF-1 secretion, which is regulated by the JAK2-STAT5 system. Male pattern GH secretion tends to stimulate increased expression of growth-promoting pathways (such as IGF-1), leading to more overall body growth in mice. Mouse models have also shown that STAT5b is linked to male body growth, specifically, while STAT5a affects the growth of both sexes, indicating that estrogen is essential for growth and development irrespective of sex (Fernández-Pérez et al., 2016; Lichanska and Waters, 2008).

Studies have shown that the use of exogenous sex hormones impacts GH. Oral estrogen has been shown to increase GH binding protein and inhibit IGF-1 messenger RNA (mRNA) expression in the liver. Due to decreased feedback inhibition secondary to the decline in IGF-1 levels, concentrations of GH then increase. Additionally, oral estrogen reduces levels of the IGF-binding protein complex, reducing circulating IGF-1 levels (Kam et al., 2000). These effects are not seen with transdermal estrogen, probably due to avoiding the first-pass effect through the liver (Leung et al., 2004; Weissberger et al., 1991). In cisgender males with hypogonadism, exogenous testosterone appears to have a synergistic effect with GH on protein metabolism, resulting in increased protein synthesis and decreased breakdown (Gibney et al., 2005). It is also worth noting that the liver, the target organ of GH, is also influenced by sex hormones, with hepatocytes having receptors for both estrogens and androgens. Sexual dimorphism in hepatocyte gene expression has been observed, and differential concentrations of sex hormones between the sexes also affect how the liver responds to GH (Fernández-Pérez et al., 2016).

Thyroid

Thyroid hormone plays a role in the concentrations of sex hormones by indirectly increasing levels of sex hormone–binding globulin (Selva and Hammond, 2009). As is therefore expected, thyroid dysfunction has been associated with abnormalities in the concentrations of sex hormones (Bates et al., 2020; Gabrielson et al., 2019).

All three estrogen receptor forms have been found in human thyroid tissue. It is thought that ERα plays a role in cell proliferation while ERβ promotes apoptosis (Santin and Furlanetto, 2011). This finding has prompted researchers to investigate the role of these receptors in neoplastic thyroid cells and whether neoplastic thyroid cells may have a higher ratio of ERα expression than ERβ (Chen et al., 2008; Kumar et al., 2010; Rajoria et al., 2010). Indeed, one study found increased ERα expression compared with ERβ in papillary thyroid cancer cells (Qiu et al., 2019). Androgen receptors are also found in both normal and malignant thyroid tissue. Thus, like estrogen, researchers have postulated that testosterone may play a role in abnormal thyroid cell proliferation, although further research is needed (Magri et al., 2012; Stanley et al., 2012). Oral estrogen also increases thyroid-binding globulin (TBG) levels because of first-pass metabolism through the liver (Fernández-Pérez et al., 2016). In euthyroid individuals, this does not affect the steady state of thyroid hormone; however, in hypothyroid individuals, the use of oral estrogen may change the necessary doses of thyroid hormone replacement (Mazer, 2004).

Adrenal

Sexual dimorphism of both the overall size of the adrenal glands and the size of the different adrenal cortex zones have been reported in the literature (Bielohbuby et al., 2007). In murine models, female mice have also been shown to have higher adrenal cell turnover than males, potentially related to circulating gonadal androgens (Grabek et al., 2019). Both androgen and estrogen receptors are found throughout adrenal tissue, and there is evidence that the gonadal hormones play a direct role in adrenal steroidogenesis. This concept has been particularly well studied as it pertains to glucocorticoid production. Estrogen stimulates steroidogenesis in the adrenal glands, whereas testosterone may inhibit said production (Nowak et al., 1995). Clinically, many diseases of the adrenal cortex, such as hypercortisolism due to cortisol-secreting adrenal adenomas and adrenocortical carcinomas, affect females disproportionately (Lyraki and Schedl, 2021). Given the purported effects of estrogens and androgens on the adrenal gland, it seems plausible that varying concentrations of sex hormones between the sexes may contribute to the pathogenesis of adrenal disease. Oral exogenous estrogen increases cortisol-binding globulin (CBG) and total cortisol levels. However, free cortisol levels are generally unchanged or, as in one study, lower (Brien, 1975; Qureshi et al., 2007). This effect is not seen with the use of transdermal estrogen (Qureshi et al., 2007). Spironolactone, a mineralocorticoid antagonist with antiandrogen properties, can occasionally result in excessive mineralocorticoid antagonism, resulting in electrolyte abnormalities and dehydration, which requires providers to be vigilant for side effects.

GAHT and the Endocrine System

Pituitary

Several case studies and case series have reported on occurrences of pituitary adenomas, both secretory and nonsecretory, in the TGD population (Cunha et al., 2015; Kleinschmidt-DeMasters, 2020; Nota et al., 2018; Roerink et al., 2014). Historically, exogenous estrogen has been associated with the development of hyperprolactinemia in transfeminine individuals, prompting the Endocrine Society to recommend periodic monitoring of prolactin levels in this population (Hembree et al., 2017). However, studies that have observed an association between exogenous estrogen use and rising prolactin included patients who were also using CPA as an adjunctive antiandrogen, indicating that this agent may be stimulating prolactin levels (Cunha et al., 2015; Nota et al., 2018; Raven et al., 2021). Indeed, observational data in patients using exogenous estrogen and spironolactone for feminizing GAHT have generally not been associated with elevated prolactin levels (Bisson et al., 2018; Fung et al., 2016).

In a study investigating the prevalence of pituitary adenomas in TGD individuals, three adenomas were identified among 1,373 transfeminine individuals—one prolactinoma and two somatotrophinomas (Nota et al., 2018). The prevalence of prolactinoma was not higher than the expected rate. Conversely, the two cases of somatotrophinoma would represent a significant increase from the expected prevalence, given the rarity of these tumors. As previously noted, it has been proposed that testosterone may have a stimulatory effect on somatotrophs (Nota et al., 2018; Roerink et al., 2014).

Growth Hormone

The influence of GAHT on the GH axis has mainly been assessed in the context of pubertal growth and the use of GnRH agonists. As previously noted, GH and sex hormones work in tandem to support one's growth and development. The contribution of sex hormones is clear in TGD youth who receive GnRH agonists and experience delayed skeletal growth and less change to body composition despite having an intact GH axis (Roberts and Carswell, 2021). The effect of GnRH agonists on growth and body composition is discussed in greater detail in the bone and body composition section of this review. Researchers have shown that, in transfeminine individuals who used GnRH agonists and were later transitioned to feminizing GAHT, there may be a dose-dependent effect on height, such that higher doses of estrogen may help achieve height patterns similar to cisgender females (Boogers et al., 2022; Hembree et al., 2017). The use of aromatase inhibitors or nonaromatizable agents (DHT or oxandrolone) has been considered in specific populations, such as in patients with Turner syndrome, to help augment gain in height (Keenan et al., 1993; Wickman et al., 2001; Wit and Oostdijk, 2015). There is not yet strong enough evidence to support the use of these agents in transmasculine patients to help achieve taller heights, although this is an area of active research (Grimstad et al., 2021).

Thyroid

As previously noted, sex hormones influence the levels of TBG in the body. One study suggests that the prevalence of hypothyroidism in the TGD population is higher than that in the cisgender population. However, these findings were observed in a cohort of just 54 TGD patients (Christensen et al., 2021). To date, no large study has evaluated how GAHT influences thyroid function. New evidence is emerging that those receiving feminizing GAHT have a higher prevalence of thyroid cancer. However, how much of this prevalence may be due to GAHT itself remains unknown (Christensen et al., 2023). No studies have investigated whether masculinizing GAHT affects the incidence of thyroid cancer.

Adrenal

In a study investigating whether GAHT affected cortisol levels in TGD individuals, 18 TGD individuals underwent an adrenocorticotropic hormone (ACTH) stimulation test before and after initiation of GAHT (Sofer et al., 2024). Total basal serum cortisol was noted to be increased in transfeminine individuals following initiation of GAHT, as expected, because of exogenous estrogen increasing levels of CBG. In both transmasculine and cisgender male individuals, however, ACTH-stimulated serum cortisol levels decreased. A separate study similarly noted an overall reduction in cortisol levels after starting GAHT (Colizzi et al., 2013). The literature is somewhat discordant, however, with one study showing that feminizing GAHT increased ACTH and cortisol secretion while masculinizing GAHT decreased ACTH and cortisol secretion (Fuss et al., 2019).

The link between adrenal androgens and feminizing GAHT has also been investigated. In one study, transfeminine individuals using estradiol and CPA for feminizing GAHT had adrenal androgens measured at baseline and up to 4 years of follow-up. They found that levels of adrenal androgens were suppressed after 3 months and remained suppressed through 4 years. This suppression persisted with the cessation of CPA for patients who received a gonadectomy (Cocchetti et al., 2022). This finding may be due to the LH suppression by CPA and estradiol. CPA has also been shown in some cases to cause cortisol suppression in adults and has been studied alone and in conjunction with estrogen treatment in transfeminine patients. A prior study found that the use of CPA alone does not cause cortisol suppression in transfeminine individuals (de Vries et al., 1986).

Key Points:

1. Differences in the hormonal milieu of developing adolescents result in differences in the size of the pituitary gland, with cisgender females having a larger pituitary gland than cisgender males upon reaching adulthood.
2. Somatotrophinoma has been observed in two transmasculine individuals using exogenous testosterone, while hyperprolactinemia has been associated with exogenous estrogen combined with CPA in

transfeminine individuals. The risk of prolactin elevation may exist only for those using CPA as an adjunctive antiandrogen agent.

3. Exogenous oral estrogen may increase TBG, increase CBG, and decrease IGF-1, therefore increasing GH. These effects are not observed with exogenous estrogen given via alternative ROAs.

4. Estrogen may increase steroidogenesis in the adrenal glands, whereas testosterone inhibits steroidogenesis production. Despite some discordance in the literature, GAHT appears to decrease ACTH-stimulated serum cortisol levels.

5. In addition to suppressing the production of gonadal sex steroids, feminizing GAHT appears to suppress adrenal androgens as well.

NERVOUS SYSTEM

Sex Differences in the Nervous System

Unlike many other organ systems in the human body, well-defined anatomical sexual dimorphisms in the nervous system are uncommon, with sex differences depending on a complex interplay between genetic, epigenetic, and hormone-related factors. Historically, this has been a challenging area to study, given the profound influence of environment and experiences on the human brain and behavior. However, in the decades since neuroscience was firmly established as an independent field, an explosion of research in the discipline, from animal models to functional imaging in humans, has dramatically increased understanding of sex differences in the brain.

In the mid-twentieth century, the work of Geoffrey Harris (1948) revealed that the hypothalamus controls the release of hormones from the adenohypophysis, establishing a connection between the brain and the endocrine system and setting the framework for what would become the science of neuroendocrinology (de Vries et al., 1986). Subsequent researchers identified peptide-releasing factors in hypothalamic tissue and, eventually, receptor mechanisms in the hypothalamus and pituitary gland, with structural and mechanical similarities to those observed in other peripheral tissues, including those for sex hormones (Schally et al., 1973; Stumpf and Sar, 1976). Indeed, it is now well established that the hypothalamus is a critical component of the HPG axis, responsible for regulating reproductive function, and is subject to feedback inhibition by circulating sex hormones. The intricacies of this system are discussed in more detail elsewhere in this review. These early findings inspired researchers to search for sex hormone receptors elsewhere in the central nervous system.

To examine the potential impact of sex hormones on the human brain, it is essential to recognize that the adult brain is no longer regarded as a static and unchanging organ. Building upon several decades of research on brain plasticity in animal models, more recent evidence demonstrates that the human hippocampus, a brain region involved in learning and memory, experiences significant neurogenesis throughout adulthood (Spalding et al., 2013). Aside from sex differences that may arise from the action of circulating sex hormones, differences may occur from contributions of genes on X and Y chromosomes or mitochondrial DNA. As noted, sexual dimorphisms in the brain are uncommon. It is reasonable to suspect that, when they do exist, they may be due to these genetic influences. Perhaps the most celebrated example in the mammalian brain is the sexually dimorphic nucleus (SDN) of the preoptic region, called the INAH-3 in humans, which is three to five times larger in male rats than in females (Gorski et al., 1978). Similarly, the nucleus is larger in male humans than in females, although its function remains a topic of debate (Allen et al., 1989). Generally, sex differences in the human brain are far more subtle.

Receptors for sex hormones have now been identified in many regions of the nervous system. After the hypothalamus, the hippocampus was the next brain region in which estrogen receptors were identified (McEwen and Milner, 2007). Research has found evidence for estrogen-induced synapse formation and maturation involving multiple cell types and signaling pathways in the hippocampus (McEwen and Milner, 2017). In fact, the brain appears to have the capability to locally generate estrogens, either by aromatization of androgen precursors or directly from cholesterol (Hajszan et al., 2008). Interestingly, progesterone treatment following estrogen-induced synapse formation was found to downregulate hippocampal spine synapses in rats; however, the mechanism for doing so remains unknown (Woolley and McEwen, 1993). Although less well described, androgens have also been shown to induce hippocampal spine synapses in rats, and, like estrogen, the brain may also be able to generate the androgen DHT locally (Leranth et al., 2004; Okamoto et al., 2012). Similarly, estrogen-regulated spine synapse formation and turnover have been shown to occur in the prefrontal cortex, a region of the brain implicated in executive functions such as planning, decision making, moderating social behavior, and expressing one's personality (Hao et al., 2007). Animal models have demonstrated that neurons projecting from the amygdala to the prefrontal cortex undergo dendritic expansion in females dependent on the presence of circulating estrogens, with ovariectomized females failing to show these changes (Shansky et al., 2010).

Given the inherent dichotomy between the concentration of circulating androgens and estrogens in cisgender males and that of cisgender females, differential activation of sex hormone receptors in the central nervous system results in sex-specific changes on the molecular and cellular levels. Additional research involving animal models and human subjects has endeavored to connect these findings to tangible sex differences in behavior.

Perhaps one of the more robust behavioral sex differences in humans is sexual partner preference. In one study, male rats neonatally treated with 1,4,6-androstatriene-3,17-dione (ATD), which blocks the aromatization of testosterone into estradiol, experienced either a loss of sexual preference or a reversal toward preference for mounting other male rats (Bakker et al., 1993). Additionally, the size of the SDN, which sex hormones can manipulate, has been shown to correlate with partner preference in rodents, sheep, and humans (Balthazart, 2016). Also, indirect measures of sex hormone exposure in utero correlate with partner preference in adult humans (Roselli and Balthazart, 2011). It is important to note that the observations in humans have generated considerable controversy. Indeed, given the vast array of variables that impact human brain development and behavior throughout the lifespan, it is challenging to make inferences from nonhuman mammalian models or isolated observations in humans. However, the preponderance of evidence does support a hormonal contribution to sexual preference in humans, and it is reasonable to conclude that humans, as with other mammalian species, exhibit sexual differentiation of the brain.

Increasingly, neuroimaging techniques such as functional MRI (fMRI) and diffusion tensor imaging (DTI) have allowed for new inferences to be made regarding how men and women differ in their response to stimuli and how brain connectivity varies between sexes. fMRI studies have suggested sex differences in distributed brain activation during phonological and spatial processing. During phonological processing, where cisgender females tend to perform better than cisgender males, brain activation in cisgender males has been shown to be predominately left lateralized, whereas the pattern of activation in cisgender females is more diffuse (Shaywitz et al., 1995). Conversely, cisgender females showed less right-lateralized brain activation than cisgender males for spatial tasks, where cisgender males tend to perform better than cisgender females (Gur et al., 2000). In one study of 949 youths modeling the structural connectome using DTI, the authors concluded that the brains of cisgender male individuals are structured to facilitate connectivity between perception and coordinated action. In contrast, the brains of cisgender females are structured to facilitate communication between analytical and intuitive processing modes (Ingalhalikar et al., 2014). These studies, however, have also generated controversy, with some expressing concerns related to implicit bias; reverse inference; and technical considerations, such as the role of brain size and movement in the scanner (McCarthy, 2016).

Investigating sex differences in the human brain through the lens of certain health conditions has provided additional insight. In their studies of cisgender girls with congenital adrenal hyperplasia (CAH), a condition that results in prenatal androgen exposure due to a genetic anomaly, researchers found that cisgender girls with CAH were less responsive than unaffected cisgender girls to information that particular objects (i.e., toys) are "for girls" (Hines et al., 2016). This research suggests that prenatal sex hormone exposure may influence subsequent behavior in part by impacting an individual's sensitivity to socializing cues, rather than inducing permanent changes in the brain. The menopausal transition also provides an opportunity to observe how changes in the concentration of circulating sex hormones may impact the central nervous system.

Independent of normal aging, modest declines in delayed verbal recall have been shown to occur early in the menopausal transition, with immediate recall declining late in the transition (Epperson et al., 2013). Importantly, abrupt loss of estrogen with oophorectomy appears to have a much more profound impact on cognition than the gradual decline of estrogen that occurs with natural menopause (Burger et al., 1999). Data are conflicting on whether initiation of HRT for menopausal cisgender female individuals impacts global cognitive function. Still, there is some consensus that the later that hormone replacement is initiated relative to the age of menopause, the less likely it is to have a beneficial impact on scales of cognitive function (Hara et al., 2015). Interestingly, animal studies using ovariectomized female nonhuman primates have shown that cyclical unopposed estrogen treatments improved synaptic health and cognitive performance, while chronic estrogen or combination estrogen–progesterone did not (Hara et al., 2015).

GAHT and the Nervous System

Given what we know about the role of hormones in modulating sex differences in the central nervous system, it is reasonable to assume that the provisioning of GAHT may impact the brain's structure and function. Indeed, as with cisgender individuals, advances in functional imaging have provided insight into the potential influence of GAHT on brain structure and activity in TGD individuals. While the available data are heterogeneous, studies generally indicate an anabolic and anticatabolic effect of testosterone on brain volumes. In contrast, estradiol and adjunct antiandrogen treatment seem to have the opposite effect (Kranz et al., 2020). In a recent study, investigators examined hypothalamic volume before and after 4 months of GAHT in TGD individuals. They found significant volume reductions only in those using estrogen and adjunctive antiandrogens (Konadu et al., 2022). Task-based fMRI studies involving participants on GAHT are expanding but remain scarce. A recent study leveraging fMRI to investigate how GAHT in transmasculine individuals may influence emotional perception found that, while the neural pattern in transmasculine individuals was like that of cisgender females before GAHT, after 6–10 months of receiving testosterone, the neural pattern resembled the pattern of cisgender males (Kiyar et al., 2022). While, to the authors' knowledge, no similar fMRI study exists for transfeminine individuals before and after initiation of GAHT, investigators examining the impact of GAHT following gonadectomy in transfeminine individuals concluded that lower serum estradiol levels were associated with cortical thickening. In contrast, higher levels were associated with cortical thinning, although no appreciable relationship to cognitive function was observed (Schneider et al., 2020).

Researchers have employed additional techniques, including genomic sequencing and positron emission tomography (PET), to investigate the effect of GAHT on sexual differentiation of the brain. In one study, investigators sought to examine whether methylation of region III of the estrogen receptor alpha (ESR1) promoter—the promoter of a gene implicated in brain sex differences—is involved in the biological basis of gender incongruence (Fernández et al., 2020). They found that, before GAHT, TGD individuals showed a characteristic methylation profile that differed from both cisgender males and cisgender females and that, following GAHT, the methylation patterns became more like that of their cisgender counterparts who share their gender identity. Research using PET indicates that GAHT may influence serotonergic neurotransmission, with investigators showing that serum testosterone levels are positively correlated with serotonin reuptake transporter (SERT) binding in transmasculine individuals, and, although SERT levels decline after 4 months of estradiol and adjunct antiandrogen therapy in transfeminine individuals, estradiol levels are also positively correlated with SERT binding (Kranz et al., 2015).

Although hypotheses related to behavior and cognition may stem from examining the effect of GAHT on the structure and function of the nervous system, studies employing cognitive and psychological testing have been even more informative. In general, the extant literature supports an enhancing role of postpubertal GAHT on visuospatial ability in transmasculine individuals. There is less consensus regarding the effect of GAHT on cognitive scales in transfeminine individuals. Moreover, the evidence does not support an adverse impact of GAHT on cognitive function for TGD individuals (Karalexi et al., 2020). In terms of psychological health, GAHT appears to have an overwhelmingly positive effect, reducing symptoms of anxiety and depression, lowering social distress, and improving quality of life and self-esteem in TGD individuals (Nguyen et al., 2018). Prior research in this area was reinforced by a recent prospective cohort study of TGD individuals, in which investigators found a significant reduction in symptoms of depression and a nonsignificant decrease in symptoms of anxiety after 18 months of GAHT (Aldridge et al., 2021). More research is needed to investigate the impact of GAHT on executive function, which would provide more insight into how GAHT might affect the day-to-day functioning of TGD people.

Outside of the improvement in symptoms of depression and anxiety, there is, to the authors' knowledge, no known correlation between GAHT and diseases of the nervous system in the United States. Historically, the use of exogenous sex hormones has been implicated in the development of meningiomas, a class of common intracranial tumors. Indeed, the use of high-dose CPA in transfeminine individuals appears to be associated with an increased risk of meningioma (Millward et al., 2022). This medication is often used as part of GAHT in Europe but is not commercially available in the United States. Of all the agents commonly used as part of GAHT in this country, none have been definitively associated with an increased risk of meningioma in the TGD population. It is worth noting that evidence from cisgender females does not seem to support an increased risk of meningiomas with the use of oral contraceptive pills, and data are conflicting concerning HRT in menopausal patients (Hage et al., 2022). The risk of thromboembolic disease with the use of GAHT, a topic of great interest and controversy, which may impact the cerebrovascular system in the case of ischemic stroke, is discussed in the cardiovascular section of this review. Similarly, hyperprolactinemia, a disease state of the adenohypophysis, has been associated with adjunctive CPA as part of feminizing GAHT and is discussed in the endocrine system section of this review.

In summarizing the extant literature on GAHT and its effect on the brain, there appears to be a consensus that GAHT has a positive impact on the psychological health of TGD patients and, albeit with less consensus, a neutral effect on cognitive function, with some investigators noting an enhancement in visuospatial ability in transmasculine individuals using testosterone. Further research could stratify these potential effects by the dose, ROA, and duration of GAHT. Aside from data reporting an increased incidence of meningioma in users of CPA, no association has been made between the use of GAHT and neurologic disease. Importantly, however, data from cisgender females have shown a potential protective effect on cognition when HRT is initiated closer to the time of menopause (Hara et al., 2015). This surrogate data may help inform providers caring for TGD individuals who could consider prompt initiation or resumption of GAHT following GAS.

Key Points:
1. Research involving mammalian animal models supports a hormonal contribution to sexual differentiation of the brain.
2. Functional imaging in humans suggests that the brains of cisgender males are structured to facilitate more connectivity between perception and coordinated action. In contrast, the brains of cisgender females are designed to facilitate more communication between analytical and intuitive processing modes.

3. Exogenous testosterone appears to have an anabolic and anticatabolic effect on brain volumes, whereas exogenous estradiol and antiandrogens appear to have the opposite effect.
4. Exogenous testosterone may enhance visuospatial ability in transmasculine individuals, whereas exogenous estrogen does not clearly affect cognitive ability in transfeminine individuals.
5. GAHT, whether feminizing or masculinizing, does not appear to have an adverse impact on cognitive function in TGD individuals and has an overwhelmingly positive effect on psychological health.

PULMONARY SYSTEM

Sex Differences in the Pulmonary System

The pulmonary system is a network of tissues and organs crucial for respiration; it includes the airways, lungs, and blood vessels. Variations between the sexes have been established regarding morphology, lung volumes, airway sizes, and responses to exercise (Bellemare et al., 2003; LoMauro and Aliverti, 2021; Townsend et al., 2012). Cisgender males have larger luminal airways, higher total lung volumes and capacity, and a larger number of alveoli in their respiratory tracts. However, relative lung volumes and capacities are the same between the sexes. The ratio of functional residual capacity to total lung capacity remains consistent between cisgender males and cisgender females, indicating that elastic recoil properties are independent of sex (Dominelli and Molgat-Seon, 2022; LoMauro and Aliverti, 2018).

Regarding exercise, cisgender females exhibit lower minute ventilation (Ve) and tidal volume (Vt) during maximal exertion than do cisgender males. However, the extent of increase in both Ve and Vt after exercise is similar in both sexes. Cisgender females allocate a greater proportion of maximal ventilation, or VO2, to respiratory muscles than do cisgender males. Additionally, they experience a higher work of breathing than cisgender males, influenced by factors such as the prismatic shape of the natal female rib cage, body mass, and hemoglobin concentration (Dominelli et al., 2019; Torres-Tamayo et al., 2018). Recent evidence also suggests that cisgender females have a higher incidence of exercise-induced arterial hypoxemia compared with cisgender males (Ansdell et al., 2020; Dominelli et al., 2019). The heightened oxygen expenditure in cisgender females during breathing suggests that a substantial portion of their oxygen intake and cardiac output is allocated to respiratory muscles, impacting their exercise performance (Dominelli et al., 2015).

Sex hormones may also influence pulmonary pathophysiology. One study found that TRT may slow down the progression of chronic obstructive pulmonary disease (COPD) in cisgender males, as measured by a relative decrease in respiratory hospitalizations over time. Additionally, both estrogen and androgen receptors are present in bronchial airways, and some evidence suggests that, in patients with asthma, elevated levels of bronchial androgen receptors and higher serum androgen levels are linked to reduced hyperreactivity; fewer symptoms; and lower fractional exhaled nitric oxide, a byproduct of inflammation and biomarker for asthma (Han et al., 2020; Mikkonen et al., 2010; Millas and Duarte Barros, 2021; Zein et al., 2021). Fractional exhaled nitric oxide level is positively correlated to progesterone levels and inversely correlated to 17β-estradiol levels (Mandhane et al., 2009). This might explain why asthma exacerbations are seen more frequently in menstrual cycle phases corresponding to high progesterone levels (Chowdhury et al., 2021). Indeed, a murine model demonstrated that female sex hormones enhance the proinflammatory response in the lung when exposed to allergens (Fuentes and Silveyra, 2018). Asthma prevalence shifts toward cisgender females in adulthood and suggests a sex difference in airway reactivity after puberty (Shah and Newcomb, 2018). Furthermore, up to 40 percent of cisgender females with asthma report premenstrual worsening of symptoms, and 20 percent of female asthmatics experience an exacerbation during pregnancy, supporting the role of female sex hormones as proinflammatory in the lung (Rao et al., 2013; Tan and Thomson, 2000).

GAHT and the Pulmonary System

A recent cross-sectional study compared the cardiopulmonary capacity of 15 nonathlete transfeminine individuals who received GAHT for a median of 14.4 years, with 14 cisgender males and 13 cisgender females. The volume of oxygen at peak flow and the mean expiratory volumes for transfeminine individuals on GAHT were found to be higher than that of cisgender females and lower than that of cisgender males. Importantly, relative cardiopulmonary capacity adjusted for fat-free mass was unchanged between the groups (Alvares et al., 2022). Hemoglobin concentration can also affect exercise performance and aerobic capacity, and research has shown that hemoglobin is reduced by 11–14 percent in transfeminine individuals on GAHT (Wiik et al., 2020). Still, other factors contribute to the VO2, including total blood volume and cardiac contractility, which may lead to differences in the aerobic capacity of transfeminine individuals compared with cisgender females (Hilton and Lundberg, 2021).

A recent review attempted to address the question of athletic advantage for TGD individuals. Researchers concluded that in nonathletic transfeminine individuals, after a year of feminizing GAHT, there was a roughly 30 percent increase in fat mass and a 5 percent drop in muscle mass. After 3 years, the percentage of muscle mass had steadily reduced. Although transfeminine individuals still have higher absolute lean mass, their relative percentages of fat mass, lean mass, hemoglobin, and VO2 peak, when corrected for weight, were like those of cisgender females. No benefit was seen in the physical performance of transfeminine individuals as determined by running time after 2 years of GAHT (Cheung et al., 2024).

From a practical standpoint, spirometry is used to diagnose obstructive and restrictive lung disease. A study of 17 TGD people out of a cohort of 303 aimed to identify the appropriate gender reference to use for the interpretation of spirometry in TGD individuals (Foer et al., 2021). Of the 17 participants, 15 had complete pulmonary function tests available (5 were transmasculine, 8 were transfeminine, and 2 identified as gender nonbinary). The FEV_1 (forced expiratory volume in the first minute) and FVC (forced vital capacity) values were interpreted differently when the gender reference not matching the individual's gender identity was used. These results imply that applying cisgender male projected FEV_1 and FVC values for a female-sized body may give a false diagnosis of restriction, while the opposite may conceal a real restriction. That said, the authors found that obstructive lung disease diagnosis was not impacted by gender reference (Foer et al., 2021). Another study investigating the use of gender identity, rather than sex recorded at birth, for the analysis of spirometry values found that for transfeminine individuals, the percent predicted FEV_1 and FVC was higher if cisgender male range values were used, while for transmasculine individuals, the percent predicted for FEV_1 and FVC was lower if cisgender male range values were used (Haynes and Stumbo, 2018). The authors concluded that spirometry interpretation was affected for a total of 45 percent of cisgender males and 70 percent of cisgender females when employing gender identity as the reference (Haynes and Stumbo, 2018).

Sex steroids likely play a role in the pathogenesis and symptomatology of chronic lung diseases. For example, HRT use in a large group of Danish postmenopausal cisgender female individuals was associated with a 63 percent heightened risk of new-onset asthma (Hansen et al., 2021). Additionally, other studies have shown that higher serum testosterone levels are associated with a lower risk of asthma in both sexes (Bulkhi et al., 2020; Han et al., 2020). A small case series on TGD individuals revealed the resolution of obstructive sleep apnea (OSA) in a transfeminine individual on estrogen and a new diagnosis of OSA in several transmasculine individuals who started on testosterone (Robertson et al., 2019). Some studies in cisgender males have shown TRT to be a risk factor for the development of OSA (La Vignera et al., 2020; Payne et al., 2021). Contrary to this observation, in hypogonadal cisgender males, studies have shown testosterone deficiency to be a risk factor for OSA (Gambineri et al., 2003; Kim and Cho, 2019). It is therefore recommended to monitor sleep function in individuals prescribed testosterone.

A 2018 cross-sectional study revealed that 29.6 percent of Medicare beneficiaries who identified as TGD had a diagnosis of asthma, compared with 13.6 percent of cisgender individuals. Of note, the risk was highest for transfeminine individuals but was also significantly higher than the cisgender cohort for transmasculine individuals (Dragon et al., 2017). Similarly, the prevalence of COPD among transgender beneficiaries was 27.3 versus 20.8 percent in cisgender beneficiaries. Cisgender males have 1.5 times the risk of developing COPD compared with cisgender females, even without a smoking history, and it is speculated that this may be related to sex hormones (Pinkerton et al., 2015). Further research is needed to elucidate the role of sex steroid hormones on the development or progression of reactive airway disease.

In conclusion, sexual dimorphism exists in the respiratory system; those recorded female at birth have smaller airways and different responses to exercise. There is minimal research regarding the role of GAHT in the progression of chronic lung disease. Nascent research indicates that the relative cardiopulmonary capacity adjusted for fat-free mass was not significantly changed with GAHT. Finally, spirometry tests need to be adapted to take gender identity into account to diagnose restrictive lung disease more accurately in TGD individuals.

Key Points:
1. Sex hormone receptors are present throughout the respiratory system and contribute to sexual dimorphism in the structure and function of the lungs. However, relative lung volumes and capacities are the same between sexes.
2. Estrogen and progesterone may exhibit proinflammatory effects in the lung, whereas androgens are associated with reduced airway hyperreactivity.
3. While TGD individuals on GAHT may exhibit peak flow and mean expiratory volumes that differ from their cisgender counterparts, relative cardiopulmonary capacity adjusted for fat-free mass remains unchanged and no apparent benefit to physical performance has been observed.
4. The reference curves of one's gender identity should be considered when interpreting spirometry in TGD individuals to avoid falsely diagnosing or, conversely, missing a diagnosis of restrictive lung disease.
5. Exogenous testosterone has been associated with an increased risk of OSA in transmasculine individuals, so it is prudent to monitor for changes in sleep pattern and quality in these patients.
6. Asthma appears to occur with an increased prevalence in TGD individuals compared with the cisgender population. However, this is likely multifactorial, and additional research is needed to elucidate the role of sex hormones in the pathogenesis of asthma.

RENAL SYSTEM

Sex Differences in the Renal System

The renal system is responsible for the excretion of metabolic waste and maintenance of acid–base and electrolyte balance, and contributes to stable blood pressure. It is well established that, in general, blood pressure runs higher in cisgender males than in cisgender females at similar ages until menopause, at which point blood pressure in cisgender females may increase to levels even higher than those seen in cisgender males (Sandberg and Ji, 2012). Researchers have proposed sexual dimorphism in renal structure and physiology as a potential contributing factor to the observed differences in blood pressure. Indeed, one may assume that some degree of sexual dimorphism must be present to maintain homeostasis in the face of fluid and electrolyte flux that occurs when females experience pregnancy and lactation, whereas males have virtually static renal function throughout adulthood.

Experimental animal models have identified sexually dimorphic patterns of renal transporter expression and salt handling. For example, female rats have lower sodium and water transporters and lower fractional reabsorption in the proximal nephron coupled with more abundant transporters in the distal nephron than do male rats (Veiras et al., 2017). These differences, if present in humans, would have significant implications for renal function and could be responsible for the adaptations in fluid retention required during pregnancy and lactation, as well as the "female advantage" regarding blood pressure observed in premenopausal cisgender females. Mouse models have also provided evidence for sexual dimorphism in renal ammonia metabolism, an essential process for maintaining acid–base homeostasis, associated with fundamental structural differences and differences in the expression of proteins involved in renal ammonia and transport (Harris et al., 2018).

Much of the observed sexual dimorphism in renal structure and function is likely driven by inherent sex chromosome differences. There is evidence to suggest that gonadal hormones play a role in mediating these differences. Androgen receptors are expressed exclusively throughout the proximal tubule in the kidneys of both sexes, whereas estrogen receptors are detected in both proximal and distal tubules (Ransick et al., 2019). In a study using male mice, orchiectomy was found to decrease kidney and proximal tubule size while increasing ammonia excretion, effects that were all reversible with testosterone replacement (Harris et al., 2020). Data from animal studies indicate that estrogen may have renoprotective effects, decreasing glomerulosclerosis and risk of ischemia-reperfusion injury (Elliot et al., 2003; Hutchens et al., 2012). Additionally, estrogen contributes to vasodilation by increasing nitric oxide activity, which may increase renal blood flow and, thus, glomerular filtration rate (GFR) (Issa et al., 2015). Testosterone, on the other hand, has been associated with worsening albuminuria and glomerulosclerosis in mouse models (Long et al., 2013). If the effects of sex steroids on the renal system in mice can be extrapolated to humans, then one might expect a decline in renal function with the loss of estrogen in cisgender females. Indeed, in a population-based cohort study of cisgender females who underwent bilateral oophorectomy before age 50, a higher risk of developing chronic kidney disease (CKD) was noted even after adjusting for multiple chronic conditions and other possible confounders (Kattah et al., 2018).

Serum creatinine is a commonly used biomarker to estimate one's GFR. Creatinine is a chemical waste product of creatine that is formed during the digestion of protein or the breakdown of skeletal muscle tissue and cleared by the renal system. Therefore, serum creatinine levels outside the normal range may indicate a change in kidney function, diet, or medications.

Epidemiologic research has shown that cisgender males have higher mean serum creatinine, findings that have prompted the development of sex-distinct reference ranges for what is considered normal serum creatinine (Jones et al., 1998). This is likely due, at least in part, to sex differences in body composition—cisgender males tend to have more lean mass, whereas cisgender females have more fat mass (Bredella, 2017).

GAHT and the Renal System

GAHT may influence body composition, with testosterone-based masculinizing GAHT increasing lean mass and estrogen-based feminizing GAHT decreasing lean mass (Klaver et al., 2017). The influence of GAHT on body composition is explored in more detail in this review's bone and body composition section. Because one's serum creatinine level is partly a reflection of skeletal muscle breakdown and GAHT may either increase or decrease lean mass, it is crucial to understand the impact of GAHT on serum creatinine to allow for accurate interpretation of these laboratory values.

Researchers have explored the relationship between GAHT and measures of renal function in a systematic review and meta-analysis of nine studies involving a total of 488 transmasculine individuals and 593 transfeminine individuals (Krupka et al., 2022). In transmasculine individuals, serum creatinine increased significantly after 12 months of GAHT, whereas transfeminine individuals experienced a nonsignificant decline in serum creatinine. Two studies included in the meta-analysis reported on 24-hour urine creatinine excretion, with similar changes again noted in transmasculine but not transfeminine individuals at 12 months. These findings are supported by a subsequent retrospective chart review of 108 adult TGD patients initiated on GAHT at the Mayo Clinic (Maheshwari et al., 2022). In that study, creatinine levels were found to be significantly decreased in transfeminine and increased in transmasculine individuals as early as 3 months and to have reached a new baseline around 6 months, with changes persisting at 12 months. To investigate the effect of hormonal preparations and dose on serum creatinine, those on feminizing GAHT were further stratified by ROA, dose, and serum estradiol level. No significant differences were observed.

However, the authors noted more prominent serum creatinine level changes in those transfeminine individuals who achieved a serum estradiol level of more than 100 pg/mL and who were on higher doses of estradiol therapy. This analysis was not performed in those on masculinizing GAHT, as there were too few in the study.

Sexual dimorphism exists regarding the structure and function of the renal system, and some of these differences are likely mediated by gonadal sex steroids, with estrogen appearing to be somewhat renoprotective. Researchers have detected significant changes in creatinine levels with the use of GAHT. Still, it remains unclear whether these changes represent alterations in renal function or are surrogate markers for changes in body composition. To answer this question, further research needs to examine the effect of GAHT on other biomarkers of renal function, such as cystatin C and measured GFR. There is also a need to explore this effect in TGD individuals with CKD and pediatric TGD individuals, as there is currently a dearth of research involving these populations whose age, etiology of kidney disease, and other factors may modify the effect. Lastly, additional research is needed to determine whether various doses, formulations, and durations—as well as the use of antiandrogen adjunctive agents—modify the impact of both feminizing and masculinizing GAHT on renal function.

Until more robust data are available, providers caring for transgender individuals should be mindful of the potential impact of GAHT on biomarkers of renal function and be wary of relying on the estimated GFR in isolation, particularly in those with borderline renal function, before the initiation of GAHT. A modifier for "female sex" exists to account for expected sex differences in creatinine when estimating GFR. However, this must be interpreted in the context of one's gender-affirming care to avoid potential harms associated with an imprecise estimated GFR. Based on the extant literature, it would seem reasonable to reassess serum creatinine 6–12 months after initiating GAHT to establish a new baseline and to use the individual's gender identity when calculating estimated GFR. In situations of ambiguity when estimating GFR, a measured GFR may be appropriate (Mohottige and Tuot, 2022).

Key Points:

1. Cisgender males have higher mean serum creatinine than cisgender females.
2. Exogenous testosterone may result in an increase in serum creatinine in transmasculine individuals, whereas exogenous estrogen may result in a decrease in serum creatinine in transfeminine individuals.
3. The ROA and dose of exogenous estrogen used as part of feminizing GAHT in transfeminine individuals do not appear to have a significant effect on the magnitude of change in serum creatinine.
4. Clinicians should consider reassessing serum creatinine 6–12 months after initiating GAHT to establish a new baseline and use an individual's gender identity when calculating estimated GFR.

INTEGUMENTARY SYSTEM

Sex Differences in the Integumentary System

The skin, the largest organ in the body, serves a crucial role as the protective barrier between an individual and their environment. Androgens and estrogens are known to affect the pilosebaceous unit of the skin, with receptors for both expressed in sebocytes and the hair follicle dermal papilla (Choudhry et al., 1992; Hasselquist et al., 1980). There are notable sex differences in the structure and function of the skin, in part driven by sex hormones known to influence skin thickness, hair quality and distribution, and sebum production by sebaceous glands. Additionally, sex hormones drive sex differences in immunology, with potential dermatologic implications, discussed in more detail in the immune system section of this review.

Cisgender males have thicker skin than cisgender females and, with aging, cisgender females experience more thinning than cisgender males (Aubert et al., 1985). Evidence from human and animal research suggests that estrogen plays a crucial role in maintaining skin thickness. Menopause is associated with a marked decrease in skin thickness in cisgender females, and ovariectomy has been associated with skin thinning. In contrast, exogenous estrogen administration has been shown to thicken the skin (Bolognia et al., 1989; Punnonen, 1971). Similar findings have been observed in studies of gonadectomized mice, wherein estrogen seems to have a role in regulating epidermal thickness, while androgens regulate dermal thickness (Azzi et al., 2005).

The role of sex hormones in modulating hair growth is complex, involving an interplay among estrogens, androgens, and potentially progesterone.

Androgenetic alopecia is the most common form of hair loss, irrespective of sex. In cisgender males, it usually involves progressive hair thinning in the frontal and temporal areas of the scalp, beginning after puberty and continuing throughout adult life. This process is driven by DHT, a sex hormone that results from the conversion of testosterone by the 5a-reductase enzyme found in the pilosebaceous unit, resulting in a transformation of thick terminal hair follicles into thin villus-like hair follicles on the scalp while stimulating hair growth on the face and body (Makrantonaki and Zouboulis, 2009). In contrast, androgenetic alopecia in cisgender females generally begins after age 30, involves the frontal and parietal scalp, and is not clearly related to androgens, as most patients have normal serum levels (Olsen, 2001).

Sebum production by sebaceous glands plays a role in the development of acne, which may be increased by androgens and decreased by estrogens (Strauss et al., 1962). Male mice have larger sebaceous glands than those of female mice, and gonadectomy has been shown to cause atrophy of sebaceous glands in male mice and growth in female mice, suggesting a role for sex hormone stimulation in the maintenance of sebaceous glands (Azzi et al., 2005). Clinical observations in humans, too, support the role of androgens in the development of acne, as conditions causing androgen excess—including PCOS, adrenal/ovarian tumors, and CAH—can all cause acne (Chen et al., 2011). Conversely, acne generally does not occur before adrenarche, when levels of dehydroepiandrosterone sulfate rise, and neither acne nor sebum production occurs in cisgender males with androgen insensitivity (Imperato-McGinley et al., 1993). Estrogens and antiandrogens, on the other hand, have been shown to decrease sebum production, resulting in an improvement in acne (Lemay and Poulin, 2002).

Beyond structure, sex hormones appear to influence the function of the skin by changing the epidermal permeability barrier, with implications for wound healing. Animal studies have been informative here as well, as estrogen appears to accelerate barrier development in fetal rat skin while testosterone slows it, with male rats having slower barrier formation than females (Hanley et al., 1996).

While sex differences in the epidermal permeability barrier have not been demonstrated in humans, abnormal wound healing predominates in cisgender males over cisgender females, particularly if they are of advanced age (Fimmel and Zouboulis, 2005). Treatment with topical estrogens has been shown to accelerate wound healing in both sexes (Ashcroft et al., 1999). Interestingly, however, the effect is attenuated in cisgender males compared with their cisgender female counterparts, possibly due to an antagonistic effect of testosterone (Fimmel and Zouboulis, 2005).

GAHT and the Integumentary System

For the most part, the dermatologic effects of GAHT may be readily anticipated, given what we know about how testosterone and estrogen affect the skin in all forms. In transmasculine individuals using testosterone, rapid increases in facial and back acne have been observed within the first 6 months of treatment before stabilizing somewhat after 2 years of therapy (Cocchetti et al., 2022; Rutnin et al., 2023; Wierckx et al., 2014b). Testosterone esters have been shown to dramatically increase the severity of acne compared with other preparations (Cocchetti et al., 2022). Testosterone also appears to reliably increase the growth rate and density of facial and body hair within 6–12 months of treatment, remaining steady after 2 years (Cocchetti et al., 2022; Rutnin et al., 2023; Wierckx et al., 2014b). While all testosterone preparations effectively increase hair distribution, IM injections have shown superior outcomes compared with transdermal administration (Cocchetti et al., 2022). Androgenetic alopecia can be expected to occur with testosterone therapy in a subset of transmasculine individuals, ranging in severity, with studies reporting one-third to one-half developing a mild form and one-fourth to one-third developing a moderate to severe form (Rutnin et al., 2023; Wierckx et al., 2014b). When this occurs, it generally happens within 2–5 years of GAHT initiation (Moreno-Arrones et al., 2017).

In transfeminine individuals using estrogen, improvement in facial and back acne is seen in almost all individuals, usually within 3–6 months of initiation, and is accentuated with the addition of an antiandrogen (Radi et al., 2022; Rutnin et al., 2023). Melasma, a common skin condition that generally presents as symmetric hyperpigmentation, has been associated with circulating estrogen in cisgender females, who experience this condition at about twice the rate of cisgender males (Goandal et al., 2022). In one study, melasma was found in one-third of transfeminine individuals on GAHT, a proportion like that seen in cisgender female individuals (Handel et al., 2014; Rutnin et al., 2023). Feminizing GAHT also appears to change facial and body hair patterns, decreasing terminal hair growth rate and density, generally within 6 months, and remaining mostly constant after that (Cocchetti et al., 2022; Giltay and Gooren, 2000; Rutnin et al., 2023). Importantly, a large proportion of individuals continue to experience some level of hirsutism on long-term feminizing GAHT, prompting many to seek cosmetic treatment (Cocchetti et al., 2022). Consensus has not been reached regarding the likelihood of androgenetic alopecia with feminizing GAHT. One study noted an increase in the proportion of individuals with androgenetic alopecia from 0 percent at baseline to 16 percent after 2 years of feminizing GAHT (Rutnin et al., 2023). This is a surprising finding, as estrogens have been postulated to extend the anagen phase of the hair cycle, aiding hair growth during pregnancy, for example (Desai et al., 2021). It may be that this observation represents a distinct variant of androgenetic alopecia, one that results from an increased estrogen-to-androgen ratio and that has been observed in cisgender men with hypotestosteronemia (Kerkemeyer et al., 2021). The effect of variations in the preparation and ROA of feminizing GAHT on dermatologic changes has not been assessed.

Key Points:
1. Sex hormones drive sex differences in skin thickness, hair quality and distribution, and sebum production.
2. Use of exogenous testosterone in transmasculine individuals increases facial and back acne, increases the growth rate and density of facial and body hair, and may contribute to androgenetic alopecia in a subset of individuals.
3. Use of exogenous estrogen in transfeminine individuals improves facial and back acne, decreases terminal hair growth rate and density, and may increase one's likelihood of melasma.
4. Variations in dose, preparation, and ROA of GAHT have an unclear effect on the integumentary system, although IM testosterone appears to increase hair distribution more effectively than does transdermal administration.

FERTILITY

Sex Differences in Fertility

Fertility is defined as the capacity of humans to produce offspring. Accordingly, infertility is defined as the inability of two individuals, one cisgender male and one cisgender female, to conceive after 1 year of unprotected intercourse. Successful fertilization involves a sperm cell meeting an ovum, leading to the formation of a zygote. Infertility affects approximately 15 percent of couples in the United States and can be attributed to factors related to one or both sexes (Leslie et al., 2023). A study conducted by the World Health Organization (WHO) found that in 35 percent of infertility cases, both male and female factors were involved (Walker and Tobler, 2023). Since the average human lifespan has increased and rates of infertility increase with age, many tests and gamete quality metrics have been developed to address fertility issues.

Semen analysis is used to assess the reproductive capabilities of cisgender males. This involves measuring total sperm count, total progressive motility, total motility (progressive and nonprogressive), and sperm morphology. The WHO established minimum threshold values that are associated with a higher likelihood of male fertility (Sunder and Leslie, 2022).

Abnormalities in these metrics are attributed to a multitude of factors, including those related to sex hormones. Spermatogenesis is stimulated by testosterone, and the absence of this hormone prevents spermatogonium from developing into spermatids. However, the effects of low testosterone levels on fertility are currently still equivocal.

In one retrospective cohort study of infertile cisgender males, no statistically significant association was found between lower testosterone levels and abnormal sperm parameters (Di Guardo et al., 2020). The authors noted that the absolute number of abnormalities was higher in the low testosterone group, and the nonsignificance could be attributed to a lack of statistical power. Interestingly, while low testosterone may adversely affect reproductive capabilities, studies suggest that TRT may also lead to infertility (Patel et al., 2019). Spermatogenesis is carried out by Sertoli cells, and their proper functioning requires adequate levels of follicle-stimulating hormone (FSH) in addition to testosterone. Exogenous testosterone may hinder this process, as it can negatively feed back on the anterior pituitary, preventing the production of FSH. Indeed, studies have shown that testosterone therapy may have weak contraceptive effects, as patients on therapy produce sperm with altered, albeit reversible, morphologies (Patel et al., 2019). While testosterone is the most abundant sex hormone in cisgender males, estrogen can also influence their fertility; however, much of the existing knowledge is speculative and observational.

In murine models, inhibition of the aromatase gene was associated with infertility (Robertson et al., 1999). Authors noted that aromatase knockout mice exhibited germ cells that could not mature into spermatids. Additionally, they reported an increased frequency of germ cell apoptosis and abnormalities during acrosomal development. While estrogen may be necessary for spermatogenesis, high levels of the hormone have also been associated with infertility. One study of infertile men at a Chinese academic hospital showed inverse associations between estrogen levels and sperm parameters (Luo et al., 2021). Specifically, high serum estrogen levels were associated with low sperm concentration, lower rates of progressively motile sperm, and lower rates of normal sperm morphology. The authors also reported that patients with normal sperm morphology had lower concentrations of estrogen and ERα. Overall, while the relationship between estrogen and fertility in cisgender males needs to be further elucidated, current studies suggest that estrogen is essential for proper reproductive functioning. Still, higher levels of the hormone may lead to infertility.

Among cisgender females, fertility is assessed by characterizing an individual's ovarian reserves. This entails testing serum levels of anti-Müllerian hormone (AMH) and FSH and counting the number of antral follicles (Deadmond et al., 2000). These tests provide information about the number of remaining follicles but do not indicate oocyte quality. Females are born with a set number of follicles and their ovarian reserves decrease with age. It is likely that the oocyte quality also decreases with age. Indeed, in a clinical study of infertile cisgender females, the authors reported that while both groups had diminished ovarian reserves, younger women had higher-quality oocytes that led to more successful cycles of in vitro fertilization (IVF) and intracytoplasmic sperm injection (Chang et al., 2018). While age is a significant factor in determining fertility in cisgender female individuals, sex hormones also have notable influences. For example, adequate estrogen levels are essential for proper progression through the menstrual cycle and endometrial thickening for successful embryo implantation. Indeed, low estrogen levels have been associated with endometrial thinning, which can be reversed with estrogen replacement therapy (Liu et al., 2015). Murine models also highlight the importance of estrogen, as low estrogen levels have been associated with abnormal oogenesis (Liu et al., 2022). While estrogen is present at higher levels than testosterone in cisgender females, the latter hormone is still important for fertility.

Elevated testosterone levels have historically been associated with infertility in cisgender females. An early research study examining testosterone levels among cisgender female partners of infertile couples showed that the cohort's testosterone levels were much higher than that of the general cisgender female population (Steinberger et al., 1979). The authors reported that higher testosterone levels were associated with prolonged follicular phase, as well as higher rates of amenorrhea and anovulation. Many of the participants were determined to have hyperandrogenism, and all were treated with prednisone, a glucocorticoid that suppresses androgen levels. In this study, treatment led to adequate androgen suppression among 80 percent of the participants and approximately half of those who had sufficient suppression were able to achieve conception (Steinberger et al., 1979).

One might conclude from this study that high testosterone levels adversely affect fertility in cisgender female individuals. An explanation for this association is testosterone's inhibitory effect on GnRH release, which is important for FSH production in the anterior pituitary. Indeed, an in vitro study showed that high testosterone levels arrested follicular development and that supplementation with FSH reversed this effect (Liu et al., 2015). Overall, these studies suggest that high levels of testosterone may contribute to infertility in cisgender females. It is worth noting, however, that a complete lack of testosterone would also adversely affect their fertility.

Animal studies highlight the important role of testosterone in folliculogenesis. An in vitro study of follicles from fetal calves and baboons showed that testosterone could promote differentiation of primary follicles into secondary follicles (Yang and Fortune, 2006). When the researchers added an androgen receptor (AR) blocker, this differentiation was not seen, which suggests that testosterone's effect on folliculogenesis is mediated by

ARs localized in follicles. Indeed, the authors reported that an immunohistochemistry study of ARs showed increased immunoreactivity as follicles matured (Yang and Fortune, 2006). Another study corroborated this, showing increased AR mRNA expression during early follicular development in bovine models (Hampton et al., 2004). Finally, IVF studies also highlight the therapeutic capabilities of testosterone in treating infertility, as testosterone therapy has been associated with fertility success among cisgender females who initially had poor ovarian responses while undergoing IVF (Noventa et al., 2019; Saharkhiz et al., 2018).

GAHT and Fertility

Extensive research has increased knowledge on how estrogen and testosterone affect the fertility of cisgender males and cisgender females; this gives us insight into how GAHT may affect the fertility of TGD individuals.

The use of feminizing GAHT among transfeminine individuals has been associated with poor sperm parameters. In two cohort studies involving transfeminine individuals who provided semen samples, authors noted that participants who were using hormone therapy had higher rates of abnormalities such as lower sperm motility, concentrations, and total sperm count (Adeleye et al., 2019; Rodriguez-Wallberg, 2021). An explanation for these results is exogenous estrogen's inhibitory effect on GnRH production. It is important to note that other studies have found a positive association between behavioral factors, such as tucking and wearing tight undergarments, and abnormal sperm parameters (de Nie et al., 2022). Indeed, Rodriguez-Wallberg and colleagues (2021) found that, while transfeminine individuals who were not on hormone therapy had lower rates of abnormal sperm parameters than those who used exogenous estrogen, they still had higher rates of abnormalities than did cisgender populations. While many studies suggest that estrogen adversely affects the fertility of transfeminine individuals, other research suggests that its effects on fertility are multifaceted and may be reversible.

A cross-sectional study examining testes samples from transfeminine individuals who had been on hormone therapy for more than a year showed that approximately 80 percent of samples had germ cells and 33 percent exhibited signs of spermatogenesis (Jiang et al., 2019). Interestingly, authors noted that those who were older were more likely to have germ cells in their semen samples, which suggests that initiation of hormone therapy at an earlier age may impact fertility negatively. Next, two studies showed that spermatogenesis can be restored in many cases after cessation of estrogen therapy and that the semen quality can be adequate for successful fertilization (de Nie, 2022; Yau and Safer, 2023). It should be noted that these are preliminary findings, and more research is needed to understand the factors that predict success in fertility restoration.

Considering these data, clinicians should encourage early sperm banking for transfeminine individuals before initiation of hormone therapy, when feasible. Additionally, clinicians who are helping transfeminine individuals restore fertility should consider temporarily withholding estrogen therapy and encourage their patients to avoid behaviors that may negatively affect their fertility.

Among transmasculine individuals who use testosterone therapy, much of the current research suggests that they can still be fertile after prolonged testosterone usage. One study showed that despite long-term testosterone usage, TGD participants without PCOS had AMH levels that mirrored those of the general non-TGD population (Yaish et al., 2021). This suggests that, while exogenous testosterone may disrupt the menstrual cycle, it does not affect the number of follicles available for retrieval. The viability and quality of oocytes in transmasculine individuals are also likely unaffected, as previous studies have shown that oocytes recovered from individuals on testosterone can be successfully fertilized and developed into embryos that can be implanted (Greenwald et al., 2022; Leung et al., 2019). Overall, these studies suggest testosterone is not detrimental to oocytes, and fertility can be achieved in many transmasculine individuals utilizing testosterone, especially with the advancement of assisted reproductive technology.

Key Points:
1. Absolute deficiency of endogenous testosterone in cisgender males results in infertility due to the cessation of spermatogenesis, although a milder deficiency may not affect fertility. Exogenous testosterone use in cisgender males may also hinder spermatogenesis through negative feedback on the pituitary, reducing the production of FSH.
2. While some endogenous estrogen is likely necessary for fertility in cisgender male individuals, high levels may lead to infertility.
3. In cisgender female individuals, estrogen is critical for proper progression through the menstrual cycle and endometrial thickening for successful embryo implantation. Relative estrogen deficiencies are associated with abnormal oogenesis.
4. While some endogenous testosterone is likely necessary for fertility in cisgender female individuals, possibly because of the role this hormone plays in normal folliculogenesis, excess levels of testosterone are associated with infertility.
5. In transfeminine individuals, feminizing GAHT results in decreased sperm count and motility, likely because of exogenous estrogen's inhibition of GnRH production. Therefore, early sperm banking, ideally before initiation of GAHT, is recommended. These effects appear most pronounced for those who initiate GAHT earlier,

and they appear to be at least partially reversible when estrogen is withheld.

6. Transmasculine individuals often remain fertile with prolonged masculinizing GAHT, suggesting that while exogenous testosterone may disrupt the menstrual cycle, its effect on the follicles themselves is less pronounced.

SEXUAL FUNCTION

Sex Differences in Sexual Function

Sexual function is multidimensional. The International Index of Erectile Function and the Female Sexual Function Index are validated questionnaires frequently employed to measure sexual function in the cisgender male and cisgender female populations, respectively (Lukacs, 2001; Rosen, 2000). Both surveys include general questions to assess one's libido, arousal, and satisfaction while also aiming to measure certain anatomical aspects of sexual function, such as erectile performance in cisgender men and lubrication in cisgender women. It is estimated that sexual dysfunction affects 31 percent of cisgender male and 43 percent of cisgender female individuals (Rosen, 2000). While biopsychosocial factors influence healthy sexual functioning, this review will focus on the impact of sex hormones—testosterone and estrogen—on sexual function.

Many studies have shown that testosterone is essential for proper sexual functioning in cisgender males. In a survey of hypogonadism in middle-aged and elderly cisgender males, researchers showed that low levels of testosterone were associated with low libido and erectile dysfunction (Wu et al., 2010). Sexual dysfunction was also present in individuals with chromosomal abnormalities associated with hypogonadism. Indeed, in a meta-analysis investigating the association between Klinefelter syndrome and sexual dysfunction, authors reported that lower serum testosterone levels were associated with low libido (Barbonetti et al., 2021). It is worth noting that low endogenous testosterone was not associated with erectile dysfunction in this study.

Current treatment recommendations for sexual dysfunction depend on patients' symptoms. In patients with erectile dysfunction, for instance, treatment depends on the pathology underlying their condition. Individuals with milder forms of erectile dysfunction and those experiencing decreased libido with demonstrated low serum testosterone levels would likely benefit from testosterone replacement therapy. Conversely, those with more severe erectile dysfunction and those who have erectile dysfunction in the context of vasculopathy, often with intact libido, might be more suitable for treatment with phosphodiesterase type 5 inhibitors, which increase blood flow to the penis, along with lifestyle modifications (Corona et al., 2017; Rizk et al., 2017). In addition to testosterone, current studies suggest that estrogen may influence sexual function in cisgender males.

In two studies that compared treatment outcomes of bicalutamide, an antiandrogen, with scrotal castration among patients with advanced prostate cancer, researchers reported that patients in the bicalutamide group had higher sexual interest and functioning. Given that castration leads to lower endogenous estrogen and the use of antiandrogen does not have as profound an effect on estrogen levels, these findings suggest that estrogen may promote sexual function in the context of depleted testosterone levels (Kacker et al., 2012). In cisgender males with normal levels of testosterone, however, blocking estrogen receptor signaling was not associated with any change in sexual function (Gooren, 1985). Additionally, in another study that induced hypogonadal changes in healthy cisgender males using GnRH antagonists, authors reported similar improvements in sexual functioning in groups receiving TRT, irrespective of whether they received testolactone, an aromatase inhibitor (Bagatell et al., 1994). However, these results contrast with murine model studies that suggest that estrogen plays a vital role in sexual behavior. Indeed, the authors reported that the knockout of estrogen receptors or aromatase enzymes was associated with decreased sexual behavior in male mice (Brooks et al., 2020; Ogawa et al., 2000). Taken together, these studies suggest that in the context of profoundly suppressed testosterone levels, estrogen may alleviate sexual dysfunction (Kacker et al., 2012). However, under conditions of normal serum testosterone, estrogen may not significantly impact sexual function.

Studies of sexual functioning in postmenopausal cisgender females highlight the connection between estrogen deficiency and sexual dysfunction. The importance of estrogen in supporting normal sexual function is suggested by the presence of estrogen receptors throughout urogenital tissues (Simon, 2011). Indeed, declining estrogen levels have been associated with vulvovaginal atrophy, decreased vaginal lubrication, lowered vaginal blood flow, and reduced orgasmic functions (Clayton, 2003; Simon, 2011). Estrogen deficiency leads to vaginal atrophy through decreased collagen levels and muscular bundle thinning (Da Silva Lara et al., 2009). Additionally, since vaginal lubrication depends on sufficient genital engorgement and estrogen deficiency leads to delayed vasocongestion in the genitalia, individuals with low endogenous estrogen commonly report vaginal dryness, itching, and pain from intercourse due to lack of lubrication (Simon, 2011). These symptoms, however, are usually reversible through estrogen treatment. Indeed, a study of 169 healthy postmenopausal cisgender females found that oral and vaginal estradiol were able to enhance sexual desire and orgasm, increase vaginal lubrication, and decrease vaginal irritation (Cayan et al., 2008). In addition to estrogen, testosterone also influences female sexual functioning, specifically by influencing libido levels.

Androgen deficiency is common among postmenopausal cisgender females and has been associated with decreased energy, low libido, and fatigue in this population (Khera, 2015). Additionally, lack of androgen is implicated in sexual dysfunction symptoms related to genitourinary tissues, including vaginal atrophy and decreased lubrication (Maseroli and Vignozzi, 2020). These symptoms may improve with TRT, as was evident in a study of postmenopausal cisgender females with low serum testosterone levels, in which investigators reported that transdermal testosterone treatment was associated with an improvement in sexual function (Davis et al., 2006). The magnitude of improvement was the same regardless of whether participants were treated with an aromatase inhibitor, implying that androgens likely directly affect sexual function through AR signaling in different tissues.

GAHT and Sexual Function

While sexual dysfunction is a common problem among transfeminine individuals, the influence of estrogen therapy may be less than what has been assumed historically. In a longitudinal study of TGD individuals' sexual desire after hormone therapy, authors reported decreases in sexual desire inventory (SDI) scores among transfeminine individuals in the first 3 months after initiation of feminizing GAHT (Defreyne et al., 2020). This score eventually stabilized and then began increasing after 1 year. After 3 years, participants' SDI scores were higher than their baseline scores, suggesting that hormone therapy may indirectly improve sexual desire among transfeminine individuals. It is also possible that estrogen therapy may be protective of sexual dysfunction attributed to adjunct antiandrogens, echoing results from aforementioned studies investigating the effects of estrogen on biological men with prostate cancer (Bales and Chodak, 1996; Tyrrell et al., 1998). Finally, while estrogen therapy may lead to a reduction in nocturnal erections, studies have shown that estrogen likely does not affect sexually stimulated erections (Bettocchi et al., 2004; Kwan et al., 1985).

Among transmasculine individuals, testosterone therapy has been associated with increased sexual desire. Indeed, one study showed that TGD individuals experienced increases in SDI scores shortly after hormone initiation (Defreyne et al., 2020). On average, scores increased until 12 months after initiation and decreased after that. SDI scores were still above baseline at 3 years, but the difference was not statistically significant. Despite these observations, some have postulated that the use of exogenous testosterone in transmasculine individuals may be associated with decreased estrogen levels in the vagina, resulting in vulvovaginal atrophy and decreased lubrication, thereby increasing the risk of discomfort with sexual activity (Tordoff et al., 2023). More research is needed to better delineate these effects and how they may change over time. In the meantime, it is reasonable to offer topical estrogen, applied to the vaginal tissues, for transmasculine patients who may be experiencing the bothersome effects of decreased lubrication.

Key Points:
1. Sexual dysfunction in cisgender males is associated with testosterone deficiency and, in specific clinical contexts, estrogen deficiency. These effects are partially reversible with TRT.
2. Sexual dysfunction in cisgender females is associated with both estrogen and testosterone deficiencies. These effects are partially reversible with estrogen replacement therapy.
3. Sexual desire in transfeminine individuals appears to decrease with initiation of feminizing GAHT but increases above baseline after several years of therapy.
4. Sexual desire in transmasculine individuals appears to increase shortly after initiation of masculinizing GAHT. Still, the effects are transient, and sexual desire seems to regress to baseline after several years of therapy.

CONCLUSION

Sex differences in the human body are widespread and complex, with circulating sex hormones playing a pivotal role in developing and maintaining dimorphisms throughout the lifespan. Like endogenous sex hormones, exogenous sex hormones have the potential to modify one's underlying physiology, exhibiting protective effects against disease in some cases and increasing the propensity for disease in others. Gender-affirming care for TGD individuals regularly involves the provisioning of GAHT, often for many years, and clinicians must understand how these treatments may affect a patient's underlying physiology, predisposition to pathophysiology, and key biomarkers. While there is a need for larger-scale prospective clinical research in this area, the current body of literature is mostly reassuring. TGD individuals who desire gender-affirming care are likely to derive significant benefits from these therapies, and the potential adverse outcomes associated with such therapies may, for the most part, be readily mitigated with appropriate risk stratification and close monitoring.

REFERENCES

Abou-Ismail, M. Y., D. Citla Sridhar, and L. Nayak. 2020. Estrogen and thrombosis: A bench to bedside review. *Thrombosis Research* 192:40–51.

Adeleye, A. J., G. Reid, C. N. Kao, E. Mok-Lin, and J. F. Smith. 2019. Semen parameters among transgender women with a history of hormonal treatment. *Urology* 124:136–141.

Aldridge, Z., S. Patel, B. Guo, E. Nixon, W. Pierre Bouman, G. L. Witcomb, and J. Arcelus. 2021. Long-term effect of gender-affirming hormone treatment on depression and anxiety symptoms in transgender people: A prospective cohort study. *Andrology* 9(6):1808–1816.

Allen, L. S., M. Hines, J. E. Shryne, and R. A. Gorski. 1989. Two sexually dimorphic cell groups in the human brain. *Journal of Neuroscience* 9(2):497–506.

Allen, A. N., R. Jiao, P. Day, P. Pagels, N. Gimpel, and J. A. SoRelle. 2021. Dynamic impact of hormone therapy on laboratory values in transgender patients over time. *The Journal of Applied Laboratory Medicine* 6(1):27–40.

Almeida, M., M. R. Laurent, V. Dubois, F. Claessens, C. A. O'Brien, R. Bouillon, D. Vanderschueren, and S. C. Manolagas. 2017. Estrogens and androgens in skeletal physiology and pathophysiology. *Physiological Reviews* 97(1):135–187.

Alvares, L. A. M., L. M. Santos, M. R. Santos, F. R. Souza, V. P. Almeida, B. B. Mendonca, E. M. F. Costa, M.-J. N. N. Alves, and S. Domenice. 2021. Body composition of transgender women after long-term hormone therapy—A cross-sectional study. *Journal of the Endocrine Society* 5(S1):A788–A788.

Alvares, L. A. M., M. R. Santos, F. R. Souza, L. M. Santos, B. B. Mendonca, E. M. F. Costa, M. Alves, and S. Domenice. 2022. Cardiopulmonary capacity and muscle strength in transgender women on long-term gender-affirming hormone therapy: A cross-sectional study. *British Journal of Sports Medicine* 56(22):1292–1298.

Alzahrani, T., T. Nguyen, A. Ryan, A. Dwairy, J. McCaffrey, R. Yunus, J. Forgione, J. Krepp, C. Nagy, R. Mazhari, and J. Reiner. 2019. Cardiovascular disease risk factors and myocardial infarction in the transgender population. *Circulation: Cardiovascular Quality & Outcomes* 12(4):e005597.

Anagnostis, P., K. Christou, A. M. Artzouchaltzi, N. K. Gkekas, N. Kosmidou, P. Siolos, S. A. Paschou, M. Potoupnis, E. Kenanidis, E. Tsiridis, I. Lambrinoudaki, J. C. Stevenson, and D. G. Goulis. 2019. Early menopause and premature ovarian insufficiency are associated with increased risk of type 2 diabetes: A systematic review and meta-analysis. *European Journal of Endocrinology* 180(1):41–50.

Angum, F., T. Khan, J. Kaler, L. Siddiqui, and A. Hussain. 2020. The prevalence of autoimmune disorders in women: A narrative review. *Cureus* 12(5):e8094.

Ansdell, P., K. Thomas, K. M. Hicks, S. K. Hunter, G. Howatson, and S. Goodall. 2020. Physiological sex differences affect the integrative response to exercise: Acute and chronic implications. *Experimental Physiology* 105(12):2007–2021.

Antun, A., Q. Zhang, S. Bhasin, A. Bradlyn, W. D. Flanders, D. Getahun, T. L. Lash, R. Nash, D. Roblin, M. J. Silverberg, V. Tangpricha, S. Vupputuri, and M. Goodman. 2020. Longitudinal changes in hematologic parameters among transgender people receiving hormone therapy. *Journal of the Endocrine Society* 4(11):bvaa119.

Apostolov, R., E. Gianatti, D. Wong, N. Kutaiba, P. Gow, M. Grossmann, and M. Sinclair. 2022. Testosterone therapy reduces hepatic steatosis in men with type 2 diabetes and low serum testosterone concentrations. *World Journal of Hepatology* 14(4):754–765.

Armeni, E., and I. Lambrinoudaki. 2022. Menopause, androgens, and cardiovascular ageing: A narrative review. *Therapeutic Advances in Endocrinology and Metabolism* 13:20420188221129946.

Arrington-Sanders, R., N. T. Connell, D. Coon, N. Dowshen, A. L. Goldman, Z. Goldstein, F. Grimstad, N. M. Javier, E. Kim, M. Murphy, T. Poteat, A. Radix, A. Schwartz, C. St Amand, C. G. Streed, Jr., V. Tangpricha, M. Toribio, and R. H. Goldstein. 2023. Assessing and addressing the risk of venous thromboembolism across the spectrum of gender affirming care: A review. *Endocrine Practice* 29(4):272–278.

Ashcroft, G. S., T. Greenwell-Wild, M. A. Horan, S. M. Wahl, and M. W. Ferguson. 1999. Topical estrogen accelerates cutaneous wound healing in aged humans associated with an altered inflammatory response. *American Journal of Pathology* 155(4):1137–1146.

Aubert, L., P. Anthoine, J. D. Rigal, and J. L. Leveque. 1985. An in vivo assessment of the biomechanical properties of human skin modifications under the influence of cosmetic products. *International Journal of Cosmetic Science* 7(2):51–59.

Azzi, L., M. El-Alfy, C. Martel, and F. Labrie. 2005. Gender differences in mouse skin morphology and specific effects of sex steroids and dehydroepiandrosterone. *Journal of Investigative Dermatology* 124(1):22–27.

Bachman, E., R. Feng, T. Travison, M. Li, G. Olbina, V. Ostland, J. Ulloor, A. Zhang, S. Basaria, T. Ganz, M. Westerman, and S. Bhasin. 2010. Testosterone suppresses hepcidin in men: A potential mechanism for testosterone-induced erythrocytosis. *Journal of Clinical Endocrinology & Metabolism* 95(10):4743–4747.

Bagatell, C. J., J. R. Heiman, J. E. Rivier, and W. J. Bremner. 1994. Effects of endogenous testosterone and estradiol on sexual behavior in normal young men. *The Journal of Clinical Endocrinology & Metabolism* 78(3):711–716.

Bain, B. J. 1996. Ethnic and sex differences in the total and differential white cell count and platelet count. *Journal of Clinical Pathology* 49(8):664–666.

Bain, B. J., and J. M. England. 1975. Normal haematological values: Sex difference in neutrophil count. *British Medical Journal* 1(5953):306–309.

Bakker, J., T. Brand, J. van Ophemert, and A. K. Slob. 1993. Hormonal regulation of adult partner preference behavior in neonatally ATD-treated male rats. *Behavioral Neuroscience* 107(3):480–487.

Bales, G. T., and G. W. Chodak. 1996. A controlled trial of bicalutamide versus castration in patients with advanced prostate cancer. *Urology* 47(1A Suppl):38–43.

Balthazart, J. 2016. Sex differences in partner preferences in humans and animals. *Philosophical Transactions of the Royal Society B* 371(1688):20150118.

Barbonetti, A., S. D'Andrea, W. Vena, A. Pizzocaro, G. Rastrelli, F. Pallotti, R. Condorelli, A. E. Calogero, D. Pasquali, and A. Ferlin. 2021. Erectile dysfunction and decreased libido in Klinefelter syndrome: A prevalence meta-analysis and meta-regression study. *The Journal of Sexual Medicine* 18(6):1053–1064.

Basu, R., C. Dalla Man, M. Campioni, A. Basu, G. Klee, G. Toffolo, C. Cobelli, and R. A. Rizza. 2006. Effects of age and sex on postprandial glucose metabolism: Differences in glucose turnover, insulin secretion, insulin action, and hepatic insulin extraction. *Diabetes* 55(7):2001–2014.

Bates, J. N., T. P. Kohn, and A. W. Pastuszak. 2020. Effect of thyroid hormone derangements on sexual function in men and women. *Sexual Medicine Reviews* 8(2):217–230.

Bellemare, F., A. Jeanneret, and J. Couture. 2003. Sex differences in thoracic dimensions and configuration. *American Journal of Respiratory and Critical Care Medicine* 168(3):305–312.

Bettocchi, C., F. Palumbo, L. Cormio, P. Ditonno, M. Battaglia, and F. P. Selvaggi. 2004. The effects of androgen depletion on human erectile function: A prospective study in male-to-female transsexuals. *International Journal of Impotence Research* 16(6):544–546.

Bhasin, S., and K. Herbst. 2003. Testosterone and atherosclerosis progression in men. *Diabetes Care* 26(6):1929–1931.

Bielohuby, M., N. Herbach, R. Wanke, C. Maser-Gluth, F. Beuschlein, E. Wolf, and A. Hoeflich. 2007. Growth analysis of the mouse adrenal gland from weaning to adulthood: Time- and gender-dependent alterations of cell size and number in the cortical compartment. *American Journal of Physiology-Endocrinology and Metabolism* 293(1):E139–E146.

Bilezikian, J. P., A. Morishima, J. Bell, and M. M. Grumbach. 1998. Increased bone mass as a result of estrogen therapy in a man with aromatase deficiency. *New England Journal of Medicine* 339(9):599–603.

Birzniece, V., A. Sata, S. Sutanto, and K. K. Ho. 2010. Paracrine regulation of growth hormone secretion by estrogen in women. *Journal of Clinical Endocrinology & Metabolism* 95(8):3771–3776.

Bisson, J. R., K. J. Chan, and J. D. Safer. 2018. Prolactin levels do not rise among transgender women treated with estradiol and spironolactone. *Endocrine Practice* 24(7):646–651.

Blaak, E. 2001. Gender differences in fat metabolism. *Current Opinion in Clinical Nutrition and Metabolic Care* 4(6):499–502.

Black, D. M., and C. J. Rosen. 2016. Clinical practice. Postmenopausal osteoporosis. *New England Journal of Medicine* 374(3):254–262.

Boekhout-Berends, E. T., C. M. Wiepjes, N. M. Nota, H. H. Schotman, A. C. Heijboer, and M. den Heijer. 2023. Changes in laboratory results in transgender individuals on hormone therapy—A retrospective study and practical approach. *European Journal of Endocrinology* 188(5):457–466.

Bolognia, J. L., I. M. Braverman, M. E. Rousseau, and P. M. Sarrel. 1989. Skin changes in menopause. *Maturitas* 11(4):295–304.

Bonora, E., G. Formentini, F. Calcaterra, S. Lombardi, F. Marini, L. Zenari, F. Saggiani, M. Poli, S. Perbellini, A. Raffaelli, V. Cacciatori, L. Santi, G. Targher, R. Bonadonna, and M. Muggeo. 2002. Homa-estimated insulin resistance is an independent predictor of cardiovascular disease in type 2 diabetic subjects: Prospective data from the Verona Diabetes Complications Study. *Diabetes Care* 25(7):1135–1141.

Boogers, L. S., C. M. Wiepjes, D. T. Klink, I. Hellinga, A. S. P. van Trotsenburg, M. den Heijer, and S. E. Hannema. 2022. Transgender girls grow tall: Adult height is unaffected by GnRH analogue and estradiol treatment. *Journal of Clinical Endocrinology & Metabolism* 107(9):e3805–e3815.

Bredella, M. A. 2017. Sex differences in body composition. *Advances in Experimental Medicine and Biology* 1043:9–27.

Brien, T. G. 1975. Cortisol metabolism after oral contraceptives: Total plasma cortisol and the free cortisol index. *British Journal of Obstetrics and Gynaecology* 82(12):987–991.

Brooks, D. C., J. S. Coon V, C. M. Ercan, X. Xu, H. Dong, J. E. Levine, S. E. Bulun, and H. Zhao. 2020. Brain aromatase and the regulation of sexual activity in male mice. *Endocrinology* 161(10):bqaa137.

Brouillette, J., K. Rivard, E. Lizotte, and C. Fiset. 2005. Sex and strain differences in adult mouse cardiac repolarization: Importance of androgens. *Cardiovascular Research* 65(1):148–157.

Bulkhi, A. A., K. V. Shepard, 2nd, T. B. Casale, and J. C. Cardet. 2020. Elevated testosterone is associated with decreased likelihood of current asthma regardless of sex. *Journal of Allergy and Clinical Immunology* 8(9):3029–3035.e4.

Bunderen, C. C. V., J. Leentjens, and S. Middeldorp. 2022. Transgender medicine and risk of venous thromboembolism. *Hamostaseologie* 42(5):301–307.

Burger, H. G., E. C. Dudley, J. L. Hopper, N. Groome, J. R. Guthrie, A. Green, and L. Dennerstein. 1999. Prospectively measured levels of serum follicle-stimulating hormone, estradiol, and the dimeric inhibins during the menopausal transition in a population-based cohort of women. *Journal of Clinical Endocrinology & Metabolism* 84(11):4025–4030.

Campbell, S. E., and M. A. Febbraio. 2002. Effect of the ovarian hormones on GLUT4 expression and contraction-stimulated glucose uptake. *American Journal of Physiology-Endocrinology and Metabolism* 282(5):E1139–E1146.

Carey, V. J., E. E. Walters, G. A. Colditz, C. G. Solomon, W. C. Willett, B. A. Rosner, F. E. Speizer, and J. E. Manson. 1997. Body fat distribution and risk of non-insulin-dependent diabetes mellitus in women. The Nurses' Health Study. *American Journal of Epidemiology* 145(7):614–619.

Carmina, E., S. Bucchieri, A. Esposito, A. Del Puente, P. Mansueto, F. Orio, G. Di Fede, and G. Rini. 2007. Abdominal fat quantity and distribution in women with polycystic ovary syndrome and extent of its relation to insulin resistance. *Journal of Clinical Endocrinology & Metabolism* 92(7):2500–2505.

Çayan, F., U. Dilek, Ö. Pata, and S. Dilek. 2008. Comparison of the effects of hormone therapy regimens, oral and vaginal estradiol, estradiol+ drospirenone and tibolone, on sexual function in healthy postmenopausal women. *The Journal of Sexual Medicine* 5(1):132–138.

Ceolin, C., A. Scala, M. Dall'Agnol, C. Ziliotto, A. Delbarba, P. Facondo, A. Citron, B. Vescovi, S. Pasqualini, S. Giannini, V. Camozzi, C. Cappelli, A. Bertocco, M. De Rui, A. Coin, G. Sergi, A. Ferlin, A. Garolla, and Gender Incongruence Interdisciplinary Group. 2023. Bone health and body composition in transgender adults before gender-affirming hormonal therapy: Data from the comet study. *Journal of Endocrinological Investigation* 47(2):401–410.

Chakrabarti, S., J. S. Morton, and S. T. Davidge. 2014. Mechanisms of estrogen effects on the endothelium: An overview. *Canadian Journal of Cardiology* 30(7):705–712.

Chang, Y., J. Li, X. Li, H. Liu, and X. Liang. 2018. Egg quality and pregnancy outcome in young infertile women with diminished ovarian reserve. *Medical Science Monitor: International Medical Journal of Experimental and Clinical Research* 24:7279–7284.

Chen, D., L. Simons, E. K. Johnson, B. A. Lockart, and C. Finlayson. 2017. Fertility preservation for transgender adolescents. *Journal of Adolescent Health* 61(1):120–123.

Chen, G. G., A. C. Vlantis, Q. Zeng, and C. A. van Hasselt. 2008. Regulation of cell growth by estrogen signaling and potential targets in thyroid cancer. *Current Cancer Drug Targets* 8(5):367–377.

Chen, W., B. Obermayer-Pietsch, J. B. Hong, B. C. Melnik, O. Yamasaki, C. Dessinioti, Q. Ju, A. I. Liakou, S. Al-Khuzaei, A. Katsambas, J. Ring, and C. C. Zouboulis. 2011. Acne-associated syndromes: Models for better understanding of acne pathogenesis. *Journal of the European Academy of Dermatology and Venerology* 25(6):637–646.

Cheung, A. S., S. Zwickl, K. Miller, B. J. Nolan, A. F. Q. Wong, P. Jones, and N. Eynon. 2024. The impact of gender-affirming hormone therapy on physical performance. *Journal of Clinical Endocrinology & Metabolism* 109(2):e455–e465.

Chitturi, S., and G. C. Farrell. 2013. Adverse effects of hormones and hormone antagonists on the liver. In *Drug-induced liver disease* (3rd ed.), edited by N. Kaplowitz and L. D. DeLeve. Boston: Academic Press. Pp. 605–619.

Choudhry, R., M. B. Hodgins, T. H. Van der Kwast, A. O. Brinkmann, and W. J. Boersma. 1992. Localization of androgen receptors in human skin by immunohistochemistry: Implications for the hormonal regulation of hair growth, sebaceous glands and sweat glands. *Journal of Endocrinology* 133(3):467–475.

Chowdhury, N. U., V. P. Guntur, D. C. Newcomb, and M. E. Wechsler. 2021. Sex and gender in asthma. *European Respiratory Review: An Official Journal of the European Respiratory Society* 30(162):210067.

Christensen, J. D., C. Davidge-Pitts, M. R. Castro, and P. Caraballo. 2021. Characterization of thyroid disease prevalence among transgender and gender-diverse patients. *Journal of the Endocrine Society* 5(S1):A837–A838.

Christensen, J., H. Basheer, and J. Lado-Abeal. 2023. Late breaking abstracts. *Thyroid®* 33(S1):A-125–A-171.

Cirillo, D. J., R. B. Wallace, R. J. Rodabough, P. Greenland, A. Z. LaCroix, M. C. Limacher, and J. C. Larson. 2005. Effect of estrogen therapy on gallbladder disease. *Journal of the American Medical Association* 293(3):330–339.

Cirrincione, L. R., and R. R. Narla. 2021. Gender-affirming hormone therapy and bone health: Do different regimens influence outcomes in transgender adults? A narrative review and call for future studies. *Journal of Applied Laboratory Medicine* 6(1):219–235.

Clayton, A. H. 2003. Sexual function and dysfunction in women. *Psychiatric Clinics North America* 26(3):673–682.

Clegg, D. J., L. M. Brown, J. M. Zigman, C. J. Kemp, A. D. Strader, S. C. Benoit, S. C. Woods, M. Mangiaracina, and N. Geary. 2007. Estradiol-dependent decrease in the orexigenic potency of ghrelin in female rats. *Diabetes* 56(4):1051–1058.

Cocchetti, C., G. Castellini, D. Iacuaniello, A. Romani, M. Maggi, L. Vignozzi, T. Schreiner, M. den Heijer, G. T'Sjoen, and A. D. Fisher. 2021. Does gender-affirming hormonal treatment affect 30-year cardiovascular risk in transgender persons? A two-year prospective European study (ENIGI). *Journal of Sexual Medicine* 18(4):821–829.

Cocchetti, C., A. Romani, S. Collet, Y. Greenman, T. Schreiner, C. Wiepjes, M. den Heijer, G. T'Sjoen, and A. D. Fisher. 2022. The ENIGI (European Network for the Investigation of Gender Incongruence) Study: Overview of acquired endocrine knowledge and future perspectives. *Journal of Clinical Medicine* 11(7):1784.

Colizzi, M., R. Costa, V. Pace, and O. Todarello. 2013. Hormonal treatment reduces psychobiological distress in gender identity disorder, independently of the attachment style. *Journal of Sexual Medicine* 10(12):3049–3058.

Colizzi, M., R. Costa, F. Scaramuzzi, C. Palumbo, M. Tyropani, V. Pace, L. Quagliarella, F. Brescia, L. C. Natilla, G. Loverro, and O. Todarello. 2015. Concomitant psychiatric problems and hormonal treatment induced metabolic syndrome in gender dysphoria individuals: A 2 year follow-up study. *Journal of Psychosomatic Research* 78(4):399–406.

Cooper, A. J., S. R. Gupta, A. F. Moustafa, and A. M. Chao. 2021. Sex/gender differences in obesity prevalence, comorbidities, and treatment. *Current Obesity Reports* 10(4):458–466.

Corona, G., G. Rastrelli, A. Morgentaler, A. Sforza, E. Mannucci, and M. Maggi. 2017. Meta-analysis of results of testosterone therapy on sexual function based on international index of erectile function scores. *European Urology* 72(6):1000–1011.

Cosman, F., S. J. de Beur, M. S. LeBoff, E. M. Lewiecki, B. Tanner, S. Randall, R. Lindsay, and F. National Osteoporosis. 2014. Clinician's guide to prevention and treatment of osteoporosis. *Osteoporosis International: A journal established as a result of cooperation between the European Foundation for Osteoporosis and The National Osteoporosis Foundation of the USA* 25(10):2359–2381.

Cui, X., C. Zhang, F. Wang, X. Zhao, S. Wang, J. Liu, D. He, C. Wang, F. C. Yang, S. Tong, and Y. Liang. 2023. Latexin regulates sex dimorphism in hematopoiesis via gender-specific differential expression of microrna 98-3p and thrombospondin 1. *Cell Reports* 42(3):112274.

Cunha, F. S., S. Domenice, V. L. Camara, M. H. Sircili, L. J. Gooren, B. B. Mendonca, and E. M. Costa. 2015. Diagnosis of prolactinoma in two male-to-female transsexual subjects following high-dose cross-sex hormone therapy. *Andrologia* 47(6):680–684.

Cushman, M., L. H. Kuller, R. Prentice, R. J. Rodabough, B. M. Psaty, R. S. Stafford, S. Sidney, F. R. Rosendaal, and Women's Health Initiative Investigators. 2004. Estrogen plus progestin and risk of venous thrombosis. *Journal of the American Medical Association* 292(13):1573–1580.

Da Silva Lara, L. A., B. Useche, R. A. Ferriani, R. M. Reis, M. F. S. De Sá, M. M. S. De Freitas, J. C. R. e Silva, and A. C. J. De Sá Rosa e Silva. 2009. The effects of hypoestrogenism on the vaginal wall: Interference with the normal sexual response. *The Journal of Sexual Medicine* 6(1):30–39.

Davis, S. R., R. Goldstat, M. A. Papalia, S. Shah, J. Kulkarni, S. Donath, and R. J. Bell. 2006. Effects of aromatase inhibition on sexual function and well-being in postmenopausal women treated with testosterone: A randomized, placebo-controlled trial. *Menopause* 13(1):37–45.

de Blok, C. J., C. M. Wiepjes, D. M. van Velzen, A. S. Staphorsius, N. M. Nota, L. J. Gooren, B. P. Kreukels, and M. den Heijer. 2021. Mortality trends over five decades in adult transgender people receiving hormone treatment: A report from the Amsterdam Cohort of Gender Dysphoria. *Lancet Diabetes & Endocrinology* 9(10):663–670.

De Bree, L., R. Janssen, P. Aaby, R. van Crevel, L. A. Joosten, C. S. Benn, and M. G. Netea. 2018. The impact of sex hormones on BCG-induced trained immunity. *Journal of Leukocyte Biology* 104(3):573–578.

de Nie, I., J. Asseler, A. Meissner, I. A. C. Voorn-de Warem, E. H. Kostelijk, M. den Heijer, J. Huirne, and N. M. van Mello. 2022. A cohort study on factors impairing semen quality in transgender women. *American Journal of Obstetrics and Gynecology* 226(3):390. e1-390.e10.

De Sanctis, V., A. T. Soliman, S. Di Maio, N. Soliman, and H. Elsedfy. 2019. Long-term effects and significant adverse drug reactions (ADRS) associated with the use of gonadotropin-releasing hormone analogs (GNRHA) for central precocious puberty: A brief review of literature. *Acta Biomedica* 90(3):345–359.

de Vries, C. P., L. J. Gooren, and E. A. van der Veen. 1986. The effect of cyproterone acetate alone and in combination with ethinylestradiol on the hypothalamic pituitary adrenal axis, prolactin and growth hormone release in male-to-female transsexuals. *Hormone and Metabolic Research* 18(3):203–205.

Deadmond, A., C. A. Koch, and J. P. Parry. 2000. Ovarian reserve testing [Updated 2022 December 21]. In *Endotext [Internet]*. South Dartmouth, MA: MDText.com.

Deenadayalu, V., Y. Puttabyatappa, A. T. Liu, J. N. Stallone, and R. E. White. 2012. Testosterone-induced relaxation of coronary arteries: Activation of BKCA channels via the CGMP-dependent protein kinase. *American Journal of Physiology-Heart and Circulatory* 302(1):H115–H123.

Defreyne, J., B. Vantomme, E. Van Caenegem, K. Wierckx, C. J. M. De Blok, M. Klaver, N. M. Nota, D. Van Dijk, C. M. Wiepjes, M. Den Heijer, and G. T'Sjoen. 2018. Prospective evaluation of hematocrit in gender-affirming hormone treatment: Results from European Network for the Investigation of Gender Incongruence. *Andrology* 6(3):446–454.

Defreyne, J., E. Elaut, B. Kreukels, A. D. Fisher, G. Castellini, A. Staphorsius, M. Den Heijer, G. Heylens, and G. T'Sjoen. 2020. Sexual desire changes in transgender individuals upon initiation of hormone treatment: Results from the longitudinal European Network for the Investigation of Gender Incongruence. *Journal of Sexual Medicine* 17(4):812–825.

Deischinger, C., D. Slukova, I. Just, U. Kaufmann, J. Harreiter, M. van Trotsenburg, S. Trattnig, M. Krssak, A. Kautzky-Willer, R. Klepochova, and L. Kosi-Trebotic. 2022. Effects of gender-affirming hormone therapy on cardiovascular risk factors focusing on glucose metabolism in an Austrian Transgender Cohort. *International Journal of Transgender Health* 24(4):499–509.

DeLoughery, T. G. 2022. Hematologic concerns in transgender patients. *Clinical Advances in Hematology and Oncology* 20(8):516–523.

Desai, K., B. Almeida, and M. Miteva. 2021. Understanding hormonal therapies: Overview for the dermatologist focused on hair. *Dermatology* 237(5):786–791.

Deswal, A., and B. Bozkurt. 2006. Comparison of morbidity in women versus men with heart failure and preserved ejection fraction. *American Journal of Cardiology* 97(8):1228–1231.

Di Guardo, F., V. Vloeberghs, E. Bardhi, C. Blockeel, G. Verheyen, H. Tournaye, and P. Drakopoulos. 2020. Low testosterone and semen parameters in male partners of infertile couples undergoing IVF with a total sperm count greater than 5 million. *Journal of Clinical Medicine* 9(12):3824.

Dias, S. P., M. C. Brouwer, and D. van de Beek. 2022. Sex and gender differences in bacterial infections. *Infection and Immunity* 90(10):e0028322.

Dominelli, P. B., J. N. Render, Y. Molgat-Seon, G. E. Foster, L. M. Romer, and A. W. Sheel. 2015. Oxygen cost of exercise hyperpnoea is greater in women compared with men. *Journal of Physiology* 593(8):1965–1979.

Dominelli, P. B., Y. Molgat-Seon, and A. W. Sheel. 2019. Sex differences in the pulmonary system influence the integrative response to exercise. *Exercise and Sport Sciences Reviews* 47(3):142–150.

Dominelli, P. B., and Y. Molgat-Seon. 2022. Sex, gender and the pulmonary physiology of exercise. *European Respiratory Review* 31(163):210074.

dos Santos, R. L., F. B. da Silva, R. F. Ribeiro, Jr., and I. Stefanon. 2014. Sex hormones in the cardiovascular system. *Hormone Molecular Biology and Clinical Investigation* 18(2):89–103.

Drake, M. T., and S. Khosla. 2013. The role of sex steroids in the pathogenesis of osteoporosis. In *Primer on the metabolic bone diseases and disorders of mineral metabolism*. Hoboken, NJ: John Wiley & Sons, Ltd. Pp. 367–375.

Dragon, C. N., P. Guerino, E. Ewald, and A. M. Laffan. 2017. Transgender medicare beneficiaries and chronic conditions: Exploring fee-for-service claims data. *LGBT Health* 4(6):404–411.

Duan, Y., T. J. Beck, X. F. Wang, and E. Seeman. 2003. Structural and biomechanical basis of sexual dimorphism in femoral neck fragility has its origins in growth and aging. *Journal of Bone and Mineral Research* 18(10):1766–1774.

Elamin, M. B., M. Z. Garcia, M. H. Murad, P. J. Erwin, and V. M. Montori. 2010. Effect of sex steroid use on cardiovascular risk in transsexual individuals: A systematic review and meta-analyses. *Clinical Endocrinology (Oxford)* 72(1):1–10.

Elbers, J. M., H. Asscheman, J. C. Seidell, J. A. Megens, and L. J. Gooren. 1997. Long-term testosterone administration increases visceral fat in female to male transsexuals. *Journal of Clinical Endocrinology & Metabolism* 82(7):2044–2047.

Elbers, J. M., E. J. Giltay, T. Teerlink, P. G. Scheffer, H. Asscheman, J. C. Seidell, and L. J. Gooren. 2003. Effects of sex steroids on components of the insulin resistance syndrome in transsexual subjects. *Clinical Endocrinology (Oxford)* 58(5):562–571.

Elliot, S. J., M. Karl, M. Berho, M. Potier, F. Zheng, B. Leclercq, G. E. Striker, and L. J. Striker. 2003. Estrogen deficiency accelerates progression of glomerulosclerosis in susceptible mice. *American Journal of Pathology* 162(5):1441–1448.

Emi, Y., M. Adachi, A. Sasaki, Y. Nakamura, and M. Nakatsuka. 2008. Increased arterial stiffness in female-to-male transsexuals treated with androgen. *Journal of Obstetrics and Gynaecology Research* 34(5):890–897.

English, K. M., R. D. Jones, T. H. Jones, A. H. Morice, and K. S. Channer. 2002. Testosterone acts as a coronary vasodilator by a calcium antagonistic action. *Journal of Endocrinological Investigation* 25(5):455–458.

Epperson, C. N., M. D. Sammel, and E. W. Freeman. 2013. Menopause effects on verbal memory: Findings from a longitudinal community cohort. *Journal of Clinical Endocrinology & Metabolism* 98(9):3829–3838.

Fang, H., J. Xu, H. Wu, H. Fan, and L. Zhong. 2016. Combination of Klinefelter syndrome and acromegaly: A rare case report. *Medicine* 95(17):e3444.

Fernandez, J. D., and L. R. Tannock. 2016. Metabolic effects of hormone therapy in transgender patients. *Endocrine Practice* 22(4):383–388.

Fernández, R., E. Delgado-Zayas, K. Ramírez, J. Cortés-Cortés, E. Gómez-Gil, I. Esteva, M. C. Almaraz, A. Guillamon, and E. Pásaro. 2020. Analysis of four polymorphisms located at the promoter of the estrogen receptor alpha ESR1 gene in a population with gender incongruence. *Sexual Medicine* 8(3):490–500.

Fernández-Pérez, L., M. de Mirecki-Garrido, B. Guerra, M. Díaz, and J. C. Díaz-Chico. 2016. Sex steroids and growth hormone interactions. *Endocrinologia y Nutricion* 63(4):171–180.

Fighera, T. M., E. da Silva, J. D. Lindenau, and P. M. Spritzer. 2018. Impact of cross-sex hormone therapy on bone mineral density and body composition in transwomen. *Clinical Endocrinology* 88(6):856–862.

Fimmel, S., and C. C. Zouboulis. 2005. Influence of physiological androgen levels on wound healing and immune status in men. *Aging Male* 8(3–4):166–174.

Fink, A. L., K. Engle, R. L. Ursin, W. Y. Tang, and S. L. Klein. 2018. Biological sex affects vaccine efficacy and protection against influenza in mice. *Proceedings of the National Academy of Sciences of the United States of America* 115(49):12477–12482.

Finkelstein, J. S., H. Lee, B. Z. Leder, S. A. Burnett-Bowie, D. W. Goldstein, C. W. Hahn, S. C. Hirsch, A. Linker, N. Perros, A. B. Servais, A. P. Taylor, M. L. Webb, J. M. Youngner, and E. W. Yu. 2016. Gonadal steroid-dependent effects on bone turnover and bone mineral density in men. *Journal of Clinical Investigation* 126(3):1114–1125.

Finlayson, C., D. Styne, and J. Jameson. 2016. Endocrinology of sexual maturation and puberty. In *Endocrinology: Adult and Pediatric.* Philadelphia, PA: Saunders. Pp. 2119–2129.e2112.

Florencio-Silva, R., G. R. Sasso, E. Sasso-Cerri, M. J. Simoes, and P. S. Cerri. 2015. Biology of bone tissue: Structure, function, and factors that influence bone cells. *BioMed Research International* 2015:421746.

Foer, D., D. Rubins, A. Almazan, P. G. Wickner, D. W. Bates, and O. R. Hamnvik. 2021. Gender reference use in spirometry for transgender patients. *Annals of the American Thoracic Society* 18(3):537–540.

Folsom, A. R., S. A. Kaye, T. A. Sellers, C. P. Hong, J. R. Cerhan, J. D. Potter, and R. J. Prineas. 1993. Body fat distribution and 5-year risk of death in older women. *Journal of the American Medical Association* 269(4):483–487.

Freier, E., L. Kassel, J. Rand, and B. Chinnakotla. 2021. Estrogen-induced gallstone pancreatitis in a transgender female. *American Journal of Health-System Pharmacy* 78(18):1674–1680.

Fuentes, N., and P. Silveyra. 2018. Endocrine regulation of lung disease and inflammation. *Experimental Biology and Medicine (Maywood)* 243(17–18):1313–1322.

Fung, R., M. Hellstern-Layefsky, C. Tastenhoye, I. Lega, and L. Steele. 2016. Differential effects of cyproterone acetate vs spironolactone on serum high-density lipoprotein and prolactin concentrations in the hormonal treatment of transgender women. *Journal of Sexual Medicine* 13(11):1765–1772.

Fuss, J., L. Claro, M. Ising, S. V. Biedermann, K. Wiedemann, G. K. Stalla, P. Briken, and M. K. Auer. 2019. Does sex hormone treatment reverse the sex-dependent stress regulation? A longitudinal study on hypothalamus-pituitary-adrenal (HPA) axis activity in transgender individuals. *Psychoneuroendocrinology* 104:228–237.

Gabrielson, A. T., R. A. Sartor, and W. J. G. Hellstrom. 2019. The impact of thyroid disease on sexual dysfunction in men and women. *Sexual Medicine Reviews* 7(1):57–70.

Gambineri, A., C. Pelusi, and R. Pasquali. 2003. Testosterone levels in obese male patients with obstructive sleep apnea syndrome: Relation to oxygen desaturation, body weight, fat distribution and the metabolic parameters. *Journal of Endocrinological Investigation* 26(6):493–498.

Gava, G., I. Mancini, S. Cerpolini, M. Baldassarre, R. Seracchioli, and M. C. Meriggiola. 2018. Testosterone undecanoate and testosterone enanthate injections are both effective and safe in transmen over 5 years of administration. *Clinical Endocrinology* 89(6):878–886.

Getahun, D., R. Nash, W. D. Flanders, T. C. Baird, T. A. Becerra-Culqui, L. Cromwell, E. Hunkeler, T. L. Lash, A. Millman, V. P. Quinn, B. Robinson, D. Roblin, M. J. Silverberg, J. Safer, J. Slovis, V. Tangpricha, and M. Goodman. 2018. Cross-sex hormones and acute cardiovascular events in transgender persons: A cohort study. *Annals of Internal Medicine* 169(4):205–213.

Gibney, J., T. Wolthers, G. Johannsson, A. M. Umpleby, and K. K. Ho. 2005. Growth hormone and testosterone interact positively to enhance protein and energy metabolism in hypopituitary men. *American Journal of Phsyiology-Endocrinology and Metabolism* 289(2):E266–E271.

Giltay, E. J., and L. J. Gooren. 2000. Effects of sex steroid deprivation/administration on hair growth and skin sebum production in transsexual males and females. *Journal of Clinical Endocrinology & Metabolism* 85(8):2913–2921.

Glintborg, D., K. H. Rubin, T. G. Petersen, O. Lidegaard, G. T'Sjoen, M. Hilden, and M. S. Andersen. 2022. Cardiovascular risk in Danish transgender persons: A matched historical cohort study. *European Journal of Endocrinology* 187(3):463–477.

Goandal, N. F., J. Rungby, and K. E. Karmisholt. 2022. The role of sex hormones in the pathogenesis of melasma. *Ugeskr Laeger* 184(6):V10210769.

Godwin, M. D., A. Aggarwal, Z. Hilt, S. Shah, J. Gorski, and S. J. Cameron. 2022. Sex-dependent effect of platelet nitric oxide: Production and platelet reactivity in healthy individuals. *JACC Basic to Translational Science* 7(1):14–25.

Gooren, L. 1985. Human male sexual functions do not require aromatization of testosterone: A study using tamoxifen, testolactone, and dihydrotestosterone. *Archives of Sexual Behavior* 14:539–548.

Gorski, R. A., J. H. Gordon, J. E. Shryne, and A. M. Southam. 1978. Evidence for a morphological sex difference within the medial preoptic area of the rat brain. *Brain Research* 148(2):333–346.

Grabek, A., B. Dolfi, B. Klein, F. Jian-Motamedi, M. C. Chaboissier, and A. Schedl. 2019. The adult adrenal cortex undergoes rapid tissue renewal in a sex-specific manner. *Cell Stem Cell* 25(2):290–296.e292.

Greenwald, P., B. Dubois, J. Lekovich, J. H. Pang, and J. Safer. 2022. Successful in vitro fertilization in a cisgender female carrier using oocytes retrieved from a transgender man maintained on testosterone. *AACE Clinical Case Reports* 8(1):19–21.

Greiman, A. K., and T. E. Keane. 2017. Approach to androgen deprivation in the prostate cancer patient with pre-existing cardiovascular disease. *Current Urology Reports* 18(6):41.

Grimstad, F. W., M. M. Knoll, and J. D. Jacobson. 2021. Oxandrolone use in trans-masculine youth appears to increase adult height: Preliminary evidence. *LGBT Health* 8(4):300–306.

Grossmann, M. 2014. Testosterone and glucose metabolism in men: Current concepts and controversies. *Journal of Endocrinology* 220(3):R37–R55.

Guo, W., E. Bachman, M. Li, C. N. Roy, J. Blusztajn, S. Wong, S. Y. Chan, C. Serra, R. Jasuja, T. G. Travison, M. U. Muckenthaler, E. Nemeth, and S. Bhasin. 2013. Testosterone administration inhibits hepcidin transcription and is associated with increased iron incorporation into red blood cells. *Aging Cell* 12(2):280–291.

Gur, R. C., D. Alsop, D. Glahn, R. Petty, C. L. Swanson, J. A. Maldjian, B. I. Turetsky, J. A. Detre, J. Gee, and R. E. Gur. 2000. An fMRI study of sex differences in regional activation to a verbal and a spatial task. *BrainLang* 74(2):157–170.

Hage, M., O. Plesa, I. Lemaire, and M. L. Raffin Sanson. 2022. Estrogen and progesterone therapy and meningiomas. *Endocrinology* 163(2):bqab259.

Hajszan, T., N. J. MacLusky, and C. Leranth. 2008. Role of androgens and the androgen receptor in remodeling of spine synapses in limbic brain areas. *Hormones and Behavior* 53(5):638–646.

Hampton, J., M. Manikkam, D. Lubahn, M. Smith, and H. Garverick. 2004. Androgen receptor mRNA expression in the bovine ovary. *Domestic Animal Endocrinology* 27(1):81–88.

Han, Y. Y., Q. Yan, G. Yang, W. Chen, E. Forno, and J. C. Celedon. 2020. Serum free testosterone and asthma, asthma hospitalisations and lung function in British adults. *Thorax* 75(10):849–854.

Handel, A. C., L. D. Miot, and H. A. Miot. 2014. Melasma: A clinical and epidemiological review. *Anais Brasileiros de Dermatologia* 89(5):771–782.

Hanley, K., U. Rassner, Y. Jiang, D. Vansomphone, D. Crumrine, L. Komuves, P. M. Elias, K. R. Feingold, and M. L. Williams. 1996. Hormonal basis for the gender difference in epidermal barrier formation in the fetal rat. Acceleration by estrogen and delay by testosterone. *Journal of Clinical Investigation* 97(11):2576–2584.

Hansen, E. S. H., K. Aasbjerg, A. L. Moeller, E. J. Gade, C. Torp-Pedersen, and V. Backer. 2021. Hormone replacement therapy and development of new asthma. *Chest* 160(1):45–52.

Hao, J., P. R. Rapp, W. G. Janssen, W. Lou, B. L. Lasley, P. R. Hof, and J. H. Morrison. 2007. Interactive effects of age and estrogen on cognition and pyramidal neurons in monkey prefrontal cortex. *Proceedings of the National Academy of Sciences of the United States of America* 104(27):11465–11470.

Hara, Y., E. M. Waters, B. S. McEwen, and J. H. Morrison. 2015. Estrogen effects on cognitive and synaptic health over the life course. *Physiological Reviews* 95(3):785–807.

Harper, S., and J. Lynch. 2007. Trends in socioeconomic inequalities in adult health behaviors among U.S. states, 1990–2004. *Public Health Reports* 122(2):177–189.

Harris, A. N., H. W. Lee, G. Osis, L. Fang, K. L. Webster, J. W. Verlander, and I. D. Weiner. 2018. Differences in renal ammonia metabolism in male and female kidney. *American Journal of Physiology—Renal Physiology* 315(2):F211–F222.

Harris, A. N., H. W. Lee, J. W. Verlander, and I. D. Weiner. 2020. Testosterone modulates renal ammonia metabolism. *American Journal of Physiology—Renal Physiology* 318(4):F922–F935.

Harris, G. W. 1948. Neural control of the pituitary gland. *Physiological Reviews* 28(2):139–179.

Harvey, R. E., K. E. Coffman, and V. M. Miller. 2015. Women-specific factors to consider in risk, diagnosis and treatment of cardiovascular disease. *Womens Health* 11(2):239–257.

Hashemi, L., Q. Zhang, D. Getahun, G. K. Jasuja, C. McCracken, J. Pisegna, D. Roblin, M. J. Silverberg, V. Tangpricha, S. Vupputuri, and M. Goodman. 2021. Longitudinal changes in liver enzyme levels among transgender people receiving gender affirming hormone therapy. *Journal of Sexual Medicine* 18(9):1662–1675.

Hasselquist, M. B., N. Goldberg, A. Schroeter, and T. C. Spelsberg. 1980. Isolation and characterization of the estrogen receptor in human skin. *Journal of Clinical Endocrinology & Metabolism* 50(1):76–82.

Hattori, K., Y. Tahara, K. Moji, K. Aoyagi, and T. Furusawa. 2004. Chart analysis of body composition change among pre- and post-adolescent Japanese subjects assessed by underwater weighing method. *International Journal of Obesity and Related Metabolic Disorders* 28(4):520–524.

Haynes, J. M., and R. W. Stumbo. 2018. The impact of using non-birth sex on the interpretation of spirometry data in subjects with air-flow obstruction. *Respiratory Care* 63(2):215–218.

Hembree, W. C., P. T. Cohen-Kettenis, L. Gooren, S. E. Hannema, W. J. Meyer, M. H. Murad, S. M. Rosenthal, J. D. Safer, V. Tangpricha, and G. G. T'Sjoen. 2017. Endocrine treatment of gender-dysphoric/gender-incongruent persons: An endocrine society clinical practice guideline. *Journal of Clinical Endocrinology & Metabolism* 102(11):3869–3903.

Herring, M. J., P. M. Oskui, S. L. Hale, and R. A. Kloner. 2013. Testosterone and the cardiovascular system: A comprehensive review of the basic science literature. *Journal of the American Heart Association* 2(4):e000271.

Hilton, E. N., and T. R. Lundberg. 2021. Transgender women in the female category of sport: Perspectives on testosterone suppression and performance advantage. *Sports Medicine* 51(2):199–214.

Hines, M., V. Pasterski, D. Spencer, S. Neufeld, P. Patalay, P. C. Hindmarsh, I. A. Hughes, and C. L. Acerini. 2016. Prenatal androgen exposure alters girls' responses to information indicating gender-appropriate behaviour. *Philosophical Transactions of the Royal Society B* 371(1688):20150125.

Howard, B. V., and J. E. Rossouw. 2013. Estrogens and cardiovascular disease risk revisited: The Women's Health Initiative. *Current Opinion in Lipidology* 24(6):493–499.

Hou, J., and W. F. Zheng. 1988. Effect of sex hormones on NK and ADDC activity of mice. *International Journal of Immunopharmacology* 10(1):15–22.

Hutchens, M. P., T. Fujiyoshi, R. Komers, P. S. Herson, and S. Anderson. 2012. Estrogen protects renal endothelial barrier function from ischemia-reperfusion in vitro and in vivo. *American Journal of Physiology—Renal Physiology* 303(3):F377–F385.

Imperato-McGinley, J., T. Gautier, L. Q. Cai, B. Yee, J. Epstein, and P. Pochi. 1993. The androgen control of sebum production. Studies of subjects with dihydrotestosterone deficiency and complete androgen insensitivity. *Journal of Clinical Endocrinology & Metabolism* 76(2):524–528.

Ingalhalikar, M., A. Smith, D. Parker, T. D. Satterthwaite, M. A. Elliott, K. Ruparel, H. Hakonarson, R. E. Gur, R. C. Gur, and R. Verma. 2014. Sex differences in the structural connectome of the human brain. *Proceedings of the National Academy of Sciences of the United States of America* 111(2):823–828.

Irwig, M. S. 2017. Testosterone therapy for transgender men. *The Lancet Diabetes & Endocrinology* 5(4):301–311.

Islam, N., R. Nash, Q. Zhang, L. Panagiotakopoulos, T. Daley, S. Bhasin, D. Getahun, J. Sonya Haw, C. McCracken, M. J. Silverberg, V. Tangpricha, S. Vupputuri, and M. Goodman. 2022. Is there a link between hormone use and diabetes incidence in transgender people? Data from the strong cohort. *Journal of Clinical Endocrinology & Metabolism* 107(4):e1549–e1557.

Issa, Z., E. W. Seely, M. Rahme, and G. El-Hajj Fuleihan. 2015. Effects of hormone therapy on blood pressure. *Menopause* 22(4):456–468.

Jacobsen, H., and S. L. Klein. 2021. Sex differences in immunity to viral infections. *Frontiers in Immunology* 12:720952.

Jensen, M. D. 2008. Role of body fat distribution and the metabolic complications of obesity. *Journal of Clinical Endocrinology & Metabolism* 93(11 Suppl 1):S57–S63.

Jiang, D. D., E. Swenson, M. Mason, K. R. Turner, D. D. Dugi, J. C. Hedges, and S. L. Hecht. 2019. Effects of estrogen on spermatogenesis in transgender women. *Urology* 132:117–122.

Jiao, L., J. O. Machuki, Q. Wu, M. Shi, L. Fu, A. O. Adekunle, X. Tao, C. Xu, X. Hu, Z. Yin, and H. Sun. 2020. Estrogen and calcium handling proteins: New discoveries and mechanisms in cardiovascular diseases. *American Journal of Physiology-Heart and Circulatory* 318(4):H820–H829.

Jones, C. A., G. M. McQuillan, J. W. Kusek, M. S. Eberhardt, W. H. Herman, J. Coresh, M. Salive, C. P. Jones, and L. Y. Agodoa. 1998. Serum creatinine levels in the U.S. population: Third national health and nutrition examination survey. *American Journal of Kidney Disease* 32(6):992–999.

Jones, R. D., P. J. Pugh, T. H. Jones, and K. S. Channer. 2003. The vasodilatory action of testosterone: A potassium-channel opening or a calcium antagonistic action? *British Journal of Pharmacology* 138(5):733–744.

Jones, T. H., S. Arver, H. M. Behre, J. Buvat, E. Meuleman, I. Moncada, A. M. Morales, M. Volterrani, A. Yellowlees, J. D. Howell, K. S. Channer, and T. Investigators. 2011. Testosterone replacement in hypogonadal men with type 2 diabetes and/or metabolic syndrome (the Times2 Study). *Diabetes Care* 34(4):828–837.

Kacker, R., A. M. Traish, and A. Morgentaler. 2012. Estrogens in men: Clinical implications for sexual function and the treatment of testosterone deficiency. *The Journal of Sexual Medicine* 9(6):1681–1696.

Kam, G. Y., K. C. Leung, R. C. Baxter, and K. K. Ho. 2000. Estrogens exert route- and dose-dependent effects on insulin-like growth factor (IGF)-binding protein-3 and the acid-labile subunit of the IGF ternary complex. *Journal of Clinical Endocrinology & Metabolism* 85(5):1918–1922.

Karalexi, M. A., M. K. Georgakis, N. G. Dimitriou, T. Vichos, A. Katsimpris, E. T. Petridou, and F. C. Papadopoulos. 2020. Gender-affirming hormone treatment and cognitive function in transgender young adults: A systematic review and meta-analysis. *Psychoneuroendocrinology* 119:104721.

Karastergiou, K., S. R. Smith, A. S. Greenberg, and S. K. Fried. 2012. Sex differences in human adipose tissues—The biology of pear shape. *Biology of Sex Differences* 3(1):13.

Karim, R., R. M. Dell, D. F. Greene, W. J. Mack, J. C. Gallagher, and H. N. Hodis. 2011. Hip fracture in postmenopausal women after cessation of hormone therapy: Results from a prospective study in a large health management organization. *Menopause* 18(11):1172–1177.

Kasarinaite, A., M. Sinton, P. T. K. Saunders, and D. C. Hay. 2023. The influence of sex hormones in liver function and disease. *Cells* 12(12):1604.

Kattah, A. G., C. Y. Smith, L. Gazzuola Rocca, B. R. Grossardt, V. D. Garovic, and W. A. Rocca. 2018. Ckd in patients with bilateral oophorectomy. *Clinical Journal of the American Society of Nephrology* 13(11):1649–1658.

Kautzky-Willer, A., M. Leutner, and J. Harreiter. 2023. Sex differences in type 2 diabetes. *Diabetologia* 66(6):986–1002.

Keenan, B. S., G. E. Richards, S. W. Ponder, J. S. Dallas, M. Nagamani, and E. R. Smith. 1993. Androgen-stimulated pubertal growth: The effects of testosterone and dihydrotestosterone on growth hormone and insulin-like growth factor-I in the treatment of short stature and delayed puberty. *Journal of Clinical Endocrinology & Metabolism* 76(4):996–1001.

Kerkemeyer, K. L., L. T. de Carvalho, R. Jerjen, J. John, R. D. Sinclair, J. Pinczewski, and B. Bhoyrul. 2021. Female pattern hair loss in men: A distinct clinical variant of androgenetic alopecia. *Journal of the American Academy of Dermatology* 85(1):260–262.

Khalid, S., G. Laput, K. Khorfan, and M. Roytman. 2023. Development of liver cancers as an unexpected consequence of anabolic androgenic steroid use. *Cureus* 15(1):e34357.

Khera, M. 2015. Testosterone therapy for female sexual dysfunction. *Sexual Medicine Reviews* 3(3):137–144.

Khosla, S., L. J. Melton, 3rd, and B. L. Riggs. 2011. The unitary model for estrogen deficiency and the pathogenesis of osteoporosis: Is a revision needed? *Journal of Bone and Mineral Research* 26(3):441–451.

Kim, S. D., and K. S. Cho. 2019. Obstructive sleep apnea and testosterone deficiency. *World Journal of Men's Health* 37(1):12–18.

Kiyar, M., M. A. Kubre, S. Collet, T. Van Den Eynde, G. T'Sjoen, A. Guillamon, and S. C. Mueller. 2022. Gender-affirming hormonal treatment changes neural processing of emotions in trans men: An fMRI study. *Psychoneuroendocrinology* 146:105928.

Klaver, M., M. Dekker, R. de Mutsert, J. W. R. Twisk, and M. den Heijer. 2017. Cross-sex hormone therapy in transgender persons affects total body weight, body fat and lean body mass: A meta-analysis. *Andrologia* 49(5):e12660.

Klein, S. L., and K. L. Flanagan. 2016. Sex differences in immune responses. *Nature Reviews Immunology* 16(10):626–638.

Kleinschmidt-DeMasters, B. K. 2020. Pituitary adenomas in transgender individuals? *Journal of Neuropathology and Experimental Neurology* 79(1):62–66.

Kline, L. W., and E. Karpinski. 2008. Testosterone and dihydrotestosterone inhibit gallbladder motility through multiple signaling pathways. *Steroids* 73(11):1174–1180.

Klink, D., M. Caris, A. Heijboer, M. van Trotsenburg, and J. Rotteveel. 2015. Bone mass in young adulthood following gonadotropin-releasing hormone analog treatment and cross-sex hormone treatment in adolescents with gender dysphoria. *Journal of Clinical Endocrinology & Metabolism* 100(2):E270–E275.

Konadu, M. E., M. B. Reed, U. Kaufmann, P. A. Handschuh, M. Spies, B. Spurny-Dworak, M. Klöbl, V. Ritter, G. M. Godbersen, R. Seiger, P. Baldinger-Melich, G. S. Kranz, and R. Lanzenberger. 2022. Changes to hypothalamic volume and associated subfields during gender-affirming hormone treatment in gender dysphoria. *medRxiv (Cold Spring Harbor Laboratory)*. Pre-print.

Kosmas, C. E., D. Silverio, A. Sourlas, P. D. Montan, and E. Guzman. 2018. Role of spironolactone in the treatment of heart failure with preserved ejection fraction. *Annals of Translational Medicine* 6(23):461.

Kovats, S. 2015. Estrogen receptors regulate innate immune cells and signaling pathways. *Cell Immunology* 294(2):63–69.

Kranz, G. S., W. Wadsak, U. Kaufmann, M. Savli, P. Baldinger, G. Gryglewski, D. Haeusler, M. Spies, M. Mitterhauser, S. Kasper, and R. Lanzenberger. 2015. High-dose testosterone treatment increases serotonin transporter binding in transgender people. *Biological Psychiatry* 78(8):525–533.

Kranz, G. S., B. B. B. Zhang, P. Handschuh, V. Ritter, and R. Lanzenberger. 2020. Gender-affirming hormone treatment—A unique approach to study the effects of sex hormones on brain structure and function. *Cortex* 129:68–79.

Krishnamurthy, N., D. J. Slack, M. Kyweluk, O. Cullen, J. Kirkley, and J. D. Safer. 2023. Erythrocytosis is rare with exogenous testosterone in gender-affirming hormone therapy. *Journal of Clinical Endocrinology & Metabolism* 109(5):1285–1290.

Krupka, E., S. Curtis, T. Ferguson, R. Whitlock, N. Askin, A. C. Millar, M. Dahl, R. Fung, S. B. Ahmed, and N. Tangri. 2022. The effect of gender-affirming hormone therapy on measures of kidney function: A systematic review and meta-analysis. *Clinical Journal of the American Society of Nephrology* 17(9):1305–1315.

Kumar, A., C. M. Klinge, and R. E. Goldstein. 2010. Estradiol-induced proliferation of papillary and follicular thyroid cancer cells is mediated by estrogen receptors alpha and beta. *International Journal of Oncology* 36(5):1067–1080.

Kwan, M., J. VanMaasdam, and J. M. Davidson. 1985. Effects of estrogen treatment on sexual behavior in male-to-female transsexuals: Experimental and clinical observations. *Archives of Sexual Behavior* 14(1):29–40.

La Vignera, S., A. E. Calogero, R. Cannarella, R. A. Condorelli, C. Magagnini, and A. Aversa. 2020. Obstructive sleep apnea and testosterone replacement therapy. *Androgens: Clinical Research and Therapeutics* 1(1):10–14.

Lapidus, L., C. Bengtsson, B. Larsson, K. Pennert, E. Rybo, and L. Sjostrom. 1984. Distribution of adipose tissue and risk of cardiovascular disease and death: A 12 year follow up of participants in the population study of women in Gothenburg, Sweden. *British Medical Journal (Clinical Research Edition)* 289(6454):1257–1261.

Lee, J. Y., C. Finlayson, J. Olson-Kennedy, R. Garofalo, Y. M. Chan, D. V. Glidden, and S. M. Rosenthal. 2020. Low bone mineral density in early pubertal transgender/gender diverse youth: Findings from the trans youth care study. *Journal of the Endocrine Society* 4(9):bvaa065.

Lee, J. Y., B. Fan, G. Montenegro, R. K. Long, S. Sanda, G. Capodanno, A. L. Schafer, A. J. Burghardt, S. M. Rosenthal, and E. B. Fung. 2022. Interpretation of bone mineral density z-scores by dual-energy x-ray absorptiometry in transgender and gender diverse youth prior to gender-affirming medical therapy. *Journal of Clinical Densitometry* 25(4):559–568.

Leemaqz, S. Y., M. Kyinn, K. Banks, E. Sarkodie, D. Goldstein, and M. S. Irwig. 2023. Lipid profiles and hypertriglyceridemia among transgender and gender diverse adults on gender-affirming hormone therapy. *Journal of Clinical Lipidology* 17(1):103–111.

Lemay, A., and Y. Poulin. 2002. Oral contraceptives as anti-androgenic treatment of acne. *Journal of Obstetrics and Gynecology Canada* 24(7):559–567.

Leranth, C., T. Hajszan, and N. J. MacLusky. 2004. Androgens increase spine synapse density in the CA1 hippocampal subfield of ovariectomized female rats. *Journal of Neuroscience* 24(2):495–499.

Leslie, S., T. Soon-Sutton, and M. A. Khan. 2024. *Male infertility* [Updated 2024 February 25], StatPearls. Treasure Island, FL: StatPearls Publishing.

Leung, A., D. Sakkas, S. Pang, K. Thornton, and N. Resetkova. 2019. Assisted reproductive technology outcomes in female-to-male transgender patients compared with cisgender patients: A new frontier in reproductive medicine. *Fertility and Sterility* 112(5):858–865.

Leung, K. C., G. Johannsson, G. M. Leong, and K. K. Ho. 2004. Estrogen regulation of growth hormone action. *Endocrine Reviews* 25(5):693–721.

Liu, B., J. Wang, Y.-y. Li, K.-p. Li, and Q. Zhang. 2023. The association between systemic immune-inflammation index and rheumatoid arthritis: Evidence from NHANES 1999–2018. *Arthritis Research & Therapy* 25(1):34.

Liu, T., Y.-q. Cui, H. Zhao, H.-b. Liu, S.-d. Zhao, Y. Gao, X.-l. Mu, F. Gao, and Z.-j. Chen. 2015. High levels of testosterone inhibit ovarian follicle development by repressing the FSH signaling pathway. *Journal of Huazhong University of Science and Technology [Medical Sciences]* 35(5):723–729.

Liu, Y., F. Kong, W. Wang, J. Xin, S. Zhang, J. Chen, X. Ming, X. Wu, W. Cui, H. Wang, and W. Li. 2022. Low estrogen level in aged mice leads to abnormal oogenesis affecting the quality of surrounded nucleolus-type immature oocytes. *Reproduction, Fertility, and Development* 34(15):991–1001.

Lichanska, A. M., and M. J. Waters. 2008. How growth hormone controls growth, obesity and sexual dimorphism. *Trends in Genetics* 24(1):41–47.

Lincoff, A. M., S. Bhasin, P. Flevaris, L. M. Mitchell, S. Basaria, W. E. Boden, G. R. Cunningham, C. B. Granger, M. Khera, I. M. Thompson, Jr., Q. Wang, K. Wolski, D. Davey, V. Kalahasti, N. Khan, M. G. Miller, M. C. Snabes, A. Chan, E. Dubcenco, X. Li, T. Yi, B. Huang, K. M. Pencina, T. G. Travison, S. E. Nissen, and TRAVERSE Study Investigators. 2023. Cardiovascular safety of testosterone-replacement therapy. *New England Journal of Medicine* 389(2):107–117.

Lizardi-Cervera, J., L. Cuéllar-Gamboa, and D. Motola-Kuba. 2006. Focal nodular hyperplasia and hepatic adenoma: A review. *Annals of Hepatology* 5(3):206–211.

LoMauro, A., and A. Aliverti. 2018. Sex differences in respiratory function. *Breathe* 14(2):131–140.

LoMauro, A., and A. Aliverti. 2021. Sex and gender in respiratory physiology. *European Respiratory Review* 30(162):210038.

Long, D. A., M. Kolatsi-Joannou, K. L. Price, C. Dessapt-Baradez, J. L. Huang, E. Papakrivopoulou, M. Hubank, R. Korstanje, L. Gnudi, and A. S. Woolf. 2013. Albuminuria is associated with too few glomeruli and too much testosterone. *Kidney International* 83(6):1118–1129.

Loomba-Albrecht, L. A., and D. M. Styne. 2009. Effect of puberty on body composition. *Current Opinion in Endocrinology, Diabetes and Obesity* 16(1):10–15.

Lotter, H., E. Helk, H. Bernin, T. Jacobs, C. Prehn, J. Adamski, N. González-Roldán, O. Holst, and E. Tannich. 2013. Testosterone increases susceptibility to amebic liver abscess in mice and mediates inhibition of IFNγ secretion in natural killer T cells. *PLoS ONE* 8(2):e55694.

Lovejoy, J. C., C. M. Champagne, L. de Jonge, H. Xie, and S. R. Smith. 2008. Increased visceral fat and decreased energy expenditure during the menopausal transition. *International Journal of Obesity* 32(6):949–958.

Lovejoy, J. C., A. Sainsbury, and Stock Conference Working Group. 2009. Sex differences in obesity and the regulation of energy homeostasis. *Obesity Reviews* 10(2):154–167.

Lukacs, B. 2001. Assessment of male sexual function. *Prostate Cancer Prostatic Diseases* 4(S1):S7–S11.

Luo, H., Y. Huang, M. Han, Y. Pang, P. Yu, Y. Tang, H. Yuan, J. Li, and W. Chen. 2021. Associations of serum estradiol level, serum estrogen receptor-alpha level, and estrogen receptor-alpha polymorphism with male infertility: A retrospective study. *Medicine* 100(29):e26577.

Lyraki, R., and A. Schedl. 2021. The sexually dimorphic adrenal cortex: Implications for adrenal disease. *International Journal of Molecular Sciences* 22(9):4889.

MacMaster, F. P., M. Keshavan, Y. Mirza, N. Carrey, A. R. Upadhyaya, R. El-Sheikh, C. J. Buhagiar, S. P. Taormina, C. Boyd, M. Lynch, M. Rose, J. Ivey, G. J. Moore, and D. R. Rosenberg. 2007. Development and sexual dimorphism of the pituitary gland. *Life Sciences* 80(10):940–944.

Madsen, M. C., D. van Dijk, C. M. Wiepjes, E. B. Conemans, A. Thijs, and M. den Heijer. 2021. Erythrocytosis in a large cohort of trans men using testosterone: A long-term follow-up study on prevalence, determinants, and exposure years. *Journal of Clinical Endocrinology & Metabolism* 106(6):1710–1717.

Magri, F., V. Capelli, M. Rotondi, P. Leporati, L. La Manna, R. Ruggiero, A. Malovini, R. Bellazzi, L. Villani, and L. Chiovato. 2012. Expression of estrogen and androgen receptors in differentiated thyroid cancer: An additional criterion to assess the patient's risk. *Endocrine-Related Cancer* 19(4):463–471.

Maheshwari, A., V. Dines, D. Saul, T. Nippoldt, A. Kattah, and C. Davidge-Pitts. 2022. The effect of gender-affirming hormone therapy on serum creatinine in transgender individuals. *Endocrine Practice* 28(1):52–57.

Makrantonaki, E., and C. C. Zouboulis. 2009. Androgens and ageing of the skin. *Current Opinion in Endocrinology, Diabetes and Obesity* 16(3):240–245.

Malkin, C. J., P. J. Pugh, R. D. Jones, D. Kapoor, K. S. Channer, and T. H. Jones. 2004. The effect of testosterone replacement on endogenous inflammatory cytokines and lipid profiles in hypogonadal men. *The Journal of Clinical Endocrinology & Metabolism* 89(7):3313–3318.

Mandhane, P. J., S. E. Hanna, M. D. Inman, J. M. Duncan, J. M. Greene, H. Y. Wang, and M. R. Sears. 2009. Changes in exhaled nitric oxide related to estrogen and progesterone during the menstrual cycle. *Chest* 136(5):1301–1307.

Maraka, S., N. Singh Ospina, R. Rodriguez-Gutierrez, C. J. Davidge-Pitts, T. B. Nippoldt, L. J. Prokop, and M. H. Murad. 2017. Sex steroids and cardiovascular outcomes in transgender individuals: A systematic review and meta-analysis. *Journal of Clinical Endocrinology & Metabolism* 102(11):3914–3923.

Martinez, C., R. Rikhi, T. Haque, A. Fazal, M. Kolber, B. E. Hurwitz, N. Schneiderman, and T. T. Brown. 2020. Gender identity, hormone therapy, and cardiovascular disease risk. *Current Problems in Cardiology* 45(5):100396.

Maseroli, E., and L. Vignozzi. 2020. Testosterone and vaginal function. *Sexual Medicine Reviews* 8(3):379–392.

Masumori, N., and M. Nakatsuka. 2023. Cardiovascular risk in transgender people with gender-affirming hormone treatment. *Circulation Reports* 5(4):105–113.

Mauvais-Jarvis, F. 2015. Sex differences in metabolic homeostasis, diabetes, and obesity. *Biology of Sex Differences* 6(1):14.

Mauvais-Jarvis, F., D. J. Clegg, and A. L. Hevener. 2013. The role of estrogens in control of energy balance and glucose homeostasis. *Endocrine Reviews* 34(3):309–338.

Mauvais-Jarvis, F., J. E. Manson, J. C. Stevenson, and V. A. Fonseca. 2017. Menopausal hormone therapy and type 2 diabetes prevention: Evidence, mechanisms, and clinical implications. *Endocrine Reviews* 38(3):173–188.

Maynard, L. M., W. Wisemandle, A. F. Roche, W. C. Chumlea, S. S. Guo, and R. M. Siervogel. 2001. Childhood body composition in relation to body mass index. *Pediatrics* 107(2):344–350.

Mazer, N. A. 2004. Interaction of estrogen therapy and thyroid hormone replacement in postmenopausal women. *Thyroid* 14 Suppl 1:S27–S34.

McCarthy, M. M. 2016. Multifaceted origins of sex differences in the brain. *Philosophical Transaction of the Royal Society, Series B, Biological Sciences* 371(1688):20150106.

McEwan, S., H. Kwon, A. Tahiri, N. Shanmugarajah, W. Cai, J. Ke, T. Huang, A. Belton, B. Singh, L. Wang, Z. P. Pang, E. Dirice, E. A. Engel, and A. El Ouaamari. 2021. Deconstructing the origins of sexual dimorphism in sensory modulation of pancreatic beta cells. *Molecular Metabolism* 53:101260.

McEwen, B. S., and T. A. Milner. 2007. Hippocampal formation: Shedding light on the influence of sex and stress on the brain. *Brain Research Reviews* 55(2):343–355.

McEwen, B. S., and T. A. Milner. 2017. Understanding the broad influence of sex hormones and sex differences in the brain. *Journal of Neuroscience Research* 95(1–2):24–39.

McKenzie, J., B. M. Fisher, A. J. Jaap, A. Stanley, K. Paterson, and N. Sattar. 2006. Effects of HRT on liver enzyme levels in women with type 2 diabetes: A randomized placebo-controlled trial. *Clinical Endocrinology* 65(1):40–44.

Medina, K. L., A. Strasser, and P. W. Kincade. 2000. Estrogen influences the differentiation, proliferation, and survival of early b-lineage precursors. *Blood* 95(6):2059–2067.

Mikkonen, L., P. Pihlajamaa, B. Sahu, F. P. Zhang, and O. A. Janne. 2010. Androgen receptor and androgen-dependent gene expression in lung. *Molecular & Cellular Endocrinology* 317(1–2):14–24.

Millas, I., and M. Duarte Barros. 2021. Estrogen receptors and their roles in the immune and respiratory systems. *Anatomical Record* 304(6):1185–1193.

Millward, C. P., S. M. Keshwara, A. I. Islim, M. D. Jenkinson, A. F. Alalade, and C. E. Gilkes. 2022. Development and growth of intracranial meningiomas in transgender women taking cyproterone acetate as gender-affirming progestogen therapy: A systematic review. *Transgender Health* 7(6):473–483.

Mitsuhashi, K., T. Senmaru, T. Fukuda, M. Yamazaki, K. Shinomiya, M. Ueno, S. Kinoshita, J. Kitawaki, M. Katsuyama, M. Tsujikawa, H. Obayashi, N. Nakamura, and M. Fukui. 2016. Testosterone stimulates glucose uptake and glut4 translocation through LKB1/AMPK signaling in 3T3-l1 adipocytes. *Endocrine* 51(1):174–184.

Mode, A., and J. A. Gustafsson. 2006. Sex and the liver—A journey through five decades. *Drug Metabolism Reviews* 38(1–2):197–207.

Mohammad, I., I. Starskaia, T. Nagy, J. Guo, E. Yatkin, K. Väänänen, W. T. Watford, and Z. Chen. 2018. Estrogen receptor α contributes to T cell-mediated autoimmune inflammation by promoting T cell activation and proliferation. *Science Signaling* 11(526):eaap9415.

Mohammed, K., A. M. Abu Dabrh, K. Benkhadra, A. Al Nofal, B. G. Carranza Leon, L. J. Prokop, V. M. Montori, S. S. Faubion, and M. H. Murad. 2015. Oral vs transdermal estrogen therapy and vascular events: A systematic review and meta-analysis. *Journal of Clinical Endocrinology & Metabolism* 100(11):4012–4020.

Mohottige, D., and D. S. Tuot. (2022). Advancing kidney health equity. *Clinical Journal of the American Society of Nephrology* 17(9):1281–1283.

Møller, N., and J. O. Jørgensen. 2009. Effects of growth hormone on glucose, lipid, and protein metabolism in human subjects. *Endocrine Reviews* 30(2):152–177.

Molloy, E. J., A. J. O'Neill, J. J. Grantham, M. Sheridan-Pereira, J. M. Fitzpatrick, D. W. Webb, and R. W. Watson. 2003. Sex-specific alterations in neutrophil apoptosis: The role of estradiol and progesterone. *Blood* 102(7):2653–2659.

Montano, L. M., E. Calixto, A. Figueroa, E. Flores-Soto, V. Carbajal, and M. Perusquia. 2008. Relaxation of androgens on rat thoracic aorta: Testosterone concentration dependent agonist/antagonist l-type CA2+ channel activity, and 5beta-dihydrotestosterone restricted to l-type CA2+ channel blockade. *Endocrinology* 149(5):2517–2526.

Moreno-Arrones, O. M., A. Becerra, and S. Vano-Galvan. 2017. Therapeutic experience with oral finasteride for androgenetic alopecia in female-to-male transgender patients. *Clinical and Experimental Dermatology* 42(7):743–748.

Murphy, W. G. 2014. The sex difference in haemoglobin levels in adults—Mechanisms, causes, and consequences. *Blood Reviews* 28(2):41–47.

Murphy, W. G., E. Tong, and C. Murphy. 2010. Why do women have similar erythropoietin levels to men but lower hemoglobin levels? *Blood* 116(15):2861–2862.

Muscogiuri, G., L. Verde, C. Vetrani, L. Barrea, S. Savastano, and A. Colao. 2023. Obesity: A gender-view. *Journal of Endocrinological Investigation* 47(2):299–306.

Nahrendorf, M., S. Frantz, K. Hu, C. von zur Muhlen, M. Tomaszewski, H. Scheuermann, R. Kaiser, V. Jazbutyte, S. Beer, W. Bauer, S. Neubauer, G. Ertl, B. Allolio, and F. Callies. 2003. Effect of testosterone on post-myocardial infarction remodeling and function. *Cardiovascular Research* 57(2):370–378.

Nguyen, H. B., A. M. Chavez, E. Lipner, L. Hantsoo, S. L. Kornfield, R. D. Davies, and C. N. Epperson. 2018. Gender-affirming hormone use in transgender individuals: Impact on behavioral health and cognition. *Current Psychiatry Reports* 20(12):110.

Nolan, B. J., S. Y. Leemaqz, O. Ooi, P. Cundill, N. Silberstein, P. Locke, M. Grossmann, J. D. Zajac, and A. S. Cheung. 2021. Prevalence of polycythaemia with different formulations of testosterone therapy in transmasculine individuals. *Internal Medicine Journal* 51(6):873–878.

Nota, N. M., C. M. Wiepjes, C. J. M. de Blok, L. J. G. Gooren, S. M. Peerdeman, B. P. C. Kreukels, and M. den Heijer. 2018. The occurrence of benign brain tumours in transgender individuals during cross-sex hormone treatment. *Brain* 141(7):2047–2054.

Nota, N. M., C. M. Wiepjes, C. J. M. de Blok, L. J. G. Gooren, B. P. C. Kreukels, and M. den Heijer. 2019. Occurrence of acute cardiovascular events in transgender individuals receiving hormone therapy. *Circulation* 139(11):1461–1462.

Noventa, M., A. Vitagliano, A. Andrisani, M. Blaganje, P. Viganò, E. Papaelo, M. Scioscia, F. Cavallin, G. Ambrosini, and M. Cozzolino. 2019. Testosterone therapy for women with poor ovarian response undergoing IVF: A meta-analysis of randomized controlled trials. *Journal of Assisted Reproduction and Genetics* 36:673–683.

Nowak, K. W., G. Neri, G. G. Nussdorfer, and L. K. Malendowicz. 1995. Effects of sex hormones on the steroidogenic activity of dispersed adrenocortical cells of the rat adrenal cortex. *Life Sciences* 57(9):833–837.

Oakes, M., A. Arastu, C. Kato, J. Somers, H. D. Holly, B. K. Elstrott, G. W. Dy, T. C. L. Kohs, R. R. Patel, O. J. T. McCarty, T. G. DeLoughery, C. Milano, V. Raghunathan, and J. J. Shatzel. 2021. Erythrocytosis and thromboembolic events in transgender individuals receiving gender-affirming testosterone. *Thrombosis Research* 207:96–98.

Ogawa, S., A. E. Chester, S. C. Hewitt, V. R. Walker, J.-Å. Gustafsson, O. Smithies, K. S. Korach, and D. W. Pfaff. 2000. Abolition of male sexual behaviors in mice lacking estrogen receptors α and β (αβerko). *Proceedings of the National Academy of Sciences* 97(26):14737–14741.

Ohtani, M., A. García, A. B. Rogers, Z. Ge, N. S. Taylor, S. Xu, K. Watanabe, R. P. Marini, M. T. Whary, and T. C. Wang. 2007. Protective role of 17β-estradiol against the development of helicobacter pylori-induced gastric cancer in INS-GAS mice. *Carcinogenesis* 28(12):2597–2604.

Okamoto, M., Y. Hojo, K. Inoue, T. Matsui, S. Kawato, B. S. McEwen, and H. Soya. 2012. Mild exercise increases dihydrotestosterone in hippocampus providing evidence for androgenic mediation of neurogenesis. *Proceedings of the National Academy of Sciences of the United States of America* 109(32):13100–13105.

Olié, V., M. Canonico, and P. Y. Scarabin. 2010. Risk of venous thrombosis with oral versus transdermal estrogen therapy among postmenopausal women. *Current Opinion in Hematology* 17(5):457–463.

Olsen, E. A. 2001. Female pattern hair loss. *Journal of the American Academy of Dermatology* 45(S3):S70–S80.

Olson-Kennedy, J., V. Okonta, L. F. Clark, and M. Belzer. 2018. Physiologic response to gender-affirming hormones among transgender youth. *Journal of Adolescent Health* 62(4):397–401.

Oskarsson, V., N. Orsini, O. Sadr-Azodi, and A. Wolk. 2014. Postmenopausal hormone replacement therapy and risk of acute pancreatitis: A prospective cohort study. *Canadian Medical Association Journal* 186(5):338–344.

Ott, J., U. Kaufmann, E. K. Bentz, J. C. Huber, and C. B. Tempfer. 2010. Incidence of thrombophilia and venous thrombosis in transsexuals under cross-sex hormone therapy. *Fertility and Sterility* 93(4):1267–1272.

Ott, J., S. Aust, R. Promberger, J. C. Huber, and U. Kaufmann. 2011. Cross-sex hormone therapy alters the serum lipid profile: A retrospective cohort study in 169 transsexuals. *Journal of Sexual Medicine* 8(8):2361–2369.

Panagiotakopoulos, L. 2018. Transgender medicine—Puberty suppression. *Reviews in Endocrine and Metabolic Disorders* 19(3):221–225.

Patel, A. S., J. Y. Leong, L. Ramos, and R. Ramasamy. 2019. Testosterone is a contraceptive and should not be used in men who desire fertility. *The World Journal of Men's Health* 37(1):45–54.

Payne, K., L. I. Lipshultz, J. M. Hotaling, and A. W. Pastuszak. 2021. Obstructive sleep apnea and testosterone therapy. *Sexual Medicine Reviews* 9(2):296–303.

Pecina, H. I., T. C. Pecina, V. Vyroubal, I. Kruljac, and M. Slaus. 2017. Age and sex related differences in normal pituitary gland and fossa volumes. *Frontiers in Bioscience-Elite* 9(2):204–213.

Perez, P. A., J. P. Petiti, F. Picech, C. B. Guido, L. dV Sosa, E. Grondona, J. H. Mukdsi, A. L. De Paul, A. I. Torres, and S. Gutierrez. 2018. Estrogen receptor beta regulates the tumoral suppressor PTEN to modulate pituitary cell growth. *Journal of Cellular Physiology* 233(2):1402–1413.

Perez-Luis, J., B. Gomez-Alvarez, and P. Guirado-Pelaez. 2019. *Predictive factors of testosterone-induced erythrocytosis on transgender males.* Paper read at 21st European Congress of Endocrinology (ECE 2019), Lyon, France.

Pham, T. V., E. A. Sosunov, E. P. Anyukhovsky, P. Danilo, Jr., and M. R. Rosen. 2002. Testosterone diminishes the proarrhythmic effects of dofetilide in normal female rabbits. *Circulation* 106(16):2132–2136.

Pietzak, E., and P. Mucksavage. 2016. Bone health in prostate cancer. In *Prostate cancer*. Cambridge, MA: Academic Press. Pp. 491–507.

Pinkerton, K. E., M. Harbaugh, M. K. Han, C. Jourdan Le Saux, L. S. Van Winkle, W. J. Martin, 2nd, R. J. Kosgei, E. J. Carter, N. Sitkin, S. M. Smiley-Jewell, and M. George. 2015. Women and lung disease. Sex differences and global health disparities. *American Journal of Respiratory and Critical Care Medicine* 192(1):11–16.

Polan, M. L., A. Daniele, and A. Kuo. 1988. Gonadal steroids modulate human monocyte interleukin-1 (IL-1) activity. *Fertility and Sterility* 49(6):964–968.

Polderman, K. H., L. J. Gooren, H. Asscheman, A. Bakker, and R. J. Heine. 1994. Induction of insulin resistance by androgens and estrogens. *Journal of Clinical Endocrinology & Metabolism* 79(1):265–271.

Pontes, L. T., D. T. Camilo, M. R. De Bortoli, R. S. S. Santos, and W. M. Luchi. 2018. New-onset lupus nephritis after male-to-female sex reassignment surgery. *Lupus* 27(13):2166–2169.

Pothuri, V. S., M. Anzelmo, E. Gallaher, Y. Ogunlana, S. Aliabadi-Wahle, B. Tan, J. S. Crippin, and C. W. Hammill. 2023. Transgender males on gender-affirming hormone therapy and hepatobiliary neoplasms: A systematic review. *Endocrine Practice* 29(10):822–829.

Prabhavathi, K., K. T. Selvi, K. N. Poornima, and A. Sarvanan. 2014. Role of biological sex in normal cardiac function and in its disease outcome—A review. *Journal of Clinical and Diagnostic Research* 8(8):BE01–BE04.

Punnonen, R. 1971. On the effect of castration and peroral estrogen therapy on the skin. *Acta Obstetricia et Gynecologica Scandinavica* 9(S21):Suppl 9:32.

Qiu, Y. B., L. Y. Liao, R. Jiang, M. Xu, L. W. Xu, G. G. Chen, and Z. M. Liu. 2019. PES1 promotes the occurrence and development of papillary thyroid cancer by upregulating the ERalpha/ERbeta protein ratio. *Science Reports* 9(1):1032.

Qureshi, A. C., A. Bahri, L. A. Breen, S. C. Barnes, J. K. Powrie, S. M. Thomas, and P. V. Carroll. 2007. The influence of the route of oestrogen administration on serum levels of cortisol-binding globulin and total cortisol. *Clinical Endocrinology* 66(5):632–635.

Radi, R., S. Gold, J. P. Acosta, J. Barron, and H. Yeung. 2022. Treating acne in transgender persons receiving testosterone: A practical guide. *American Journal of Clinical Dermatology* 23(2):219–229.

Rajoria, S., R. Suriano, A. Shanmugam, Y. L. Wilson, S. P. Schantz, J. Geliebter, and R. K. Tiwari. 2010. Metastatic phenotype is regulated by estrogen in thyroid cells. *Thyroid* 20(1):33–41.

Ramaekers, D., H. Ector, A. E. Aubert, A. Rubens, and F. Van de Werf. 1998. Heart rate variability and heart rate in healthy volunteers. Is the female autonomic nervous system cardioprotective? *European Heart Journal* 19(9):1334–1341.

Ransick, A., N. O. Lindstrom, J. Liu, Q. Zhu, J. J. Guo, G. F. Alvarado, A. D. Kim, H. G. Black, J. Kim, and A. P. McMahon. 2019. Single-cell profiling reveals sex, lineage, and regional diversity in the mouse kidney. *Developmental Cell* 51(3):399–413.e397.

Rao, C. K., C. G. Moore, E. Bleecker, W. W. Busse, W. Calhoun, M. Castro, K. F. Chung, S. C. Erzurum, E. Israel, D. Curran-Everett, and S. E. Wenzel. 2013. Characteristics of perimenstrual asthma and its relation to asthma severity and control: Data from the severe asthma research program. *Chest* 143(4):984–992.

Raven, L. M., M. Guttman-Jones, and C. A. Muir. 2021. Hyperprolactinemia and association with prolactinoma in transwomen receiving gender affirming hormone treatment. *Endocrine* 72(2):524–528.

Rettew, J. A., Y. M. Huet-Hudson, and I. Marriott. 2008. Testosterone reduces macrophage expression in the mouse of toll-like receptor 4, a trigger for inflammation and innate immunity. *Biology of Reproduction* 78(3):432–437.

Rizk, P. J., T. P. Kohn, A. W. Pastuszak, and M. Khera. 2017. Testosterone therapy improves erectile function and libido in hypogonadal men. *Current Opinion in Urology* 27(6):511–515.

Roberts, S. A., and J. M. Carswell. 2021. Growth, growth potential, and influences on adult height in the transgender and gender-diverse population. *Andrology* 9(6):1679–1688.

Robertson, B. D., B. S. Lerner, J. F. Collen, and P. R. Smith. 2019. The effects of transgender hormone therapy on sleep and breathing: A case series. *Journal of Clinical Sleep Medicine* 15(10):1529–1533.

Robertson, K. M., L. O'Donnell, M. E. Jones, S. J. Meachem, W. C. Boon, C. R. Fisher, K. H. Graves, R. I. McLachlan, and E. R. Simpson. 1999. Impairment of spermatogenesis in mice lacking a functional aromatase (CYP 19) gene. *Proceedings of the National Academy of Sciences of the United States of America* 96(14):7986–7991.

Robinson, G. A., J. Peng, H. Peckham, G. Butler, I. Pineda-Torra, C. Ciurtin, and E. C. Jury. 2022. Investigating sex differences in T regulatory cells from cisgender and transgender healthy individuals and patients with autoimmune inflammatory disease: A cross-sectional study. *Lancet Rheumatology* 4(10):e710–e724.

Roden, A. C., M. T. Moser, S. D. Tri, M. Mercader, S. M. Kuntz, H. Dong, A. A. Hurwitz, D. J. McKean, E. Celis, B. C. Leibovich, J. P. Allison, and E. D. Kwon. 2004. Augmentation of T cell levels and responses induced by androgen deprivation. *Journal of Immunology* 173(10):6098–6108.

Rodriguez-Wallberg, K. A., J. Haljestig, S. Arver, A. L. V. Johansson, and F. E. Lundberg. 2021. Sperm quality in transgender women before or after gender affirming hormone therapy—A prospective cohort study. *Andrology* 9(6):1773–1780.

Roerink, S., D. Marsman, A. van Bon, and R. Netea-Maier. 2014. A missed diagnosis of acromegaly during a female-to-male gender transition. *Archives of Sexual Behavior* 43(6):1199–1201.

Roselli, C., and J. Balthazart. 2011. Sexual differentiation of sexual behavior and its orientation. *Frontiers in Neuroendocrinology* 32(2):109.

Rosen, H. N., O. R. Hamnvik, U. Jaisamrarn, A. O. Malabanan, J. D. Safer, V. Tangpricha, L. Wattanachanya, and S. S. Yeap. 2019. Bone densitometry in transgender and gender non-conforming (TGNC) individuals: 2019 ISCD official position. *Journal of Clinical Densitometry* 22(4):544–553.

Rosen, R. C. 2000. Prevalence and risk factors of sexual dysfunction in men and women. *Current Psychiatry Reports* 2(3):189–195.

Rothman, M. S., and S. J. Iwamoto. 2019. Bone health in the transgender population. *Clinical Reviews in Bone and Mineral Metabolism* 17(2):77–85.

Roubinian, J., N. Talal, J. Greenspan, J. Goodman, and P. Siiteri. 1978. Effect of castration and sex hormone treatment on survival, anti-nucleic acid antibodies, and glomerulonephritis in NZB/NZW F1 mice. *The Journal of Experimental Medicine* 147(6):1568–1583.

Rutnin, S., P. Suchonwanit, C. Kositkuljorn, C. Pomsoong, S. Korpaisarn, J. Arunakul, and T. Rattananukrom. 2023. Characterizing dermatological conditions in the transgender population: A cross-sectional study. *Transgender Health* 8(1):89–99.

Saeedi, P., I. Petersohn, P. Salpea, B. Malanda, S. Karuranga, N. Unwin, S. Colagiuri, L. Guariguata, A. A. Motala, K. Ogurtsova, J. E. Shaw, D. Bright, R. Williams, and IDF Diabetes Atlas Committee. 2019. Global and regional diabetes prevalence estimates for 2019 and projections for 2030 and 2045: Results from the *International Diabetes Federation Diabetes Atlas*, 9th edition. *Diabetes Research and Clinical Practice* 157:107843.

Safer, J. D., and V. Tangpricha. 2019. Care of transgender persons. *New England Journal of Medicine* 381(25):2451–2460.

Saharkhiz, N., S. Zademodares, S. Salehpour, S. Hosseini, L. Nazari, and H. G. Tehrani. 2018. The effect of testosterone gel on fertility outcomes in women with a poor response in in vitro fertilization cycles: A pilot randomized clinical trial. *Journal of Research in Medical Sciences* 23(1):3.

Sandberg, K., and H. Ji. 2012. Sex differences in primary hypertension. *Biology of Sex Differences* 3(1):7.

Santin, A. P., and T. W. Furlanetto. 2011. Role of estrogen in thyroid function and growth regulation. *Journal of Thyroid Research* 2011:875125.

Scarabin, P. Y., E. Oger, G. Plu-Bureau, EStrogen and THromboEmbolism Risk Study Group. 2003. Differential association of oral and transdermal oestrogen-replacement therapy with venous thromboembolism risk. *Lancet* 362(9382):428–432.

Schagen, S. E., P. T. Cohen-Kettenis, H. A. Delemarre-van de Waal, and S. E. Hannema. 2016. Efficacy and safety of gonadotropin-releasing hormone agonist treatment to suppress puberty in gender dysphoric adolescents. *Journal of Sexual Medicine* 13(7):1125–1132.

Schagen, S. E. E., F. M. Wouters, P. T. Cohen-Kettenis, L. J. Gooren, and S. E. Hannema. 2020. Bone development in transgender adolescents treated with GnRH analogues and subsequent gender-affirming hormones. *Journal of Clinical Endocrinology & Metabolism* 105(12):e4252–e4263.

Schally, A. V., A. Arimura, and A. J. Kastin. 1973. Hypothalamic regulatory hormones. *Science* 179(4071):341–350.

Scheres, L. J. J., N. L. D. Selier, N. M. Nota, J. J. K. van Diemen, S. C. Cannegieter, and M. den Heijer. 2021. Effect of gender-affirming hormone use on coagulation profiles in transmen and transwomen. *Thrombosis and Haemostasis* 19(4):1029–1037.

Scheuer, J., A. Malhotra, T. F. Schaible, and J. Capasso. 1987. Effects of gonadectomy and hormonal replacement on rat hearts. *Circulation Research* 61(1):12–19.

Schneider, M. A., P. M. Spritzer, J. S. Suh, L. Minuzzi, B. N. Frey, K. Schwarz, A. B. Costa, D. C. da Silva, C. C. G. Garcia, A. M. V. Fontanari, M. Anes, J. U. Castan, F. R. Cunegatto, F. A. Picon, E. Luders, and M. I. R. Lobato. 2020. The link between estradiol and neuroplasticity in transgender women after gender-affirming surgery: A bimodal hypothesis. *Neuroendocrinology* 110(6):489–500.

Schutte, M. H., R. Kleemann, N. M. Nota, C. M. Wiepjes, J. M. Snabel, G. T'Sjoen, A. Thijs, and M. den Heijer. 2022. The effect of transdermal gender-affirming hormone therapy on markers of inflammation and hemostasis. *PLoS ONE* 17(3):e0261312.

Segal, J. B., and A. R. Moliterno. 2006. Platelet counts differ by sex, ethnicity, and age in the United States. *Annals of Epidemiology* 16(2):123–130.

Selva, D. M., and G. L. Hammond. 2009. Thyroid hormones act indirectly to increase sex hormone-binding globulin production by liver via hepatocyte nuclear factor-4alpha. *Journal of Molecular Endocrinology* 43(1):19–27.

Shadid, S., K. Abosi-Appeadu, A. S. De Maertelaere, J. Defreyne, L. Veldeman, J. J. Holst, B. Lapauw, T. Vilsboll, and G. T'Sjoen. 2020. Effects of gender-affirming hormone therapy on insulin sensitivity and incretin responses in transgender people. *Diabetes Care* 43(2):411–417.

Shah, M. S., C. Lee, L. Guo, A. Bryant, J.-M. Ragunton, L. Caldwell, L. Xu, T. Onodera, R. Gordillo, P. E. Scherer, and K. Soe. 2022. PMON280 effect of gender affirming hormone therapy (GAHT) on adipose tissue morphology and metabolism in transgender individuals. *Journal of the Endocrine Society* 6(S1):A706–A707.

Shah, R., and D. C. Newcomb. 2018. Sex bias in asthma prevalence and pathogenesis. *Frontiers in Immunology* 9:2997.

Shansky, R. M., C. Hamo, P. R. Hof, W. Lou, B. S. McEwen, and J. H. Morrison. 2010. Estrogen promotes stress sensitivity in a prefrontal cortex-amygdala pathway. *Cerebral Cortex* 20(11):2560–2567.

Sharula, C. Chekir, Y. Emi, F. Arai, Y. Kikuchi, A. Sasaki, M. Matsuda, K. Shimizu, K. Tabuchi, Y. Kamada, Y. Hiramatsu, and M. Nakatsuka. 2012. Altered arterial stiffness in male-to-female transsexuals undergoing hormonal treatment. *Journal of Obstetrics and Gynaecology Research* 38(6):932–940.

Shaywitz, B. A., S. E. Shaywitz, K. R. Pugh, R. T. Constable, P. Skudlarski, R. K. Fulbright, R. A. Bronen, J. M. Fletcher, D. P. Shankweiler, and L. Katz. 1995. Sex differences in the functional organization of the brain for language. *Nature* 373(6515):607–609.

Shepherd, R., A. S. Cheung, K. Pang, R. Saffery, and B. Novakovic. 2021. Sexual dimorphism in innate immunity: The role of sex hormones and epigenetics. *Frontiers in Immunology* 11:604000.

Shipley, L. C., D. T. Steele, C. M. Wilcox, and C. M. Burski. 2020. A rare cause of acute pancreatitis in a transgender female. *Journal of Investigative Medicine High Impact Case Reports* 8:2324709620921333.

Simon, J. A. 2011. Identifying and treating sexual dysfunction in postmenopausal women: The role of estrogen. *Journal of Womens Health* 20(10):1453–1465.

Singer, K., N. Maley, T. Mergian, J. DelProposto, K. W. Cho, B. F. Zamarron, G. Martinez-Santibanez, L. Geletka, L. Muir, P. Wachowiak, C. Demirjian, and C. N. Lumeng. 2015. Differences in hematopoietic stem cells contribute to sexually dimorphic inflammatory responses to high fat diet-induced obesity. *Journal of Biological Chemistry* 290(21):13250–13262.

Singh-Ospina, N., S. Maraka, R. Rodriguez-Gutierrez, C. Davidge-Pitts, T. B. Nippoldt, L. J. Prokop, and M. H. Murad. 2017. Effect of sex steroids on the bone health of transgender individuals: A systematic review and meta-analysis. *Journal of Clinical Endocrinology & Metabolism* 102(11):3904–3913.

Sisk-Hackworth, L., S. T. Kelley, and V. G. Thackray. 2023. Sex, puberty, and the gut microbiome. *Reproduction* 165(2):R61–R74.

Slack, D. J., and J. D. Safer. 2021. Cardiovascular health maintenance in aging individuals: The implications for transgender men and women on hormone therapy. *Endocrine Practice* 27(1):63–70.

Sloan, A., P. Gona, and A. D. Johnson. 2015. Cardiovascular correlates of platelet count and volume in the Framingham Heart Study. *Annals of Epidemiology* 25(7):492–498.

Sofer, Y., E. Osher, W. Abu Ahmad, M. Yacobi Bach, N. Even Zohar, D. Zaid, N. Golani, Y. Moshe, K. Tordjman, N. Stern, and Y. Greenman. 2024. Gender-affirming hormone therapy effect on cortisol levels in trans males and trans females. *Clinical Endocrinology* 100(2):164–169.

Spalding, K. L., O. Bergmann, K. Alkass, S. Bernard, M. Salehpour, H. B. Huttner, E. Bostrom, I. Westerlund, C. Vial, B. A. Buchholz, G. Possnert, D. C. Mash, H. Druid, and J. Frisen. 2013. Dynamics of hippocampal neurogenesis in adult humans. *Cell* 153(6):1219–1227.

Spanos, C., I. Bretherton, J. D. Zajac, and A. S. Cheung. 2020. Effects of gender-affirming hormone therapy on insulin resistance and body composition in transgender individuals: A systematic review. *World Journal of Diabetes* 11(3):66.

St Pierre, S. R., M. Peirlinck, and E. Kuhl. 2022. Sex matters: A comprehensive comparison of female and male hearts. *Frontiers in Physiology* 13:831179.

Stangl, T. A., C. M. Wiepjes, J. Defreyne, E. Conemans, D. F. A, T. Schreiner, G. T'Sjoen, and M. den Heijer. 2021. Is there a need for liver enzyme monitoring in people using gender-affirming hormone therapy? *European Journal of Endocrinology* 184(4):513–520.

Stanley, J. A., M. M. Aruldhas, M. Chandrasekaran, R. Neelamohan, E. Suthagar, K. Annapoorna, S. Sharmila, J. Jayakumar, G. Jayaraman, N. Srinivasan, and S. K. Banu. 2012. Androgen receptor expression in human thyroid cancer tissues: A potential mechanism underlying the gender bias in the incidence of thyroid cancers. *Journal of Steroid Biochemistry & Molecular Biology* 130(1–2):105–124.

Steinberger, E., K. D. Smith, R. K. Tcholakian, and L. J. Rodriguez-Rigau. 1979. Testosterone levels in female partners of infertile couples: Relationship between androgen levels in the woman, the male factor, and the incidence of pregnancy. *American Journal of Obstetrics and Gynecology* 133(2):133–138.

Straub, R. H. 2007. The complex role of estrogens in inflammation. *Endocrine Reviews* 28(5):521–574.

Strauss, J. S., A. M. Kligman, and P. E. Pochi. 1962. The effect of androgens and estrogens on human sebaceous glands. *Journal of Investigative Dermatology* 39(2):139–155.

Streed, C. G., Jr., L. B. Beach, B. A. Caceres, N. L. Dowshen, K. L. Moreau, M. Mukherjee, T. Poteat, A. Radix, S. L. Reisner, V. Singh, on behalf of the American Heart Association Council on Peripheral Vascular Disease; Council on Arteriosclerosis, Thrombosis and Vascular Biology; Council on Cardiovascular and Stroke Nursing; Council on Cardiovascular Radiology and Intervention; Council on Hypertension; and Stroke Council. 2021. Assessing and addressing cardiovascular health in people who are transgender and gender diverse: A scientific statement from the American Heart Association. *Circulation* 144(6):e136–e148.

Stumpf, W. E., and M. Sar. 1976. Steroid hormone target sites in the brain: The differential distribution of estrogin, progestin, androgen and glucocorticosteroid. *Journal of Steroid Biochemistry* 7(11–12):1163–1170.

Sunder, M., and S. W. Leslie. 2022. *Semen analysis.* In *StatPearls* [Internet]. Treasure Island, FL: StatPearls Publishing; 2024 Jan-.

Suppakitjanusant, P., Y. Ji, M. O. Stevenson, P. Chantrapanichkul, R. C. Sineath, M. Goodman, J. A. Alvarez, and V. Tangpricha. 2020. Effects of gender affirming hormone therapy on body mass index in transgender individuals: A longitudinal cohort study. *Journal of Clinical & Translational Endocrinology* 21:100230.

Tan, K. S., and N. C. Thomson. 2000. Asthma in pregnancy. *American Journal of Medicine* 109(9):727–733.

Tella, S. H., and J. C. Gallagher. 2014. Prevention and treatment of postmenopausal osteoporosis. *Journal of Steroid Biochemistry & Molecular Biology* 142:155–170.

Tilling, L., J. Hunt, B. Jiang, T. A. Sanders, B. Clapp, and P. Chowienczyk. 2013. Endothelial function does not relate to haemoglobin or serum erythropoietin concentrations and these do not explain the gender difference in endothelial function in healthy middle-aged men and women. *European Journal of Clinical Investigation* 43(3):225–230.

Tirthani, E., M. Said, B. Neupane, and M. Quartuccio. 2021. An unusual case of the "terrible triad" in a transgender woman. *Cureus* 13(8):e16869.

Tordoff, D. M., M. R. Lunn, B. Chen, A. Flentje, Z. Dastur, M. E. Lubensky, M. Capriotti, and J. Obedin-Maliver. 2023. Testosterone use and sexual function among transgender men and gender diverse people assigned female at birth. *American Journal of Obstetrics & Gynecology* 229(6):669.e661–669.e617.

Torres-Tamayo, N., D. Garcia-Martinez, S. Lois Zlolniski, I. Torres-Sanchez, F. Garcia-Rio, and M. Bastir. 2018. 3D Analysis of sexual dimorphism in size, shape and breathing kinematics of human lungs. *Journal of Anatomy* 232(2):227–237.

Toth, M. J., A. Tchernof, C. K. Sites, and E. T. Poehlman. 2000. Effect of menopausal status on body composition and abdominal fat distribution. *International Journal of Obesity and Related Metabolic Disorders* 24(2):226–231.

Townsend, E. A., V. M. Miller, and Y. Prakash. 2012. Sex differences and sex steroids in lung health and disease. *Endocrine Reviews* 33(1):1–47.

Trigunaite, A., J. Dimo, and T. N. Jorgensen. 2015. Suppressive effects of androgens on the immune system. *Cell Immunology* 294(2):87–94.

T'Sjoen, G., S. Weyers, Y. Taes, B. Lapauw, K. Toye, S. Goemaere, and J. M. Kaufman. 2009. Prevalence of low bone mass in relation to estrogen treatment and body composition in male-to-female transsexual persons. *Journal of Clinical Densitometry* 12(3):306–313.

Tyrrell, C. J., A. V. Kaisary, P. Iversen, J. B. Anderson, L. Baert, T. Tammela, M. Chamberlain, A. Webster, and G. Blackledge. 1998. A randomised comparison of 'casodex' (bicalutamide) 150 mg monotherapy versus castration in the treatment of metastatic and locally advanced prostate cancer. *European Urology* 33(5):447–456.

Uhler, M. L., J. W. Marks, B. J. Voigt, and H. L. Judd. 1998. Comparison of the impact of transdermal versus oral estrogens on biliary markers of gallstone formation in postmenopausal women. *Journal of Clinical Endocrinology & Metabolism* 83(2):410–414.

Vaccarino, V., L. Parsons, N. R. Every, H. V. Barron, and H. M. Krumholz. 1999. Sex-based differences in early mortality after myocardial infarction. National registry of myocardial infarction. *New England Journal of Medicine* 341(4):217–225.

Van Caenegem, E., K. Wierckx, Y. Taes, D. Dedecker, F. Van de Peer, K. Toye, J. M. Kaufman, and G. T'Sjoen. 2012. Bone mass, bone geometry, and body composition in female-to-male transsexual persons after long-term cross-sex hormonal therapy. *Journal of Clinical Endocrinology & Metabolism* 97(7):2503–2511.

Van Caenegem, E., Y. Taes, K. Wierckx, S. Vandewalle, K. Toye, J. M. Kaufman, T. Schreiner, I. Haraldsen, and G. T'Sjoen. 2013. Low bone mass is prevalent in male-to-female transsexual persons before the start of cross-sex hormonal therapy and gonadectomy. *Bone* 54(1):92–97.

Van Caenegem, E., K. Wierckx, Y. Taes, T. Schreiner, S. Vandewalle, K. Toye, J. M. Kaufman, and G. T'Sjoen. 2015a. Preservation of volumetric bone density and geometry in trans women during cross-sex hormonal therapy: A prospective observational study. *Osteoporosis International* 26(1):35–47.

Van Caenegem, E., K. Wierckx, Y. Taes, T. Schreiner, S. Vandewalle, K. Toye, B. Lapauw, J. M. Kaufman, and G. T'Sjoen. 2015b. Body composition, bone turnover, and bone mass in trans men during testosterone treatment: 1-year follow-up data from a prospective case-controlled study (ENIGI). *European Journal of Endocrinology* 172(2):163–171.

van der Loos, M. A., I. Hellinga, M. C. Vlot, D. T. Klink, M. den Heijer, and C. M. Wiepjes. 2021. Development of hip bone geometry during gender-affirming hormone therapy in transgender adolescents resembles that of the experienced gender when pubertal suspension is started in early puberty. *Journal of Bone and Mineral Research* 36(5):931–941.

van der Loos, M. A., M. C. Vlot, D. T. Klink, S. E. Hannema, M. den Heijer, and C. M. Wiepjes. 2023. Bone mineral density in transgender adolescents treated with puberty suppression and subsequent gender-affirming hormones. *JAMA Pediatrics* 177(12):1332–1341.

van der Sluis, I. M., A. M. Boot, E. P. Krenning, S. L. Drop, and S. M. de Muinck Keizer-Schrama. 2002. Longitudinal follow-up of bone density and body composition in children with precocious or early puberty before, during and after cessation of GnRH agonist therapy. *Journal of Clinical Endocrinology & Metabolism* 87(2):506–512.

van Velzen, D. M., A. Paldino, M. Klaver, N. M. Nota, J. Defreyne, G. K. Hovingh, A. Thijs, S. Simsek, G. T'Sjoen, and M. den Heijer. 2019. Cardiometabolic effects of testosterone in transmen and estrogen plus cyproterone acetate in transwomen. *Journal of Clinical Endocrinology & Metabolism* 104(6):1937–1947.

van Velzen, D., C. Wiepjes, N. Nota, D. van Raalte, R. de Mutsert, S. Simsek, and M. den Heijer. 2022. Incident diabetes risk is not increased in transgender individuals using hormone therapy. *Journal of Clinical Endocrinology & Metabolism* 107(5):e2000–e2007.

Vanderschueren, D., M. R. Laurent, F. Claessens, E. Gielen, M. K. Lagerquist, L. Vandenput, A. E. Borjesson, and C. Ohlsson. 2014. Sex steroid actions in male bone. *Endocrine Reviews* 35(6):906–960.

Veiras, L. C., A. C. C. Girardi, J. Curry, L. Pei, D. L. Ralph, A. Tran, R. C. Castelo-Branco, N. Pastor-Soler, C. T. Arranz, A. S. L. Yu, and A. A. McDonough. 2017. Sexual dimorphic pattern of renal transporters and electrolyte homeostasis. *Journal of the American Society of Nephrology* 28(12):3504–3517.

Vinogradova, Y., C. Coupland, and J. Hippisley-Cox. 2019. Use of hormone replacement therapy and risk of venous thromboembolism: Nested case-control studies using the Qresearch and CPRD databases. *British Medical Journal* 364:k4810.

Vlot, M. C., D. T. Klink, M. den Heijer, M. A. Blankenstein, J. Rotteveel, and A. C. Heijboer. 2017. Effect of pubertal suppression and cross-sex hormone therapy on bone turnover markers and bone mineral apparent density (BMAD) in transgender adolescents. *Bone* 95:11–19.

Vlot, M. C., C. M. Wiepjes, R. T. de Jongh, G. T'Sjoen, A. C. Heijboer, and M. den Heijer. 2019. Gender-affirming hormone treatment decreases bone turnover in transwomen and older transmen. *Journal of Bone and Mineral Research* 34(10):1862–1872.

von Schoultz, B. 2009. Oestrogen therapy: Oral versus non-oral administration. *Gynecological Endocrinology* 25(9):551–553.

Walker, M., and K. Tobler. 2023. *Female infertility.* [Updated 2022 December 19], Statpearls. Treasure Island, FL: StatPearls Publishing.

Walecki, M., F. Eisel, J. Klug, N. Baal, A. Paradowska-Dogan, E. Wahle, H. Hackstein, A. Meinhardt, and M. Fijak M. 2015. Androgen receptor modulates Foxp3 expression in CD4+CD25+Foxp3+ regulatory T-cells. *Molecular Biology of the Cell* 26(15):2845–2857.

Wang, A., N. Karunasinghe, L. Plank, S. Zhu, S. Osborne, K. Bishop, C. Brown, T. Schwass, J. Masters, M. Holmes, R. Huang, C. Keven, L. Ferguson, and R. Lawrenson. 2017. Effect of androgen deprivation therapy on bone mineral density in a prostate cancer cohort in New Zealand: A pilot study. *Clinical Medicine Insights: Oncology* 11:1179554917733449.

Weissberger, A. J., K. K. Ho, and L. Lazarus. 1991. Contrasting effects of oral and transdermal routes of estrogen replacement therapy on 24-hour growth hormone (GH) secretion, insulin-like growth factor I, and GH-binding protein in postmenopausal women. *Journal of Clinical Endocrinology & Metabolism* 72(2):374–381.

Wickman, S., I. Sipila, C. Ankarberg-Lindgren, E. Norjavaara, and L. Dunkel. 2001. A specific aromatase inhibitor and potential increase in adult height in boys with delayed puberty: A randomised controlled trial. *Lancet* 357(9270):1743–1748.

Wiepjes, C. M., M. C. Vlot, M. Klaver, N. M. Nota, C. J. de Blok, R. T. de Jongh, P. Lips, A. C. Heijboer, A. D. Fisher, T. Schreiner, G. T'Sjoen, and M. den Heijer. 2017. Bone mineral density increases in trans persons after 1 year of hormonal treatment: A multicenter prospective observational study. *Journal of Bone and Mineral Research* 32(6):1252–1260.

Wiepjes, C. M., R. T. de Jongh, C. J. de Blok, M. C. Vlot, P. Lips, J. W. Twisk, and M. den Heijer. 2019. Bone safety during the first ten years of gender-affirming hormonal treatment in transwomen and transmen. *Journal of Bone and Mineral Research* 34(3):447–454.

Wiepjes, C. M., C. J. de Blok, A. S. Staphorsius, N. M. Nota, M. C. Vlot, R. T. de Jongh, and M. den Heijer. 2020. Fracture risk in trans women and trans men using long-term gender-affirming hormonal treatment: A nationwide cohort study. *Journal of Bone and Mineral Research* 35(1):64–70.

Wierckx, K., E. Elaut, E. Declercq, G. Heylens, G. De Cuypere, Y. Taes, J. Kaufman, and G. T'Sjoen. 2013. Prevalence of cardiovascular disease and cancer during cross-sex hormone therapy in a large cohort of trans persons: A case–control study. *European Journal of Endocrinology* 169(4):471–478.

Wierckx, K., E. Van Caenegem, T. Schreiner, I. Haraldsen, A. D. Fisher, K. Toye, J. M. Kaufman, and G. T'Sjoen. 2014a. Cross-sex hormone therapy in trans persons is safe and effective at short-time follow-up: Results from the European network for the investigation of gender incongruence. *Journal of Sexual Medicine* 11(8):1999–2011.

Wierckx, K., F. Van de Peer, E. Verhaeghe, D. Dedecker, E. Van Caenegem, K. Toye, J. M. Kaufman, and G. T'Sjoen. 2014b. Short- and long-term clinical skin effects of testosterone treatment in trans men. *Journal of Sexual Medicine* 11(1):222–229.

Wiik, A., T. R. Lundberg, E. Rullman, D. P. Andersson, M. Holmberg, M. Mandic, T. B. Brismar, O. Dahlqvist Leinhard, S. Chanpen, J. N. Flanagan, S. Arver, and T. Gustafsson. 2020. Muscle strength, size, and composition following 12 months of gender-affirming treatment in transgender individuals. *Journal of Clinical Endocrinology & Metabolism* 105(3):e805–e813.

Wilkinson, N. M., H. C. Chen, M. G. Lechner, and M. A. Su. 2022. Sex differences in immunity. *Annual Review of Immunology* 40(1):75–94.

Wilson, R., A. Spiers, J. Ewan, P. Johnson, C. Jenkins, and S. Carr. 2009. Effects of high dose oestrogen therapy on circulating inflammatory markers. *Maturitas* 62(3):281–286.

Wit, J. M., and W. Oostdijk. 2015. Novel approaches to short stature therapy. *Best Practice & Research Clinical Endocrinology & Metabolism* 29(3):353–366.

Wojtys, E. M. 2020. Bone health. *Sports Health* 12(5):423–424.

Woolley, C. S., and B. S. McEwen. 1993. Roles of estradiol and progesterone in regulation of hippocampal dendritic spine density during the estrous cycle in the rat. *Journal of Comparative Neurology* 336(2):293–306.

Wu, F. C., A. Tajar, J. M. Beynon, S. R. Pye, A. J. Silman, J. D. Finn, T. W. O'Neill, G. Bartfai, F. F. Casanueva, and G. Forti. 2010. Identification of late-onset hypogonadism in middle-aged and elderly men. *New England Journal of Medicine* 363(2):123–135.

Yaish, I., K. Tordjman, H. Amir, G. Malinger, Y. Salemnick, G. Shefer, M. Serebro, F. Azem, N. Golani, Y. Sofer, N. Stern, and Y. Greenman. 2021. Functional ovarian reserve in transgender men receiving testosterone therapy: Evidence for preserved anti-Müllerian hormone and antral follicle count under prolonged treatment. *Human Reproduction* 36(10):2753–2760.

Yang, M., and J. Fortune. 2006. Testosterone stimulates the primary to secondary follicle transition in bovine follicles in vitro. *Biology of Reproduction* 75(6):924–932.

Yau, M., and J. D. Safer. 2023. The return of spermatogenesis in transgender women ceasing gender-affirming hormone therapy. *Cell Reports Medicine* 4(1).

Zeng, S. M., J. Yankowitz, J. A. Widness, and R. G. Strauss. 2001. Etiology of differences in hematocrit between males and females: Sequence-based polymorphisms in erythropoietin and its receptor. *Journal of Gender-Specific Medicine* 4(1):35–40.

Zhao, J., S. Zhu, L. Sun, F. Meng, L. Zhao, Y. Zhao, H. Tian, P. Li, and Y. Niu. 2014. Androgen deprivation therapy for prostate cancer is associated with cardiovascular morbidity and mortality: A meta-analysis of population-based observational studies. *PLoS ONE* 9(9):e107516.

Zhu, Y., Z. Bian, P. Lu, R. H. Karas, L. Bao, D. Cox, J. Hodgin, P. W. Shaul, P. Thoren, O. Smithies, J. A. Gustafsson, and M. E. Mendelsohn. 2002. Abnormal vascular function and hypertension in mice deficient in estrogen receptor beta. *Science* 295(5554):505–508.

Zein, J. G., J. M. McManus, N. Sharifi, S. C. Erzurum, N. Marozkina, T. Lahm, O. Giddings, M. D. Davis, M. D. DeBoer, and S. A. Comhair. 2021. Benefits of airway androgen receptor expression in human asthma. *American Journal of Respiratory and Critical Care Medicine* 204(3):285–293.

Ziegler, S., and M. Altfeld. 2016. Sex differences in HIV-1-mediated immunopathology. *Current Opinion in HIV and AIDS* 11(2):209–215.